DeVita, Hellman, and Rosenberg's

Cancer
Principles & Practice of Oncology
Review

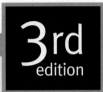

3rd edition

Vincent T. DeVita, Jr., MD
Samuel Hellman, MD
Steven A. Rosenberg, MD, PhD

EDITOR

Ramaswamy Govindan, MD

Professor
Department of Medicine
Division of Medical Oncology
Washington University School of Medicine
St. Louis, Missouri

ASSISTANT EDITORS

Saiama N. Waqar, MBBS

Instructor in Medicine
Department of Medicine
Division of Medical Oncology
Washington University School of Medicine
St. Louis, Missouri

Janakiraman Subramanian, MD

Instructor in Medicine
Department of Medicine
Division of Medical Oncology
Washington University School of Medicine
St. Louis, Missouri

Daniel Morgensztern, MD

Assistant Professor
Department of Medicine
Division of Medical Oncology
Yale University School of Medicine
New Haven, Connecticut

Wolters Kluwer | Lippincott Williams & Wilkins
Health
Philadelphia · Baltimore · New York · London
Buenos Aires · Hong Kong · Sydney · Tokyo

Senior Executive Editor: Jonathan Pine
Product Manager: Ryan Shaw
Vendor Manager: Bridgett Dougherty
Senior Manufacturing Manager: Benjamin Rivera
Senior Marketing Manager: Caroline Foote
Design Coordinator: Stephen Druding
Production Service: Aptara, Inc.

Library of Congress Cataloging-in-Publication Data
Devita, Hellman, and Rosenberg's cancer: principles & practice of oncology
review/editor, Ramaswamy Govindan; assistant editors, Maria
Q. Baggstrom, Thomas H. Fong, Janakiraman Subramanian. — 3rd ed.
   p. ; cm.
   Cancer
   Based on: DeVita, Hellman, and Rosenberg's cancer/editors, Vincent
T. DeVita Jr., Theodore S. Lawrence, Steven A. Rosenberg. 9th ed. © 2011.
   Includes bibliographical references and index.
   ISBN 978-1-4511-1639-7 (alk. paper)
   I. Govindan, Ramaswamy.   II. DeVita, Hellman, and Rosenberg's cancer.   III. Title: Cancer.
   [DNLM: 1. Neoplasms–Examination Questions. QZ 18.2]
   616.99′40076—dc23

                                                        2011040557

Care has been taken to confirm the accuracy of the information presented and to describe generally accepted practices. However, the authors, editors, and publisher are not responsible for errors or omissions or for any consequences from application of the information in this book and make no warranty, expressed or implied, with respect to the currency, completeness, or accuracy of the contents of the publication. Application of the information in a particular situation remains the professional responsibility of the practitioner.

The authors, editors, and publisher have exerted every effort to ensure that drug selection and dosage set forth in this text are in accordance with current recommendations and practice at the time of publication. However, in view of ongoing research, changes in government regulations, and the constant flow of information relating to drug therapy and drug reactions, the reader is urged to check the package insert for each drug for any change in indications and dosage and for added warnings and precautions. This is particularly important when the recommended agent is a new or infrequently employed drug.

Some drugs and medical devices presented in the publication have Food and Drug Administration (FDA) clearance for limited use in restricted research settings. It is the responsibility of the health care provider to ascertain the FDA status of each drug or device planned for use in their clinical practice.

To purchase additional copies of this book, call our customer service department at (800) 638-3030 or fax orders to (301) 223-2320. International customers should call (301) 223-2300.

Visit Lippincott Williams & Wilkins on the Internet: at LWW.com. Lippincott Williams & Wilkins customer service representatives are available from 8:30 am to 6 pm, EST.

TO
   MICHAEL C. PERRY
A GREAT PHYSICIAN, MENTOR, COLLEAGUE, AND ABOVE ALL—A FINE HUMAN BEING.

Camille N. Abboud, MD, FACP

Professor
Department of Internal Medicine
Division of Oncology
Washington University School of Medicine
St. Louis, Missouri

Douglas R. Adkins, MD

Associate Professor
Fellowship Program Director
Department of Internal Medicine
Division of Medical Oncology
Washington University School of Medicine
Siteman Cancer Center
St. Louis, Missouri

Rebecca Aft, MD, PhD

Professor of Surgery
Department of Surgery
Washington University
St. Louis, Missouri

Vorachart Auethavekiat, MD

Assistant Professor
Department of Medicine
Division of Hematology/Oncology
VA Medical Center
Washington University School of Medicine
    at St. Louis
St. Louis, Missouri

Maria Q. Baggstrom, MD

Assistant Professor of Medicine
Division of Oncology
Washington University School of Medicine
St. Louis, Missouri

Sanjeev Bhalla, MD

Associate Professor
Division of Diagnostic Radiology
Mallinckrodt Institute of Radiology
Washington University at St. Louis
St. Louis, Missouri

Leigh M. Boehmer, PharmD, BCOP

Clinical Pharmacist
Medical Oncology
Barnes Jewish Hospital
St. Louis, Missouri

Sara K. Butler, PharmD, BCPS, BCOP

Clinical Pharmacist
Medical Oncology
Barnes-Jewish Hospital
St. Louis, Missouri

Kenneth R. Carson, MD

Assistant Professor of Medicine
Department of Internal Medicine
Washington University School of Medicine
St. Louis, Missouri

Amanda F. Cashen, MD

Assistant Professor
Division of Oncology
Washington University School of Medicine
St. Louis, Missouri

Ravi Chhatrala, MD

Resident
Division of Internal Medicine
Department of Medicine
University at Buffalo
Buffalo, New York

L. Chinsoo Cho, MD, MS

Associate Professor
Department of Radiation Oncology
University of Minnesota Medical Center
Minneapolis, Minnesota

Hak Choy, MD

Professor & Chairman
Nancy B. and Jake L. Hamon Distinguished
    Chair in Therapeutic Oncology Research
Department of Radiation Oncology
UT Southwestern Medical Center
Dallas, Texas

Alex E. Denes, MD

Associate Professor of Medicine
Division of Medical Oncology
Washington University School of
    Medicine
St. Louis, Missouri

Thomas H. Fong, MD
Divisions of Hematology and Oncology
Southern California Permanente Medical Group
Fontana, California

Shirish M. Gadgeel, MD
Associate Professor
Department of Oncology
Karmanos Cancer Institute/Wayne State
    University
Detroit, Michigan

Feng Gao, MD, PhD
Division of Biostatistics
Washington University School of Medicine
St. Louis, Missouri

Mouhammed Amir Habra, MD
Assistant Professor
Department of Endocrine Neoplasia and
Hormonal Disorders
The University of Texas MD Anderson
    Cancer Center
Houston, Texas

Rami Y. Haddad, MD, FACP
Associate Professor of Medicine Chair
Division of Hematology/Oncology
Chicago Medical School
Captain James A Lovell Federal Health
    Care Center
Rosalind Franklin University of Medicine
    and Science
North Chicago, Illinois

Jennifer Ivanovich, MS
Research Assistant Professor
Department of Surgery
Washington University School of Medicine
St. Louis, Missouri

Renuka Iyer, MD
Associate Professor of Oncology
Roswell Park Cancer Institute
Buffalo, New York

Cylen Javidan-Nejad, MD
Mallinckrodt Institute of Radiology
Section of Cardiothoracic Imaging
Washington University at St. Louis
St. Louis, Missouri

Gregory Kalemkerian, MD
Professor
Department of Internal Medicine
University of Michigan
Ann Arbor, Michigan

Jason D. Keune, MD, MBA
Resident in General Surgery
Washington University School of Medicine
St. Louis, Missouri

Nikhil Khushalani, MD
Assistant Professor of Oncology
Section Chief
Soft Tissue and Melanoma
Director, High-Dose IL-2 Program
Department of Medicine
Roswell Park Cancer Institute
Buffalo, New York

C. Daniel Kingsley, MD, FACP
Clearview Cancer Institute
Clinical Assistant Professor of Internal Medicine
Department of Internal Medicine
UAB School of Medicine
Huntsville, Alabama

Robert Kratzke, MD
Associate Professor
Department of Medicine
University of Minnesota Medical School
Minneapolis, Minnesota

David I. Kuperman, MD
Hematologist/Oncologist
St. Luke's Hospital
Chesterfield, Missouri

Gerald P. Linette, MD, PhD
Division of Oncology
Washington University
St. Louis, Missouri

Kathy D. Miller, MD
Associate Professor of Medicine
Sheila D Ward Scholar
Indiana University Melvin and Bren Simon
    Cancer Center
Indianapolis, Indiana

James C. Mosley, MD

Physician
Hematology/Oncology
Southeast Cancer Center
Cape Girardeau, Missouri

Sujatha Murali, MD

Assistant Professor
Department of Hematology and Medical
    Oncology at Emory University
Winship Cancer Institute
Emory University School of Medicine
Atlanta, Georgia

David G. Mutch, MD

Judith and Ira Gall Professor
Director of the Division of Gynecology
    and Oncology
Washington University School of
    Medicine
St. Louis, Missouri

Michael C. Perry, MD, MS, MACP*

Professor of Medicine
Divisions of Hematology and Oncology
Department of Internal Medicine
Ellis Fischel Cancer Center
University of Missouri
Columbia, Missouri

Matthew A. Powell, MD

Assistant Professor
Department of Obstetrics and
    Gynecology
Washington University School of
    Medicine
St. Louis, Missouri

Toni B. Rachocki, MD

Kumar Rajagopalan, MD

Assistant Professor
Department of Medicine
Cooper Medical School at Rowan
    University
Camden, New Jersey

Suresh Ramalingam, MD

Associate Professor
Director
Division of Medical Oncology
Emory University
Winship Cancer Institute
Atlanta, Georgia

Giridharan Ramsingh, MD

Instructor
Department of Medicine
Division of Internal Medicine
Washington University School of Medicine
Saint Louis, Missouri

Lee Ratner, MD, PhD

Professor of Medicine and Molecular
    Microbiology
Co-Director
Medical & Molecular Oncology
Washington University School of Medicine
St. Louis, Missouri

Kaunteya Reddy, MD

Gastroenetrology Fellow
University at Buffalo
Buffalo, New York

Anna Roshal, MD

Assistant Professor
Medical Oncology
Washington University
St. Louis, Missouri

Bruce J. Roth, MD

Professor of Medicine
Division of Oncology
Washington University in St. Louis
St. Louis, Missouri

Mark A. Schroeder, MD

Research Instructor in Medicine
Department of Internal Medicine
Division of Oncology
Washington University School of Medicine
St. Louis, Missouri

Shalini Shenoy, MD

Medical Director, Pediatric Stem Cell Transplant
    Program
Associate Professor of Pediatrics
Washington University School of Medicine
St. Louis Children's Hospital
St. Louis, Missouri

*Deceased

George R. Simon, MD
Associate Professor
Department of Hematology and Oncology
Medical University of South Carolina
Charleston, South Carolina

Sunit Srivastava, MD

Walter Stadler, MD, FACP
Fred C. Buffett Professor of Medicine & Surgery
Sections of Hematology/Oncology & Urology
University of Chicago
Chicago, Illinois

Thomas E. Stinchcombe, MD
Associate Professor
Division of Hematology and oncology
University of North Carolina at Chapel Hill
Chapel Hill, North Carolina

Keith Stockerl-Goldstein, MD
Associate Professor of Medicine
Department of Medicine
Division of Oncology
Washington University in St. Louis and Siteman
   Cancer Center
St. Louis, Missouri

Janakiraman Subramanian, MBBS
Instructor
Department of Medicine
Division of Oncology
Washington Unversity School of Medicine
Saint Louis, Missouri

Benjamin Tan, MD
Associate Professor
Department of Internal Medicine
Washington University School of
   Medicine
St. Louis, Missouri

David D. Tran, MD, PhD
Instructor
Department of Medicine
Division of Oncology
Washington Unversity School of
   Medicine
Saint Louis, Missouri

Kathryn Trinkaus
Research Statistician
Division of Biostatistics
Washington University School of
   Medicine
St. Louis, Missouri

Brian Van Tine, MD
Assistant Professor of Medicine
Department of Internal Medicine
Division of Medical Oncology
Sarcoma Program Director
Barnes and Jewish Hospital
Washington University in St. Louis
St. Louis, Missouri

Vamsidhar Velcheti, MD
Medical Oncology
Yale University School of Medicine
New Haven, Connecticut

Ravi Vij, MD
Associate Professor
Section of BMT and Leukemia
Washington University School of
   Medicine
St Louis, Missouri

Andrea Wang-Gillam, MD, PhD
Division of Oncology
Washington University in St. Louis
St. Louis, Missouri

Muhammad Atif Waqar, MD
Hospice/Palliative Care &
   Geriatrics Fellow
Department of Internal Medicine
Division of Geriatrics
University of Nevada School of
   Medicine
Reno, Nevada

John Welch, MD, PhD
Assistant Professor of Medicine
Division of Oncology
Washington University
St. Louis, Missouri

Peter Westervelt, MD, PhD
Associate Professor of Medicine
Washington University School of
  Medicine
St. Louis, Missouri

Megan E. Wren, MD, FACP
Associate Professor
Division of Medical Education
Department of Medicine
Washington University School of Medicine
St. Louis, Missouri

The past decade has witnessed numerous advances in cancer therapy. Even since the publication of the previous edition of *Cancer: Principles and Practice of Oncology (PPO)*, or simply known as the "DeVita book," several new drugs have been approved for cancer therapy. Cancer Genome Sequencing projects are going ahead full steam. Molecular mechanisms that underline the course of several cancer types and responses to specific therapies are understood better than before. This companion review book, now in its third edition, is an attempt to cull out the key learning points from the massive tome of "the DeVita book" that captures all these advances in a timely manner. While these review books are often seen as "study-aids" for last minute cramming for the board examinations, we hope this book would serve to highlight key points from each chapter of *PPO*. Each chapter in the review book corresponds to one or more chapters in the main textbook just as they were in the first two editions. We hope you find this book useful and informative. Please do not hesitate to contact me with comments, criticisms, and suggestions. You can reach me by email at rgovinda@dom.wustl.edu.

Ramaswamy Govindan

At the outset, I want to thank the contributors for their diligence, time, and patience. I thank my dear colleagues Dr. Saiama Waqar, Dr. Janakiraman Subramanian, and Dr. Daniel Morgensztern for their hard work, dedication, and commitment to make this project successful. As assistant editors, they worked tirelessly to procure and edit the chapters to keep our production schedule more or less on time. Special thanks to Dr. Waqar who took additional responsibilities. As always, Jonathan Pine from Wolters Kluwer supported this idea and shepherded this to a reality by keeping a constant pressure on all of us. Ryan Shaw from Wolters Kluwer kept the project moving along very well. Needless to say, these projects take a sizeable amount of time away from the family. I will always be grateful to my wife Prabha and my two very adorable children, Ashwin and Akshay.

Finally I want to say a few words about my long-term friend, mentor and guide Dr. Michael C Perry. Mike passed away a few months ago. Mike was a remarkable man— intelligent, thoughtful, hard-working, creative and yet humble and gentle. He knew how to guide individuals early in their career better than anyone I know. I learnt a lot from him even though we never worked at the same institution. I would miss him very much. It is my honor to dedicate this edition to Mike. The world will be a better place if only we had more individuals like Mike.

Ramaswamy Govindan

CONTENTS

CHAPTER 1 MOLECULAR BIOLOGY OF CANCER ■ PART 1

ROBERT A. KRATZKE

DIRECTIONS Each of the numbered items below is followed by lettered answers. Select the ONE lettered answer that is BEST in each case unless instructed otherwise.

QUESTIONS

Question 1.1.   Completion of the Human Genome Project has revealed that human cells have a repertoire of genes of which approximate number?

A. 2500 genes
B. 25,000 genes
C. 250,000 genes
D. 2,500,000 genes

Question 1.2.   One of the reasons to use cancer cell culture experiments in preclinical studies of cancers is:

A. Allows evaluation of cancer cell interaction with the tumor microenvironment.
B. Cell cultures are amenable to easily manipulated experimental techniques.
C. Adaptation of cancer cells to growth in culture corresponds exactly to cancer cell growth in vivo.
D. Allows evaluation of cancer cell interaction with the native immune system.

Question 1.3.   Which of the following is false with regard to genetic mutations in cancer?

A. Gain-of-function mutations (oncogenes) are generally dominant at the cellular level.
B. Loss-of-functions mutations (tumor suppressor genes) are generally recessive at the cellular level.
C. One percent of the estimated total number of genes may contribute to some form of cancer.
D. Ninety percent of germ line mutations in familial cancer syndromes are in tumor suppressor genes.

Corresponding Chapters in *Cancer: Principles & Practice of Oncology,* Ninth Edition: 1 (The Cancer Genome), 2 (Mechanisms of Genomic Instability), 3 (Epigenetics of Cancer), 4 (Telomeres, Telomerase, and Cancer), and 5 (Cell Signaling Growth Factors and Their Receptors).

Question 1.4.   Which of the following proteins has inhibitory activity in the cell cycle?

A. Cyclin D1
B. E2F
C. p16INK4a
D. Cyclin-dependent kinase 4

Question 1.5.   All of the following contribute to suppression of cancer progression, EXCEPT:

A. Autophagy
B. Apoptosis
C. Senescence
D. Angiogenesis

Question 1.6.   Which of the following does successful invasion and metastasis NOT depend on?

A. Senescence
B. Angiogenesis
C. Evasion of apoptosis
D. Self-sufficiency in growth signals

Question 1.7.   Which of the following best describes the term "protooncogene"?

A. A normal cellular gene that has been transduced by a retrovirus that is then mutated following viral replication.
B. A homologue of a known oncogenic element identified in prehistoric specimens.
C. A transforming viral gene that can cause malignant transformation in fibroblasts in vitro.
D. The first oncogene discovered to be associated with human cancer.
E. A viral oncogene that, following infection, is the direct causative agent of human cancer.

Question 1.8.   The DNA damage checkpoints are located in which phase of the cell cycle?

A. G1/S
B. S/G2
C. M
D. All of the above

Question 1.9.   Which of the following is a potential flaw in microarray studies?

A. Inadequate controls
B. Biased estimation of prediction accuracy
C. Correlation between clusters and clinical outcome
D. All of the above

Question 1.10.   **Which of the following about miRNAs is false?**

    A. Are too small to be active inside a cell
    B. Consist of RNA 19 to 24 nucleotides in length
    C. Can be evaluated in array format as part of clinical studies
    D. May downregulate gene expression and protein translation

Question 1.11.   **The proteome is which of the following:**

    A. The set of all expressed gene products at a given time
    B. The proteins expressed preferentially in malignant cells
    C. The set of all proteins potentially expressed by the genome
    D. The set of protonated peptides subject to matrix-assisted laser desorption ionization-time of flight analysis

Question 1.12.   **Information obtained for molecular profiling using gene arrays and proteomics includes the following, EXCEPT:**

    A. Gene arrays can predict protein–protein interactions.
    B. Protein levels and protein function do not correspond directly with gene transcript levels.
    C. Polymerase chain reaction can be used to amplify biopsy material for use in gene arrays, whereas no signal amplification technology is standard in protein arrays.
    D. Proteomics can be used to investigate posttranslationally modified proteins.

Question 1.13.   **All is true about the peptidome, EXCEPT:**

    A. Consists of fragments of larger proteins.
    B. Included peptides must be less than 1000 daltons.
    C. May be amplified in the circulation.
    D. Many of the peptide fragments bind high-concentration blood proteins such as albumin.

Question 1.14.   **Which of the following statements regarding microsatellite instability is correct?**

    A. Hereditary nonpolyposis colon cancer syndrome (HNPCC) is associated with a 25% lifetime risk of developing colorectal cancer.
    B. Approximately 10% of all cases of colorectal cancer are associated with HNPCC.
    C. Microsatellite instability is associated with resistance to 5-fluorouracil chemotherapy.
    D. None of the above.

Question 1.15.   **Which of the following drugs is NOT a histone deacetylase inhibitor?**

    A. Suberoylanilide hydroxamic acid (SAHA)
    B. 5-Azacytidine
    C. Depsipeptide
    D. A and C

Question 1.16. The presence of mutations in p53 has been associated with which of the following properties on cells:

A. Loss of the G2 checkpoint following treatment with DNA-damaging agents

B. Enhanced capacity to undergo apoptosis following exposure to radiation

C. Increased capacity for DNA amplification

D. A and C

Question 1.17. Which of the following is an example of gene amplification found in cancer?

A. N-myc amplification in neuroblastoma

B. C-myc amplification in small cell lung cancer

C. Her2/neu amplification in breast cancer

D. All of the above

Question 1.18. Which of the following is true regarding microsatellite instability in colon cancer?

A. Approximately 15% of patients with hereditary nonpolyposis coli have mutations in MLH1 or MSH2.

B. There is potential resistance to 5-fluorouracil.

C. It has a less favorable prognosis.

D. Evidence is in favor of it occurring only late in sporadic colon cancer cases.

Question 1.19. Which of the following is false about excision repair mechanisms?

A. Reduced expression of ERCC1 in nonsmall cell lung cancer is associated with response to cisplatin.

B. There are two nucleotide excision repair pathways.

C. Base excision repair is involved in response to damage from chemicals and radiographs.

D. Numerous abnormalities in base excision repair machinery in multiple inherited cancers have been described.

Question 1.20. ATR/CHK1 signaling is associated with all of the following, EXCEPT:

A. Bone marrow failure

B. Predisposition to squamous cell carcinoma

C. Predisposition to acute leukemias

D. Decreased sensitivity to cisplatin

Question 1.21. Which of the following syndromes are associated with abnormalities in the double-strand repair?

A. Xeroderma pigmentosa

B. Fanconi anemia

C. Lynch syndrome

D. Bloom syndrome

Question 1.22.   Overexpression of Aurora B kinase could lead to all of the following, EXCEPT:

A. Inability for sister chromatids to separate before anaphase
B. Rapid cell division
C. Aneuploidy
D. Increased disassembly of kinetochore proteins

Question 1.23.   Which of the following characterizes cytogenetic abnormalities in most human cancers?

A. Universal (monoclonal) population of cells containing identical cyto-genetic abnormalities
B. Completely normal karyotype
C. Heterogenous complex karyotypes
D. Complete loss of X or Y chromosomes

Question 1.24.   The "Hayflick phenomenon," which is the name given to the limited replicative potential of cells, is thought to arise from which of the following?

A. The sequential loss of genetic material from the ends of chromosomes (telomeres) with each round of division
B. The gradual accumulation of uncorrected genetic defects passed on during division leading to senescence or malignancy
C. The activation of telomerase in aging cells leading to enzymatic loss of genetic material from telomeres
D. Dividing eukaryotic cells outgrowing their vascular supply

Question 1.25.   Which of the following statements is NOT accurate regarding telomerase?

A. It has both an RNA and a protein component.
B. It is a DNA polymerase.
C. Overexpression of telomerase is found in all cancer specimens.
D. Telomerase protects the integrity of the chromosomal ends.

Question 1.26.   Senescence can be induced by all of the following, EXCEPT:

A. Telomere shortening
B. Prolonged DNA damage
C. High-density growth
D. Oncogene activation

Question 1.27.   All of the following is evidence for senescence as a tumor suppressor mechanism, EXCEPT:

A. Several "tumor suppressor" proteins that are involved in senescence pathways (e.g., p16INK4a) are mutated in familial cancer syndromes.
B. Mice and humans with impaired p16INK4a and p53 function develop normally other than an age-dependent decrease in cancer and decreased susceptibility to cancer in response to carcinogen exposure.
C. Reestablishment of p53 activity in sarcoma and hepatocellular carcinoma has led to cessation of tumor growth.
D. Growth arrest in lung epithelium has been demonstrated in response to oncogenic events.

Question 1.28.   All of the following are potential therapeutic strategies to induce senescence in cancer cells, EXCEPT:

A. Restoration of p16INK4a activity via gene therapy
B. Restoration of p16INK4a activity via inhibition of DNA methyltransferases
C. Inhibition of MDM2
D. Inhibition of p16INK4a-p53 interactions

Question 1.29.   Breakage-fusion-bridge cycles lead to all of the following, EXCEPT:

A. Methylation
B. Aneuploidy
C. Amplifications
D. Deletions

Question 1.30.   Telomerase-null mice are associated with which of the following?

A. Decreased sensitivity to radiation
B. Decreased sensitivity to chemotherapy that induces double-strand breaks (DSBs)
C. Decreased genomic stability in the presence of p53 deficiency
D. Decreased rate of spontaneous malignancy

Question 1.31.   All of the following are receptor tyrosine kinases, EXCEPT:

A. Platelet-derived growth factor receptor
B. Insulin-like growth factor receptor 1
C. Kit
D. Akt

Question 1.32.   Which of the following is TRUE about receptor tyrosine kinases?

A. They are always monomeric.
B. Activation always requires tyrosine phosphorylation in all classes.
C. Different types of ligands can activate the same class of receptors.
D. Different types of ligands induce the same receptor conformational changes on binding.

Question 1.33. Which of the following is FALSE about receptor phosphotyrosine phosphatases?

    A. No true ligands for these have been described.
    B. They always function to antagonize tyrosine kinases.
    C. Activation could increase intracellular phosphorylation under certain circumstances.
    D. Most receptor phosphatases contain two catalytic domains.

Question 1.34. Which of the following statement regarding the epigenetic process is FALSE?

    A. Most CpG islands are not methylated.
    B. The level of acetylation correlates with the level of gene expression.
    C. The CpG dinucleotides are symmetrically distributed in the human DNA.
    D. The X-chromosome inactivation occurs through methylation.

Question 1.35. Which of the following is TRUE about GTP-binding proteins?

    A. GDP hydrolysis leads to a conformational change.
    B. All are lipid modified.
    C. Ras-like proteins exist in trimers.
    D. Gαi stimulates adenylate cyclase.

Question 1.36. Protein kinase A is the target of which of the following second messengers?

    A. Cyclic adenosine monophosphate (cAMP).
    B. Phospholipase C
    C. Diacylglycerol
    D. B and C

Question 1.37. Regulation of protein levels can be affected by:

    A. Signal transduction
    B. Translation
    C. Proteolysis
    D. All of the above

Question 1.38. Inhibition of the addition of a lipid moiety to Ras would potentially lead to:

    A. Increase in activation Raf
    B. Decrease in cell proliferation
    C. Increase in activation of MEK
    D. A and C

ANSWERS

Answer 1.1.   **The answer is B.**

One of the surprising findings of analysis of the sequenced human genome is the presence of only approximately 25,000 expressed genes in human cells. However, only a few thousand of these seem to be expressed at any given time. Previous estimates, based on the known approximate size of human chromosomes, were that there were up to 100,000 or more individual genes expressed in human cells.

Answer 1.2.   **The answer is B.**

Preclinical and clinical studies into cancer cell pathogenesis and response to potential treatments can be guided initially with cell culture experiments because these experiments can be manipulated in a reproducible manner. However, cell culture experiments do not allow for evaluation of the interaction between cancer cells and the tumor microenvironment. Some techniques such as cellular assays that evaluate for cellular migration and invasion through a Matrigel can mimic the tumor microenvironment, but they cannot replicate all of the cellular–environmental interactions. In addition, cancer cells can acquire genetic changes through multiple passages in culture such that they may not completely reflect in vivo cancer cell–host interactions.

Answer 1.3.   **The answer is D.**

Ninety percent of germ line mutations in familial cancer syndromes are in tumor suppressor genes. It is thought that many dominant oncogene mutations likely cause fetal demise and therefore do not arise in familial cancer syndromes. Dominant mutations in cancer genes denote oncogenes and make up 90% of all cancer genes.

Answer 1.4.   **The answer is C.**

The cell cycle is composed of the phases G0, G1, S, G2 and M. Regulation of the cell cycle depends on an interplay of multiple proteins. Cyclin-dependent kinases are serine/threonine kinases that are ubiquitous in the cell cycle. They generally require phosphorylation and association with cyclins for activity. Cyclin-dependent kinase 4 phosphorylates retinoblastoma protein, allowing depression of transcription factors (of which E2F is an example) essential to progression of the cell cycle. A series of inhibitors (INK4 family) act to decrease the activity of cyclins, of which p16INK4a is a member.

Answer 1.5.   **The answer is D.**

Angiogenesis encompasses a cascade of events that allow a tumor's vascular supply to be enhanced, thereby increasing cellular proliferation. Apoptosis and autophagy are two distinct mechanisms of cell death. Apoptosis is regulated via caspase cascades and mitochondrial-mediated pathways. Autophagy often is induced via nutrient starvation (as sensed by the mTor kinase) and involves autodigestion of intracellular organelles. Senescence, the permanent arrest of cell division, is regulated via the ARF-p53 and p16INK4a-retinoblastoma pathways.

Answer 1.6.　　　**The answer is A.**

Senescence is the permanent arrest of cell division, which would not contribute to cancer progression via invasion and metastasis. The other choices are all required for such progression. In addition, insensitivity to growth inhibitory signals and limitless replicative potential is also necessary for the complex processes of invasion and metastasis.

Answer 1.7.　　　**The answer is A.**

It has been known for almost a century that certain viruses can cause malignant transformation. The responsible genetic elements identified in the viral genomes are called viral oncogenes (v-oncogenes). It was found that homologues of these v-oncogenes existed in the eukaryotic genome from which they had likely originated. These normal human genetic elements were given the name protooncogene. One of the first of these, src, was identified in the avian Rous sarcoma virus that had been studied as a transforming virus decades earlier. In most human cancers, mutations or aberrant expressions of oncogenes have been identified.

Answer 1.8.　　　**The answer is A.**

There are three major DNA checkpoints, occurring at G1/S, G2/M, and S. These pathways promote cell cycle arrest and coordinate the recruitment of repair proteins to the sites of DNA damage.

Answer 1.9.　　　**The answer is D.**

Microarray technology is dependent on unbiased and rigorous statistical analysis, and as such, is susceptible to user bias. To help address the continuing need for standardization guidelines in the clinical use of microarray technology, the Minimum Information About A Microarray Experiment (MIAME) was published as a demonstration that microarray data can be independently verified, thereby reducing bias. The answers listed all may contribute to flawed interpretation of microarray data.

Answer 1.10.　　　**The answer is A.**

MicroRNA (miRNA) consists of an RNA sequence of 19 to 24 nucleotides in length and participates in cell processes such as apoptosis and development via the effect on gene expression and protein translation. Recently, miRNA array signatures have been evaluated in clinical samples from patients with lung cancer, chronic lymphocytic leukemia, and breast cancer. In a recent lung cancer study, the miRNA profile correlated with survival.

Answer 1.11.   **The answer is C.**

The term "proteome" is generally taken to refer to all potentially expressed proteins encoded by the genome. However, many operational definitions specify only those proteins expressed at a given time or under certain conditions, so answer "A" denotes a relatively common use of the term as well. Increasingly, the term "proteome" is used in conjunction with a modifier such as "serum," cellular," or even "malignant" to denote a more limited set of conditions. Protonation is a preparative step before proteomic evaluation by current means. Most proteomic analyses require cleavage of the proteins in the samples followed by protonation of the resulting peptides before matrix-assisted laser desorption ionization-time of flight analysis.

Answer 1.12.   **The answer is A.**

Current gene array technology is focused mostly around the detection of gene transcript levels. Small quantities of nuclear material from minimal biopsy material can be amplified via polymerase chain reaction. However, protein–protein interactions and posttranslational processing cannot be predicted. Multiple technologies have been used to detect "proteomic signatures," which include two-dimensional gel electrophoresis, affinity tagging, liquid chromatography coupled with mass spectrometry, and antibody arrays. Limitations of proteomic technologies include disruption of the native three-dimensional protein conformations in addition to the need for larger amounts of biopsy material needed compared with genomic arrays. This requires sensitive proteomic technology, such as antibodies in the femtomolar range.

Answer 1.13.   **The answer is B.**

The term "peptidome" refers to the low-molecular-weight range of the proteome that consists of peptides or protein fragments generally less than 50,000 daltons. It is thought that these peptide fragments are secreted from various tumors and exist in the circulation bound to carrier proteins. Studies are under way to determine if the secreted pattern of such fragments can be correlated with disease states. A confounding factor in peptidome analysis may be the susceptibility of peptides to protease degradation in the blood after secretion from the tumor. It remains to be seen if consistent patterns can be determined after protease degradation.

Answer 1.14.   **The answer is C.**

HNPCC is associated with a 60% to 80% lifetime risk of developing colorectal cancer and accounts for 2% to 5% of all cases of colorectal cancer. In both sporadic and HNPCC cases, microsatellite instability has been associated with a more favorable prognosis but potential resistance to 5-fluorouracil chemotherapy.

Answer 1.15.   **The answer is B.**

SAHA and depsipetide are examples of histone deacetylase inhibitors whereas 5-azacytidine and 5-Aza-2′-deoxycytidine are DNA hypomethylating agents.

Answer 1.16.   **The answer is D.**

Mutations of p53 are among the most commonly identified in human cancers. Wild-type p53 has a function in signaling cells with damaged DNA to undergo programmed cell death (apoptosis). In the presence of an inactivating mutation of p53, commonly used genotoxic agents, such as radiation and chemotherapy, may prove less effective with the intact p53 signal. This has been demonstrated in preclinical models and correlates with some human clinical trial data. It must be noted, however, that many common malignancies harboring p53 mutations, such as small cell lung cancer and ovarian cancer, are sensitive to chemotherapy and radiation. The capacity of p53 to trigger apoptosis is associated with the cell-cycle checkpoints that have been identified as critical nodal moments at which the cell may "choose" to continue to divide or, if sufficiently damaged, progress down a path to cell death and deletion of the potentially damaged clone. Interestingly, p53 mutant transgenic mice are viable and develop normally. However, they have an accelerated rate of tumor formation under certain tumorigenic stimuli.

Answer 1.17.   **The answer is D.**

Gene amplification as a mechanism resulting in overexpression of gene products involved in tumorigenesis or tumor progression has been reported in several cancers. It is known that N-myc amplification in neuroblastoma can be a useful prognostic factor aiding in designing therapy. In small cell lung cancer, c-myc amplification has been identified in up to 10% of specimens, a percentage that may increase after treatment. Her2/neu amplification occurs in up to 30% of breast cancers and is useful in predicting response to Her2/neu-targeted therapy.

Answer 1.18.   **The answer is B.**

Microsatellite instability refers to frequent mutations in regions of simple repeat sequences. Early studies in kindreds with HNPCC demonstrated mutations in MSH2 and MLH1, which are mismatch repair genes. Approximately 85% of patients with HNPCC have mutations in MSH2 and MLH1. Microsatellite instability is associated with a resistance to 5-fluorouracil treatment, more favorable prognosis, and lack of p53 mutations. The protein MSH2 complexes with MSH6 to recognize mismatched bases, and subsequent recruitment of MLH1 and PMS2 initiates the steps of repair (excision, DNA synthesis, and ligation).

Answer 1.19.   **The answer is D.**

The mismatch repair machinery of the cell includes two major pathways: nucleotide excision repair (NER) and base excision repair (BER). These pathways respond to lesions created by DNA-damaging agents, such as chemicals and radiation from numerous sources. Early discoveries in the NER pathway were made via the study of xeroderma pigmentosa, where patients exhibit extreme sun sensitivity. Two NER pathways have been described: The first involves global genome scanning for lesions, and the second detects lesions that interfere with RNA polymerases. In BER, the repair machinery responds mainly to chemical and x-ray damage and base loss by using DNA glycosylates to remove damaged bases and a complex of APEX1 endonuclease, PARP, DNA polymerase/ligase, and XRCC1 to recognize abasic sites. As of now, no inherited cancer syndromes caused by mutations in BER have been discovered.

Answer 1.20.   **The answer is D.**

DSBs can promote major cytogenetic abnormalities and are repaired via homologous recombination or nonhomologous end-joining. ATR/CHK1 signaling leads to activation of the Fanconi anemia repair pathway. Defects in Fanconi anemia lead to bone marrow failure, congenital abnormalities, predisposition to acute leukemias and squamous cell cancer, and increased sensitivity to DNA cross-linking agents such as cisplatin and mitomycin C.

Answer 1.21.   **The answer is B.**

Xeroderma pigmentosa, Lynch syndrome, and Bloom syndrome are caused by abnormalities in the nucleotide excision repair, mismatch repair, and helicase, respectively. Fanconi anemia is caused by abnormalities in *Fanc* genes, involved in the double-strand DNA repair.

Answer 1.22.   **The answer is A.**

The mitotic spindle is central to cell division, and Aurora kinase B is intricately involved in the process of cell division. The linking of sister chromatids before anaphase is lost partly because of the action of Aurora B kinase. Aurora B kinase also phosphorylates other kinetochore proteins to aid disassembly of kinetochore-microtubule attachments not under proper tension (as part of spindle checkpoint activation). Amplification of Aurora B kinase has been associated with sporadic tumors.

Answer 1.23.   **The answer is C.**

Human cancers are largely characterized by complex karyotypes with multiple different populations. In particular, solid tumors such as lung and colon cancer exhibit great heterogeneity that is likely the result of the high level of genomic instability found in cancers. Some less common malignancies, such as CML, are characterized by the relatively uniform presence of an abnormal karyotype, often with a limited number of detectable breakpoints and translocations. In fact, the presence of a uniform karyotypic abnormality raises the possibility of a germ line cytogenetic defect that may be further evaluated by examining the karyotype of noncancerous circulating lymphocytes from the same patient. The absence of any karyotypic abnormality in cancer cell populations is less common but can occur. For example, the presence of a normal karyotype is a well-recognized observation in acute myelogenous leukemia and gives important clinical information conferring an intermediate prognosis. The loss of a single X or Y chromosome is a normal variant commonly observed in older patients. It carries little clinical significance.

Answer 1.24.   **The answer is A.**

Hayflick and Moorehead documented a landmark finding of cell biology when they observed that normal eukaryotic cells would only replicate approximately 50 to 100 times before dying. This limited replicative capacity of nontransformed cells is called the "Hayflick phenomenon." It is now known that the ends of the chromosomes, called "telomeres," gradually shorten, losing 25 to 200 base pairs with each round of division. After 50 to 100 rounds of division, the telomeres reach a critically shortened length, triggering cell senescence. Telomeres can be maintained by the enzymatic activity of telomerase, which function to restore and maintain telomeres at their full length. Activation of telomerase is a key mechanism by which some cells, such as cancer cells, evade senescence. Although gene defects occur spontaneously in cells and will lead to programmed cell death, this usually occurs in the immediate generation after the defect is established. Tumor growth does require neovascularization, but the "Hayflick phenomenon" applies to programmed senescence in nontransformed cells.

Answer 1.25.   **The answer is C.**

Telomerase is the DNA polymerase that synthesizes the repeating six base pair motif (TTAGGG) that comprises the ends of all chromosomes. It is a nucleoprotein with both a protein and RNA component. With cell division, the telomere ends become progressively shorter until a critical length is reached and programmed cell death is initiated. Synthesizing and repairing the ends of the shortening telomeres allows cells to maintain the integrity of the chromosomal ends and is important for cells that need to divide without reaching senescence, such as cancer cells. In light of this, it is not surprising that the majority of cancer cells overexpress telomerase, but there are cancers that appear to have invoked alternative mechanisms to repair telomeres. Indeed, telomerase-deficient (deleted) mice can be induced to develop tumors.

Answer 1.26.   **The answer is C.**

Senescence refers to a state in cultured cells where growth arrest is permanent. Senescence differs from quiescence in that quiescent cells can reenter the cell cycle in response to appropriate mitogenic cues. Quiescence is generally induced by serum starvation, growth factor deprivation, high-density growth, and transient DNA damage. Senescence can be induced by prolonged DNA damage, oxidative stress, telomere shortening, and oncogene activation. Additional differences include uninducible c-fos expression in response to serum stimulation and increased PAI expression in senescence versus quiescence.

Answer 1.27.   **The answer is B.**

Cell-cycle inhibitors that lead to senescence include p16INK4a and p53, among others. It follows that mice and humans with impaired p16INK4a and p53 function develop normally other than an age-dependent increase in cancer and increased susceptibility to cancer in response to carcinogen exposure. Aside from the other correct answers listed, other evidence is supportive. Minimal residual disease data demonstrate frequent oncogenic events as evidence for a need for tumor suppression. Mice are highly susceptible to inactivation of p16INK4a and/or p53 as evidenced by experiments demonstrating development of primary tumors at 8 weeks of age (normal life span is approximately 100 weeks).

Answer 1.28.   **The answer is D.**

Knockout of INK4a and ARF loci separately and in combination leads to an increase in spontaneous tumors. Silencing of p16INK4a via hypermethylation has been well described and is associated with numerous types of cancers. Inhibition of methylation is thought to increase expression of p16INK4a. Gene therapy as a method to replace p16INK4a activity has been achieved in the laboratory. ARF leads to MDM2 activation and subsequent p53 degradation. Inhibition of MDM2 activity is thought to increase p53 levels and lead to apoptosis and senescence. p53 and p16INK4a do not interact directly.

Answer 1.29.   **The answer is A.**

Chromosomal rearrangements are thought to contribute to the malignant phenotype of many different cancers. Such rearrangements are the result of breakage-fusion-bridge cycles. Unprotected chromatids can fuse to form a dicentric chromosome. The fused chromosomes break during anaphase and create atelomeric chromosomes. Atelomeric chromosomes can fuse with other chromosomes and perpetuate the cycle. Amplification, deletions, and aneuploidy can arise this way. Methylation is an epigenetic phenomenon that is not thought to be directly related to chromosome fusion.

Answer 1.30.   **The answer is C.**

It is thought that one of the mechanisms of cancer pathogenesis is related to short telomeres that contribute to genomic instability followed by increased telomerase activity. Paradoxically, genomic instability can increase with decreased telomerase activity in the presence of concomitant p53 deficiency, suggesting that telomerase inhibition by itself is likely not sufficient as a cancer therapeutic. However, increased sensitivity to radiation and DSB-inducing chemotherapeutics is associated with decreased telomerase activity and suggests possible additive or synergistic effects.

Answer 1.31.   **The answer is D.**

Phosphorylation of tyrosine residues by tyrosine kinases is an important signal for cell stimulation and cancer growth. Each transmembrane tyrosine kinase is activated by its associated ligand. Increasingly, tyrosine kinases are an important target for novel therapeutics as well. Examples of this class of agents already in common use include both imatinib mesylate (Gleevec) and gefitinib (Iressa). All of the examples listed above are receptor tyrosine kinases except for Akt. Akt is a threonine/serine kinase and a key component of the downstream phosphatidylinositol 3 kinase-signaling pathway through which many of the tyrosine kinases transmit their signaling.

Answer 1.32.   **The answer is C.**

Receptor tyrosine kinases generally consist of an extracellular binding domain, a transmembrane domain, and an intracellular kinase domain. These receptors bind ligands that are usually peptides or proteins. Most are monomeric with the exception of the insulin-receptor family, which consists of heterodimers covalently bound by disulfide bonds. Six major classes exist. Activation of the receptor generally requires phosphorylation of a tyrosine on the receptor, but the insulin binding to the insulin receptor is an exception to this rule and activation is generated by an insulin-induced conformational change. Outside of this, most receptor tyrosine kinases are activated by oligomerization, which brings intracellular kinase domains into proximity to allow cross-phosphorylation. Ligands generally stimulate oligomerization. Although receptor classes have been defined by particular ligands, it is accepted that particular receptor classes may bind more than one class of ligand. A particular ligand may have different conformational changes in the same receptor, leading to distinct downstream signal pathway activation.

Answer 1.33.   **The answer is B.**

Receptor phosphotyrosine phosphatases (RPTPs) are similar in structure to receptor tyrosine kinases in that they consist of an extracellular domain, a single transmembrane domain, and an intracellular catalytic domain (generally two domains). Although no true ligands for RPTPs have been described, some RPTPs contain structural repeats that suggest adhesion molecule recognition. Although RPTPs act as phosphatases, they do not always function in opposition to tyrosine kinases. Particular phosphorylation events can be inhibitory to tyrosine kinases, and activation of phosphatase activity could then increase tyrosine kinase global activity.

Answer 1.34.   **The answer is C.**

The CpG dinucleotides are asymmetrically distributed in human DNA, with approximately half of the genes containing CpG-rich regions termed CpG island. Most of these CpG islands are not methylated. X-chromosome inactivation occurs through CpG island methylation.

Answer 1.35.   **The answer is B.**

GTP-binding proteins are well-studied mediators of signal transduction. They are organized into two main classes: (a) heterotrimeric and (b) Ras-like. These proteins act like switches and undergo conformational changes in response to the state of GTP or GDP binding. Binding of GTP induces a conformational switch that leads to increased activity. Hydrolysis of GTP to GDP leads to inactivation. All such proteins are lipid modified, which allows membrane association that is important to its downstream pathway activation. Heterotrimeric GTP-binding proteins are divided into classes based on function; two of the classes are Gas and Gai, which stimulate and inhibit adenylate cyclase, respectively.

Answer 1.36.   **The answer is A.**

Phospholipase C proteins cleave PtdIns 4.5-P_2 to generate inositol-1,4, 5-triphosphate IP3 and **diacylglycerol.** Protein kinase A is the primary target for cAMP. Binding of cAMP to protein kinase A leads to the activation of the protein kinase A catalytic unit through dissociation from the regulatory unit.

Answer 1.37.   **The answer is D.**

Myriads of cellular functions are dependent on protein–protein interactions and the concentration levels of those proteins. A single stimulus received by a cell can affect the transcription levels of hundreds of genes. Regulation of histone deacetylases, histone acetylases, nuclear receptors, and phosphorylation levels all play a role. Translation of protein from mRNA can be affected by ribosomal processing. Ubiquitination results in proteasome degradation of proteins. Lysosomes contribute to protein degradation, often after receptors are endocytosed.

Answer 1.38.   **The answer is B.**

Colocalization of proteins plays an important role in signal transduction and cell signaling pathways. Ras is a GTP-binding protein that requires the addition of a lipid moiety (generally a farnesyl group) to localize it to the membrane. There, it interacts with and activates Raf, which then interacts with MEK. Increased cell proliferation is one of the effects of signaling via this pathway, so a lack of the lipid moiety could lead to decreased cell proliferation because it is not in close proximity to the membrane and Raf. Colocalization is an important phenomenon in cell signaling and can also be achieved via protein–protein interactions (i.e., nuclear transport) and membrane localization lipid rafts.

CHAPTER 2 MOLECULAR BIOLOGY OF CANCER ▪ PART 2

SUNIT SRIVASTAVA • GEORGE R. SIMON

DIRECTIONS Each of the numbered items below is followed by lettered answers. Select the ONE lettered answer that is BEST in each case unless instructed otherwise.

QUESTIONS

Question 2.1. The correct order of mitosis is:

A. Prometaphase, metaphase, anaphase, telophase, prophase
B. Prometaphase, metaphase, prophase, anaphase, telophase
C. Prophase, prometaphase, metaphase, anaphase, telophase
D. Telophase, anaphase, prophase, metaphase, prometaphase

Question 2.2. The cyclin responsible for progressing the cell into and through mitosis is:

A. Cyclin A
B. Cyclin B
C. Cyclin D
D. Cyclin E

Question 2.3. Which of the following is NOT a means of regulating cyclin-dependent kinases (CDKs)?

A. Positive regulatory acetylation
B. Negative regulatory phosphorylation
C. CDK inhibitors
D. Cyclin availability

Question 2.4. Which of the following is necessary for the G1/S-phase transition?

A. Cyclin B-CDK1 complex accumulation
B. Cyclins E and A accumulation
C. Dephosphorylation of T14 and Y15
D. CDK1 activation along with binding of CDC20 to anaphase promoting complex/cyclosome (APC/C)

Corresponding Chapters in *Cancer: Principles & Practice of Oncology*, Ninth Edition: 6 (Cell Cycle), 7 (Mechanisms of Cell Death), 8 (Cancer Metabolism), 9 (Angiogenesis), 10 (Invasion and Metastasis), 11 (Cancer Stem Cells), and 12 (Biology of Personalized Cancer Medicine).

Question 2.5. Which of the following has no role in cell-cycle exit?

A. Downregulation of CDKs and cyclins
B. Accumulation of INK4, Cip/Kip, and pRb proteins
C. Reduction in protein synthesis
D. Activation of APC/C

Question 2.6. Activation of antimitogenic signaling involves all of the following EXCEPT:

A. Interleukin (IL)-2
B. Transforming growth factor (TGF)-β
C. Interferon (IFN)-α
D. Upregulation of CDK inhibitors and downregulation of cyclins

Question 2.7. Which of the following choices is not true regarding microRNAs?

A. microRNAs encode protein kinases that regulate cell cycle.
B. They regulate mRNA expression.
C. There is at least five clusters of microRNAs targeting mRNA that encodes cell-cycle regulatory proteins.
D. miR-15a/16 cluster targets cyclin E1 and cyclin D1.

Question 2.8. Which gene is involved in both cell-cycle regulation and DNA repair?

A. TP53
B. NBS1
C. PTTG1
D. CHK2

Question 2.9. Replicative senescence is initiated by means of:

A. Downregulation of cyclins
B. p53 activation
C. Progressive telomere shortening
D. Upregulation of IFNs

Question 2.10. Genes that encode negative regulators of growth and proliferation are:

A. Protooncogenes
B. Oncogenes
C. S-phase genes
D. Tumor suppressor genes

Question 2.11. Which of the following syndromes is associated with a mutation in the gene encoding Nbs1, leading to microcephaly and a strong predisposition to lymphoid malignancies?

A. Nijmegen disease
B. Von Hippel–Lindau (VHL) syndrome
C. Familial malignant melanoma syndrome
D. Li–Fraumeni syndrome

Question 2.12.   Type I cell death is also known as:

    A. Autophagy
    B. Apoptosis
    C. Necrosis
    D. Autolysis

Question 2.13.   All of the following are ligands for the death receptor pathway EXCEPT:

    A. TNFα
    B. Fas
    C. TRAIL
    D. Noxa

Question 2.14.   Taxanes specifically target this BH3-only Bcl-2 protein:

    A. Nbk/Bik
    B. Bim
    C. Puma
    D. Bad

Question 2.15.   RAF is inhibited by which of these therapeutic agents that induce apoptosis?

    A. Sorafenib
    B. Imatinib mesylate
    C. Bortezomib
    D. Taxanes

Question 2.16.   Bcl-2 small molecule inhibitors like ABT-737 induce apoptosis by:

    A. Binding to the BH3-binding pocket
    B. Inhibiting tyrosine kinase activity of Bcr/Abl restoring Bim function
    C. Stimulating Bim expression
    D. Blocking proteosome degradation of Bim

Question 2.17.   Angiogenesis inhibitors theoretically induce apoptosis by which means?

    A. Tyrosine kinase inhibition
    B. Histone deacetylase inhibition
    C. Inhibition of antiapoptotic proteins
    D. Nutrient deprivation

Question 2.18.   Type II programmed cell death, autophagy, is regulated by:

    A. mTOR in the PI3-kinase/AKT pathway
    B. Bax/Bak
    C. BH3-only proteins
    D. APC/C

Question 2.19.   Autophagy does not have a role in:

A. Recycling of normal cellular components
B. Protection against aging
C. Cell lysis caused by surrounding inflammation
D. Innate immunity by protecting against intracellular pathogens

Question 2.20.   Which of the following is NOT a feature of necrosis?

A. Rapid cellular swelling
B. Lysosome activation
C. Loss of plasma membrane integrity
D. Release of intracellular components to the extracellular compartment

Question 2.21.   The Warburg effect describes:

A. Exponential cell growth in response to an exogenous stimulant.
B. Inefficient energy production by most cancer cells, resulting in rapid adenosine triphosphate (ATP) depletion and necrotic cell death.
C. Initiation of neoplasia requires two somatic mutations for initiation of sporadic neoplasms, and hereditary neoplasms require a genetic plus a somatic mutation.
D. Sculpting of normal human tissues as a result of cell death.

Question 2.22.   Unless tumor cells grow an adequate blood vessel supply, they will NOT grow greater than:

A. <1 mm^3
B. 1 to 2 mm^3
C. Approximately 5 mm^3
D. 1 cm^3

Question 2.23.   Bevacizumab is:

A. A monoclonal antibody to basic fibroblast growth factor (bFGF)
B. A monoclonal antibody to vascular endothelial growth factor (VEGF)
C. A monoclonal antibody to phospholipid lipid growth factor (PLGF)
D. A monoclonal antibody to epidermal growth factor receptor (EGFR)

Question 2.24.   The first step in tumor angiogenesis is:

A. A localized degradation of the surrounding basement membrane of a parental venule
B. Paracrine signaling causing increased leakiness of a parental venule's basement membrane
C. An inflammatory response causing recruitment and activation of leukocytes that mediate angiogenesis
D. Release of endothelial cell (EC) progenitors from the bone marrow

Question 2.25.   Which of the following is NOT a function of pericytes?

A. Paracrine signaling
B. Regulation of vessel diameter
C. Mediation of resistance to antiangiogenic therapy
D. All of the above

Question 2.26.   Which of the following is NOT a characteristic of tumor vasculature?

A. Increased dilation
B. Increased tortuosity
C. Increased red blood cell (RBC) flow
D. Decreased support

Question 2.27.   Which of the following is NOT considered a primary angiogenic factor?

A. Granulocyte-colony stimulating factor
B. VEGF
C. Angiopoietins
D. Notch-signaling receptors

Question 2.28.   Which of the following is NOT a function of VEGF?

A. Stimulate EC division
B. Upregulate various inhibitors of apoptosis
C. Mobilize EC progenitors
D. Create focal areas of breakdown in parental venule basement membranes

Question 2.29.   VEGF is inducible by many factors, of which the most important may be:

A. H1F1α
B. TSP-1
C. pVHL
D. p53

Question 2.30.   Which of the following is NOT thought to inhibit tumor angiogenesis?

A. TSP-1
B. IL-6, IL-8
C. DLL4
D. Vasohibin

Question 2.31.   Metronomic low-dose chemotherapy describes:

A. Continuous low-dose treatment with chemotherapeutics
B. Pulse dosing with low doses of chemotherapeutics
C. Continuous low-dose treatment with intermittent pulse dosings of chemotherapeutics
D. Treatment of refractory tumors with continuous low doses of chemotherapeutics in conjunction with metronidazole

Question 2.32. Which of the following is NOT thought to be a mechanism of antiangiogenic treatment resistance?

A. Decreased penetration of antiangiogenic molecules into tumor cells
B. Selection of hypoxia resistant cells
C. Vascular remodeling
D. Proangiogenic growth factor redundancy

Question 2.33. Which of the following is NOT an associated potential toxicity of antiangiogenic therapy?

A. Hypertension
B. Aplastic anemia
C. Bowel perforation
D. Arteriothrombotic event

Question 2.34. Which of the following is NOT associated with a risk of metastasis?

A. Tumor grade
B. Depth of invasion beyond normal cellular compartments
C. Lymphovascular invasion
D. Proper immune function

Question 2.35. What percentage of tumor cells can give rise to metastases?

A. <0.01%
B. 1%
C. 20%
D. >80%

Question 2.36. Genes that can mediate tumorigenic functions and secondarily serve metastatic-specific functions either in a general way or with particular organ selectivity are best known as:

A. Tumorigenic genes
B. Metastasis progression genes
C. Metastasis virulence genes
D. Protooncogenes

Question 2.37. Cells that mediate the breakdown of the basement membrane allowing for tumor invasion are known as:

A. Carcinoma-associated fibroblasts
B. Pericyte-derived fibroblast
C. Tumor-associated macrophages (TAMs)
D. Dendritic cells

Question 2.38. Cellular loss of this molecule leads to decreased cellular attachment and enhanced tumor invasion/motility:

A. E-cadherin
B. β-catenin
C. α-tubulin
D. Ankrin

Question 2.39.   Which of the following is NOT a selective pressure experienced by circulating tumor cells (CTCs)?

A. Shear stress
B. Nitric oxide
C. DARC
D. Nutrient deprivation

Question 2.40.   Which of the following molecules does NOT assist in the extravasation of CTCs?

A. Ezrin
B. VEGF
C. $\alpha v \beta 3$ integrin
D. CXCR4

Question 2.41.   Osteoblastic bone metastases are characteristic of which type of cancer?

A. Breast
B. Prostate
C. Lung
D. Renal cell

Question 2.42.   Which of the following does NOT typically metastasize to the liver?

A. Colon cancer
B. Breast cancer
C. Prostate cancer
D. Melanoma

Question 2.43.   The stochastic model of tumor heterogeneity is best described as:

A. Every cell has equal potential to initiate and sustain tumor growth, but most cells do not proliferate extensively because of the low cumulative probability of permissive events.
B. Cancer stem cells (CSCs) are biologically distinct from the bulk cell population, which does not possess tumor-initiating activity.
C. Tumors are heterogeneous secondary to random, acquired mutations.
D. Tumors are pressured into heterogeneity by variable pressures applied to the tumor.

Question 2.44.   The hierarchy model of tumor heterogeneity is best described as:

A. Every cell has equal potential to initiate and sustain tumor growth, but most cells do not proliferate extensively because of the low cumulative probability of permissive events.
B. CSCs are biologically distinct from the bulk cell population, which does not possess tumor-initiating activity.
C. Tumors are heterogenous secondary to random, acquired mutations.
D. Tumors are pressured into heterogeneity by variable pressures applied to the tumor.

Question 2.45.   The drug vemurafenib (PLX4032) targets which gene in MAPK/ERK pathway?

    A. RAS
    B. BRAF
    C. BIM
    D. ERK

Question 2.46.   Which of the following agents targets tumor metabolic pathways?

    A. Pemetrexed
    B. Cytarabine
    C. Temsirolimus
    D. All of the above

ANSWERS

Answer 2.1.   **The answer is C.**

Mitosis is divided into prophase, prometaphase, metaphase, anaphase, and telophase. Most of the internal membranous components of the cell are dissembled and dispersed in prophase. Prometaphase prepares the cell for metaphase by forming bivalent attachments to the spindle driving them to the cellular equator. Paired chromatids align along the spindle during metaphase, followed by anaphase where sister chromatids pull to opposite poles. During telophase, prophase is reversed. Mitosis is completed by daughter cells separating during cytokinesis.

Answer 2.2.   **The answer is B.**

Cyclins are the required positive regulatory subunits of CDKs. B-type cyclins, along with CDK1, are responsible for getting cells into and through mitosis. Cyclin B1 accumulates during S and G2 phase and then is degraded at the metaphase–anaphase transition.

Answer 2.3.   **The answer is A.**

After phosphorylation of the T loop, there is an increase in CDK-cyclin contacts and changes in the binding site. Proteins from the INK4 (p15, p16, p18, and p19), Cip/Kip (p21^{Cip1}, p27^{Kip1}, and p57^{Kip2}), and Rb (p107 and p130) families all act as inhibitors of CDKs. Function of CDKs is dependent on cellular availability of cyclins for them to have enzymatic activity. Last, nuclear import/export regulation further regulates the activity of CDKs.

Answer 2.4.   **The answer is B.**

Accumulation of cyclins E and A via transcriptional induction and interaction with CDK2 allows for entry into S phase from G1 and is regulated by proteins from the Cip/Kip family. Cyclin B-CDK1 similarly accumulates allowing for the transition into M phase from G2. Entry into M phase is signaled by the dephosphorylation of T15 and Y15 resulting in the activation of CDK1. Activation of CDK1 and binding of CDC20 to APC/C is the trigger for which sister chromatids separate and move to opposite poles during anaphase.

Answer 2.5.   **The answer is D.**

Positive cell-cycle machinery is dismantled after the reduction of CDKs and cyclins. Cell-cycle exit is also usually associated with a transient increase in the number of CDK inhibitors, such as those from the INK4, Cip/Kip, and Rb protein families. Cells in quiescence also have a reduced rate of protein synthesis. Protein synthesis is largely dependent on growth factors and mitogens activating the cell through the mitogen-activated protein kinase/extracellular signaling-regulated kinase pathway and the phosphoinositide 3 (PI3) kinase/AKT pathway.

Answer 2.6.   **The answer is A.**

TGF-β is a cytokine that binds to a class of transcription factors known as SMADs that translocate to the nucleus, where they complex with DNA-binding transcription factors and coactivators to transactivate specific genes. IFNs are another class of cytokines that have antiproliferative effects by means of upregulation of CDK inhibitors and downregulation of cyclins. INK family proteins are CDK inhibitors of which p15 specifically inhibits CDK4 and CDK6 directly and cyclin E-CDK2 and cyclin A-CDK2 indirectly. The final outcome of antimitogenic signaling involves the upregulation of CDK inhibitors and downregulation of cyclins.

Answer 2.7.   **The answer is A.**

MicroRNAs regulate mRNA expression by degradation or inhibition of translation. Some of them target mRNA encoding cell-cycle regulatory proteins but none of them directly encode proteins that regulate cell cycle.

Answer 2.8.   **The answer is B.**

All of these genes are involved in regulation of cell cycle. The *NBS1* gene regulates checkpoints in cell cycles and also is involved in DNA repair. Mutation involving the *NBS1* gene results in the Nijmegen breakage syndrome 1. Patients diagnosed with this syndrome have increased risk of developing non-Hodgkins lymphoma.

Answer 2.9.   **The answer is C.**

Secondary to the topology of telomeres and the requirements of DNA replication, each cell cycle causes progressive shortening of the telomeres. In most, if not all, somatic cells, when sufficient telomere attrition has been reached, cells enter into a chronic checkpoint response, which is the molecular basis of senescence. Germ line cells forego this checkpoint by means of a special replicase, telomerase. For a somatic cell to undergo malignant transformation, the senescence barrier must be overcome allowing for unlimited proliferative capacity.

Answer 2.10.   **The answer is D.**

Tumor suppressor genes usually encode negative regulators of growth and proliferation, thereby conferring protection to cells against malignancy. Protooncogenes encode genes in which mutations may cause gain of function or an enhanced level of function leading to malignancy. Mutations of both tumor suppressor genes and protooncogenes may lead to uncontrolled proliferation and malignancy.

Answer 2.11.   **The answer is A.**

Li–Fraumeni syndrome is caused by an inherited mutation in TP53, the gene encoding the checkpoint effector p53. Nijmegen disease is caused by mutation of the gene encoding Nbs1, which is required for the activation of Chk1 and Chk2 kinases. This disease is characterized by microcephaly, immunodeficiency, increased sensitivity to radiation, and a predisposition to lymphoid malignancies. VHL is caused by a mutation in the pVHL tumor suppressor gene causing development of sporadic hemangioblastomas and clear-cell renal carcinomas. Familial malignant melanoma syndrome is caused by mutation in CDKN4A, the gene encoding p16.

Answer 2.12.   **The answer is B.**

Apoptosis is a genetically programmed means of rapid and efficient killing of unnecessary or damaged cells. It is characterized by cell shrinkage, blebbing of the plasma membrane, chromatin condensation, and intranucleosomal DNA fragmentation without being followed by surrounding inflammation.

Answer 2.13.   **The answer is D.**

The death receptor pathway is involved in the modulation of apoptosis. It involves the ligands TNFα, Fas, TRAIL, and their receptors. Noxa is a member of the BH3-only protein family and can induce apoptosis.

Answer 2.14.   **The answer is B.**

Taxanes specifically induce apoptosis by stimulating Bim expression. Nbk/Bik stimulates apoptosis by inhibiting protein synthesis. Puma and Noxa mediate apoptosis by p53 activation. After growth factor withdrawal, Bad stimulates apoptosis.

Answer 2.15.   **The answer is A.**

Sorafenib directly inhibits RAF, thereby causing MAP kinase inhibition and restoring apoptotic function. Imatinib mesylate, by means of blocking the constitutively active tyrosine kinase activity of the Bcr/Abl fusion gene, restores Bim and Bad apoptotic function. Bortezomib is a proteosome inhibitor that blocks Bim degradation, knowing it to induce apoptosis. Taxanes induce apoptosis by stimulating Bim expression.

Answer 2.16.   **The answer is A.**

Bcl-2 inhibitors like ABT-737 binds to the BH3-binding pocket of Bcl-2, Bcl-xL, and Bcl-w, thereby blocking the antiapoptotic effect of Bcl-2. ABT-737 exhibits some activity against some human lymphomas and small cell lung cancers in vitro. Inhibition of the tyrosine kinase activity of Bcr/Abl is accomplished through imatinib mesylate. Taxanes stimulate Bim expression, restoring apoptosis. Bortezomib blocks the proteosomal degradation of Bim.

Answer 2.17.   **The answer is D.**

Tumor cells generally have a reduced metabolic capacity that is frequently coupled with high-energy demand sustaining rapid cell growth. One means for specifically targeting tumor cells is through therapeutic nutrient deprivation. This is the basis for the use of angiogenesis inhibitors.

Answer 2.18.   **The answer is A.**

Autophagy is regulated by mTOR in the PI3-kinase/AKT pathway that functions to link nutrient availability to cellular metabolism. Defective autophagy has been implicated in carcinogenesis in certain human breast, ovarian, and prostate tumors. Type I programmed cell death, apoptosis, is regulated by Bax/Bak and BH3-only proteins. APC/C is the anaphase promoting complex/cyclosome that regulates sister chromatid separation in mitosis.

Answer 2.19.   **The answer is C.**

Autophagy is involved in recycling normal cellular constituents, damaged protein/organelle removal, innate immunity by removal of cells infected by intracellular pathogens, acquired immunity by promoting T-cell survival/proliferation, and protection against aging. Cell lysis secondary to surrounding inflammation or insult is a feature of necrosis.

Answer 2.20.   **The answer is B.**

Lysosome activation is a feature of apoptosis, as is cell shrinkage, blebbing of the plasma membrane, chromatin condensation, and intranucleosomal DNA fragmentation without being followed by surrounding inflammation. Necrosis is characterized by rapid swelling of the cell, loss of plasma membrane integrity, and release of intracellular components into the extracellular compartment resulting in an acute inflammatory response.

Answer 2.21.   **The answer is B.**

The Warburg effect describes an observation where most cancer cells produce energy by anerobic glycolycis even when oxygen is plentiful. This is an inefficient way of producing energy. Generating less ATPs per mode of glucose metabolized explaining the high glucose requirement by tumors.

Answer 2.22.   **The answer is B.**

For tumor cells to support their vast metabolic demands, they must induce and sustain a supply of new blood vessels through the process of angiogenesis. This is the basis of antiangiogenic therapy as a means of cancer treatment.

Answer 2.23.   **The answer is B.**

Bevacizumab is the first successful antiangiogenic agent that has shown activity in randomized phase III trials. It is a monoclonal antibody to VEGF. It has been shown to be effective in combination with chemotherapy for the treatment of metastatic colorectal cancer, breast cancer, renal cell carcinoma, and nonsmall cell lung cancer.

Answer 2.24.   **The answer is A.**

Tumor angiogenesis is first mediated by several proteolytic enzymes, such as matrix metalloproteinases, and urokinase plasminogen activator, causing a focal degradation of a venule's basement membrane. This is likely a consequence of various proangiogenic growth factors secreted by the tumor cell population or reactive stromal cells.

Answer 2.25.   **The answer is D.**

The single layer of periendothelial smooth muscle cells is formed by pericytes. These cells modulate EC function and are critical for the development of a mature vessel network. In addition to regulation of vessel diameter and permeability, they provide mechanical support and survival of ECs through paracrine signaling. Because of their ability to maintain EC survival, they have become an important target for antiangiogenic therapy and it is hypothesized that they may mediate resistance to this therapy.

Answer 2.26.   **The answer is C.**

The vasculature of solid tumors has several notable abnormalities. These vessels are classically much dilated with little to no basement membrane and have excessive tortuosity. A decreased number of pericytes portrays a relative lack of support and excessive vascular leakiness. These features contribute to the highly heterogeneous and often sluggish flow through solid tumors and create areas of relative nutrient deprivation and hypoxia. The increased leak from these vessels also allows for extravasation of high-molecular-weight plasma proteins, leading to areas of elevated interstitial fluid pressures.

Answer 2.27.   **The answer is D.**

VEGF promotes tumor angiogenesis is various ways, including stimulation of EC division, inducing EC locomotion/migration, enhancing EC survival by upregulating various inhibitors of apoptosis, and mobilizing endothelial progenitor cells from the bone marrow to sites of angiogenesis. Further, VEGF is approximately 50,000 times more potent than histamine in increasing vascular permeability. VEGF is expressed in most if not all of human cancers, and increased levels carry a poor prognosis.

Answer 2.28.   **The answer is D.**

There are at least four proposed mechanisms of how VEGF may promote tumor angiogenesis. VEGF can stimulate EC division, induce EC locomotion/migration, and enhance EC survival by upregulating different inhibitors of apoptosis and mobilizing endothelial progenitor cells from the bone marrow to sites of angiogenesis. The necessary breakdown of the basement membrane of a parental venule is most likely mediated by proangiogenic growth factors secreted by the tumor cells themselves.

Answer 2.29.   **The answer is A.**
H1F1α is upregulated by hypoxia. H1F1α then, in turn, activates numerous other genes, of which VEGF may be the most important.

Answer 2.30.   **The answer is B.**

IL-6/8 is thought to be secondarily angiogenic. TSP-1, DLL4, and vaso-hibin are all shown to inhibit angiogenesis. Embryologic studies have shown that Notch/DLL4 is important in early angiogenesis; however, in the adult, it has been shown to be an inhibitor of tumor angiogenesis.

Answer 2.31.   **The answer is A.**

The effectiveness of antiangiogenic therapy is profoundly reversed during episodes of drug-free breaks. This is thought to be mediated by the rapid mobilization and homing of ECs to the drug-treated tumors. This has led to the concept of metronomic low-dose chemotherapy. By reducing or eliminating altogether drug-free periods with continuous low-dose chemotherapy, the rapid reversal of antiangiogenic therapy may be prevented.

Answer 2.32.   **The answer is A.**

There are four currently proposed mechanisms by which tumors overcome antiangiogenic therapy. Tumors possess proangiogenic growth factor redundancy, so targeting one pathway of angiogenesis may not completely eliminate the ability of tumors to produce new vasculature. Decreasing the ability of the tumor to develop new vessels may also select for mutant/variant tumor subpopulations that are more resistant to hypoxia. Further, antiangiogenic therapy targets newly formed blood vessels. Tumors may exploit existing organ vasculature to obtain necessary oxygen and nutrients. Lastly, targeting newly forming blood vessels may accelerate the maturation and remodeling of already existing blood vessels. This may produce a more stable vascularity in tumors.

Answer 2.33.   **The answer is B.**

Antiangiogenic therapy is not without side effects. Anti-VEGF therapy has been shown to lead to specific toxicities, such as hypertension, proteinuria, bowel perforation, hemorrhage, arteriothrombotic events, and others. Among these, aplastic anemia has not been documented.

Answer 2.34.   **The answer is D.**

Tumor grade, depth of invasion, and lymphovascular invasion all carry a higher risk of metastasis. Proper immune function would hinder the development of metastasis because CTCs would be targeted for destruction.

Answer 2.35.   **The answer is B.**

By using radioactive nucleotides incorporated into tumor DNA, it has been shown that less than 0.01% of tumor cells can give rise to metastases.

Answer 2.36.   **The answer is B.**

Metastasis progression genes promote tumor metastases among other functions. Tumorigenic genes are genes that promote primary tumor growth. Metastasis virulence genes confer protection to tumor cells in the distant environment but confer no protection to the primary tumor.

Answer 2.37.   **The answer is C.**

TAMs can comprise a large percentage of the bulk of a tumor mass. Through secretion of FGF, EGF receptor ligands, and PDGF, they can stimulate tumor cell growth and motility. Furthermore, by producing uPA, MMP7, and MMP9, TAMs help degrade basement membrane allowing tumor cells to invade and metastasize.

Answer 2.38.   **The answer is A.**

Invasion starts with loss of cellular adhesion. This is largely mediated by loss of E-cadherin, the prototypic protein of the cadherin family. Cadherins are transmembrane glycoproteins that mediate cellular attachment. They anchor the cell through attachments to the actin cytoskeleton via another family of proteins called the catenins.

Answer 2.39.   **The answer is D.**

CTCs experience multiple stressors in the circulation, leading to a short half-life. Of these, physical stressors such as shear forces or mechanical injury may limit CTC life span. Also, EC-mediated stressors such as nitric oxide may induce apoptosis in CTCs. DARC, a Duffy blood group glycoprotein, interacts with KAI1 expressed on CTCs causing them to undergo senescence.

Answer 2.40.   **The answer is C.**

Ezrin links the cell membrane to the actin cytoskeleton and has been found to assist in extravasation of CTCs via activation of the MAPK pathway. VEGF has been shown to assist in CTC extravasation by causing disruptions in EC junctions and increased vascular permeability. CTC expression of CXCR4 interacts with CXCL12 expressed on certain organs, such as lung, liver, bone, and lymph nodes, allows for selective extravasation.

Answer 2.41.   **The answer is B.**

Breast, lung, and kidney cancer typically cause osteolytic lesions on metastasizing to bone. Unlike these lesions, prostate cancer causes osteoblastic lesions on metastases to bone. In contrast with osteolytic metastasis, osteoblastic lesions result from the preferential stimulation of osteoblasts or the inhibition of osteoclasts. This is mediated through many different molecules, including bone morphogenetic proteins such as WNT, TGF-β, IGF, PDGF, FGF, and VEGF.

Answer 2.42.   **The answer is C.**

Because of the microenvironment the liver provides and the dual blood supply (from the portal vein and hepatic artery), the liver is a common site of metastasis. Colon cancer generally seeds the liver via the portal system, whereas breast, lung, and melanoma approach the liver via the systemic circulation through the hepatic artery.

Answer 2.43.   **The answer is A.**

In the stochastic model of tumor heterogeneity, every cell within the tumor has equal potential but low probability of initiating tumor growth.

Answer 2.44.   **The answer is B.**

The hierarchy model of tumor heterogeneity hypothesizes the existence of functionally distinct classes of cells within the tumor, and only those with unique self-renewal ability produce new tumor growth.

Answer 2.45.   **The answer is B.**

PLX4032 is an orally available inhibitor of the mutated *BRAF* gene. It has shown activity in patients with malignant melanoma that carry the BRAF V600E mutation. About 60% of all patients with melanomas have the V600E BRAF mutation.

Answer 2.46.   **The answer is D.**

Pemetrexed is a folate antimetabolite that targets enzymes involved in purine and pyrimidine synthesis. 5-Fluorouracil is an antimetabolite that targets thymidylate synthase. Temsirolimus is mammalian target of rapamycin (mTOR) inhibitor that targets the PI3-kinase pathway. The PI3-kinase pathway is involved in regulation of glucose metabolism.

CHAPTER 3 ETIOLOGY OF CANCER ■ PART 1

SHIRISH M. GADGEEL

DIRECTIONS   Each of the numbered items below is followed by lettered answers. Select the ONE lettered answer that is BEST in each case unless instructed otherwise.

QUESTIONS

Question 3.1.   All the following statements regarding the relationship between cigarette smoking and lung cancer are correct, EXCEPT:

A. The duration of smoking is the strongest determinant of lung cancer in smokers.
B. Smoking increases the risk of all histologic types of lung cancer.
C. The risk of developing lung cancer in ex-smokers drops to the level of never smokers two years after smoking cessation.
D. The risk of developing lung cancer increases with the number of cigarettes smoked.

Question 3.2.   The role of specific tobacco product carcinogens in specific tumors is characterized by the following, EXCEPT:

A. Polycyclic aromatic hydrocarbons are major causative factors in lung cancer.
B. Aromatic amines are a major cause of bladder cancer.
C. N-nitrosamines are important causative factors in esophageal cancer.
D. Nicotine is an important carcinogen in the causation of laryngeal cancer.

Question 3.3.   The following enzymes are involved in metabolic activation of the carcinogens in cigarette smoke:

A. P450 enzyme 1A1 and 1A2
B. Glutathione-S-transferases and uridine diphosphate-glucuronosyl transferases
C. Nucleotide excision repair enzymes
D. None of the above

Corresponding Chapters in *Cancer: Principles & Practice of Oncology*, Ninth Edition: 13 (Tobacco), 14 (Cancer Susceptibility Syndromes), 15 (DNA Viruses), 16 (RNA Viruses), and 17 (Inflammation).

Question 3.4. Mechanisms of tumor induction by carcinogens in tobacco products include the following, EXCEPT:

A. Bonds formed between carcinogens and DNA, resulting in DNA adducts.

B. Nicotine and nitrosamines bind to cellular receptors, resulting in activation of the pathways that enhance growth and suppress apoptosis.

C. Enzymatic methylation of gene promoters, resulting in gene silencing.

D. Inhibition of DNA repair enzymes.

Question 3.5. Which of the following cancers is caused by smokeless tobacco use?

A. Cancer of the oral cavity

B. Esophageal cancer

C. Pancreatic cancer

D. All of the above

Question 3.6. Knudson's hypothesis regarding cancer susceptibility:

A. Postulates that predisposition to cancer arises as the result of a heterozygous germ line mutation, which then requires a second acquired mutation in the unaffected allele for tumor to develop.

B. Was validated by observations in patients with neuroblastoma.

C. Postulates that different genes are involved in familial and sporadic forms of a tumor.

D. None of the above.

Question 3.7. All of the following are true regarding genetic changes that are involved in cancer initiation, EXCEPT:

A. Changes in genes regulating cell cycle can be involved in cancer initiation.

B. Changes in genes that maintain DNA integrity can be involved in cancer initiation.

C. Genetic mutations involved with cancer initiation only occur in the tissue of origin.

D. Changes in genes regulating cellular functions, such as angiogenesis, can be involved in cancer initiation.

Question 3.8. Current American Society of Clinical Oncology (ASCO) guidelines recommend testing for cancer susceptibility syndromes in the following, EXCEPT:

A. The general population should be tested for the common cancer susceptibility syndromes.

B. In individuals suspected to have familial syndrome.

C. Genetic test can be adequately interpreted.

D. Genetic test results will aid management of individuals undergoing the test.

Question 3.9.   Retinoblastoma protein, Rb1, is characterized by the following, EXCEPT:

A. Involved in maintaining the integrity of the retina
B. A central regulator of cell cycle
C. Binds to E2F transcription proteins
D. A 105-kDa protein that undergoes phosphorylation during cell cycle

Question 3.10.   Hereditary nonpolyposis colon cancer (HNPCC) syndrome is characterized by:

A. Mutations in genes that regulate cellular proliferation
B. Autosomal-recessive inheritance
C. Greater penetrance in women
D. Mutations in genes that are involved in DNA mismatch repair

Question 3.11.   Which of the following is characteristic of HNPCC or Lynch syndrome?

A. HNPCC is inherited in autosomal-dominant pattern with increased penetrance in males.
B. Multiple polyps are seen on colonoscopy, preceding the diagnosis of colon cancer.
C. Annual colonoscopy is recommended for family members of patients with HNPCC, starting at age 40.
D. Patients with HNPCC have germ line mutations in the *APC* gene.

Question 3.12.   Impaired activity of BRCA 1 and BRCA 2 proteins affects:

A. Repair of double-stranded DNA breaks
B. Cell-cycle regulation
C. Microtubule stabilization
D. Angiogenesis

Question 3.13.   BRCA1 mutation carriers typically develop which of the following types of breast cancer?

A. High grade, ER positive, Her2/neu positive, invasive ductal carcinoma
B. High grade, ER negative, Her2/neu negative, invasive ductal carcinoma
C. Low grade, ER positive, Her2/neu negative, invasive ductal carcinoma
D. Low grade, ER negative, Her2/neu positive, invasive ductal carcinoma

Question 3.14.   All of the following statements regarding neurofibromatosis Type 1(NF1) are correct, EXCEPT:

A. NF1 is inherited in an autosomal-dominant pattern, with 100% penetrance for neurofibroma.
B. 70 different mutations in NF1 have been reported, most of which result in a truncated neurofibromin protein.
C. Mutations in *SPRED1* gene can give rise to an NF1-like phenotype.
D. Genetic testing for NF1 significantly impacts clinical management.

Question 3.15. Familial adenomatous polyposis (FAP) syndrome is characterized by the following, EXCEPT:

A. It results from mutations in the *APC* gene.
B. There is an almost 100% risk of developing colon cancer by age 40 years.
C. Increased risk of desmoid tumors.
D. Nonsteroidal anti-inflammatory drugs (NSAIDs) can be recommended in place of prophylactic colectomy to reduce the risk of colon cancer.

Question 3.16. p53 protein is characterized by the following, EXCEPT:

A. It is a DNA-binding transcription factor.
B. Is activated in response to cellular stress.
C. Mutations of p53 are common in hereditary cancer syndromes but rare in sporadic cancers.
D. Germ line mutations of p53 are the cause of Li–Fraumeni syndrome.

Question 3.17. Hereditary cancer syndromes more commonly:

A. Result from gain-of-function mutations
B. Result from loss-of-function mutations
C. Result from abnormality of genes that promote angiogenesis
D. None of the above

Question 3.18. Von Hippel–Lindau (VHL) gene:

A. Encodes a ubiquitin ligase to target HIF 1a and HIF 2a for degradation
B. Enhances angiogenesis
C. Is mutated in renal cell cancers in patients with VHL syndrome but not in sporadic renal cell cancers
D. None of the above

Question 3.19. Alteration in PTEN gene and cancer susceptibility are characterized by the following, EXCEPT:

A. Loss of one PTEN allele can lead to cancer, but loss of both alleles is anticancer.
B. Patients inherit a mutation in the *PTEN* gene and then require a second hit to the normal allele to develop cancer.
C. Variations in PTEN expression rather than complete loss may lead to carcinogenesis.
D. Pharmacologic manipulation toward complete loss of PTEN expression in cancer cells may help in cancer prevention and/or therapy.

Question 3.20.   **Retroviruses are:**

A. RNA viruses that have the capacity to synthesize double-stranded DNA from single-stranded viral RNA genome
B. DNA viruses that have the capacity to synthesize double-stranded RNA from single-stranded viral DNA genome
C. Dependent on host nucleotide synthesis enzymes to replicate the viral genome
D. Viruses that cause oncogenic transformation in humans only through a direct transforming effect

Question 3.21.   **Retroviruses participate in oncogenic transformation through the following mechanisms, EXCEPT:**

A. By causing insertional mutagenesis
B. By affecting the expression of cellular growth and differentiation genes
C. Acutely transforming viruses that insert an oncogene in the infected cells
D. By inducing an inflammatory response in the tissue

Question 3.22.   **Which of the following features does the human T-cell lymphotropic virus type I (HTLV1) have in common with human immunodeficiency virus (HIV)?**

A. Both HIV and HTLV1 lead to induction of syncytia in cultured T cells.
B. Both retroviruses have a tropism for CD4+ T lymphocytes, and result in marked cellular immunodeficiency.
C. Significant viremia is detected in individuals infected with either HTLV-1 or HIV.
D. All of the above.

Question 3.23.   **Pathogenesis of adult T-cell leukemia (ATL) from HTLV1 infection is related to:**

A. Insertion of the viral genome at specific locations in the T-cell genome
B. Presence of host-derived oncogene in the viral genome
C. The viral protein Tax transactivating many cellular genes, particularly interleukin (IL)-2 and IL-2 receptor
D. HTLV1 infection increasing susceptibility of T cells to other transforming viruses

Question 3.24.   **HTLV2 is a retrovirus with the following characteristics, EXCEPT:**

A. It is closely related to HTLV 1.
B. HTLV2 can also cause ATL-like HTLV1.
C. It is transmitted by the same routes as HTLV1, such as sexual intercourse, contaminated blood, and breastfeeding.
D. Convincing data for an etiologic role for HTLV2 in human disease are lacking.

Question 3.25.   Pathogenesis of increased risk of cancer in HIV-infected patients is characterized by the following:

A. HIV infection leads to the insertion of the viral genome at critical locations of the cellular genome leading to chimeric proteins that are procarcinogenic.
B. HIV genome contains oncogenes that are transcribed in the infected cells causing cancers.
C. HIV infection causes immune deficiency in infected patients, which contributes to the development of cancer.
D. HIV reverse transcriptase activates many cellular oncogenes during viral replication.

Question 3.26.   Acquired immune deficiency syndrome (AIDS)-related Kaposi's sarcoma (KS) is characterized by the following, EXCEPT:

A. Immune deficiency caused by HIV is involved in the pathogenesis of KS.
B. HHV-8 infection in HIV-infected patients is the etiologic agent of KS.
C. Tat protein secreted by the infected HIV cells increases the level of various cytokines and contributes to the pathogenesis of KS.
D. Mutation induced by HIV in infected endothelial cells contributes to the pathogenesis of KS.

Question 3.27.   Pathogenesis of lymphomas in patients with HIV is linked to all the following, EXCEPT:

A. Epstein–Barr virus (EBV) in patients with HIV
B. Immune deficiency caused by HIV
C. Lymphomas that arise in the HIV-infected CD4+ T cells
D. HIV-induced cytokine dysregulation

Question 3.28.   Hepatitis C virus (HCV) is:

A. An RNA virus that is transmitted by percutaneous routes
B. A retrovirus that is transmitted by percutaneous route
C. A DNA virus that is transmitted by the fecal–oral route
D. None of the above

Question 3.29.   Which of the following statements is correct regarding the association between HCV infection and hepatocellular carcinoma (HCC)?

A. Approximately 1% to 5% of patients with chronic HCV infection will develop HCC.
B. The incidence of HCC has decreased during the last few decades, due to better screening of blood products for HCV.
C. Vaccination against HCC is an effective means for preventing HCC.
D. All of the above.

Question 3.30.   Association between HCV and HCC includes the following, EXCEPT:

A. Alcohol consumption or coinfection with hepatitis B virus (HBV) in a patient with HCV increases the risk of HCC.
B. Treatment of patients with HCV with interferon and ribavirin eliminates the risk of HCC in these patients.
C. There is a 20- to 30-year lag period between HCV infection and the development of HCC.
D. Inflammatory changes resulting from HCV infection are primarily responsible for development of HCC in HCV-infected patients.

Question 3.31.   HBV has the following characteristics, EXCEPT:

A. DNA virus that belongs to the hepadnavirus family.
B. In 95% of individuals who become infected with HBV, the infection resolves with clearance of the virus.
C. Twenty-five percent of individuals infected with HBV develop HCC.
D. HBV-infected patients who develop chronic hepatitis are at an increased risk of developing HCC.

Question 3.32.   Human papilloma virus (HPV) has been linked with the following cancers, EXCEPT:

A. Cervical cancer
B. Penile cancer
C. Oropharyngeal cancers
D. Esophageal cancers

Question 3.33.   Pathogenesis of cervical cancer from HPV infection is characterized by the following, EXCEPT:

A. E6 and E7 viral proteins are most closely related to the transforming potential of HPV.
B. Every person infected with HPV eventually develops cancer.
C. Smoking is identified as a risk factor and can increase the risk of cervical cancer in HPV-infected patients.
D. Cell-cycle regulatory proteins p53 and RB (retinoblastoma protein) are important targets of HPV oncoproteins.

Question 3.34.   The following type of HPV has a strong association with cervical cancer:

A. HPV-6
B. HPV-11
C. HPV-16
D. None of the above

Question 3.35.   The recently approved HPV vaccine:

A. Is a quadrivalent vaccine containing virus-like particles (VLPs) from four different types of HPV
B. Protects all types of HPV-causing cervical cancer
C. Is recommended for all sexually active men and women
D. Eliminates the need for routine cervical cancer screening 2 years after completing the vaccination schedule

Question 3.36.   The role of EBV in cancer is characterized by the following, EXCEPT:

A. EBV nuclear proteins target transcription factor RBPJk/CBF1.
B. Membrane protein LMP1 activates IKK alpha and enhances cellular proliferation and survival.
C. Involvement in minority of the gastric cancers.
D. Involvement in all Hodgkin's lymphoma.

Question 3.37.   The risk of KS in patients with HIV is highest:

A. In homosexual men
B. In pediatric patients with AIDS
C. In heterosexual men
D. In patients with AIDS related to blood transfusions

Question 3.38.   Human herpes virus 8 (HHV8) infection is characterized by:

A. HHV8 sequences are detected only in tumors of patients with KS who are HIV positive.
B. Five to seven percent of the US general population is infected with HHV8.
C. In patients with HIV, coinfection with EBV infection is necessary for development of KS.
D. HHV8 infection is transmitted only through sexual contact.

Question 3.39.   The role of polyomaviruses in human cancers is characterized by:

A. A double-blind study has confirmed the correlation of SV40 with human cancers.
B. SV40 DNA or antigen has been observed in some human cancers, such as osteosarcomas, mesotheliomas, and brain tumors.
C. BK and JC viruses are recognized etiologic factors in human brain tumors.
D. Epidemiologic data have confirmed the association of SV40-contaminated polio vaccines with human cancers.

Question 3.40.   Which of the following sentences best describes immune surveillance of tumors?

A. Innate immunity has no effective role in immune surveillance of tumors.

B. A standard mechanism of immune surveillance is involved for all tumors.

C. Immune surveillance of tumors is based on expression of appropriate tumor antigens.

D. Both innate and adaptive immune cells, along with their effector molecules, are important in immune surveillance of tumors.

Question 3.41.   All the following statements are true regarding immune surveillance of tumors, EXCEPT:

A. The presence of tumor-infiltrating lymphocytes in tumors, such as colon and ovarian cancer, is associated with improved prognosis.

B. In patients with paraneoplastic neurologic syndromes, the autoimmune response also controls tumor progression.

C. Among the skin cancers, melanoma risk is increased the most in immune-suppressed individuals.

D. Acute infections with bacteria could induce regressions of cancers.

Question 3.42.   Evidence that supports the association of inflammation and cancer include the following, EXCEPT:

A. An ulcerative lesion resulting from chronic inflammation after skin thermal injury can undergo malignant transformation.

B. Inflammatory cells are frequently present in tumor stroma.

C. Changes induced by acute bronchitis can lead to lung cancer.

D. Risk of colon cancer is increased in patients with inflammatory bowel disease.

Question 3.43.   Infectious agents can cause cancers by:

A. Transformation of infected cells

B. Establishing a chronic inflammatory microenvironment in the infected tissues

C. None of the above

D. Both A and B

Question 3.44.   All statements regarding tumor necrosis factor (TNF) and cancer are true, EXCEPT:

A. TNF can induce apoptosis of tumor and endothelial cells.

B. TNF can induce production of matrix metalloproteinase (MMP)-9 and activation of nuclear factor (NF)-kB.

C. TNF can promote carcinogenesis.

D. None of the above.

Question 3.45.   Which of the following is TRUE regarding cyclooxygenase (COX)-2 and cancer?

A. COX-2 inhibitors can reduce the incidence of colon cancer only in individuals with FAP.
B. COX inhibitors not only reduce colon cancers but also decrease the number of colonic polyps.
C. COX-2 inhibitors can prevent only colon cancers associated with inflammatory conditions such as ulcerative colitis.
D. None of the above.

Question 3.46.   Cancer-associated stromal fibroblasts (CAFs) are characterized by:

A. Lack of expression of vimentin unlike other fibroblasts
B. Consistently demonstrate genetic alterations and have undergone transformation
C. Their ability to better support tumor progression than other fibroblasts
D. Their ability to inhibit tumor progression

Question 3.47.   Dendritic cells (DCs) are characterized by the following, EXCEPT:

A. DCs rapidly respond to alterations in tissue homeostasis.
B. DCs secrete proinflammatory cytokines, including IL-12 and TNF.
C. DCs present antigens in the context of major histocompatibility complex class I and II to T cells.
D. DCs are activated in tumors and contribute to immune surveillance of tumors.

Question 3.48.   Tumor-associated macrophages (TAMs):

A. Have no role in tumor growth or tumor destruction
B. Only promote angiogenesis and tumor progression
C. Have reduced antitumor effects in the presence of IL-10
D. Produce high levels of proinflammatory cytokines and therefore are only associated with tumor destruction

Question 3.49.   Toll-like receptors (TLRs) are:

A. A family of at least 12 different pattern recognition receptors.
B. TLRs, along with other pattern-recognizing receptors, are important in microbial sensing.
C. TLR triggering in tumor cells may result in tumor apoptosis, but activation of TLRs in tumor-infiltrating cells results in tumor promotion.
D. All the above.

ANSWERS

Answer 3.1.   **The answer is C.**

Smoking increases the risk of developing all histologic types of lung cancer, including adenocarcinoma, squamous cell carcinoma, large cell carcinoma, and small cell carcinoma. The strongest determinant of lung cancer in smokers is duration of smoking. The risk also increases with the number of cigarettes smoked. Cessation of smoking avoids the further increase in risk of lung cancer caused by continued smoking. However, the risk of developing lung cancer in ex-smokers remains elevated for years after cessation, compared to that of never smokers.

Answer 3.2.   **The answer is D.**

Cigarette smoke consists of many carcinogens. Data from carcinogenicity studies, product analyses, and biochemical and molecular biological investigations support a significant role for certain carcinogens in specific types of tobacco-induced cancers. In this regard, evidence suggests a significant role for polycyclic aromatic hydrocarbons and *N*-nitrosamines as causative factors in lung cancer. Evidence also supports the role of aromatic amines as a cause of bladder cancer and a role for *N*-nitrosamines as a cause for esophageal cancer. Nicotine itself is not known to initiate cancer formation, but recent evidence suggests that nicotine through nicotinic receptors may promote cellular proliferation.

Answer 3.3.   **The answer is A.**

Many cigarette smoke carcinogens are not active and require metabolic activation to transform them into active carcinogens. Cytochrome P450 enzymes convert these compounds into electrophilic entities that can covalently bind to DNA-forming DNA adducts. P-450 enzymes 1A1 and 1A2 are particularly important in the metabolic activation of some of the carcinogens in cigarette smoke. Other P450 enzymes involved in this process include 1B1, 2A13, 2E1, and 3A4. 1A1 and 1B2 are induced by compounds in cigarette smoke, and the induction of these enzymes may be a critical aspect of cancer susceptibility in smokers. The cigarette smoke carcinogens can undergo detoxification by glutathione-S-transferases and uridine diphosphate -glucuronosyl transferases. Therefore, cancer susceptibility may be determined by the balance achieved between activation of the carcinogens in cigarette smoke and their detoxification. In addition, polymorphisms in genes encoding these enzymes may influence an individual's risk of cancer from these carcinogens. Cellular repair systems can remove the DNA adducts formed by smoke carcinogens and repair the DNA, but they are not involved in metabolic activation of carcinogens in cigarette smoke. Nucleotide excision repair enzymes are a component of these repair systems.

Answer 3.4.   **The answer is D.**

Formation of bonds between smoke carcinogens and DNA resulting in DNA adducts is an important aspect of the carcinogenicity of cigarette smoke. DNA adducts that are not removed result in miscoding during replication leading to mutations. Mutations have been frequently observed in the KRAS oncogene in lung cancer and in the TP53 tumor suppressor gene in various cigarette smoke-induced cancers. Processes, other than formation of DNA adducts, that contribute to cancer formation are activation of cellular receptors by *N*-nitrosamines and nicotine and the silencing of certain genes through methylation of the gene promoters. Nucleotide excision repair enzymes are part of the cellular repair systems that remove DNA adducts and repair the DNA. There are no data to suggest that carcinogens in cigarette smoke inhibit these enzymes.

Answer 3.5.   **The answer is D.**

Various carcinogens have been detected in smokeless tobacco products. The most abundant are *N*-nitrosamines 4-(methylnitrosamino)-1-(3-pyridyl)-1-butanone (NNK) and *N*-nitrosonornicotine (NNN). Smokeless tobacco use is known to cause three cancers: pancreatic cancer, esophageal cancer, and cancer of the oral cavity. Based on animal studies, the most probable carcinogens causing these cancers in smokeless tobacco users are NNN for esophageal cancer, NNK for pancreatic cancer, and both NNN and NNK for cancers of the oral cavity.

Answer 3.6.   **The answer is A.**

More than 30 years ago, Alfred Knudson postulated that predisposition to cancer arises as the result of a heterozygous germ line mutation, which then requires a second acquired mutation in the unaffected allele for tumor to develop, also called the "two-hit hypothesis." The hypothesis was validated in patients with retinoblastoma. These individuals inherit a mutated *Rb* gene and then acquire mutation in the normal allele of the gene leading to cancer. Further studies also revealed that the genes involved in carcinogenesis of the familial form of the cancer can also be involved in the sporadic forms of that cancer.

Answer 3.7.   **The answer is C.**

For cancer to initiate, the cancerous cell has to eventually acquire the ability to proliferate or abrogate apoptosis. It is recognized that two classes of tumor suppressors may cooperate in tumor formation: (a) those that control proliferation and survival through control of the cell cycle and (b) those that are involved in the control of genomic integrity. Loss of genes involved in maintaining genomic integrity may lead to mutations in genes that control proliferation or apoptosis. Apart from alterations in genes involved with cellular functions of proliferation and survival, changes in genes involved in other cellular functions such as angiogenesis may be the driving force for carcinogenesis. In addition, even though genetic changes in tissue of origin are generally the cause of cancer initiation, in some cases the genetic changes may occur in the stromal cells resulting in aberrant stromal–parenchymal interactions, leading to carcinogenesis.

Answer 3.8.   **The answer is A.**

The ASCO guidelines state that screening for cancer susceptibility syndromes is not warranted in the general population but is recommended for individuals with a suspected familial syndrome. In addition, the guidelines recommend that the testing should be done if the results can be easily interpreted and will influence the management of the individuals being tested.

Answer 3.9.   **The answer is A.**

Rb1 protein is a central regulator of the cell cycle. It is a 105-kDa protein that undergoes phosphorylation at specific points in the cell cycle. During the G0 and G1 phases of the cell cycle, hypophosphorylated Rb1 protein binds to E2F transcription factors. Cyclin D-CDK4 phosphorylates Rb1 protein when the cell cycle transitions to the S phase. Phosphorylated RB1 protein dissociates from the E2F transcription factors, which then allows these factors to recruit and activate other cell-cycle genes.

Answer 3.10.   **The answer is D.**

HNPCC, originally known as Lynch syndrome, is the most common cancer susceptibility disease and is responsible for at least 2% to 3% of total colon cancer cases in the United States. HNPCC can be caused by a germ line mutation in one of five genes: *MLH1, MSH2, MSH6, PMS1,* or *PMS2.* All five genes function in DNA mismatch repair, and so mutations in these genes affect genomic integrity. HNPCC is inherited in an autosomal-dominant fashion with a penetrance of approximately 90%. Men are affected at a higher penetrance, with women being less affected but at an additional risk of endometrial cancer.

Answer 3.11.   **The answer is A.**

HNPCC accounts for 2% to 3% of total colon cancer cases, and is caused by a germ line mutation in one of six DNA mismatch repair genes: *MLH1, MSH2, MSH3, MSH6, PMS1,* or *PMS2.* HNPCC is inherited in an autosomal-dominant manner with a penetrance of about 90%. Males are affected at a higher penetrance. Patients with HNPCC have increased risk of stomach, ovary, small intestine, ureter, and kidney cancers. Patients typically present with colon cancer at a younger average age than patients with sporadic colon cancer. In contrast to other familial colon cancer syndromes, patients with HNPCC rarely exhibit polyps, making early detection difficult. Family members of patients with HNPCC should undergo annual screening colonoscopy starting at approximately age 20 years. In addition, women should undergo yearly pelvic examinations and ultrasound.

Answer 3.12.   **The answer is A.**

BRCA1 and BRCA2 proteins function in DNA damage repair. BRCA1 and BRCA2 proteins are recruited to the site of double-stranded DNA breaks along with other proteins. These complexes function to repair the double-stranded break, although the precise role of BRCA1 and BRCA2 in these complexes remains unclear. These proteins have no known role in cell-cycle regulation, microtubule stabilization, or angiogenesis.

Answer 3.13.   **The answer is B.**

BRCA1 mutation carriers typically develop high grade, ER negative, and Her2/neu negative invasive ductal carcinoma of the breast. On the other hand, tumors in BRCA2 mutation carriers typically show a wider spectrum of histological features.

Answer 3.14.   **The answer is D.**

NF1 is inherited in an autosomal-dominant manner with a 100% penetrance for neurofibromas, resulting from mutations in the *NF1* gene. NF1 encodes the neurofibromin protein, a GTPase activating protein for the Ras family of proteins. Over 70 different mutations in NF1 have been reported, with 70% of these mutations resulting in a truncated neurofibromin protein. Mutations in *SPRED1* gene can give rise to a NF1-like phenotype. Patients with NF1 syndrome develop neurofibromas and have an increased risk for glioblastomas, pheochromocytomas, and myeloid leukemias. Café au lait spots are found in 100% of patients with NF1 syndrome and increase in size and frequency with age. Genetic testing is available but typically does not impact clinical management because the disorder is readily identified by phenotype.

Answer 3.15.   **The answer is D.**

FAP is caused by germ line mutations in the *APC* gene on chromosome 5q that are inherited in an autosomal-dominant fashion. The characteristic feature of FAP syndrome is the presence of numerous adenomatous polyps. Development of colon cancer by the age of 40 years is a certainty. Patients with FAP also have an increased risk of desmoids tumors and malignancies of the upper gastrointestinal tract. Prophylactic colectomy is recommended in these individuals to reduce the risk of colon cancer. Nonsteroidal anti-inflammatory drugs can reduce the size and number of the polyps in patients with FAP through the inhibition of COX-2 pathway but are not recommended in place of surgery to reduce the risk of colon cancer.

Answer 3.16.   **The answer is C.**

p53 protein is a labile DNA-binding transcription factor that is not expressed at high levels during normal cellular homeostasis. In response to cellular stress, including hypoxia and DNA damage, p53 protein is stabilized and activates transcription of growth arrest genes that halt the cell in G1. The G1 arrest halts the cell until damage can be repaired. If the damage persists, the cells remain in an irreversible G1 arrest or undergo apoptosis. Mutations in p53 are found in the majority of sporadic cancers, and it is hypothesized that p53 function may be compromised in some way in all cancers. p53 mutations are the cause of Li–Fraumeni syndrome. The most common cancers found in patients with Li–Fraumeni are sarcomas, breast cancer, and brain tumors.

Answer 3.17.   **The answer is B.**

Hereditary cancer syndromes more commonly occur as a result of mutations that result in loss of function. Thus, Li–Fraumeni syndrome, HNPCC syndrome, FAP, BRCA1, and BRCA2 are caused by mutations that result in the loss of function of the gene. It is hypothesized that most oncogenic gain-of-function mutations are incompatible with embryonic development, explaining their rarity in hereditary cancer syndromes. Examples of hereditary cancer syndromes resulting from gain-of-function mutations are multiple endocrine neoplasia type 2, which results from mutations of the receptor tyrosine kinase RET; hereditary papillary renal cancer resulting from mutations in the *MET* gene; and hereditary gastrointestinal stromal tumor resulting from mutations in the *KIT* gene. Mutations in genes that regulate angiogenesis may also lead to hereditary cancer syndromes. VHL is a genetic disorder that results from loss-of-function mutation of the *VHL* gene leading to increased expression of angiogenic factors. Hereditary leiomyomatosis and renal cancer is another familial cancer syndrome that might result from genes affecting angiogenesis.

Answer 3.18.   **The answer is A.**

VHL gene encodes a ubiquitin ligase to target HIF 1α and HIF 2α for degradation under normoxic conditions. In hypoxic conditions, the expression of VHL is downregulated, resulting in accumulation of HIF 1α and HIF 2α, which act as transcription factors, and the expression of angiogenic factors, such as vascular endothelial growth factor, is upregulated. In VHL syndrome, mutations in the *VHL* gene result in loss of function of the VHL protein, resulting in accumulation of HIF 1α and HIF 2α even under normoxic conditions. Individuals with VHL syndrome have an increased risk of developing renal cysts, renal cancer, and hemangioblastomas of the central nervous system. VHL function is also altered in 70% to 80% of the clear cell renal carcinomas.

Answer 3.19.   **The answer is B.**

PTEN operates as a haploinsufficient tumor suppressor to oppose tumor initiation. Cancer can develop in individuals with loss of one PTEN allele resulting in cellular proliferation and survival advantages. However, complete PTEN loss is detrimental to the cancer cell because it triggers a "cellular senescence" response. This cellular senescence response to complete loss of PTEN is being evaluated for cancer chemoprevention and therapy. Many tumor suppressor genes have been found to be haploinsufficient for specific functions. The PTEN paradigm also highlights the importance of subtle incremental variations in the expression levels of tumor suppressor genes, which then can lead to devastating consequences resulting in distinct outcomes in distinct tissues. The haploinsufficient tumor suppressors contrast with the retinoblastoma paradigm or the Knudson's hypothesis. In retinoblastoma, individuals inherit a mutation in one of the alleles of the RB gene and require a "second hit" to the other allele to develop cancer.

Answer 3.20.   **The answer is A.**

Among the animal viruses, retroviruses are unique in having an RNA genome that replicates through a DNA intermediate. Once the retrovirus infects the cell, the single-stranded viral genome is converted to double-stranded DNA by an RNA-dependent DNA polymerase or reverse transcriptase. The double-stranded DNA then is integrated into a host cell chromosome. Retroviruses in animals can transform the infected cell by integrating the viral DNA close to cellular oncogenes, integrating a protooncogene in the host cell genome, or altering the cellular gene expression or function. In humans, HTLV1 is the only retrovirus that has been shown to have a direct transforming effect. HIV, the other retrovirus, is more likely to cause malignant transformation in humans through an indirect effect of immune suppression.

Answer 3.21.   **The answer is D.**

Retroviruses transform cells through either an acute process or a slow transforming process. Acutely transforming viruses insert a viral oncogene into the host cell genome leading to malignant transformation. The slowly transforming viruses cause cellular transformation either by inserting the viral DNA adjacent to a cellular protooncogene (insertional mutagenesis) or altering the expression of cellular gene expression and function by viral proteins. Inflammation and its consequences are not known to be an important cause of retrovirus-induced cellular transformation.

Answer 3.22.   **The answer is A.**

HTLV-1 shares a number of features with HIV: a complex genetic structure, tropism for CD4 T lymphocytes, induction of syncytia in cultured T cells, and similar routes of transmission (blood transfusions, sexual contact, needle sharing, and breastfeeding). However, HTLV-1 infection is not associated with marked cellular immunodeficiency unless ATL develops. Unlike HIV, where infection by free virions is typical, with high levels of viremia detected in HIV-1-infected individuals, a significant viremia is not detected in individuals with HTLV-1. In patients with HTLV-1, the virus spreads to uninfected cells by cell-to-cell transmission of the virus. In addition, the number of HTLV-1-infected cells within an individual increases by simple mitosis of virus-containing T cells.

Answer 3.23.   **The answer is C.**

HTLV1 protein Tax activates viral gene expression by interacting with cellular transcription proteins. Subsequently through this interaction with cellular transcription proteins, Tax leads to activation of several cellular gene promoters. IL-2 and IL-2 receptor are the most relevant genes activated by Tax. Adult T cells constitutively express the alpha chain of IL-2 receptor at high levels, and this can stimulate proliferation of infected cells. The site of integration of the viral genome is random and different from patient to patient, indicating that insertional mutagenesis does not play a role in the transforming effect of HTLV1. The long latency period between the onset of the infection and the development of the malignancy suggests that HTLV1 genome does not contain an acutely transforming oncogene. Unlike HIV, HTLV1 does not have an immuno-suppressive effect.

Answer 3.24.   **The answer is B.**

HTLV2 shares 70% homology at the amino acid level with HTLV1. The virus was isolated from a patient with atypical T-cell variant hairy cell leukemia, but convincing epidemiologic data for an etiologic role for HTLV2 in any human disease do not exist. HTLV2 is also transmitted by the same routes as HTLV1 and is found in 0.01% of blood donors and in a larger proportion of intravenous drug users.

Answer 3.25.   **The answer is C.**

HIV, unlike HTLV1, the other retrovirus with transforming effects in humans, does not have a direct oncogenic effect. None of the HIV proteins have a directly transforming effect, and none of the proteins are known to enhance the expression of any of the cellular oncogenes. Rarely, insertional mutagenesis resulting in T-cell lymphomas has been reported in HIV-infected patients. However, this disease does not occur disproportionately in HIV-infected patients, making the observation of insertional mutagenesis in some patients with T-cell lymphomas as a random event rather than a specific oncogenic transforming effect of the virus. Many of the malignancies observed in HIV-infected patients, including the AIDS-defining cancers such as cervical cancer or non-Hodgkin's lymphoma, are associated with coinfection by DNA viruses. Infection with these viruses and the subsequent transforming effect are facilitated by the state of immune suppression induced by the HIV infection.

Answer 3.26.   **The answer is D.**

KS tumors are histologically complex tumors. The predominant cell and the most likely candidate tumor cell of KS is the spindle cell, but the tumor also consists of inflammatory cells and angiogenic cells. A polyclonal, multicentric proliferative process seems to occur, which is reflected in the frequently observed waxing and waning clinical course of KS. HHV-8 is the primary etiologic agent of KS in HIV-infected and noninfected patients. The role of HIV in the pathogenesis of KS is related to its ability to suppress immunity. In addition to the immune suppression, secretion of Tat protein by HIV-infected cells contributes to the production of cytokines, such as vascular endothelial growth factor, and these factors enhance the proliferation of the endothelial cells. HIV does not have any direct transforming effect on endothelial cells.

Answer 3.27.   **The answer is C.**

HIV-infected patients are at an increased risk of developing non-Hodgkin's lymphoma, including Burkitt's or Burkitt's-like lymphomas. The majority of these lymphomas are B-cell lymphomas, and many are associated with EBV. In addition to the immunosuppression, it has been theorized that HIV may contribute to lymphomagenesis via dysregulation of cytokine production and subsequent alteration of B-cell growth regulation. HIV does not have a transforming effect on the infected CD4+ T cells.

Answer 3.28.   **The answer is A.**

HCV is an RNA virus that belongs to the Hepacivirus genus of the Flaviviridae family of viruses. HCV is transmitted in a majority of the cases by a percutaneous route. Before 1989, when screening for HCV began, transfusion of contaminated blood products was the most important cause of HCV infection. Use of contaminated needles by intravenous drug users remains an important source of the infection. It can also be transmitted perinatally and via sexual routes. In 10% of the cases, risk factors for transmission are not identified. The fecal–oral route is not known to be a route for infection with HCV.

Answer 3.29.   **The answer is A.**

Approximately 1% to 5% of the patients with chronic HCV infection will develop HCC. The incidence of HCV infection has decreased with improved screening of blood products for HCV; however, there is a 10- to 20-year lag between HCV infection and cirrhosis, and a 20- to 30-year lag to developing HCC. This has resulted in the rising incidence of HCC in previously infected patients. An effective HCV vaccine is not available.

Answer 3.30.   **The answer is B.**

Alcohol consumption or coinfection with HBV greatly increases the risk of developing HCC in HCV-infected patients. The role of HCV in the pathogenesis of HCC remains to be fully clarified. The inflammatory response caused by the HCV infection leads to hepatocyte destruction, regeneration, and fibrosis. Cellular turnover as a result of the inflammatory response could have a transforming effect leading to the pathogenesis of HCC. A direct oncogenic role of HCV is unlikely, although there have been results suggesting that the HCV core protein may have an oncogenic effect. In addition, infection with different strains of the virus may pose a different level of risk for development of HCC. Treatment with interferon and ribavirin can reduce the risk of HCC from HCV infection but cannot eliminate it.

Answer 3.31.   **The answer is C.**

HBV is a small DNA virus classified as a member of the hepadnavirus family (for hepatotropic DNA viruses). HBV is the only human virus in this family. Primary HBV infection produces a subclinical infection or acute liver injury, but 95% of such infections resolve with clearance of the virus. However, 5% of patients develop persistent hepatic infection, and these individuals are at risk of developing HCC. Patients with the highest levels of HBV viremia display the highest HCC risk. Patients with persistent infection can develop chronic active hepatitis and cirrhosis. These events, through hepatocyte injury, regeneration, and inflammation, lead to increased cellular turnover and increased risk of replicative errors that could then lead to a transforming effect. A more direct oncogenic effect of HBV is suggested by the presence of integrated HBV genomes in most hepatoma cells. However, the abundance of data suggests that a direct oncogenic effect by HBV may be relevant in only a few cases.

Answer 3.32.   **The answer is D.**

Among the different human cancers, HPV has the greatest association with cervical cancer. HPV-16 and HPV-18 are associated with 70% of all cervical cancers, with other HPV strains associated with the remaining 30%. HPV is associated with penile cancers. HPV has also been linked to some head and neck cancers, and most of the HPV-associated head and neck cancers occur in the oral pharynx. Esophageal cancers in humans have not been convincingly shown to be associated with HPV.

Answer 3.33.   **The answer is B.**

Molecular studies of cervical cancer reveal that the HPV DNA is usually integrated into the cellular genome. Integration of viral DNA is generally not at specific sites. In HPV-positive cancers, there appears to be a selection for the integration of E6 and E7 coding regions and the upstream regulatory regions. This leads to E6 and E7 genes being regularly expressed in these cancers. The E6 and E7 proteins are oncoproteins and lead to cellular transformation at least partly by binding the cell-cycle regulatory proteins p53 and Rb. Only a small fraction of those individuals infected with HPV will develop cancer, and the time interval between infection and development of cervical cancer can be decades. It appears that HPV infection, though essential, is not sufficient to lead to cervical cancer, and other factors are essential for progression to invasive cancer. Epidemiologic studies suggest that smoking may be such a factor because it is associated with an increased risk of cervical cancer.

Answer 3.34.   **The answer is C.**

HPV types 16 and 18 are the two most frequent HPV types associated with cervical cancer and have been demonstrated in approximately 70% of the cervical cancers. Among the other HPV types associated with cervical cancer are HPV-31, HPV-33, HPV-39, and HPV-42, respectively. HPV-6 and HPV-11 are rarely associated with genital tract cancers.

Answer 3.35.   **The answer is A.**

Recently approved vaccine for HPV consists of VLPs from HPV-16, HPV-18, HPV-6, and HPV-11. The expression in yeast and insect cells of the major HPV capsid protein L1, either alone or together with L2, leads to the assembly of VLPs that are morphologically identical to native virion particles. These VLPs present the epitopes that are necessary for the development of a high titer neutralizing antisera. HPV-16 and HPV-18 are associated with approximately 70% of cervical cancers and HPV-6 and HPV-11 are associated with 90% of anogenital warts. There are HPV types other than HPV-16 and 18 that can cause cervical cancer, and therefore vaccinated individuals at risk should continue to receive cervical cancer screening. In addition, the duration of protection for the specific HPV types is unknown. The vaccine has been evaluated in women and therefore for now is recommended in women only.

Answer 3.36.   **The answer is D.**

EBV is associated with many cancers. EBV nuclear proteins, particularly EBNA2, target the transcription factor RBPJk/CBF1. It is through this transcription factor that EBV nuclear proteins regulate viral LMP1 promoter and the cellular C-myc promoter. EBV viral protein LMP1 engages the TNF receptor cytoplasmic factors and the death domain proteins, including TRADD and RIP, which may activate downstream proteins inducing cellular proliferation and survival. EBV is detected in approximately 50% of Hodgkin's lymphoma. EBV is also associated with many Burkitt's lymphomas, nasopharyngeal cancers, and some gastric cancers.

Answer 3.37.   **The answer is A.**

Among patients with AIDS, KS risk is highest in homosexual men. The risk is much lower among AIDS cases related to blood transfusion and in pediatric AIDS cases. This difference in the risk of KS is a result of higher prevalence of HHV8 infection, a known cause of KS, among homosexual men. This infection could then be transmitted among homosexual patients with AIDS, placing these patients at a higher risk for KS. The prevalence of this infection among women and prepubertal children is very low.

Answer 3.38.   **The answer is B.**

HHV8 (also KS's associated virus KSHV) sequences are found in tumors of every patient with KS, irrespective of whether the patient is HIV infected or not. The prevalence of this virus is high in countries whereas classic KS is common and ranges from 20% in Italy to 60% in sub-Saharan Africa. In the United States, which has a low incidence of classic KS, the prevalence of HHV8 infection is 5% to 7%. HHV8 is transmitted by the sexual route, particularly in homosexual men. However, in countries with a high incidence of classic KS, seroprevalence is detected in children, suggesting that other routes of transmission exist. The nonsexual routes involved in the transmission of this virus are not well defined. The rarity of KS in the United States, despite the HHV8 prevalence rate of 5%, suggests that other factors are essential for the development of KS. In patients with AIDS-KS, the HIV infection is the other factor, but the cofactors in classic KS are not yet identified. EBV is not a cofactor in the development of KS in AIDS or classic KS.

Answer 3.39.   **The answer is B.**

SV40 DNA or antigens have been detected in some human cancers, including mesotheliomas, osteosarcomas, and brain tumors. The major source for human exposure to this virus was through contaminated poliovirus vaccines administered from 1955 to 1963. However, there is no epidemiologic evidence that individuals exposed to these contaminated vaccines have increased risk of cancer. In the only double-blind study conducted, there was no correlation found between SV40 and human tumors. Human polyomaviruses BK and JC are ubiquitous, and there have been occasional reports linking these viruses to human cancers. However, comprehensive analysis of the data suggests no convincing evidence of an association.

Answer 3.40.   **The answer is D.**

Both innate and adaptive immunity play a role in immune surveillance of tumors. Adaptive immune cells, T and B lymphocytes, along with their effector molecules, innate immunity cells (e.g., natural killer cells), and proinflammatory cytokines (e.g., IL-12) are all important for immune surveillance of tumors. In animal models, deficiency of different inflammatory or immune mediators leads to different tumors, suggesting that the immune surveillance mechanisms differ for tumors arising in different tissues. Immune surveillance of tumors may or may not be dependent on antigens expressed on the tumor. In addition, antigens expressed on tumor stroma or certain self-antigens may be relevant for immune surveillance.

Answer 3.41.   **The answer is C.**

More than a century ago, studies showed that infection with inflammation-causing bacteria induced dramatic regressions of cancers. An important role for immune surveillance of tumors is suggested by increased incidence of certain tumors in organ transplant recipients receiving immunosuppressive therapy. Nonmelanoma skin cancers are increased 50-fold in these patients, but the risk of melanoma is increased only modestly. Immunosuppressive therapy has a differential effect on various aspects of the immune system, and different components of the immune system are relevant for surveillance of the various tumors. This differential effect may account for the differences in the risk for the various tumors in immune-suppressed patients. The presence of tumor-infiltrating lymphocytes, particularly T cells in tumors such as melanomas, colon cancers, and ovarian cancers, is associated with improved prognosis supporting the role of immune surveillance in limiting tumor progression. Tumor progression is also controlled in many patients by the autoimmune response that leads to paraneoplastic neurologic syndromes.

Answer 3.42.   **The answer is C.**

Many lines of evidence support the association of inflammation and cancer. In general, acute inflammation has a greater capacity to eradicate tumors, whereas chronic smoldering inflammatory conditions that lead to infiltration of the tissue stroma by inflammatory cells could be associated with tumor initiation and progression. Thus, in conditions such as inflammatory bowel disease or chronic inflammation associated with a nonhealing ulcer, inflammatory factors could have antiapoptotic, proangiogenic, prometastatic, and immunosuppressive effects. All these can then lead to tumor formation and tumor progression. The ability of COX-2 inhibitors to reduce human cancers, particularly colon cancers, supports this association between inflammation and cancer.

Answer 3.43.   **The answer is D.**

Approximately 15% of human cancers have an association with an infectious agent. Although some infectious agents, particularly viruses, can induce cellular transformation, many infections give rise to cancers as a result of the chronic inflammation that develops in response to these infections. Chronic hepatitis that occurs in response to HCV can result in HCC. Similarly, *Helicobacter pylori* infection results in chronic gastric inflammation that then can lead to gastric cancer.

Answer 3.44.   **The answer is D.**

Inflammatory factors could be involved in procarcinogenic or antitumor effects, and some factors could have both effects. TNF is a cytokine released by inflammatory cells in response to an inflammatory stimulus. TNF can have an apoptotic effect on tumor calls and endothelial cells. However, by activating NFkB and inducing the production of MMP-9, it can have procarcinogenic effects. The balance between these effects leads to TNF being a procarcinogenic or antitumor factor in a particular tumor.

Answer 3.45.   **The answer is B.**

The observation that COX inhibitors can reduce the incidence of cancers was one of the initial indicators of the role of inflammation in cancer formation and progression. COX-2 inhibitors can reduce the numbers of polyps and prevent cancers in individuals with FAP and patients with inflammatory bowel disease, and can reduce the number of polyps in individuals with adenomatous polyps.

Answer 3.46.   **The answer is C.**

CAFs are better able to support tumor progression than fibroblasts from normal tissue. CAFs have characteristics like the other fibroblasts, such as expression of vimentin. These cells have not undergone transformation, and only few studies have found genetic alterations in these cells. The pro-tumor effects of CAFs are mediated by soluble factors released by these cells that include SDF-1/CXCL12, transforming growth factor (TGF)-β, several growth factors, and MMP-9. The soluble factors released by CAFs can induce tumor formation in adjacent epithelial cells without the presence of other carcinogenic stimuli.

Answer 3.47.   **The answer is D.**

DCs are characterized by an ability to rapidly respond to alteration of tissue homeostasis because of the presence of pattern-recognizing receptors, such as the TLRs. Once activated, these cells secrete many proinflammatory cytokines such as IL-12, TNF, and IL-6. The activated DCs migrate to the regional lymph nodes and present antigens acquired in the tissues to T cells in the context of major histocompatibility complex class I and II antigens. Thus, through the production of cytokines and activation of T cells, DCs activate both innate and adaptive immunity in response to changes in the tissue homeostasis. DCs in tumors are generally hyporesponsive because of their interaction with other inflammatory cells or the tumor cells and therefore are not involved in immune surveillance. Activation of DCs is one of the immune strategies being pursued in the treatment of some cancers.

Answer 3.48.   **The answer is C.**

TAMs are derived from monocytes and monocyte precursors from the blood. TAMs have the capacity to induce either cytotoxic and antitumor or protumor and proangiogenic effects. In most progressing tumors, TAMs mediate protumor effects They favor tumor growth by producing growth factors, angiogenic cytokines, and expression of MMPs, TGFβ, and TNF that help tumor invasion and metastasis. IL-10 produced by inflammatory cells, including the TAMs, has an immunosuppressive effect on TAMs that impair the antitumor effects of these cells.

Answer 3.49.   **The answer is D.**

TLRs are evolutionary conserved molecules that are a family of at least 12 different pattern-recognizing receptors. TLRs are important in recognition of microbes, pathogens, and endogenous ligands that have a role in regulation of inflammation. The role of TLRs and other pattern-recognizing receptors in tumor-associated inflammation remains to be defined. TLRs expressed on tumor cells can cause apoptosis, but activation of TLRs on tumor-infiltrating cells may promote tumor progression.

NIKHIL I. KHUSHALANI • KAUNTEYA REDDY

DIRECTIONS   Each of the numbered items below is followed by lettered answers. Select the ONE lettered answer that is BEST in each case unless instructed otherwise.

QUESTIONS

Question 4.1.   Cancer in humans is:

A.   A genetically determined sequela of aging
B.   A manifestation of individual exposure to carcinogens
C.   A combination of a genetically susceptible individual and exposure to carcinogen
D.   An unknown mechanism of development

Question 4.2.   Which of the following has been implicated in increased cancer risk?

A.   Tobacco and alcohol
B.   Diet
C.   Sexual behavior
D.   All of the above

Question 4.3.   Match the following agents most commonly involved with cancer of that particular organ:

A.   Lung   1. Asbestos
B.   Pleura   2. Benzene
C.   Urinary bladder 3. Tobacco
D.   Liver   4. Cadmium
E.   Bone marrow   5. Ultraviolet (UV) light
F.   Prostrate   6. Phenacetin
G.   Skin   7. Aflatoxin

Question 4.4.   Which of the following statements is TRUE?

A.   Interaction of genotoxic carcinogens is random.
B.   Interaction of genotoxic carcinogens is selective based on their class.
C.   Genotoxic carcinogens can cause base mispairing and small deletions, but not large deletions.
D.   All toxins implicated in cancers are genotoxic.

Corresponding Chapters in *Cancer: Principles & Practice of Oncology*, Ninth Edition: 18 (Chemical Factors), 19 (Physical Factors), 20 (Dietary Factors), and 21 (Obesity and Physical Activity).

Question 4.5.   Studies in animal models have led to which of the following conclusions?

A. Carcinogenic agents activate oncogenes.
B. Carcinogenic agents inactivate tumor suppressor genes.
C. Carcinogenic agents cause genomic changes that are required for production of malignant phenotype.
D. All of the above.

Question 4.6.   Which of the following statements is FALSE regarding fundamental principles of molecular epidemiology?

A. Carcinogenesis is a multistage process.
B. Carcinogenesis involves numerous genetic events at each stage.
C. Human response to carcinogen exposure is homogeneous.
D. There is a wide range of interindividual variation in carcinogen exposure.

Question 4.7.   Which of the following components are involved in the estimation of dose and corresponding risk in epidemiological studies?

A. Measurement of external and internal exposure
B. Biomarkers estimating the biologically effective dose
C. Biomarkers of harm
D. All of the above

Question 4.8.   Which of the following statements about benzene is NOT true?

A. Benzene is metabolized in the liver by CYP2E1 (P-4502E1).
B. Benzene oxide and hydroquinone are reactive metabolites of benzene.
C. Presence of functional polymorphisms of myeloperoxidase in humans may have a protective role against toxicity of benzene to bone marrow.
D. There exists a perfect dose-response relationship of benzene in humans, and genetically susceptible individuals can be easily identified.

Question 4.9.   Which of the following statements is NOT TRUE?

A. UVC light is the most damaging to DNA compared to UVA or UVB.
B. UVA can induce reactive oxygen species leading to single-strand breaks and base lesions.
C. Living organisms are mostly exposed to UVA and UVC.
D. UVB and UVC induce predominantly pyrimidine dimers.

Question 4.10.   Which of the following is TRUE about UV light?

A. Proliferating skin cells are very vulnerable to UV light because UV lesions block DNA replication.
B. The risk of melanoma is related to the cumulative lifetime exposure to UV light.
C. The risk of nonmelanoma skin cancers is related to high sunlight exposure during childhood.
D. All of the above.

Question 4.11.   Radiation was used to treat which of the following disease conditions?

A. Enlarged thymus glands
B. Peptic ulcers
C. Ankylosing spondylitis
D. All of the above

Question 4.12.   Which of the following statements is TRUE about radiation exposure, tissue sensitivity, and latent period?

A. Evidence suggests that acute and chronic myelogenous leukemias are very sensitive to induction after radiation exposure.
B. Latent period is defined as the period of time between radiation exposure and the appearance of radiation-induced tumors.
C. The peak incidence for the development of radiation-induced leukemia occurs between 0 and 2 years after exposure.
D. Both A and B.

Question 4.13.   Which of the following is TRUE regarding theoretic models of radiation interaction?

A. Linear and linear-quadratic models have been described.
B. Cancer risk is directly proportional to radiation dose in the linear model.
C. Cancer risk is directly proportional to radiation dose at low dose and a function of square of the dose at higher dose in the linear-quadratic model.
D. All of the above.

Question 4.14.   In regard to high linear energy transfer (LET) radiation, which of the following is NOT true?

A. Ionization tracks through an individual cell are few.
B. Because of the high density of this type of exposure, the probability of producing complex effects is high.
C. The dose response in this case is nonlinear.
D. None of the above.

Question 4.15.   Which of the following regarding radon is TRUE?

A. Radon is a major source of high LET radiation to the general population.
B. Radon is chemically active and charged.
C. Radon exposure is not a risk factor for lung cancer.
D. Bystander effect is not true with radon exposure.

Question 4.16.   Match the following:

A. Younger age of exposure   1. High risk of cancer induction
B. Middle age at exposure   2. Low risk of cancer induction
C. High penetrance genes   3. Ataxia-telangiectasia
D. Breast cancer   4. High probability of cancer induction

Question 4.17.   Which of the following plays a role in second cancers after radiation therapy?

A.   Age of exposure
B.   Body size
C.   Genetic susceptibility
D.   All of the above

Question 4.18.   Which of the following is a mechanism of radiation-induced cancer?

A.   DNA double-strand break induction
B.   Telomere dysfunction and instability
C.   Cytogenetic damage in progeny of irradiated cells
D.   All of the above

Question 4.19.   Which of the following influences development of skin cancer?

A.   Presence of skin pigment
B.   Latitude of location on earth
C.   Family history of skin cancer
D.   All of the above

Question 4.20.   Which of the following statements is TRUE regarding malignant melanoma?

A.   Malignant melanoma is more a result of chronic exposure to sunlight than acute exposure.
B.   History of sunburns does not predispose one to malignant melanoma.
C.   Melanoma development is independent of tumor suppressor gene pathways and mutated oncogenes.
D.   Familial form of malignant melanoma involves deletions or mutations in CDKN2A.

Question 4.21.   Which of the following is NOT TRUE regarding asbestos?

A.   Asbestos and tobacco act in synergy to induce lung cancer.
B.   Approximately 5% of all lung cancers are attributable to exposure to asbestos.
C.   p53 mutations are common in mesothelioma.
D.   B and C.

Question 4.22.   Obesity is defined as a body mass index (BMI) (Quetelet's Index) greater than which of the following values?

A.   24 kg/m^2
B.   26 kg/m^2
C.   28 kg/m^2
D.   30 kg/m^2

Question 4.23.   Case-control studies examining the role of diet in the cause of cancer do not suffer from recall bias.

    A. True
    B. False

Question 4.24.   Which of the following instruments is the most widely used in population-based studies of dietary intake?

    A. Food-frequency questionnaire
    B. 24-hour recall record
    C. 7-day diet record
    D. None of the above

Question 4.25.   In the American Cancer Society Cohort Study from 1982 to 1998 examining the relation of BMI in 1982 and the risk of death from all cancers, obese individuals had a higher risk of cancer-related mortality from all of the following cancers, EXCEPT:

    A. Pancreas cancer
    B. Colorectal cancer
    C. Brain cancer
    D. Kidney cancer

Question 4.26.   Which of the following statements regarding alcohol consumption is NOT True?

    A. Consumption of alcohol increases the risk of breast and colorectal carcinomas.
    B. In most cancers, there are significant differences in risk of cancer development according to the type of alcoholic beverage.
    C. Acetaldehyde is the main metabolite of alcohol and a known carcinogen.
    D. In the developed world, approximately 75% of laryngeal cancers are attributed to alcohol and tobacco.

Question 4.27.   There is clear association between dietary fat consumption and the risk of developing breast cancer in women.

    A. True
    B. False

Question 4.28.   Regular consumption of red meat is associated with an increased risk of which of the following cancers?

    A. Larynx cancer
    B. Colorectal cancer
    C. Liver cancer
    D. Esophagus cancer

Question 4.29.   What is the relationship between consumption of soy products and the risk of breast cancer?

    A. No relation noted
    B. Increase in risk of breast cancer
    C. Decrease in risk of breast cancer

Question 4.30.   Which of the following statements regarding the consumption of fruits and vegetables is TRUE?

    A. High consumption of fruits is associated with decreased risk of invasive breast carcinoma.
    B. High intake of fruits and vegetables is associated with decreased incidence of lung cancer.
    C. High consumption of fruits and vegetables is associated with a decreased incidence of colorectal cancer.
    D. None of the above.

Question 4.31.   Obesity and physical inactivity are established risk factors for which of the following cancers?

    A. Colon cancer
    B. Postmenopausal breast cancer
    C. Both A and B
    D. Neither A or B

Question 4.32.   Convincing evidence exists for the association between obesity and all of the following cancers, EXCEPT:

    A. Adenocarcinoma of the esophagus
    B. Kidney cancer
    C. Ovarian cancer
    D. Endometrial cancer

ANSWERS

Answer 4.1.   **The answer is C.**

The development of cancer is a multistage process. It depends not only on genetic predispositions but is also influenced by the environment, diet, occupation, and lifestyle of an individual. Therefore, cancer results from a combination of hereditary susceptibility and individual exposure to either endogenous or exogenous factors.

Answer 4.2.   **The answer is D.**

All of the listed factors are implicated in cancer development. Exposure to chemicals can result in DNA damage and mutations. These genotoxic events can occur directly from exposure or indirectly through the generation of intermediate compounds that disrupt normal cellular function. Tobacco and alcohol are well known to predispose humans to numerous cancers, including cancers of the oral cavity, oropharynx, larynx, lung, and esophagus. Common examples of diet-related carcinogenesis include smoked or pickled foods (stomach cancer) and red meat (colon cancer). The relationship between human papilloma virus and cancer of the cervix is an example of cancer associated with sexual behavior.

Answer 4.3.   **The answers are (A) 3, (B) 1, (C) 6, (D) 7, (E) 2, (F) 4, (G) 5.**

Tobacco is the single most important risk factor in lung cancer. Although it does increase the risk of lung cancer, asbestos is a major risk factor in the development of pleural mesothelioma. Studies have shown the association between liver cancer and exposure to aflatoxins. Benzene has been well studied in the causation of leukemia. UV light exposure directly correlates to the development of skin cancer.

Answer 4.4.   **The answer is B.**

Genotoxic carcinogens are potent mutagens. They interact with DNA and cause base mispairing, deletions, both small and large, and are capable of causing direct chromosomal breaks. Each class of genotoxic agent reacts selectively with purine and pyrimidine targets within a nucleotide sequence. The mechanism of action of nongenotoxic carcinogens is less clear and believed to be mediated through direct cell death, deregulated hyperplasia, induction of endogenous toxic radical production, and so forth.

Answer 4.5.   **The answer is D.**

Studies in animal models have shown that carcinogenic agents act in a variety of different ways. They can activate oncogenes directly and inactivate tumor suppressor genes. They cause genomic changes that help propagate the malignant phenotype that manifests as unregulated growth, resistance to apoptosis, and potential for metastatic spread.

Answer 4.6. **The answer is C.**

Carcinogenesis is a multistage process involving several genetic events at each stage. There is a wide interindividual variation in humans to carcinogen exposure. Herein lies the difficulty in using in vitro models to mimic human cellular response. Experimental studies that involve a single clone being exposed to a particular carcinogen to study a particular gene might not be representative of the population. It does allow the investigation of specific mechanisms that may be involved in carcinogenesis.

Answer 4.7. **The answer is D.**

There are four components in the estimation of dose and effect in epidemiologic studies. Measurements of internal and external exposure, markers of the biologically effective dose, and markers of damage are all important, and these components help quantify the exposure at the cellular level. When assessing these surrogate markers, their sensitivity and specificity, reproducibility, and general applicability for human use should be taken into appropriate consideration.

Answer 4.8. **The answer is D.**

Benzene is metabolized in the liver by CYP2E1 into active metabolites. These metabolites are known to bind to DNA in the bone marrow cells. Myeloperoxidase is involved in the production of active metabolites of benzene (benzoquinone). Functional polymorphisms in myeloperoxidase might play a protective role by reduced enzyme expression in some individuals. Currently, the dose response of benzene needs further evaluation.

Answer 4.9. **The answer is C.**

UVC light, the most damaging to DNA, has most of its emission from the sun absorbed by the ozone layer, with living organisms exposed mainly to UVA and UVB. UVB and UVC induce predominantly covalent pyrimidine dimers, whereas UVA induces reactive oxygen species.

Answer 4.10. **The answer is A.**

Proliferating skin cells are very vulnerable to UV light because UV lesions block DNA replication. Although there is a strong link between UV exposure and skin cancers, the mechanism appears to be different, with the risk of melanoma linked to childhood exposure and nonmelanomas to cumulative lifetime exposure.

Answer 4.11. **The answer is D.**

All the disease conditions listed above were treated with radiation in the past. Other examples include tinea capitis, tonsillar enlargement, benign breast, and gynecologic disease. Studies in these cohorts have contributed toward the understanding of radiation-related acute and chronic toxicity, as well as the development of radiation-related cancers such as thyroid cancer and breast cancer.

Answer 4.12.   **The answer is D.**

The latent period is defined as the time between the radiation exposure and the development of a radiation-induced tumor. Acute and chronic myelogenous leukemias are sensitive to induction and their peak latent period is usually around 4 to 8 years, although cases as early as 2 years have also been reported. For solid tumors, the latent period is typically longer and can even exceed two decades.

Answer 4.13.   **The answer is D.**

Studies at the molecular and cellular levels and epidemiological data have helped derive two dose-response models of radiation interaction. First is the linear model wherein cancer risk is directly proportional to radiation dose. In the linear-quadratic model, the risk is proportional to dose at low dose and rapidly increases with high doses.

Answer 4.14.   **The answer is C.**

High LET results in few energy tracks in the cell. Although few, they have a high density that is sufficient to produce complex effects. The dose-response relationship in this case is linear because of the higher effectiveness of this type of radiation. Radon exposure (e.g., in uranium mines) is an example of high LET.

Answer 4.15.   **The answer is B.**

Radon is a naturally occurring high LET radiation found in rocks and soil. It is chemically inert and uncharged, but spontaneous decay results in its progeny, which are radioactive and electrically charged. The latter can attach to ambient dust particles, which when inhaled can result in lung irradiation. This is a well-defined etiologic factor in the development of lung cancer. Bystander effect is an interesting feature observed with radon wherein the cells exposed to radon send out signals to adjacent cells, which are not exposed. These signals result in mutagenic and oncogenic changes.

Answer 4.16.   **The answers are (A) 1, (B) 2, (C) 4, (D) 3.**

The age at time of exposure plays a critical role in cancer induction. Younger age at exposure increases the risk substantially when compared with middle age of exposure. Good examples are breast cancer and thyroid cancer. When compared with middle-aged women, young children and adolescents have a higher risk of developing breast cancer after exposure to radiation. The defects involved in ataxia-telangiectasia may be involved in radiation-induced breast cancer secondary to increased radiation sensitivity.

Answer 4.17.   **The answer is D.**

Age plays an important role in induction of second cancers because children are more susceptible to radiation. Because children have a smaller body size, multiple organs may be exposed, as the area exposed to radiation is large. Genetic susceptibility is an important factor in induction of second cancers. Common second cancers after radiation include those of the breast, thyroid, esophagus, and lung, as well as leukemia.

Answer 4.18.   **The answer is D.**

Induction of DNA double-strand breaks, telomere instability, and dysfunction are all effects of radiation exposure. It was initially believed that the mutagenic and cytogenetic effects of ionizing radiation occurred in the first few cell divisions after exposure, but it is now thought that this kind of damage can occur in several generations in progeny of radiation-exposed cells.

Answer 4.19.   **The answer is D.**

Individuals who lack skin pigment have a history of sunburn, have a family history of skin cancer, and live closer to the equator have a higher risk of developing skin cancer. The development of malignant melanoma is less dependent on the total exposure of sunlight; rather, acute exposures causing sunburn is of greater concern. A history of five or more sunburns in adolescence doubles the risk of developing melanoma. In addition, the site of development does not seem to be related to the site of chronic exposure in melanoma.

Answer 4.20.   **The answer is D.**

In the familial form of malignant melanoma, deletions and mutations of CDKN2A are most often seen. CDKN2A encodes p16INK4A and p14ARF, both tumor suppressors. Oncogene activation involving the RAS pathway is also seen in melanoma. Clinically, its development seems to be related to acute, repeated sunburn rather than chronic exposure.

Answer 4.21.   **The answer is C.**

Asbestos is responsible for approximately 5% to 7% of all lung cancers and acts in synergy with tobacco in smokers. Mutations in p53 are fairly rare in mesotheliomas.

Answer 4.22.   **The answer is D.**

Quetelet's Index (or BMI) is calculated as the weight (in kilograms) divided by the square of the height (in meters). Being overweight is defined as a BMI of 25.0 to 29.9 kg/m^2, whereas a BMI greater than 30 kg/m^2 constitutes being obese. Approximately one-third of the US population in 2000 met this definition of obesity with physical inactivity being the likely cause.

Answer 4.23.   **The answer is B.**

Recall bias is commonly encountered in case-control studies examining the effect of dietary factors in causing cancer. Another type of bias seen is control selection bias. Individuals under study (cases) may overemphasize their consumption of foods traditionally considered unhealthy, which may skew the results observed.

Answer 4.24.   **The answer is A.**

The food frequency questionnaire requests subjects to recall and report their average intake of a variety of food over the preceding year. Although this instrument tends to overrepresent foods considered healthy (vegetables and fruits, so-called social desirability bias), it is the most widely used in large studies of dietary pattern reporting in large studies. The 24-hour recall method offers too narrow a window to accurately reflect dietary patterns, and the 7-day diary record is cumbersome for data transfer and extraction.

Answer 4.25.   **The answer is C.**

In this study of more than 900,000 individuals who were cancer free at enrollment in 1982, an increased BMI was associated with an increased risk of cancer-related death. Cancers of the esophagus, pancreas, liver, gall bladder, colorectal, kidney, breast, uterus, and cervix were among those in which this association was noted, whereas no such relation was found for cancers of the brain and bladder and for melanoma. The relative risk of death from cancer was 1.52 and 1.62 in men and women, respectively, who had a BMI greater than 40, compared with individuals of normal weight. Elevated levels of endogenous estrogen, insulin, and proinflammatory factors, and decreased levels of sex hormone binding proteins and insulin-like growth factor, are believed to contribute to the increased risk of cancer in overweight individuals.

Answer 4.26.   **The answer is B.**

Acetaldehyde is a known carcinogen that increases the proliferation of epithelial cell and forms DNA adducts. Alcohol consumption has been associated with development of breast and colorectal malignancies. In the developed world, approximately 75% of the esophageal and head and neck malignancies are associated with alcohol and tobacco consumption, which have a synergistic carcinogen effect. For most malignancies, there are no significant differences regarding the type of alcoholic beverage, suggesting the pivotal role of alcohol in carcinogenesis.

Answer 4.27.   **The answer is B.**

Initial case-control studies examining the relation of breast cancer in women to the consumption of dietary fat suggested a positive correlation with a pooled relative risk of 1.35 in a meta-analysis of 12 studies. This risk was greater in postmenopausal women. However, cohort studies have failed to confirm these findings, including the large Nurses' Health Study and the Women's Health Initiative Randomized Controlled Dietary Modification Trial.

Answer 4.28.   **The answer is B.**

Several studies have demonstrated an increased risk of colorectal cancer with the regular consumption of red meat, with a stronger association with processed meat. A meta-analysis of prospective studies examining this subject confirms these findings with a relative risk of 1.24.

Answer 4.29.   **The answer is C.**

Available evidence suggests that there is a decreased risk of breast cancer associated with consumption of soy products. This hypothesis was borne from initial observations of lower incidences of breast cancer in women in Asia, where soy consumption is high. Soybeans contain genistein and daidzein, whose metabolites have several biologic effects, including inhibition of the epidermal growth factor receptor tyrosine kinase activity and competition with estrogen for the estrogen receptor. In a meta-analysis of 18 studies, a modest decrease (odds ratio, 0.86) in the risk of breast cancer was noted with high soy intake.

Answer 4.30.   **The answer is D.**

Large studies including the Nurses' Health Study and the Health Professionals' follow-up study showed no impact of high consumption of fruits and vegetables in the prevention of cancer.

Answer 4.31.   **The answer is C.**

There is good evidence suggesting an increased risk of colon cancer and postmenopausal breast cancer in individuals who are obese or physically inactive. This relation has not been established for rectal cancer. In colon cancer, postulated mechanisms of obesity-related carcinogenesis include insulin resistance, elevated levels of insulin and insulin-like growth factor, and inflammation. These contribute to cellular proliferation, DNA damage, and tumor growth. Improved colonic transit time in subjects who are physically active is another possible mechanism contributing to decreased risk of colon cancer in this cohort. The effects of obesity and physical inactivity have been more pronounced in men compared with women.

Please refer to Question 4.30 for a more detailed discussion on the relationship between these factors and postmenopausal breast cancer.

Answer 4.32.   **The answer is C.**

An etiologic association exists between high BMI and cancers of the esophagus (adenocarcinoma), endometrium, kidney, colon, and breast (postmenopausal), whereas such evidence in ovarian cancer is inconclusive. Obesity increases gastroesophageal reflux disease, which is a known risk factor for esophageal adenocarcinoma. The obesity epidemic in North America may, in part, be responsible for the dramatic increase in the incidence of this cancer during the past two decades. There is a linear risk between increasing weight and endometrial cancer, which, like breast cancer, is hormonally dependent. The mechanisms are believed to be similar as well, with an increase in circulating estrogen levels in overweight or obese women. In kidney cancer, there is a 7% increase in risk for every unit increase in the BMI. The data in ovarian cancer at this time are inconclusive, and a positive association, if any, is weak.

CHAPTER 5 EPIDEMIOLOGY OF CANCER

THOMAS E. STINCHCOMBE

DIRECTIONS Each of the numbered items below is followed by lettered answers. Select the ONE lettered answer that is BEST in each case unless instructed otherwise.

QUESTIONS

Question 5.1. **All of the following are true about prevalence and incidence, EXCEPT:**

  A. Prevalence is calculated by dividing the number of existing cases by the total population.

  B. Cumulative incidence is the proportion of people who develop the disease during a specified period of time.

  C. Prevalence is considered a more relevant measure of disease frequency for etiologic evaluation, and incidence reflects the public health burden of the disease.

  D. The quality of incidence data varies substantially depending on the accuracy of the population numbers, the completeness of reporting the diagnosis, and the degree with which the diagnosis is pursued.

Question 5.2. **Surveillance, Epidemiology, and End Results (SEER) program of the National Cancer Institute provides data on new cancer cases and cancer survival within the United States. All of the following are true about the SEER database, EXCEPT:**

  A. Geographic areas are selected for their ability to operate high-quality data reporting systems and their epidemiologically significant population subgroups.

  B. The population covered by the SEER database is comparable to the US population in regard to poverty and education.

  C. SEER data provide information on the demographic characteristics of cancer cases and cancer characteristics (site, morphology, and stage).

  D. The SEER database includes approximately 1% of the US population.

Corresponding Chapters in *Cancer: Principles & Practice of Oncology*, Ninth Edition: 22 (Epidemiologic Methods), 23 (Global Cancer Incidence and Mortality), and 24 (Trends in Cancer Mortality).

Question 5.3. All of the following are differences between molecular epidemiology and genetic epidemiology, EXCEPT:

A. Molecular epidemiology assesses genetic involvement, whereas genetic epidemiology focuses mainly on heredity.

B. Molecular epidemiology studies unrelated individuals, whereas genetic epidemiology investigates family members in the format of pedigrees.

C. Molecular epidemiology usually studies low penetrance markers that are commonly present in the general population, whereas genetic epidemiology research is often designed to identify markers with high penetrance but low prevalence in the general population.

D. Molecular epidemiology uses linkage analysis, whereas genetic epidemiology often calculates relative risks or odds ratios.

Question 5.4. For all the following analytical studies, the individual is the unit of analysis, EXCEPT:

A. Ecological

B. Cross-sectional

C. Cohort

D. Case-control

Question 5.5. Dr. Bush finds that people who carry matches are more likely to develop lung cancer. Therefore, he concludes that carrying matches increases the risk for lung cancer. This is an example of:

A. Information bias

B. Selection bias

C. Misclassification bias

D. Confounding

Question 5.6. The probability that an individual will develop or die of cancer in a lifetime is frequently reported in the media. For example, it is reported that lung cancer will affect 1 in 13 men over a lifetime. Although this statistic provides some valuable information, the problem(s) with this statistic is:

A. It underestimates the risk for individuals with certain risk factors.

B. It overestimates the risk for individuals without certain risk factors.

C. It underestimates and overestimates the risk for individuals depending on the age.

D. All of the above.

Question 5.7. To accurately portray the incidence of various cancers, the data require standardization, particularly when comparing data from different countries. The reasons why this is required are the following:

A. Different age structures between separate countries

B. Different numbers of men and women between the separate countries

C. Cohort effects

D. All the above

Question 5.8. In cohort studies, all of the following statements are true regarding relative risk EXCEPT:

A. Relative risk is ratio of the disease incidence in the exposed group and disease incidence in the unexposed group.
B. Relative risk is the difference between the disease incidence in the exposed group and disease incidence in the unexposed group.
C. Relative risk measurement is useful in establishing causality for the disease.

Question 5.9. Which of the following statements is true regarding the use of molecular markers in epidemiologic studies?

A. Genotypic markers refer to protein sequences encoded by the genomic DNA.
B. Genotypic markers do not generally change over time.
C. Single nucleotide polymorphisms (SNPs) are considered as phenotypic markers.
D. None of the above.

Question 5.10. Migrant studies have helped differentiate whether variations in cancer rates across countries and among different racial and ethnic groups are caused by environmental factors or inherited genetic factors. An example of this is the difference in death rates from selected cancers comparing Japanese in Japan with first- and second-generation Japanese in California with native California whites. All of the following are true, EXCEPT:

A. Mortality from cancers of the stomach and liver is higher among Japanese in Japan.
B. Among first-generation Japanese who migrated to California, the mortality from stomach and liver cancer is substantially lower than in Japanese in Japan and higher than in Californian whites.
C. The mortality from colon cancer approximately doubled among first-generation Japanese who moved to California and approached the rates of Californian whites by the second generation.
D. The mortality from colorectal cancer is higher among Japanese in both the United States and Japan than in Californian whites.
E. All of the above are true.

Question 5.11. There has been increasing interest in the use of computed tomography (CT) screening for lung cancer. Potential problems with CT screening for lung cancer include:

A. Lead-time bias
B. Length-time bias
C. Neither
D. Both

Question 5.12.   The recent development of molecular and molecular biomarkers has changed the development of epidemiology studies and clinical trials. Further investigation of molecular markers, especially phenotypic markers, will require which of the following issues to be addressed:

A. Reproducibility of assays
B. Versatile assays
C. Sensitive and specific assays
D. Quality assurance procedures
E. All of the above

Question 5.13.   Statistical methods are required to evaluate the role of chance. A usual way to calculate chance is to establish the upper and lower limits of a 95% confidence interval around a point estimate for relative risk (risk ratio, rate ratio, or odds ratio). All are true about confidence intervals, EXCEPT:

A. If the confidence interval does not include 1, the observed association is statistically significant.
B. The width of the confidence interval is not inversely related to the number of participants in a study or sample size.
C. The calculation of the confidence interval assumes that the only thing that would differ in hypothetical replications of the study would be statistical or chance element in the data.
D. The calculation of the confidence interval assumes that the variability in the data can be described adequately by statistical methods and that biases are nonexistent.
E. The choice of 95% is almost default in the upper and lower limits of the interval (e.g., 90% or 99%) and can be calculated and interpreted accordingly.

Question 5.14.   All of the following are true about lung cancer prevalence, EXCEPT:

A. The number of lung cancer cases in economically developing countries now exceeds the number in developed countries.
B. Globally, an estimated 85% of lung cancers in men and 47% of lung cancers in women are attributable to tobacco smoking.
C. The lung cancer incidence rate in 2002 in Chinese women is higher than that among women in France and Germany despite the low prevalence of smoking.
D. The highest rates of lung cancer are among men in Eastern Europe, North America, and the rest of Europe, reflecting differences in historical patterns of smoking.
E. All of the above are true.

Question 5.15.   SNPs in which of the following genes are associated with increased risk for developing lung cancer?

A. CHRNA3
B. FGFR2
C. JAZF1
D. SMAD7

Question 5.16.   SNPs in which of the following genes are associated with increased risk for developing pancreatic cancer?

A. MSMB
B. EIF3H
C. TACC3
D. ABO

ANSWERS

Answer 5.1.   **The answer is C.**

Prevalence reflects the public health burden of the disease (i.e., how many patients need to be treated and/or followed by the health system), and incidence is considered a more relevant measure of disease frequency for etiologic evaluation. An example would be breast cancer in women and prostate cancer in men are more prevalent, whereas lung cancer compromises only a small fraction of the prevalent cases but is the most common fatal cancer. The incidence of a disease can vary depending on the reporting to the cancer diagnosis and the presence of screening tests such as prostate-specific antigen.

Answer 5.2.   **The answer is D.**

The SEER database covers approximately 26% of the US population.

Answer 5.3.   **The answer is D.**

Both molecular epidemiology and genetic epidemiology have an emphasis on molecular analysis, but linkage analysis is usually performed in genetic epidemiology studies because participants are genetically related family members.

Answer 5.4.   **The answer is A.**

Ecological studies use groups of people as the unit and are performed when the level measures of exposure and/or outcome are available. An example would be the relationship between dietary fat intake and the incidence of a type of cancer by country.

Answer 5.5.   **The answer is D.**

Tobacco smokers are more likely to carry matches than nonsmokers. Therefore, the increased risk for lung cancer is due to tobacco smoking and not from carrying matches. This is an example of confounding where a third variable (which has not been taken into account in the study) affects the association between the exposure and disease resulting in an erroneous conclusion.

Answer 5.6.   **The answer is D.**

Although this figure is popular and useful, it significantly overestimates the risk in the never-smoking population and underestimates the risk on the smoking population. The incidence of lung cancer also increases with age, so this number overestimates the risk in younger people and underestimates the risk in older people.

Answer 5.7.   **The answer is D.**

Age standardization eliminates differences in the age structure, which is important because cancer has a higher incidence in older people, and a country with an older or younger population may have a different incidence of a cancer related to the age distribution. Gender similarly influences the incidence of cancer. A cohort effect typically results from the introduction of a risk factor that becomes established at a young age in people born in the same time period. An example would be lung cancer death rates peaked in cohorts born around the late 1920s and early 1930s, and cigarette smoking also peaked during this time period.

Answer 5.8.   **The answer is B.**

In cohort studies, relative risk is defined as the ratio between cumulative disease incidence in the exposed group and cumulative disease incidence in the unexposed group. Absolute risk is calculated as the cumulative incidence in the exposed group minus the cumulative incidence in the unexposed group. Relative risk is preferred when the focus of the cohort study is to infer on the causality of the disease.

Answer 5.9.   **The answer is B.**

Genotypic markers are defined as the nucleotide sequences of genomic DNA, and all other molecules are classified as phenotypic marker. SNPs are genotypic markers and they do not change with time or due to disease status. In the case of phenotypic markers such as protein sequence, they can be affected by the development of disease.

Answer 5.10.   **The answer is E.**

Migrant studies have helped to differentiate whether variation in cancer rates across countries and among different racial and ethnic groups is due to environmental factors or inherited factors. In this study, the increase in the mortality from colorectal cancer among Japanese migrants was presumably reflecting the changing dietary and physical activity patterns among migrants, and the rate of colorectal cancer in Japan has increased dramatically since World War II, most likely reflecting changes in lifestyle in the Japanese population. The higher rate of stomach and liver cancer among Japanese in Japan and the decline in first-generation Japanese, and the fact that the risk among second-generation Japanese and whites is similar most likely reflect the influence of an environmental exposure.

Answer 5.11.   **The answer is D.**

Lead-time bias reflects when earlier detection (lead time) did not change outcome. For example, a person receives the diagnosis of lung cancer on screening CT scan in 2008 and subsequently dies of lung cancer in 2010, whereas a person who does not undergo CT screening receives the diagnosis in 2010 and dies of lung cancer in 2010. The outcome is the same, but it would appear that the survival time has increased from 1 to 3 years. Length-time bias refers to the detection of indolent cancers by screening at a higher rate than the more aggressive cancers, resulting in an apparent survival advantage to screening.

Answer 5.12.   **The answer is E.**

The analysis of phenotypic markers, such as proteins, requires a reliable laboratory method of being quantitative (a wide range of measurable concentration), sensitive (able to detect a small amount of the analyte), specific (able to detect only the molecule of interest, no other molecules), reproducible (high precision and low variation), and versatile (easy to use). In addition, appropriate quality assurance procedures during sample processing and testing, as well as control samples in specimen analysis, will be required.

Answer 5.13.   **The answer is B.**

A larger sample size leads to less variability in the data, a tighter confidence interval, and a higher possibility in finding a statistically significant relationship.

Answer 5.14.   **The answer is E.**

The number of lung cancers cases in economically developing countries now exceeds the number in developed countries, but the proportion of all cancer deaths attributable to lung cancer is higher (22%) in developed countries than in developing countries (15%). The percentage of lung cancer cases caused by smoking among men in Europe and North American is higher (90% to 95%), where cigarette smoking has been entrenched for decades. Environmental factors such as exposure to coal smoke, indoor emissions from burning other fuels, exposure to fumes from frying foods at high temperatures, and secondhand smoke are all thought to contribute to the high rate of lung cancer among Chinese women.

Answer 5.15.   **The answer is A.**

Three large genome-wide association studies (GWAS) identified SNPs in the CHRNA3 and CHRNA5 genes to be associated with increased risk for lung cancer. These genes encode for nicotinic acetylcholine receptor subunits. Findings from two of the three GWAS studies suggest that these SNPs may increase the individual's predisposition to smoke tobacco and thereby increasing their risk for developing lung cancer.

Answer 5.16.   **The answer is D.**

ABO blood group has been long known to be associated with increased risk for developing pancreatic cancer. GWAS studies have now identified specific SNPs in the ABO gene to be associated with increased risk for pancreatic cancer.

CHAPTER 6 PRINCIPLES OF SURGICAL ONCOLOGY

REBECCA L. AFT • JASON KEUNE

DIRECTIONS   Each of the numbered items below is followed by lettered answers. Select the ONE lettered answer that is BEST in each case unless instructed otherwise.

QUESTIONS

Question 6.1.   A 45-year-old woman with breast cancer is starting adjuvant chemotherapy for breast cancer. You prescribe EMLA (lidocaine/prilocaine) cream for topical anesthesia prior to port-a-cath access. She cautions you that she is allergic to benzocaine. Which of the following statement is NOT correct?

A. She should avoid using EMLA cream given her allergy history.
B. EMLA cream contains a combination of amide local anesthetics.
C. Allergy to benzocaine is unlikely to result in cross-allergy to EMLA cream.
D. Allergy to benzocaine is a result of sensitivity to its metabolite, para-aminobenzoic acid.

Question 6.2.   Epidural anesthesia involves the injection of a local anesthetic agent:

A. Into the cerebrospinal fluid, by puncturing the dura between L2 and L4
B. Into the extradural space within the spinal canal
C. Into the space outside of the spinal canal, superficial to the ligamentum flavum
D. Into the subarachnoid space

Question 6.3.   Palliative surgery for gastric outlet obstruction in a patient with metastatic cancer of the head of the pancreas carries a mortality rate of up to:

A. 5%
B. 20%
C. 40%.
D. 60%.

Corresponding Chapter in *Cancer: Principles & Practice of Oncology*, Ninth Edition: 25 (Surgical Oncology: General Issues) and 26 (Surgical Oncology: Laparoscopic Surgery).

Question 6.4.   An 83-year-old man presents for colon resection after evaluation for microcytic anemia revealed a 3-cm villous adenoma in his cecum. Colonoscopy was performed, and the adenoma was not able to be resected. Biopsy revealed dysplastic changes. No evidence of metastatic disease was seen on computed tomography (CT) of the chest, abdomen, and pelvis. Which of the following statements is TRUE?

A. Surgery should be avoided in this patient because of the prohibitive morbidity and mortality in this octogenarian.
B. The patient's medical history and physical examination are the best determinants of preoperative risk.
C. The patient requires a cardiac stress test and possible cardiac catheterization before surgical resection.
D. No additional testing besides routine laboratory testing is required.

Question 6.5.   A 67-year-old man with poorly controlled diabetes, congestive heart failure with an ejection fraction of 14%, and Stage III chronic kidney disease is scheduled to undergo pancreaticoduodenectomy. He should be categorized as American Society of Anesthesiologists Class:

A. II
B. III
C. IV
D. V

Question 6.6.   A 42-year-old woman presents with a 4-year history of a lump on her right lateral thigh. On examination, she has a firm nodule in her right thigh, approximately 5 cm in size. The mass appears to be in the subcutaneous tissue but is not freely mobile. The patient has no associated neurologic findings. The next appropriate step in management is:

A. Perform fine-needle aspiration
B. Perform core biopsy
C. Perform excisional biopsy
D. Obtain magnetic resonance imaging

Question 6.7.   A 45-year-old woman with a body mass index of 34 is scheduled to undergo Ivor Lewis esophagectomy for a T2N0M0 adenocarcinoma of the distal esophagus. Her relative risk of pulmonary complications after surgery compared with a nonobese patient is approximately:

A. 0.8 to 1.7
B. 1.5 to 2.0
C. 1.7 to 3.0
D. 2.0 to 4.5

Question 6.8.   The same patient presents to a center regarded as very experienced in minimally invasive surgery. Her esophagectomy is performed laparoscopically. Compared with open esophagectomy, she is expected to have:

    A. No difference in either lymph node retrieval or 3-year survival
    B. No difference in lymph node retrieval but a decreased 3-year survival
    C. Decreased lymph node retrieval but no difference in 3-year survival
    D. Decreased lymph node retrieval and 3-year survival

Question 6.9.   The decreased venous return and increased transmitted intrathoracic pressure inherent in laparoscopic surgery are thought to cause which of the following physiologic changes during laparoscopic procedures?

    A. Increased heart rate
    B. Decreased cardiac index
    C. Decreased systemic vascular resistance
    D. Decreased central venous pressure

Question 6.10.   Retrospective analyses of colon resection for colon cancer have demonstrated that the difference in the rate of recurrence at laparoscopic port sites compared with the rate of recurrence in analogous open procedures is approximately:

    A. 0
    B. Greater by 10%
    C. Greater by 20%
    D. Not known

Question 6.11.   A 55-year-old man with a several-month history of hemoccult positive stools has recently been diagnosed with gastric cancer by upper endoscopy. Staging CT demonstrates no evidence of intra-abdominal disease. You recommend a staging laparoscopy before definitive resection because:

    A. CT has a high false-negative rate in the staging of most cancers.
    B. Carcinomatosis and peritoneal seeding are more accurately diagnosed with laparoscopy.
    C. Nontherapeutic laparotomies can be avoided in more than 20% of patients after staging laparoscopy.
    D. All of the above.

Question 6.12.   The benefits of laparoscopy are:

    A. Reduction in postoperative pain
    B. Decreased healing time
    C. Decreased adhesion formation
    D. All of the above

Question 6.13.   Which of the following may result from the use of general anesthetics for oncologic surgery?

    A. Bone marrow depression
    B. Alteration of the phagocytic activity of macrophages
    C. Immunosuppression
    D. All of the above

Question 6.14.   A 46-year-old man underwent hemicolectomy and adjuvant chemotherapy for stage III adenocarcinoma of the colon. 18 months after completion of therapy, he is noted to have an elevated carcinoembryonic antigen level on a routine follow-up visit. Imaging reveals a 2-cm lesion in the right lobe of the liver. Ultrasound-guided biopsy demonstrates metastatic adenocarcinoma, consistent with colon primary. Which of the following is the appropriate next step?

    A. Referral to a surgeon
    B. Observation, as he is not symptomatic
    C. Chemotherapy for metastatic disease
    D. Hospice

Question 6.15.   A 50-year-old man with a history of renal cell carcinoma, status post-nephrectomy 3 years ago, presents with slurred speech and left-sided arm weakness. Imaging of the brain reveals a right parietal mass measuring 3 cm with surrounding edema. CT scan of the chest, abdomen, and pelvis shows postsurgical changes, with no other sites of disease. He is placed on steroids to decrease cerebral edema. Which of the following is the appropriate management of this patient?

    A. Sorafenib therapy
    B. High-dose interleukin-2 therapy
    C. Resection of the brain lesion
    D. Hospice

Question 6.16.   A 40-year-old woman presents with weight loss, night sweats, and a 2-cm left neck mass. She is found to have an elevated LDH of 800. Imaging reveals extensive cervical, mediastinal, and abdominal adenopathy. You suspect lymphoma and schedule a biopsy of the neck mass for histologic diagnosis. Which of the following would be the most appropriate technique to obtain tissue for diagnosis?

    A. Fine-needle aspiration
    B. Core needle biopsy
    C. Incisional biopsy
    D. Excisional biopsy

Question 6.17.   Which of the following conditions is associated with a high incidence of cancer, which can be prevented by prophylactic surgery?

    A. Ulcerative colitis
    B. Multiple endocrine neoplasia type 2
    C. Cryptorchidism
    D. All of the above

ANSWERS

Answer 6.1.   **The answer is A.**

Benzocaine is an ester local anesthetic. Allergic reaction to ester local anesthetics (cocaine, procaine, benzocaine, tetracaine) occurs due to sensitivity to their metabolite, para-aminobezoic acid. This does not result in cross-allergy to amide local anesthetics such as lidocaine, prilocaine, and bupivacaine. Therefore, amides can be used as an alternative in patients who are allergic to esters.

Answer 6.2.   **The answer is B.**

Epidural anesthesia refers to injection of local anesthetic into the epidural or peridural space. This potential space is bounded by the dura anteriorly and the ligamentum flavum posteriorly and includes the lymphatics, areolar tissue, and epidural venous plexus. The primary site of action of the local anesthetic is on the spinal nerve roots that traverse the space.

Answer 6.3.   **The answer is B.**

Patients with widely metastatic disease undergoing palliative surgery have a mortality rate of up to 20%. The underlying disease (metastatic cancer) is the major determinant of operative risk in this case.

Answer 6.4.   **The answer is B.**

Surgery in the elderly population is decided on a case-by-case basis. Physiologic age does not always correlate with chronologic age. Approximately half of surgical morbidity is attributed to perioperative cardiac events. The American College of Cardiology has defined an algorithm to estimate risk and the need for preoperative testing. Risk is stratified on the basis of the intrinsic risk of the procedure, the patient's cardiac history, and the exercise tolerance of the patient. High-risk procedures carry a risk of cardiac morbidity greater than 4% (noncarotid vascular surgery, thoracic procedures, abdominal procedures, major head and neck procedures, and emergent procedures). Intermediate-risk procedures (1% to 4% risk of cardiac morbidity) include carotid surgery, radical prostatectomy, and orthopedic procedures. Low-risk procedures (<1% risk) include breast surgery and soft-tissue biopsies. Patient risk factors include history of congestive heart failure, diabetes, prior myocardial infarction, angina, and ventricular arrhythmia. These patients should undergo some form of preoperative risk assessment with cardiac stress testing before high-risk surgery.

Answer 6.5.   **The answer is C.**

This patient should be classified as American Society of Anesthesiologists Class IV. A patient with Class IV has an incapacitating systemic disease that is not correctable by operation, such as organic heart disease with marked signs of cardiac insufficiency.

Answer 6.6.   **The answer is D.**

Sarcoma must be considered in the differential diagnosis of soft-tissue masses. Imaging by magnetic resonance imaging can provide information on size, tumor characteristics, and relationship to adjacent structures. Subsequent tissue sampling is essential to obtain a diagnosis.

Answer 6.7.   **The answer is A.**

Several prospective cohort studies have contributed to the development of a risk index for postoperative pulmonary complications after surgical procedures. The American Society of Anesthesiologists has summarized these data. The relative risk of pulmonary complications in an obese patient undergoing a thoracic procedure is 0.8 to 1.7.

Answer 6.8.   **The answer is A.**

A prospective study of 483 patients conducted by Smithers et al. (Smithers BM, Cotley DC, Martin I, et al. Comparison of the outcomes between open and minimally invasive esophagectomy. *Ann Surg.* 2007;245(2):232–240) revealed no differences in lymph node retrieval and 3-year survival between open and laparoscopic procedures.

Answer 6.9.   **The answer is B.**

A recent study of patients undergoing laparoscopic colectomy for carcinoma demonstrated increased mean arterial pressure, central venous pressure, mean pulmonary artery pressure, pulmonary capillary wedge pressure, and systemic vascular resistance. Cardiac index and ejection fraction decreased significantly, although heart rate remained unchanged.

Answer 6.10.   **The answer is A.**

Retrospective reviews have demonstrated a wound site recurrence rate of less than 1% in patients undergoing surgery for colon cancer. Port site recurrence rates for a similar population of patients have been reported to be approximately 1%. Port site metastases have been associated with aerosolization caused by the pneumoperitoneum, tumor manipulation, and degree of tumor burden.

Answer 6.11.   **The answer is D.**

One of the most important aspects of laparoscopic staging is the exclusion of patients from undergoing a major operation by identifying metastatic or unresectable disease (e.g., carcinomatosis), which is easily missed in imaging studies. Undetected metastatic disease has been found in 13% to 57% of patients initially staged with having no metastatic disease by conventional imaging. However, laparoscopy is not yet performed as a routine procedure because many patients are often symptomatic and require palliative resection.

Answer 6.12.   **The answer is D.**

All of the above are the beneficial effects of laparoscopy. This is attributed to the use of small incisions and lack of retractors holding the incision open. In addition, exposure to CO_2 contributes to a diminished acute phase systemic response, which likely leads to decreased inflammation and pain.

Answer 6.13.   **The answer is D.**

General anesthetics can cause bone marrow depression, alteration of the phagocytic activity of macrophages, and immunosuppression.

Answer 6.14.   **The answer is A.**

Resection of isolated liver metastasis from colon cancer can be curative; therefore, he should be referred to a surgeon for possible resection of the liver lesion. Observation until he is symptomatic and hospice are inappropriate. Decisions regarding systemic chemotherapy before or after resection of the lesion should be made after consultation with the surgeon.

Answer 6.15.   **The answer is C.**

This gentleman has an isolated brain metastasis from renal cell carcinoma. Both sorafenib and interleukin-2 are approved systemic therapies for metastatic renal cell carcinoma, but surgical resection would be the most appropriate next step, with the greatest potential for cure. Hospice would not be appropriate in this setting, as he has a potentially curable condition.

Answer 6.16.   **The answer is D.**

Fine-needle aspiration involves aspiration of cells through a needle. Core biopsy uses a special needle through which a core of tissue can be obtained. Tissue obtained from a core biopsy is usually sufficient for diagnosis of most types of cancers. For suspected lymphoma, removal of an entire lymph node (excisional biopsy) is preferred, as it can provide better evaluation of the architecture of the lymph node. Incisional biopsies are used to take a small piece of tissue from a large tumor mass. In this case, the mass is small enough that it can be removed entirely.

Answer 6.17.   **The answer is D.**

Cryptorchidism is associated with a high incidence of testicular cancer, which can be prevented by prophylactic orchiopexy. Multiple endocrine neoplasia types 2 and 3 are associated with high incidence of medullary cancer of the thyroid, which can be prevented by performing prophylactic thyroidectomy. Ulcerative colitis is associated with increased risk for colon cancer, which can be prevented by prophylactic colectomy.

CHAPTER 7 PRINCIPLES OF RADIATION ONCOLOGY

HAK CHOY • NATHAN KIM

DIRECTIONS   Each of the numbered items below is followed by lettered answers. Select the ONE lettered answer that is BEST in each case unless instructed otherwise.

QUESTIONS

Question 7.1. Which of the following describes the specific pathways for the repair of double-stranded DNA breaks?

A. The repair may be by homologous recombination (HR) or nonhomologous end-joining (NHEJ) pathway.

B. The HR repair pathway functions by degrading the single strand at each side of the break and then annealing the two ends.

C. The NHEJ pathway functions by replicating the missing genetic information from the homologous DNA template.

D. NHEJ is a minor component of mechanism for repair of double-stranded DNA breaks in mammalian cells.

Question 7.2. Which of the following is NOT true about ionizing events in tissues caused by x-rays?

A. Radiation dose describes the quantity of energy deposited per mass of tissue.

B. The fast electrons produced by high-energy x-ray photons can damage deoxyribonucleic acid (DNA) by a direct action.

C. The relative biological effectiveness (RBE) describes the ratio of doses required to yield an equivalent biologic event.

D. Indirect action of ionizing radiation where hydroxyl radicals damage target tissues is not commonly seen.

Question 7.3. Which of the following statements describes the DNA damage/repair process associated with ionizing radiation?

A. Single-stranded breaks of the DNA are thought to represent the lethal event.

B. All of the radiation-induced, double-stranded breaks are rejoined in cells within 2 hours.

C. In mammalian cells, choice of repair can be biased by phase of the cell cycle and by abundance of repetitive DNA.

D. Nonhomologous end-joining (NHEJ) is effective in rejoining DNA double strand break because it is an error free process.

Corresponding Chapter in *Cancer: Principles & Practice of Oncology,* Ninth Edition: 27 (Radiation Oncology).

Question 7.4. Which of the following statements describes the dose-related cellular response to radiation?

A. In mammalian cells, there is generally a linear relationship between the cell killing and the dose given.
B. The term "D_0" describes the slope of the exponential survival curve and represents a dose required to reduce the surviving fraction to 37%.
C. Both mammalian cells and bacterial cells display "shoulder" in the low-dose region.
D. In general, postirradiation conditions that accelerate the cell division are the ones most favorable to repair of potentially lethal damage.

Question 7.5. Which of the following statements is FALSE regarding independent events (4 R's) that occur during fractionated radiotherapy?

A. Repopulation refers to spontaneous repopulation and induced cell proliferation or recruitment of cells after irradiation.
B. Repair explains the shoulder of the radiation survival curve showing that cells can repair some of the radiation damage.
C. Redistribution explains migration of cells away from an irradiation source.
D. Reoxygenation explains how the proportion of hypoxic cells present in a tumor returns to preradiation level.

Question 7.6. Which of the following acute effects is NOT related to radiation-induced cell death?

A. Cystitis
B. Esophagitis
C. Fatigue
D. Proctitis
E. None of the above

Question 7.7. Nonirradiated cells can express all of the following responses after radiation damage to neighboring cells, EXCEPT:

A. Gene induction
B. Induction of genomic instability
C. Differentiation
D. Changes in apoptotic potential
E. Double-stranded breaks in DNA

Question 7.8. Which of the following best describes the modern linear accelerator?

A. A modern linear accelerator (LINAC) can deliver energies up to 1 MeV.
B. The ^{60}Cobalt teletherapy unit is a megavoltage machine that relies on radioactive cobalt to produce an electron beam.
C. Unlike LINAC, the ^{60}Cobalt unit is always "on" and must be kept in a shielded position until the beam is needed for treatment.
D. The focal point of the gantry's rotation is called the field edge.

Question 7.9.   Which of the following statements describes the role of oxygen in radiation effects?

A. A greater dose of radiation is required for cell killing in an oxic condition compared with a hypoxic condition.

B. A randomized trial showed that epoetin b improved survival in patients with head and neck cancer.

C. Oxygen need not be present at the time of irradiation for oxygen enhancement of radiotherapy to occur.

D. Hyperbaric oxygen often shows a dramatic increase in curability with standard fractionated radiotherapy.

E. The oxygen enhancement ratio (OER) has more relevance on the exponential portion of the cell survival curve.

Question 7.10.   Which of the following best describes the concept of altered fractionation?

A. Accelerated fractionation does not reduce the overall treatment time.

B. Hyperfractionation refers to a radiotherapy schedule that uses multiple daily treatments more than 6 hours apart with reduced fraction size and increased number of fractions.

C. A Radiation Therapy Oncology Group (RTOG) 9003 randomized trial showed that standard fractionation treatment was superior to hyperfractionation and accelerated fractionation with concomitant boost used for advanced head and neck squamous cell carcinomas.

D. Continuous hyperfractionated accelerated radiation therapy (CHART) gives a higher total dose than the standard fractionated treatment.

Question 7.11.   Which of the following statements regarding interaction of chemotherapy and radiation therapy is NOT true?

A. Rationale for combining radiation therapy with radiosensitizing chemotherapy is primarily to confer an additive effect.

B. Gemcitabine is a potent radiosensitizer, however, when used concurrently with radiation therapy, radiation fields, and gemcitabine dose and scheduling must be carefully defined, as noted in experiences with pancreatic cancer clinical studies.

C. Paclitaxel in combination with radiation has demonstrated clinical benefits in treatment of locally advanced lung cancer

D. Mechanism of radiosensitization by cisplatin may be due to its ability to inhibit DNA repair of radiation induced DNA double-strand breaks.

Question 7.12.   Which of the following statements is NOT true regarding modulation of radiation by hyperthermia?

A. Localized heat treatment can be delivered with microwaves, ultrasound, or radiofrequency sources of energy.

B. The lethality of hyperthermia is thought to be in part from denaturation of proteins.

C. Similar to radiation-induced kill, lethality from heat is most pronounced when cells are in the G2/M phase.

D. The temperature 42.5°C seems to be critical, with small increments above this temperature leading to a steep increase in lethality.

Question 7.13.   Which of the following statements best describes the tissue effects from radiation?

A. Early or acute effects typically occur within months after irradiation.
B. Large a/b ratio has a small "shoulder" in the low-dose portion.
C. The frequencies of late effects depend strongly on radiation fraction size.
D. Typical human tumors and early-responding normal tissues have a small a/b ratio.

Question 7.14.   Which of the following statements is an INCORRECT description of the interaction of x-rays with biologic material?

A. In modern treatment with greater than 4 MeV photons, photoelectric effect dominates the interaction.
B. In photoelectric effect, an incoming x-ray transfers all its energy to an inner orbit electron, which is ejected from the atom. A photon is produced as an outer shell electron fills the vacant hole.
C. In Compton scattering, energy from the x-ray is both absorbed and scattered. The photon emerges with reduced energy and a change in direction.
D. In pair production, an electron and a positron are produced.

Question 7.15.   Which of the following statements describes the depth dose characteristics of radiation?

A. Higher-energy photons deposit more dose to the skin surface.
B. For a given energy, electrons generally penetrate deeper in tissue compared with photons.
C. Electron beams deposit less dose to the skin surface as the incident electron energy increases.
D. Depth of maximum dose increases as the energy of the incident beam increases.

Question 7.16.   Which of the following statements is NOT true regarding brachytherapy?

A. Isotopes with properties of long half-lives and high energy are typically used for permanent implants.
B. Brachytherapy refers to placement of radioactive sources next to or inside the tumor, or within body or surgical cavities.
C. High doses can be delivered within a few centimeters of the source.
D. A potential advantage of brachytherapy is its ability to produce conformal treatments with low normal tissue dose.

Question 7.17.   Which of the following can be a subacute toxcitiy from radiation therapy?

A. Pneumonitis
B. Myelitis.
C. Brain necrosis.
D. B and C.

Question 7.18.   Which of the following best describes the treatment planning process?

   A. At the time of image acquisition for planning, tumor motion caused by respiration must be determined.
   B. Immobilization is not important because it does not add to accuracy.
   C. Three-dimensional dose distribution in each patient is easily measured.
   D. Intensity-modulated radiation therapy (IMRT) cannot control the shaping of the dose distribution.

Question 7.19.   Which of the following is NOT true regarding charged particle beams?

   A. Charged particle beam therapy include proton and carbon based therapy.
   B. Protons have shown to confer a definite clinical benefit over photon based therapies for most clinical cancer applications.
   C. Ability of charged particles to stop at a given depth gives it a potential advantage for treatment of tumors in close proximity to critical structures.
   D. Current challenges involved with widespread use of charged particle therapy include cost involved with production and operation of such facility.

ANSWERS

Answer 7.1.   **The answer is A.**

There are two generally accepted mechanisms of repair. They are broadly known as the HR or NHEJ. HR functions by replicating the missing genetic information from the homologous DNA template. NHEJ functions by degrading the single strand at each side of the break and then annealing the two ends in a region of microhomology. The NHEJ may result in loss or gain in genetic information and is mutation prone. Some have suggested that HR and NHEJ have overlapping complementary roles. NHEJ is a dominant mechanism for repairing double-stranded DNA breaks in mammalian cells. Several investigators have demonstrated enhanced radiosensitivity of human cell lines by inhibiting the proteins required for NHEJ.

Answer 7.2.   **The answer is D.**

All other statements are true. The indirect effects of x-rays predominate the biologic effects seen with x-rays. The photons cause ejection of fast electrons. The ejected fast electrons can directly damage the DNA (direct action) or, more commonly, the fast electrons interact with plentiful water molecules to produce hydroxyl radicals (OH—), which in turn can damage the biologic target (indirect action).

Answer 7.3.   **The answer is C.**

Although single-stranded and double-stranded breaks are observed from ionizing radiation, it is the double-stranded breaks that are thought to represent the lethal event. Although the majority of the radiation-induced, double-stranded breaks are rejoined in cells within 2 hours after exposure, the process can continue for 24 hours. In mammalian cells, choice of repair is biased by phase of cell cycle and by abundance of repetitive DNA. HRR is used primarily in late S to G_2 phase of cell cycle, and NHEJ predominates in the G_1 phase of cell cycle. However, this is not an absolute, and factors in addition to cell cycle phase are important in determining which mechanism will be used to repair DNA strand breaks. NHEJ while effective is known to be highly error prone.

Answer 7.4.   **The answer is B.**

D_0 is related to the slope of the exponential survival curve and represents a dose that is required to reduce the surviving fraction to 0.37% or 37% of the original population. The smaller D_0 represents more radiosensitivity. Mammalian cell lines display a "shoulder" in the low-dose region and the exponential relation at higher doses. The "shoulder" represents a reduced efficiency of cell killing. The linear quadratic model rather than the linear model best describes the cellular response to radiation. The postirradiation conditions that suppress the cell division are the ones most favorable to potentially lethal damage repair.

Answer 7.5. **The answer is C.**

Repair explains the shoulder of the radiation survival curve showing that cells can repair some of the radiation damage. The majority of sublethal damage repair occurs within 6 hours after irradiation. Redistribution explains differences in cell-cycle radiation sensitivity, with the mitotic (M) phase being the most sensitive. Cells gradually increase in resistance as they proceed through the late G1 and S phases. Repopulation refers to spontaneous repopulation and induced cell proliferation or recruitment of cells after irradiation. This may occur in some tumors but occurs less than that in normal tissues. Reoxygenation explains how a proportion of hypoxic cells present in a tumor return to preradiation level. Some tumor cells may reoxygenate after radiotherapy, and the proportion of the hypoxic cells that was present before irradiation may be seen.

Answer 7.6. **The answer is C.**

Acute effects of radiation usually occur in organs dependent on rapid self-renewal and are mostly caused by radiation-induced cell death during mitosis. In the case of nausea and fatigue however, these toxicities are most likely related to the release of cytokines.

Answer 7.7. **The answer is E.**

The responses of nonirradiated cells appear to be cell-type dependent. This may be mediated by diffusible substances or by cell–cell contact. The double-stranded breaks are seen after cells are directly irradiated.

Answer 7.8. **The answer is C.**

A modern LINAC can deliver energies up to 25 MeV. The focal point of the gantry's rotation is called the isocenter. The ^{60}Cobalt teletherapy unit is a megavoltage machine that relies on radioactive cobalt to produce a photon beam. Unlike the LINAC, the ^{60}Cobalt unit is always "on" and must be kept in shielded position until the beam is needed for treatment.

Answer 7.9. **The answer is E.**

Greater doses of radiation are required for cell killing in hypoxic conditions. The oxygen enhancement is seen more readily during the exponential portion of the survival curve because of the reduced capacity for cells to repair sublethal damage under hypoxic conditions. Tumor cells growing in a physiologic hypoxic condition have reduced capacity to repair sublethal damage. The OER is the ratio of dose required for equivalent cell killing in the absence of oxygen compared with the dose required in the presence of oxygen. The range of OER varies from 2.5 to 3.5. Oxygen must be present at the time of irradiation for oxygen enhancement of radiotherapy to occur. OER is more important for radiation that damages cells via hydroxyl radical intermediates. Hyperbaric oxygen often does not show a dramatic increase in curability with standard fractionated radiotherapy. However, hyperbaric oxygen appears to increase curability in a small number of fractions. A meta-analysis showed that hyperbaric oxygen improves the local control of solid tumors by approximately 10%. Unfortunately, a randomized trial published recently showed that epoetin b did not improve cancer control or survival in patients with head and neck cancer.

Answer 7.10.   **The answer is B.**

Hyperfractionation refers to a radiotherapy schedule that uses multiple daily treatments more than 6 hours apart with reduced fraction size and increased number of fractions. A randomized trial performed by the European Organization for Research and Treatment of Cancer (EORTC) showed that a hyperfractionated regimen was significantly better than standard fractionation in improving local control. Accelerated fractionation reduces the overall treatment time. It delivers the same dose with the same fraction size but in a shorter overall treatment time. An RTOG 9003 randomized trial showed that standard fractionation treatment was inferior to hyperfractionation and accelerated fractionation with concomitant boost used for advanced head and neck squamous cell carcinomas. CHART, as developed at Mt. Vernon Hospital in the United Kingdom, gave a 54 Gy total dose, which is significantly lower than the standard fractionated treatment dose for lung cancer.

Answer 7.11.   **The answer is A.**

The two proposed reasons for combining chemotherapy with radiation therapy includes radiosensitization and spatial additivity. The former concept theoretically may yield synergistic effective which is greater than simply adding the two together. Gemcitabine is a potent radiosensitizer due to the induction of dATP depletion and redistribution of the cells into the early S phase. Although full dose gemcitabine can be safely combined with radiation therapy for the treatment of locally advanced pancreatic carcinoma in cases without involved lymph nodes, including the regional lymph nodes in the radiation field can be extremely toxic. Cisplatin, 5-fluorouracil, and paclitaxel are also radiosensitizers. Paclitaxel in combination with radiation (with cis- or carboplatin) has demonstrated clinical benefit in locally advanced lung therapy. Mechanism of cisplatin radiosensitization is related to its ability to cause inter- and intrastrand DNA cross links. Two possible explanation are that cisplatin inhibits repair of radiation induced DNA double-strand breaks, or increases the number of lethal radiation-induced double-strand breaks.

Answer 7.12.   **The answer is C.**

Localized heat treatment can be delivered with microwaves, ultrasound, or radiofrequency sources of energy. The temperature 42.5°C appears to be critical, with small increments above this temperature leading to a steep increase in lethality. The lethality of hyperthermia is thought to be in part from denaturation of proteins. Unlike radiation-induced kill, lethality from heat is most pronounced when cells are in the radio-resistant S phase. When hyperthermia and radiation are combined in vitro, the net effect is greater than additive lethal effect. However, in a clinical setting, the effect appears to be additive or independent.

Answer 7.13.   **The answer is C.**

Early or acute effects typically occur within weeks after irradiation. They often occur in tissues that have rapid turnover, and it is thought to result from the depletion of the clonogenic or stem cells within that tissue. The frequencies of late effects depend strongly on radiation fraction size. There are fewer late effects with smaller fraction size. Large a/b ratio has a large "shoulder" in the low-dose portion. The a/b ratio represents the dose at which the quadratic (b) and linear (a) components of cell kill are equivalent. The dose response to radiation can be described by the formula $S = \exp(-aD - bD2)$, where S is surviving fraction and D represents dose. Typical human tumors and early-responding normal tissues have large a/b ratios (9 to 13 Gy).

Answer 7.14.   **The answer is A.**

The relative probabilities of photoelectric, Compton, and pair production interaction depend on the photon energy and the atomic number of the irradiated material. In modern treatment machines with greater than 4 MeV photons, the Compton interactions and pair productions are commonly seen. At diagnostic equipment energy range (25 kvp), photoelectric effect predominates. In photoelectric effect, an incoming x-ray transfers all its energy to an inner orbit electron, which is ejected from the atom. A photon is produced as an outer shell electron fills the vacant hole. In Compton scattering, energy from the x-ray is both absorbed and scattered. The photon emerges with reduced energy and a change in direction. In pair production, an electron and a positron are produced, which then deposit energy through collisions with other electrons. The threshold energy for pair production is 1.02 MeV.

Answer 7.15.   **The answer is D.**

Higher-energy photons deposit less dose to the skin surface. Thus, it is called the skin-sparing effect of high-energy photons. Depth of maximum dose increases as the energy of the incident beam increases. It is often desirable to use high-energy photons (>10 MeV) to reach deeply located tumors. For a given energy, electrons do not penetrate deeper in tissue compared with photons. It is for this reason that electron beams are often used to treat superficially located tumors such as skin cancer. Electron beams, unlike photons, deposit more dose to the skin surface as the incident electron energy increases.

Answer 7.16.   **The answer is A.**

Isotopes with properties of very short half-lives and low energy are used for permanent implants, such as for prostate cancer treatment with iodine-125 with a half-life of 59.4 days and an x-ray energy of 27 to 35 keV. Brachytherapy is a form of treatment that uses direct placement of radioactive sources or materials within tumors (interstitial brachytherapy) or within body or surgical cavities (intracavitary brachytherapy), either permanently or temporarily. Relative to external beam therapy energies, the emitted spectra are of low energy, but high doses can be delivered within few centimeters of the source. The ability to irradiate tumors from close range can lead to conformal treatments with potentially lower normal tissue doses.

Answer 7.17.   **The answer is A.**

Radiation related adverse effects can be divided into acute, subacute and chronic (late) effects. Acute effects tend to occur in organs (typically within the field of radiation) that depend on rapid self renewal. Acute effects commonly occurs, and typically are self limiting. Examples include mucositis, esophagitis, diarrhea, and skin reaction. Subacute toxicities typically occurs 2 weeks to 3 months after radiation has been completed. Radiation-induced pneumonitis is usually a subacute toxicity. Late effects from radiation therapy are usually observed after 6 months from completion of therapy. Some examples include radiation myelitis, brain necrosis, and bowel obstruction.

Answer 7.18.   **The answer is A.**

Immobilization is critically important because it adds to the accuracy of daily setup and treatment. A planning computed tomography (CT) scan is obtained after immobilization has been completed. At the time of image acquisition for planning, tumor motion caused by respiration must be determined. The planning volume must account for respiratory movement and uncertainty of tumor position. Three-dimensional dose distribution in each patient is not easily measured, and it must be predicted from computer calculation. Intensity-modulated radiation therapy can have a high degree of control on the shaping of the dose distribution. The computer determines the intensity profiles to achieve the desired dose distribution.

Answer 7.19.   **The answer is B.**

Charged particles include protons and carbons. These particles differ from photons in that they interact only modestly with tissue until they reach the end of their path where they then deposit majority of their energy and stops (Bragg Peak). This ability to stop at given depth gives them the potential advantage of treating tumors that are close to critical structures. While proton therapy may have potential use in clinical settings demanding such characteristics, it's widespread use for all cancer is not yet warranted. Furthermore, in the era of IMRT (Intensity Modulated Radiation Therapy) and IGRT (Image Guided Radiation Therapy), despite theoretical and dosimetric advantages conferred by charged particles, whether this will allow higher dose to be delivered more safely, and yield a clinical advantage over highly conformal photon techniques is not yet fully determined. Cost of development and operation of charged particle therapy facilities has also limited its widespread development and use.

CHAPTER 8 PRINCIPLES OF MEDICAL ONCOLOGY

SUJATHA MURALI • SURESH S. RAMALINGAM

DIRECTIONS   Each of the numbered items below is followed by lettered answers. Select the ONE lettered answer that is BEST in each case unless instructed otherwise.

QUESTIONS

Question 8.1.   Historically, the first chemotherapeutic drugs used in the clinical setting were:

A. Anthracyclines
B. Epidermal growth factor receptor (EGFR) inhibitors
C. Antimetabolites
D. Alkylating agents

Question 8.2.   In children with lymphoblastic leukemia, folic acid was observed to:

A. Cause disease proliferation
B. Cause disease regression
C. Have no effect
D. Improve survival

Question 8.3.   Antimetabolite chemotherapeutic agents include all of the following, EXCEPT:

A. Gemcitabine
B. Fluoropyrimidines
C. Mitoxantrone
D. Cytarabine

Question 8.4.   In a subset of patients with advanced or metastatic disease, which of the following has curative potential with primary induction chemotherapy?

A. Germ cell cancer
B. Non-small cell lung cancer
C. Gastric cancer
D. Colorectal cancer

Corresponding Chapter in *Cancer: Principles & Practice of Oncology,* Ninth Edition: 28 (Medical Oncology) and 29 (Assessment of Clinical Response).

Question 8.5.   The goals of therapy in incurable, advanced, metastatic disease include all of the following, EXCEPT:

A. Palliate tumor-related symptoms
B. Eradicate all evidence of cancer
C. Improve quality of life
D. Prolong time to tumor progression

Question 8.6.   Neoadjuvant chemotherapy can be utilized in all of the following cancers EXCEPT:

A. Head and neck cancer
B. Non-small cell lung cancer
C. Hematologic malignancies
D. Pancreatic cancer

Question 8.7.   All of the following are true concerning the role of adjuvant chemotherapy, EXCEPT:

A. Risk reduction in local recurrence
B. Risk reduction in distant recurrence
C. Primary therapy instead of surgery and/or radiation
D. Prolongation of disease-free and overall survival in osteogenic sarcoma

Question 8.8.   Apoptosis is inhibited by the activation of the following EXCEPT:

A. Bcl-2
B. NF-κB
C. Caspases
D. Bcl-x_L

Question 8.9.   The most important indicator of the effectiveness of chemotherapy is:

A. Achievement of a minor response
B. Achievement of a partial response
C. Achievement of a complete response
D. Achievement of stable disease

Question 8.10.   A partial response is defined as:

A. At least a 50% reduction in measurable tumor mass
B. At least a 10% reduction in measurable tumor mass
C. Improvement in quality of life
D. Improvement in survival

Question 8.11.   Anticancer activity of bortezomib is due to the inhibition of:

A. Proteasome
B. Bcl-2
C. Thymidylate synthase
D. MDM2

Question 8.12.   In early-stage colon cancer treated with adjuvant chemotherapy, the majority of relapses occur:

A. Within the first 5 years
B. Within the first 3 years
C. Within the first 2 years
D. Within the first year

Question 8.13.   Gompertzian kinetics are characterized by:

A. Clinically undetectable tumors are at their lowest growth fraction.
B. The growth fraction is stable over time.
C. The growth fraction increases exponentially with time.
D. The growth fraction decreases exponentially with time.

Question 8.14.   In patients with activating mutations in the tyrosine kinase (TK) domain of EGFR, all of the following genetic changes are associated with development of resistance to tyrosine kinase inhibitors (TKI), EXCEPT:

A. T790M mutation
B. Loss of PTEN expression
C. D761Y mutation
D. MET gene mutation

Question 8.15.   All of the following are true regarding an intermittent treatment approach, EXCEPT:

A. Salvage therapies should show a good response.
B. Sufficient time is needed between the termination of induction chemotherapy and progressive disease.
C. A majority of responses should be achieved during the induction chemotherapy period.
D. Reinitiation of the induction chemotherapy is not indicated.

Question 8.16.   In patients with colorectal cancer the genetic change associated with resistance to cetuximab is:

A. BRAF mutation
B. Wild-type Kras
C. EGFR-TK mutation
D. NFκB activation

Question 8.17.   Dose-dense chemotherapy was developed after the observation that:

A. The growth of cells is significantly lower in the early part of the growth curve.
B. The log cell kill is higher in smaller volume tumors, resulting in more rapid growth between chemotherapy cycles.
C. Growth between chemotherapy cycles is halted.
D. More frequent administration of chemotherapy led to less toxicity.

Question 8.18.   In most cases, normal bone marrow and gastrointestinal (GI) precursor cells are able to counteract the effects of cytotoxic chemotherapy because:

A. They are not exposed to the chemotherapeutic agent.
B. They have intact mechanisms for apoptosis and cell-cycle arrest.
C. They have rapid turnover.
D. They possess resistance mechanisms.

Question 8.19.   All of the following are true concerning p53, EXCEPT:

A. It is a tumor suppressor gene.
B. It is a potent inducer of apoptosis.
C. It causes S phase arrest in the cell cycle.
D. It can be protective against chemotherapy cytotoxicity.

Question 8.20.   Drug resistance in advanced tumors is thought to be due to:

A. Mutations in important genes in cell-cycle regulation
B. Drug-specific spontaneous mutations
C. Wild-type p53
D. Low tumor growth rate

Question 8.21.   The final stage of the programmed cell death pathway is mediated by:

A. Bcl-2
B. p53
C. Tumor necrosis factor
D. Caspase cascade

Question 8.22.   Imatinib inhibits all of the following, EXCEPT:

A. EGFR
B. C-kit
C. Platelet-derived growth factor
D. Bcr-abl

Question 8.23.   Cetuximab use in colorectal cancer is characterized by:

A. Approval in the first-line setting
B. Limited utility as monotherapy
C. High toxicity
D. Response rates of 21% to 23% when used with irinotecan

Question 8.24.   All of the following are characteristics of a randomized discontinuation trial design, EXCEPT:

A. Phase 2 study design
B. Preferred for drugs with preexisting predictive biomarker
C. Patients with stable disease are randomized to continue or discontinue therapy
D. Primary end point could be time to progression after randomization

Question 8.25.   Cyclin-dependent kinases are inhibited by:

A. Bortezomib
B. Cetuximab
C. Flavopiridol
D. Trastuzumab

Question 8.26.   All of the following are limitations of the RECIST criteria, EXCEPT:

A. Bone-only disease is difficult to measure.
B. Partial responses are not taken into account.
C. Tumor necrosis after therapy may actually increase the size of a mass.
D. There may be several nonmeasurable sites of tumor involvement.

Question 8.27.   Computed tomography contrast perfusion and dynamic-contrast magnetic resonance imaging may be useful in evaluating:

A. Response to alkylating agents
B. Response to antiangiogenic agents
C. Degree of tumor necrosis
D. Overall survival

Question 8.28.   Which of the following is true regarding the use of time to progression as an end point in clinical trials?

A. Uses a smaller sample size when compared with using overall survival as an end point.
B. Not confounded by subsequent therapies.
C. The study can be completed in a shorter amount of time.
D. All of the above.

ANSWERS

Answer 8.1.   **The answer is D.**

Alkylating agents were first used as antineoplastic agents after observing bone marrow and lymphoid hypoplasia in soldiers exposed to nitrogen mustard in World War II.

Answer 8.2.   **The answer is A.**

Folic acid has been observed to have a significant proliferative effect in children with lymphoblastic leukemia. This led to the development of folic acid analogues as antineoplastic agents.

Answer 8.3.   **The answer is C.**

Fluoropyrimidines, gemcitabine, and cytarabine are considered antimetabolites because of their ability to inhibit the normal pathways involved in purine and pyrimidine synthesis. They are the first examples of "targeted" therapy. Mitoxantrone is an anthracycline.

Answer 8.4.   **The answer is A.**

Germ cell cancers are curable with primary induction chemotherapy in a subset of patients presenting with advanced or metastatic disease. In the metastatic setting, non-small cell lung cancer, gastric cancer, and colorectal cancer are not considered curable with conventional chemotherapy alone.

Answer 8.5.   **The answer is B.**

In most cases, the goals of chemotherapy in patients with advanced or metastatic malignancies include palliation of tumor-related symptoms, improvement in quality of life, and prolongation of time to tumor progression. Eradication of all evidence of disease, although it may occur, is not generally the goal of therapy in this setting.

Answer 8.6.   **The answer is C.**

Neoadjuvant chemotherapy is used in a variety of locally advanced solid tumors in an effort to confer possible future surgical resectability. Chemotherapy is the primary treatment modality in patients with hematologic malignancies.

Answer 8.7.   **The answer is C.**

Adjuvant chemotherapy is used as an adjunct to surgery and/or radiation to reduce the risk of local or distant recurrence from occult micrometastatic disease. Randomized Phase III data support the use of adjuvant chemotherapy in breast cancer, colorectal cancer, non-small cell lung cancer, gastric cancer, Wilms' tumor, and osteogenic sarcoma.

Answer 8.8.   **The answer is C.**

Activation of caspases leads to cell death, whereas activation of Bcl-2, Bcl-x_L, and NF-κB lead to inhibition of apoptosis.

Answer 8.9.   **The answer is C.**

The most important indicator of the effectiveness of chemotherapy is the rate of complete response. Despite improvements in response rates and overall survival in certain metastatic diseases, unless a complete response is achieved with chemotherapy, the patient is not considered cured.

Answer 8.10.   **The answer is A.**

A partial response is defined as at least a 50% improvement in measurable tumor mass. Although there are data to suggest that quality of life and survival may improve when a partial response is achieved, these are qualitative measures.

Answer 8.11.   **The answer is A.**

Bortezomib exerts its anticancer activity by inhibiting the 26S proteasome. The proteasome–ubiquitin complex degrades several intracellular regulatory proteins including IκB that is an inhibitor of NFκB. Activation of NFκB promotes cell proliferation and inhibition of apoptosis.

Answer 8.12.   **The answer is B.**

The majority of relapses in early-stage colon cancer treated with adjuvant chemotherapy occur within the first 3 years. Therefore, adjuvant trials may use 3-year disease-free survival as the primary end point.

Answer 8.13.   **The answer is D.**

Gompertzian kinetics provides a model of tumor growth whereby the growth fraction of a tumor decreases exponentially over time. Clinically undetectable tumors are at their highest growth fraction. Therefore, chemotherapy would result in a significantly higher fractional cell kill.

Answer 8.14.   **The answer is D.**

T790M mutation and MET gene amplification are the common causes for development of resistance to EGFR TKIs such as gefitinib and erlotinib in patients with activating mutations in the TK domain of the EGFR gene. In addition, loss of PTEN expression and D761Y mutation has been implicated in the development of resistance to EGFR TKI.

Answer 8.15.   **The answer is D.**

Reinitiation of the original induction chemotherapeutic agent is possible if there is a good response.

Answer 8.16.   **The answer is A.**

Both KRAS and BRAF V600E mutations are associated with development of resistance to cetuximab in the treatment of patients with colorectal cancer. EGFR-TK mutations are uncommon in patients with colorectal cancer, and NFκB activation results in pro-apoptotic signaling; however, it has not been shown to be associated with development of resistance to cetuximab in patients with colorectal cancer.

Answer 8.17.   **The answer is B.**

The growth of cells is significantly faster in the early part of the growth curve enabling chemotherapy to cause a greater log cell kill. Dose-dense chemotherapy, by administering cytotoxic drugs more frequently, can produce greater effects on smaller volume tumors.

Answer 8.18.   **The answer is B.**

Normal bone marrow and GI precursor cells possess intact genetic machinery to undergo apoptosis, repair DNA damage, and halt cell-cycle progression. Therefore, cells that have been damaged by chemotherapy undergo programmed cell death and are not allowed to continue on through the cell cycle.

Answer 8.19.   **The answer is C.**

p53 is a tumor suppressor gene that mediates apoptosis in cells with DNA damage. It plays a role in G1 and G2 arrest of the cell cycle after exposure to cytotoxic agents.

Answer 8.20.   **The answer is A.**

Recent evidence has suggested that mechanisms of drug resistance are due to gene mutations in cell-cycle regulatory pathways rather than drug-specific mutations. Wild-type p53 acts as a tumor suppressor of the mdr-1 gene. Increasing growth rates may lead to increased drug resistance as the result of more rapid entry of cells into the cell cycle.

Answer 8.21.   **The answer is D.**

Caspase activation occurs through the activity of the intrinsic and extrinsic pathways of apoptosis. Bcl-2 is involved in the intrinsic pathway, and tumor necrosis factor mediates the extrinsic pathway. p53 is a tumor suppressor gene involved in the early activation of the programmed cell death pathway.

Answer 8.22.   **The answer is A.**

Imatinib inhibits bcr-abl, platelet-derived growth factor, and c-kit. It is used to treat chronic myeloid leukemia and GI stromal tumors that express the c-kit TK.

Answer 8.23.   **The answer is D.**

Cetuximab is a chimeric antibody with promising activity in colorectal cancer and other solid tumors. Currently, it is used in the second or third-line setting, either alone or in combination with chemotherapy. In irinotecan-resistant patients, reported overall response rates with the cetuximab/irinotecan combination are 21% to 23%. Toxicity is usually manageable and is mostly related to rash.

Answer 8.24.   **The answer is B.**

Randomized discontinuation design is a novel phase 2 study design and is useful in identifying the target population for a drug. For a drug with an established predictive biomarker, there is no benefit to using this study design since the target population is already defined by the biomarker.

Answer 8.25.   **The answer is C.**

Overexpression of cyclin-dependent kinases can lead to inhibition of the Rb gene, a key tumor suppressor. Flavopiridol acts as a cyclin-dependent kinase inhibitor and may also have antiangiogenic properties.

Answer 8.26.   **The answer is B.**

The RECIST criteria use evaluation of tumor size to define a response. Limitations include the inability to measure the extent of response in sites with unmeasurable tumor, such as pleural and ascitic fluid, bone-only disease, and leptomeningeal disease.

Answer 8.27.   **The answer is B.**

Computed tomography contrast perfusion has been studied in assessing blood flow to rectal tumors treated with bevacizumab. The functionality of vascular endothelial growth factor receptor blockers has also been studied using dynamic-contrast magnetic resonance imaging. The utility of these tests in assessing response to alkylating agents, tumor necrosis, or effect on overall survival is not known.

Answer 8.28.   **The answer is D.**

Time to tumor progression as an end point for studies involving metastatic cancer has several advantages over using overall survival: Sample size may be smaller, subsequent therapies do not confound the data, and the study may be able to be completed in a shorter amount of time.

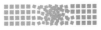

CHAPTER 9 PRINCIPLES OF IMMUNOTHERAPY

SARA K. BUTLER • SAIAMA N. WAQAR

DIRECTIONS Each of the numbered items below is followed by lettered answers. Select the ONE lettered answer that is BEST in each case unless instructed otherwise.

QUESTIONS

Question 9.1. Which of the following types of immunity is most responsible for the host response to tumor development?

A. Humoral immunity
B. B-cell–mediated immunity
C. T-cell–mediated immunity
D. Antibody-mediated immunity

Question 9.2. Currently, what is the proposed mechanism for using immunotherapy to destroy cancer cells?

A. Develop antibodies to target growth factors on cancer cells
B. Increase levels of immune lymphocytes
C. Develop antibodies to directly destroy the cancer cells
D. Increase levels of antigen-presenting cells

Question 9.3. Which of the following is NOT an approach to identify antigens involved on tumor cells?

A. Developing antibodies to identified peptides and assessing presentation on the cancer cell surface
B. Developing tumor-reactive T cells to detect identified peptides on cancer cell surface
C. Using T cells to assess cytokine release or lysis when present with cancer cells
D. Using antisera from patients with cancer to screen cancer DNA libraries

---

Corresponding Chapter in *Cancer: Principles & Practice of Oncology,* Ninth Edition: 30 (Cancer Immunotherapy).

Question 9.4. Which of the following is an example of a nonmutated melanocyte differentiation antigen?

A. gp100
B. HLA-A*1101
C. CDK4
D. NY-ESO-1

Question 9.5. Which of the following has NOT been a target for the development of reactive T cells?

A. Prostate-specific antigen (PSA)
B. Carcinoembryonic antigen (CEA)
C. p53
D. Epidermal growth factor receptor (EGFR)

Question 9.6. Expression of the Epstein-Barr virus (EBV) latent gene EBNA is seen in which of the following cancers?

A. Nasopharyngeal carcinoma
B. Burkitt's lymphoma
C. T-cell lymphoma
D. All of the above

Question 9.7. A 20 year-old sexually active woman inquires about the role of the human papilloma virus (HPV) vaccine in relation to cervical cancer. Which of the following statements regarding the HPV vaccine is correct?

A. It prevents the development of cervical cancer in all patients.
B. It induces regression of cervical cancer tumors.
C. It prevents infection with HPV16 and 18.
D. It prevents the development of cervical cancer in patients infected with HPV 16 and 18.

Question 9.8. Which of the following is the proposed mechanism for development of hepatocellular carcinoma secondary to hepatitis B or C?

A. Hepatitis B virus (HBV) produces oncogenic proteins that result in transformation into malignancy.
B. Increases in the number of somatic mutations in normal hepatocytes
C. Inhibition of normal immune responses to hepatitis infections
D. HBV or hepatitis C virus (HCV) infections lead to cirrhosis, which develops into hepatocellular carcinoma.

Question 9.9. Which of the following is TRUE of the tumor microenvironment?

A. T cells in the peripheral blood have functional impairment.
B. Expression of lysine is found in myeloid cells, which results in downregulation of T-cell receptor (TCR) zeta-chain expression.
C. Monocytes express Gr-1 molecules, leading to upregulation of T cells.
D. Tumors secrete granulocyte-macrophage colony-stimulating factor (GM-CSF), leading to an accumulation of CD34+ suppressor cells.

Question 9.10.   Which of the following is an approach to cancer immunotherapy?

    A.   Passive transfer of activated immune cells with antitumor activity
    B.   Active immunization to enhance antitumor reactions
    C.   Nonspecific stimulation of immune reactions
    D.   All of the above

Question 9.11.   Which of the following results in inhibition of T cells?

    A.   CTLA-4
    B.   CD28
    C.   B7-1
    D.   B7-2

Question 9.12.   Of 1306 vaccine treatments, what is the overall objective response rate to vaccine treatment?

    A.   3.3%
    B.   10.6%
    C.   20.4%
    D.   49.2%

Question 9.13.   Which of the following is NOT an example of active immunization?

    A.   Whole cell vaccines
    B.   Heat shock proteins
    C.   Natural killer (NK) cell vaccines
    D.   Dendritic cell vaccines

Question 9.14.   What is the purpose of adoptive cell transfer therapies?

    A.   Decreasing the number of reactive T-cells ex vivo and transfer back to the patient
    B.   Increasing the number of cytokines ex vivo and transfer back to the patient
    C.   Activating and expanding self/tumor-reactive T cells and transfer back to the patient
    D.   Modulating CD4+ tumor-specific T cells before transferring back to the patient

Question 9.15.   What is the main mechanism of the graft-versus-leukemia effect demonstrated after a donor lymphocyte infusion?

    A.   T cells within the lymphocytes recognize target antigens on residual tumor cells.
    B.   Enhancing the presence of killer inhibitory receptors (KIRs) recognized by donor NK cells
    C.   Lack of recognition of minor histocompatibility antigens within hematopoietic cells
    D.   Increases in CD8+ cells that recognize target antigens on tumor cells

Question 9.16.   **What is the major limitation of using antibody-based therapies against tumors that overexpress CEA?**

A. Delivery of the antibody to the tumor
B. Penetration of the tumor tissue
C. Invasion of normal CEA-expressing tissue
D. Stabilization of the antibody

Question 9.17.   **Which of the following most correctly defines immunoediting?**

A. Observation by the immune system for development of outgrowth of tumors
B. Selective pressure by immune systems leads to outgrowth of mutated tumor variants
C. Development of mechanisms by the tumor to prevent recognition by the immune system
D. Use of cytokine release to inhibit response by T cells

Question 9.18.   **In patients with renal cell carcinoma, which of the following factors predict response to high-dose interleukin-2 (IL-2) therapy?**

A. Presence of bone metastases
B. Relapse 3 months after nephrectomy
C. Clear cell histology
D. All of the above

Question 9.19.   **Which of the following gene products is frequently overexpressed in melanoma?**

A. PRAME
B. CDK4
C. MART-1
D. FGF5

Question 9.20.   **Which of the following is correct regarding high-dose IL-2 therapy in patients with renal cell carcinoma and melanoma?**

A. Response durations can be sustained with curative potential
B. High-dose IL-2 therapy is associated with minimal toxicity
C. Overall response rate for IL-2 in renal cell carcinoma is 70%
D. All of the above

Question 9.21.   **Which of the following is NOT an immune-mediated adverse reaction of ipilimumab?**

A. Enterocolitis
B. Dermatitis
C. Hyperthyroidism
D. Peripheral neuropathy

Question 9.22.   Which of the following is most consistent with the active immune component of Sipuleucel-T?

A. CD54+ cells activated with PAP-G-CSF
B. CD20+ cells activated with PAP-G-CSF
C. CD54+ cells activated with PAP-GM-CSF
D. CD20+ cells activated with PAP-GM-CSF

ANSWERS

Answer 9.1.   The answer is C.

Initially, it was thought that the action of antibodies or humoral immunity was mainly responsible for the response to malignant cell development. However, it has been discovered that malignant cell development is closely related to the cellular arm of the immune response, specifically a response to T cells. B cells do not play a major role in the immune response to tumor cells.

Answer 9.2.   The answer is B.

For existing malignancies, the main mechanism for immunotherapy is to try to increase the level of immune lymphocytes. These immune lymphocytes would be responsible for recognizing the cancer antigens and destroying the cancer cells. Although the development of antibodies that target growth factors on cancer cells may help in reducing the overall tumor burden, this does not work by directly destroying the cancer cells.

Answer 9.3.   The answer is A.

There are three methodologies for identifying tumor antigens that are present on the surface of the cancer cells. The first approach is using T cells that have a known ability to recognize intact cancer cells and assessing this by cytokine release or lysis in culture. The second approach is using a "reverse immunology" technique where T cells are generated by sensitization with peptides from proteins previously described. These T cells are then used to test the ability to detect intact cancer cells and to determine if the peptides are found on the surface of the cancer cell. The final approach is to use antisera from patients with known cancer and compare them with cancer DNA libraries already constructed. The development of antibodies has not been used to detect antigens on the cell surface.

Answer 9.4.   The answer is A.

Melanocyte differentiation antigens include MART-1, gp100, and tyrosinase. CDK4 and HLA-A*1101 are both mutated antigens associated with melanoma. NY-ESO-1 is a cancer testis antigen expressed in breast cancer, prostate cancer, and melanoma.

Answer 9.5.   The answer is D.

Reverse immunology has been used to develop reactive T cells to commonly overexpressed gene products found in certain types of cancer. Targets of this technique have been CEA, PSA, and Her-2/neu. p53 is often overexpressed in many cancer types. One of the difficulties in using p53 is the common mutations that are found and the wide expression of p53 in normal cellular tissues. Although epidermal growth factor receptor has been used in the development of some tyrosine kinase inhibitors, it has not been used in the development of reactive T cells.

Answer 9.6.   **The answer is D.**

Expression of the Epstein-Barr virus latent gene EBNA is seen in Burkitt's lymphoma, nasopharyngeal carcinoma, and T cell lymphoma.

Answer 9.7.   **The answer is C.**

HPV vaccines protect women from contracting the strains of HPV that are commonly associated with the development of cervical cancer: HPV 16 and 18. The quadrivalent HPV vaccine (Gardisil) also offers protection against HPV 6 and 11, which cause genital warts in 90% of cases. HPV vaccination does not prevent cervical cancer in everyone, since only 70% of cervical cancer is related to HPV. If a patient already has cervical cancer, it will not provide a tumor response, and if the patient has already contracted HPV16 or 18, it will not offer any additional protection to the patient.

Answer 9.8.   **The answer is B.**

Unlike HPV infections, HBV and HCV infections do not seem to produce oncogenic proteins that lead to transformation into carcinoma. It is thought that the majority of the liver damage results from immune responses directed against HBV-infected cells and inflammation. There is an increased cell turnover in chronic hepatitis infections that could lead to an increase in the amount of somatic mutations in the normal hepatocytes, thus leading to an increased risk of carcinoma.

Answer 9.9.   **The answer is D.**

Several models have demonstrated impairment of the immune system within the tumor microenvironment. Although the T cells within the tumor show impairment, it has been shown that peripheral T cells do not have the same dysfunctionality. Expression of arginase within myeloid cells has been shown to downregulate T-cell receptor zeta-chain expression and lead to T-cell function impairment. Myeloid suppressor cells have been discovered to secrete GM-CSF, resulting in an accumulation of CD34+ suppressor cells.

Answer 9.10.   **The answer is D.**

Three main approaches to cancer immunotherapy include nonspecific stimulation of immune reactions through stimulation of effector cells and/or inhibition of regulatory cells, active immunization using cancer vaccines, and adoptive immunotherapy, defined as the passive transfer of activated immune cells with antitumor activity.

Answer 9.11.   **The answer is A.**

When CTLA-4 is engaged on the T cell, the T-cell function is impaired. This is an example of a nonantigen-specific therapy. When CD28 is engaged, T cells are stimulated. B7-1 and B7-2 are ligands that are costimulatory on the T cells.

Answer 9.12.   **The answer is A.**

The results of treatment with cancer vaccines have been very low. Of 1306 vaccine treatments, the objective response rate is only 3.3%. The objective response rate used has been criticized by many, suggesting that the response rate may be even lower than 3.3%.

Answer 9.13.   **The answer is C.**

There are multiple active immunization approaches that have been explored for cancer therapy, such as whole cell vaccines, dendritic cell vaccines, and heat shock proteins. NK cell therapy has been explored as a passive immunological therapy.

Answer 9.14.   **The answer is C.**

Adoptive cell transfer therapies function by stimulating T cells ex vivo by activating and expanding self/tumor-reactive T cells before transfer back to the patient. CD8+ T cells have been subject to much research because they are potent effectors of the adaptive tumor response. CD4+ T cells are more controversial, because they can either help or hinder antitumor immune responses.

Answer 9.15.   **The answer is A.**

The graft-versus-leukemia effect from donor lymphocyte infusions is thought to be due to the increase in recognition of target antigens on the residual tumor cells. This will result in ultimate tumor cell kill. Lack of presence of KIRs recognized by donor NK cells confers a better response and more graft-versus-leukemia effect.

Answer 9.16.   **The answer is B.**

Antibodies directed at the glycoprotein CEA have not been successful in the treatment of solid tumors. This is mainly because of the lack of penetration of the antibody into the tumor tissue in vivo.

Answer 9.17.   **The answer is C.**

Immunoediting is a mechanism where the tumor develops mechanisms that prevent the immune system from recognizing the tumor and responding appropriately. Immunosurveillance is the process of the immune system observing for the development of malignancies. Immune escape is the process of exerting selective pressure by the immune system that leads to outgrowth of mutated tumor variants, ultimately leading to the loss of recognition by the immune system.

Answer 9.18.   **The answer is C.**

Clear cell histology predicts response to high-dose IL-2. Other predictors of response to IL-2 therapy include late relapse (occurring >6 months after nephrectomy), good performance status, and lack of bone metastases.

Answer 9.19.   **The answer is A.**

The gene product of PRAME is overexpressed in melanoma, whereas the gene product of FGF-5 is over-expressed in renal cell carcinomas, prostate cancer, and breast cancer. CDK4 is a mutated antigens expressed in melanoma, whereas the gene product of MART-1 is a melanocyte differentiation antigen expressed in melanoma.

Answer 9.20.   **The answer is A.**

The response rate of high-dose IL-2 therapy is 15% to 20% in melanoma and renal cell carcinoma. Almost half of the responses are complete, response durations can be substantial, lasting for over 10 years. High-dose IL-2 therapy is associated with significant toxicity: hypotension, cardiac arrhythmias, metabolic acidosis, fever, nausea and vomiting, dyspnea, edema, renal failure, neurotoxicity, and dermatologic complications.

Answer 9.21.   **The answer is C.**

Because of the activation and proliferation of T-cells achieved by inhibition of CTLA-4, ipilimumab is associated with many immune-mediated adverse reactions that can be fatal. Common immune-related reactions include enterocolitis, hepatitis, dermatitis, neuropathy, and endocrinopathies including hypopituitarism, adrenal insufficiency, hypogonadism, and hypothyroidism.

Answer 9.22.   **The answer is C.**

Sipuleucel-T is formulated from CD54+ cells that are activated with PAP-GM-CSF ex vivo and then infused into patients with prostate cancer in order to induce an immune response targeted against PAP.

KENNETH R. CARSON

DIRECTIONS   Each of the numbered items below is followed by lettered answers. Select the ONE lettered answer that is BEST in each case unless instructed otherwise.

QUESTIONS

Question 10.1.   **In an effort to measure the effectiveness of health care interventions in "real-world" settings, health services research frequently relies on which of the following research methods?**

A. Randomized clinical trials
B. Meta-analysis of existing clinical trials
C. Observational studies that statistically control for sources of bias
D. All of the above

Question 10.2.   **Which of the following is a common problem in the completion of health services research?**

A. Without informed consent from patients, it is difficult to obtain a representative sample.
B. It is difficult to identify confounders, patient characteristics that cannot be measured but correlate with both the outcome and the primary predictor.
C. Patients refuse to be randomized between interventions, resulting in excessive dropout from health services research studies.
D. The sample sizes obtained from administrative data sources are too small to detect a statistically significant difference between treatments.

Corresponding Chapter in *Cancer: Principles & Practice of Oncology*, Ninth Edition: 31 (Health Services Research and Economics of Cancer Care).

Question 10.3.   Which of the following is NOT true regarding the Surveillance, Epidemiology, and End Results (SEER) registry?

A. Initial patient and disease characteristics from the time of cancer diagnosis are obtained from qualified hospital registries.
B. Subsequent treatments and clinical outcomes are integrated into the SEER registry.
C. SEER data can be linked with Medicare claims to provide additional details regarding patients' treatments.
D. SEER data are correlated with population bases to allow for estimates of incidence rates.

Question 10.4.   The quality of health care is least frequently measured by which of the following:

A. Practice according to established guidelines
B. Appropriate certifications and credentialing of personnel
C. Availability of specific services or technologies
D. Clinical outcomes, such as survival or quality of life

Question 10.5.   Which of the following is TRUE regarding the association between outcomes and high-volume centers?

A. The strongest association between cancer surgery and outcomes is with low-risk procedures such as prostatectomy and colectomy.
B. Observational data often does not have sufficient information on comorbidities to control for hospital "case-mix."
C. The improvement in outcomes seen at high-volume centers is associated only with short-term outcomes, such as 30-day mortality.
D. In most cases, there are clear thresholds that differentiate high-volume from low-volume centers.

Question 10.6.   Why are patient-reported outcomes an important end point in oncology research?

A. Cancer treatments often have a large impact on overall survival.
B. Cancer treatment decisions are often straightforward.
C. Cancer treatments that are curative need to be advanced.
D. Cancer treatments often have significant toxicity.

Question 10.7.   Studies of patient-recorded outcomes require "instruments," such as surveys and symptom diaries. A good instrument should show all of the following, EXCEPT:

A. Subjectivity: Allows patients to elaborate on symptoms.
B. Variability: A broad range of responses.
C. Internal consistency: Answers to questions regarding similar symptoms correlate well with each other.
D. Reliability: Repeat administration on the same patient gives similar results.

Question 10.8.   Which of the following is TRUE regarding measurement of health-related quality of life (HRQOL)?

    A. Efforts should be made to use the same instrument across studies to allow comparisons.

    B. Validated HRQOL instruments are both precise and accurate.

    C. HRQOL instruments are easily translated into different languages.

    D. Computerized adaptive testing allows more precise measurement of HRQOL, while reducing the number of questions asked.

Question 10.9.   The burden of symptoms on a patient can be quantified by measures of "utility." Which of the following is TRUE regarding "utility" in this sense?

    A. It measures the impact of disease on a patient's independence.

    B. It numerically compares how a patient would value living with a specific disease state in comparison to perfect health.

    C. It measures the burden of relieving the symptoms on the health care system.

    D. It specifically refers to a patient's evaluation of his/her own disease.

Question 10.10.   Which of the following is NOT true regarding the costs of health care in the United States?

    A. Total annual health care expenditures are approximately $2 trillion, or $7000 per person.

    B. Approximately 30% of health care expenses occur in the last year of life.

    C. The costs associated with cancer care are estimated to be 15% of overall medical expenses and 30% of Medicare expenses.

    D. Cancer pharmaceuticals account for 40% of all Medicare pharmaceutical spending.

Question 10.11.   Which of the following is TRUE regarding comparative effectiveness research (CER) in cancer care?

    A. By definition, CER evaluates outcome differences in "real-world" settings.

    B. CER will be performed primarily through meta-analysis of existing clinical trials.

    C. CER is intended primarily to compare costs between two treatments.

    D. CER is not performed on prospectively collected data.

Question 10.12.   Which of the following is NOT true regarding methods of assessing the economic impact of medical treatments?

    A. Cost-minimization analysis takes into account the indirect costs that patients experience (e.g., changes in quality of life) and seeks to minimize these.

    B. Cost-effectiveness analysis compares cost with a relevant clinical variable, such as cost per year of life.

    C. Cost-utility analysis compares cost with quality-adjusted-life-years (QALYs) such that the toxicities of therapies and the quality of life in the setting of a chronic illness can be weighed along with the benefit.

    D. Cost-benefit analysis assigns a dollar amount to a QALY, so that two costs may be compared directly. This requires assigning a monetary value to a quality-adjusted year of life.

Question 10.13.   Assume a new drug for metastatic breast cancer is expensive, but claims to be "cost-effective." What might this mean?

    A. The new treatment is less expensive than the old treatment because it has a shorter infusion time resulting in lower administration costs.

    B. The new treatment is less toxic than the old treatment, increasing the number of QALYs compared to an older treatment.

    C. The new treatment makes patients live longer with an incremental cost of less than $50,000 for each additional year of life.

    D. All of the above.

Question 10.14.   Cost-benefit is frequently modeled as dollars per QALY. Which is NOT true regarding this method of modeling?

    A. The cost of hemodialysis ($50,000 per QALY) is frequently used as a standard for what society in the United States is willing to fund.

    B. In less affluent countries, the threshold of society support is often correlated with per capita gross domestic product.

    C. The legislation that established Medicare prohibits the consideration of cost in determining coverage.

    D. Insurers frequently incorporate these types of modeling in determining coverage.

ANSWERS

Answer 10.1.   **The answer is C.**

In an effort to assess effectiveness in a real-world setting, health services research studies are frequently observational in nature. Randomized trials typically establish efficacy of a specific intervention, and meta-analysis of randomized trials enhances the precision of efficacy (or toxicity) estimates.

Answer 10.2.   **The answer is B.**

Multivariable statistical models will not control for unmeasured variables. This can introduce confounding, which can result in abberant conclusions in an observational study. Patient consent is often not required in health services research studies, as their completion would frequently be impossible with a consent requirement. Randomization is seldom used in health services research, instead researchers must try to control for the factors that predicted the nonrandom assignment of treatment. Sample sizes from administrative databases are typically large, allowing sufficient statistical power to detect differences between groups.

Answer 10.3.   **The answer is B.**

SEER provides adequate baseline information for most observational studies and is valuable in that it can be linked to Medicare claims data for treatment details and correlated to populations to allow for estimates of incidence rates. However, one limitation of SEER is that limited longitudinal follow-up information is available in the registry.

Answer 10.4.   **The answer is D.**

Quality can be measured by "structural" metrics, which include characteristics of organizations and providers, as well as by "process" metrics, which are usually defined as adherence to established clinical guidelines. Only rarely are clinical outcome measures used to evaluate quality of care delivery.

Answer 10.5.   **The answer is B.**

One of the biggest threats to volume-outcome studies is the inability to control for hospital case-mix. In some cases, high-volume hospitals are likely selecting for better-risk patients, thereby improving survival outcomes. There are often no clear thresholds to differentiate high- and low-volume centers. Strongest associations between volume and outcome are seen with high-risk procedures. Associations are seen with both immediate and long-term outcomes.

Answer 10.6.   **The answer is D.**

Because many cancer treatments often have significant toxicity with only modest impact on overall survival, outcomes of interest to patients, including symptoms and quality of life, are important end points for clinical research. Increasing knowledge in this area can facilitate what are often complex and not straightforward treatment decisions. In areas of cancer treatment where cure is possible or clinical benefit is striking, patient-reported outcomes may play less of a role.

Answer 10.7.   **The answer is A.**

A useful instrument is sufficiently variable, internally consistent, and reliable. Subjectivity is not a desirable characteristic.

Answer 10.8.   **The answer is D.**

Computerized adaptive testing will allow more precise measurement of constructs such as quality of life, using fewer questions. Different instruments are required in different research situations. Validation does not guarantee accuracy. Translation into a new language frequently requires repeat validation in the new language.

Answer 10.9.   **The answer is B.**

"Utility" as used in health services research is synonymous with "preference" and enables comparisons between specific disease states. For example, living with chronic cancer pain can be compared with living in perfect health and assigned a numeric score. These rankings can be established by patients, families, health care workers, or others, and may vary between groups.

Answer 10.10.   **The answer is C.**

Health care expenditures in all areas have rapidly increased in the past 15 years, much faster than inflation, such that health insurance premiums are no longer affordable for many parties. The rapid accumulation of costs in the last year of life has generated considerable concern regarding the benefit of many expensive treatments. Cancer treatments costs in particular have increased, although they currently account for 5%, not 15% of overall medical expenditures, and 10%, not 30% of Medicare treatments. However, these numbers are expected to escalate as Medicare assumes more pharmaceutical costs and the cost of cancer care and the number of Medicare patients with cancer increases in concert with the aging population.

Answer 10.11.   **The answer is A.**

The purpose of CER is to understand the differences in outcomes associated with various treatments in real-world settings, hence the use of the term "effectiveness" as opposed to "efficacy." While this data can support economic analyses, the primary objective is to maximize patient outcomes regardless of cost. CER can be performed on prospectively collected data, though frequently uses observational data.

Answer 10.12.   **The answer is A.**

The various methods of comparing the benefits and costs of medical treatments have subtle but important differences. The most straightforward analysis, cost minimization, assumes equivalent outcomes, and therefore the least expensive intervention is preferred. Cost-effectiveness analysis compares cost with a relevant clinical variable, such as cost per year of life. These analyses are usually more intuitive but difficult to generalize across treatment types. Cost-utility analysis is similar but compares cost with QALYs such that the toxicities of therapies and the quality of life in the setting of a chronic illness can be weighed along with the benefit. This method has been adopted by the US Preventive Health Service Panel as the best way to account for outcomes compared with cost. Cost-benefit analysis goes one step further by assigning a dollar amount to a QALY, so that two costs may be compared directly. Because this requires assigning a monetary value to a person's life, these analyses are controversial.

Answer 10.13.   **The answer is D.**

"Cost-effective" is an imprecise term that is overutilized in the medical literature and can have many different meanings. Answer A is a cost-minimization analysis. Answer B is a cost-utility analysis. Answer C is nominally a "cost-effectivness" analysis, though this terminology has not been standardized in the medical literature.

Answer 10.14.   **The answer is D.**

Although there are multiple methods of estimating cost-effectiveness, actually implementing these analyses for decision making is problematic. One example of the application of a cost-benefit analysis is that when Congress made the decision to fund hemodialysis, the cost was considered to be approximately $50,000 per QALY. This value subsequently became an accepted standard for society's willingness to fund a particular intervention. This principle can be generalized to other countries on the basis of their annual per capita gross domestic product. Consideration of economic factors is further complicated by the fact that the original Medicare charter actually prohibits such analysis in decisions regarding coverage. Insurers are rarely inclined to consider cost-effectiveness because they are unlikely to benefit from long-term improvements in outcomes and are more concerned with current cost controls. Although cost-effectiveness analyses can be informative, practical utility of the results have rarely been realized.

CHAPTER 11 SYSTEMIC THERAPY FOR CANCER

SARA K. BUTLER • LEIGH M. BOEHMER

DIRECTIONS   Each of the numbered items below is followed by lettered answers. Select the ONE lettered answer that is BEST in each case unless instructed otherwise.

QUESTIONS

Question 11.1.   Which of the following patients would be the most likely to have the best response from treatment with 5-FU?

  A. A patient who is homozygous for 3R/3R triple repeat polymorphism resulting in decreased thymidylate synthase (TS) levels
  B. A patient who is homozygous for 2R/2R double repeat polymorphism resulting in decreased TS levels
  C. A patient who is homozygous for 3R/3R triple repeat polymorphism resulting in increased TS levels
  D. A patient who is homozygous for 2R/2R double repeat polymorphism resulting in increased TS levels

Question 11.2.   Which of the following scenarios best identifies a prognostic marker?

  A. UGT1A1*28 testing in the setting of colon cancer
  B. Dihydropyrimidine dehydrogenase (DPD) deficiency in the setting of head and neck cancer induction chemotherapy
  C. Deficiency in MMR protein expression (DNA mismatch repair gene) in colon cancer
  D. KRAS mutation testing in the setting of colon cancer

Question 11.3.   Which of the following patients would be the most appropriate candidate for high-dose methotrexate at standard doses?

  A. A patient with an elevated bilirubin at 2.1 mg/dL
  B. A patient with a moderate size left pleural effusion
  C. A patient currently receiving amoxicillin for a dental abscess
  D. A 63-year-old patient with a serum creatinine of 2.3 mg/dL

Corresponding Chapters in *Cancer: Principles & Practice of Oncology,* Ninth Edition: 32 (Pharmacokinetics and Pharmacodynamics), 33 (Pharmacogenomics), 34 (Alkylating Agents), 35 (Platinum Analogs), 36 (Antimetabolites), 37 (Topoisomerase-Interacting Agents), 38 (Antimicrotubule Agents), 39 (Targeted Therapy with Small Molecule Kinase Inhibitors), 40 (Histone Deacetylase Inhibitors and Demethylating Agents), 41 (Proteosome Inhibitors), 42 (Poly(ADP-Ribose) Polymerase Inhibitors), 43 (Miscellaneous Chemotherapeutic Agents), 44 (Interferons), 45 (Interleukin Therapy), 46 (Antisense Agents), 47 (Antiangiogenesis Agents), 48 (Monoclonal Antibodies), and 49 (Endocrine Manipulation).

Question 11.4.   Which of the following is an appropriate strategy for optimizing high-dose methotrexate elimination?

A. Initiate leucovorin rescue immediately after completion of infusion of methotrexate
B. Administer intravenous fluids prior to methotrexate infusion
C. Ensure the patient is taking folic acid 1 mg by mouth daily
D. Administer intravenous fluids with sodium bicarbonate for urine alkalinization

Question 11.5.   Which of the following medications are necessary to help minimize hematologic toxicities with pemetrexed and pralatrexate?

A. Vitamin B_6 and Vitamin B_{12}
B. Folic acid and dexamethasone
C. Vitamin B_{12} and folic acid
D. Folinic acid and Vitamin B_6

Question 11.6.   A patient with stage III colon cancer is day 10 after receiving FOLFIRI chemotherapy and presents to the hospital with a 3-day history of profuse diarrhea, severe mucositis, and an ANC of zero. Which of the following is the most likely cause of his symptoms?

A. The patient is likely homozygous for UGT1A1*28
B. Irinotecan-induced delayed diarrhea
C. DPD deficiency
D. FOLFIRI-induced myelosuppression and GI toxicity

Question 11.7.   Which one of the following chemotherapy agents requires prophylaxis against *Pneumocystis carinii*?

A. Gemcitabine
B. Fludarabine
C. Cytarabine
D. Clofarabine

Question 11.8.   Which of the following is NOT a proposed mechanism for cardiotoxicity from anthracyclines?

A. Enhanced catalysis of oxidation-reduction reactions
B. Increased susceptibility to p-glycoprotein
C. Generation of reactive oxygen species
D. Peroxidation of myocardial lipids

Question 11.9.   Which of the following is most consistent with a proposed advantage of cabazitaxel over other approved taxane chemotherapy agents?

A. It is a poor substrate for multidrug-resistant p-glycoprotein
B. There is a smaller incidence of peripheral neuropathy
C. Increased response rate with cabazitaxel over docetaxel
D. Lower incidence of febrile neutropenia

Question 11.10.   Which of the following best describes the mechanism of action for vinca alkaloids?

A. Binds to tubulin and alters the tubulin dissociation rate
B. Binds and stabilizes tubulin resulting in cell cycle arrest
C. Binds to tubulin and alters the tubulin association rate
D. Promotion of tubulin polymerization resulting in cell cycle arrest

Question 11.11.   Which of the following is NOT CORRECT with regard to therapy with azacitidine?

A. Azacitidine can be given via intravenous infusion or subcutaneous injection
B. The mechanism of action of azacitidine is via inhibition of DNA methylation
C. Azacitidine has a short stability period after reconstitution in an aqueous solution
D. Efficacy with azacitidine should be assessed after two cycles of therapy

Question 11.12.   Which of the following is CORRECT regarding hemorrhagic cystitis?

A. Bladder protection with mesna is required for all patients receiving cyclophosphamide
B. Hemorrhagic cystitis is caused by direct damage to the bladder wall by cyclophosphamide or ifosfamide
C. Mesna works by providing a free sulfhydryl group that binds to the metabolite and neutralizes it
D. Mesna should be given in divided doses to total 100% of the total dose of cyclophosphamide or ifosfamide

Question 11.13.   Which of the following is CORRECT regarding platinum analogs?

A. Carboplatin is associated with pronounced ototoxicity and should be avoided in patients with baseline hearing difficulty
B. Infusions with magnesium and calcium prior to and after oxaliplatin therapy may lessen the severity and incidence of peripheral neuropathy
C. Cisplatin is associated with an acute neuropathy exacerbated by cold food or beverages
D. Oxaliplatin is associated with significant renal toxicity and should be avoided in patients with renal insufficiency

Question 11.14. Oblimersen has been shown to reduce the expression of Bcl-2 protein using a technology known as antisense inhibition. Which of the following statements most accurately defines oblimersen's mechanism of action?

A. Oblimersen binds to its target mRNA that results in increased production of Bcl-2 and the death of cancer cells.
B. A DNA/mRNA duplex is formed that activates TNF-α, destroys the bound mRNA, and decreases production of Bcl-2.
C. The binding of oblimersen to its target mRNA forms a duplex leading to inhibition of translation of Bcl-2.
D. Oblimersen binds to its target mRNA that elicits the activity of RNase H causing increased production of Bcl-2.

Question 11.15. You are about to see a 67-year-old female with newly diagnosed multiple myeloma regarding initiation of chemotherapy. The patient's daughter is a health care worker and wants to know more about bortezomib therapy. All of the following statements are correct EXCEPT:

A. Bortezomib is approved as single-agent therapy in newly diagnosed multiple myeloma and given on days 1, 4, 8, and 11 of a 3-week cycle.
B. Thrombocytopenia and peripheral neuropathy were common adverse events in clinical trials.
C. Bortezomib inhibits chymotrypsin-like activity at the 26S proteasome leading to cell cycle arrest and apoptosis.
D. The phase III VISTA trial in patients with untreated multiple myeloma showed the addition of bortezomib significantly improved response rates in this setting.

Question 11.16. The azacytosine nucleosides possess complex dose-response characteristics. Which of the following statements is correctly paired?

A. At high concentrations, dose-dependent reversal of DNA methylation occurs.
B. At high concentrations, induction of terminal differentiation occurs in some systems.
C. At lower concentrations, DNA damage and apoptosis become more prominent.
D. At lower concentrations, inhibition of DNA methyltransferase activity predominates.

Question 11.17. Poly (ADP-ribose) polymerase (PARP) signals the presence of DNA damage and facilitates DNA repair. Each of the following is a role of PARP inhibitors in cancer treatment EXCEPT?

A. Chemotherapy and radiation sensitization
B. Serine/threonine kinase inhibition
C. Synthetic lethality with BRCA 1/2 mutations
D. Decreased hypoxia-inducible factor-1 function

Question 11.18.   The safety profile of everolimus is similar to that seen with temsirolimus. Which of the following is MOST correct regarding common side effects of therapy with everolimus?

A. Pulmonary toxicity, such as increased cough, dyspnea, and pulmonary infiltrates are a relatively common event.
B. Dry skin with acneiform skin rash can occur but it is a relatively rare event observed in about 1% of patients.
C. Hyperlipidemia and hyperglycemia occur in up to 90% of patients.
D. Venous thromboembolism is a common occurrence, and it is recommended that patients begin prophylactic anticoagulation.

Question 11.19.   Asparaginase is commonly used in combination with methotrexate as part of acute lymphoblastic leukemia treatment protocols. Which of the following statements regarding administration of these drugs is TRUE?

A. Asparaginase should be given concurrently with methotrexate in order to inhibit methotrexate's clearance and increase its cytotoxicity.
B. Asparaginase should be given immediately before methotrexate in order to decrease the risk of methotrexate neurotoxicity.
C. Asparaginase should be given 12 hours before methotrexate in order to prime cancer cells for methotrexate's antimetabolite activity.
D. Asparaginase and methotrexate should be given sequentially at least 24 hours apart secondary to methotrexate antagonism.

Question 11.20.   A 59-year-old female is admitted to the inpatient service for week one of induction interferon therapy for malignant melanoma. Her daughter is a nurse practitioner and would like to know more information about the treatment. Which of the following statements can you correctly tell her?

A. Interferons enhance the activity of the innate immune response but have little to no effect on the adaptive immune response.
B. Appetite stimulation and weight gain are typically seen with high-dose interferon for malignant melanoma.
C. Interferons exhibit antiangiogenic properties by directly inhibiting endothelial cells.
D. There are a large number of clinically significant drug–drug interactions that have been reported with interferons.

Question 11.21.   Which of the following statements regarding side effects of high-dose interferon therapy is FALSE?

A. Acute hepatic toxicity has been reported, but dose reductions are not suggested for patients who develop transaminitis during therapy.
B. Neutropenia requiring dose reduction is reported to occur in up to 60% of patients.
C. The risks and benefits of therapy should be considered carefully in patients with a history of depression or other psychiatric disorders.
D. The most common toxicities seen with all interferon therapy are constitutional, including fever, chills, headache, and fatigue.

Question 11.22.　　EC is a 61-year-old male with relapsed follicular lymphoma who is about to proceed with ibritumomab therapy. Which of the following statements regarding ibritumomab therapy is INCORRECT?

A.　Severe cutaneous and mucocutaneous skin reactions have been reported up to 4 months following ibritumomab therapy.

B.　Ibritumomab can be safely administered to patients with impaired bone marrow reserve.

C.　On day 1 of therapy only, patients receive ibritumomab complexed with indium-111 to assess biodistribution of the monoclonal antibody.

D.　Ibritumomab is a monoclonal antibody directed against the CD20 antigen used to deliver a radioactive isotope to targeted cells.

Question 11.23.　　A 45-year-old male is beginning treatment with high-dose interleukin (IL)-2 for renal cell carcinoma. He is ordered to receive 0.6 million units/kg/dose intravenously every 8 hours × 14 doses. Which of the following is TRUE?

A.　Subsequent IL-2 doses should be reduced by 25% in the setting of toxicity.

B.　For patients developing moderate-to-severe lethargy or somnolence, it is appropriate to continue treatment up to a total of 14 doses.

C.　IL-2 therapy is associated with capillary leak syndrome that may begin immediately after initiation of treatment and result in death.

D.　In the setting of IL-2-induced repetitive seizures, treatment can be resumed upon initiation of antiseizure medication and seizure cessation.

Question 11.24.　　Which of the following statements regarding antiangiogenesis agents is CORRECT?

A.　Lenalidomide was the first angiogenesis inhibitor approved by the FDA for cancer treatment.

B.　Vorinostat, celecoxib, and bortezomib may all be referred to as exclusive angiogenesis inhibitors.

C.　Proangiogenic factors include endostatin, angiostatin, and thrombospondin.

D.　Resistance to vascular endothelial growth factor inhibitors has been seen secondary to increased expression of proangiogenic factors.

Question 11.25.　　Which of the following adjuvant endocrine therapies would be the most appropriate for use in a postmenopausal woman with stage II ER/PR (+) breast cancer?

A.　Tamoxifen for 5 years

B.　Anastrozole for 5 years

C.　Goserelin for 5 years

D.　Bicalutamide for 5 years

ANSWERS

Answer 11.1.   **The answer is B.**

Patients who are homozygous for the triple repeat polymorphism were found to have two- to fourfold greater gene expression compared to double repeat polymorphism. This increase in gene expression results in increased TS levels. There is an inverse relationship between TS levels and 5-FU response; therefore, patients with higher TS levels were less likely to respond to 5-FU.

Answer 11.2.   **The answer is C.**

A prognostic marker is a genetic or molecular variation that would affect the natural history of the disease. In patients who have stage II colon cancer, a deficiency in MMR protein expression would lead to a more favorable natural course of disease and would diminish the effect of adjuvant chemotherapy. Predictive markers are more commonly seen for prediction of the likelihood of response or toxicity from a specific drug, such as KRAS mutations leading to diminished response from cetuximab.

Answer 11.3.   **The answer is A.**

Methotrexate is predominately renally cleared with about 80% to 90% excreted unchanged in the urine. Excretion is directly related to creatinine clearance, so patients with an elevated serum creatinine should either avoid methotrexate or receive a reduced dose. The renal excretion of methotrexate can be inhibited by medications such as probencid, penicillins, cephalosporins, aspirin, and NSAIDs, so these drugs need to be avoided concomitantly with methotrexate. Methotrexate distributes into third-spaces such as pleural effusions and ascites. This can cause delayed drug clearance. While methotrexate can cause elevations in bilirubin and transaminases, there are no dose reduction recommendations for bilirubin less than 3 mg/dL.

Answer 11.4.   **The answer is D.**

Leucovorin rescue is designed to provide reduced folate to normal cells and minimize the toxicity from methotrexate. This should be started about 24 hours after the infusion of methotrexate and continued until the methotrexate has cleared. Vigorous intravenous hydration is important with methotrexate, but this should also include sodium bicarbonate in order to help facilitate urine alkalinization. When the urine is acidic, methotrexate and its metabolites can precipitate within the tubules causing nephrotoxicity. Folic acid supplementation is not necessary for methotrexate infusions.

Answer 11.5.   **The answer is C.**

With both pemetrexed and pralatrexate, supplementation with Vitamin B_{12} and folic acid is required to minimize hematologic toxicities. Vitamin

B_{12} intramuscular injections (1000 mcg) should be started 1 week prior to treatment and repeated every 9 weeks. Folic acid supplementation should be initiated 1 week prior to treatment and continued daily for at least 21 days after therapy.

Answer 11.6.   **The answer is C.**

Patients receiving FOLFIRI chemotherapy commonly experience both acute and delayed diarrhea from irinotecan, but this is usually not seen in combination with mucositis and myelosuppression. Patients who are homozygous for UGT1A1*28 are at risk for developing more severe myelosuppression and diarrhea from irinotecan, and would warrant empiric dose reductions, but this would not typically be seen with severe mucositis. Patients who have DPD deficiency often present with severe diarrhea, mucositis, and myelosuppression because of the inability to metabolize 5-fluorouracil.

Answer 11.7.   **The answer is B.**

Fludarabine causes suppression of the immune system, more specifically T-cells. After initiation of fludarabine, a quick decline in CD4 positive cells occurs and often it takes greater than 1 year for recovery. During this time frame, patients are at risk for many opportunistic infections.

Answer 11.8.   **The answer is B.**

Enhanced sensitivity to p-glycoprotein and drug efflux is thought to be a major factor in development of anthracycline resistance, but not cardiotoxicity. Cardiotoxicity is thought to be multifactorial with increased oxidation–reduction reactions, generation of reactive oxygen species, and peroxidation of myocardial lipids.

Answer 11.9.   **The answer is A.**

Cabazitaxel was studied in patients who had progressed on docetaxel chemotherapy. Since it is a poor substrate for the multidrug-resistant p-glycoprotein efflux pump, it is proposed that cabazitaxel will have efficacy in chemotherapy-resistant tumors.

Answer 11.10.   **The answer is C.**

Vinca alkaloids alter the tubulin association rate constant and inhibit the assembly of microtubules thus inducing cell cycle arrest, whereas taxane chemotherapy agents alter the tubulin dissociation rate and inhibit the disassembly of microtubules. Cabazitaxel exerts it mechanism of action by stabilizing tubulin and inhibiting microtubule depolymerization. Epothilones promote tubulin polymerization and induce mitotic arrest.

Answer 11.11.   **The answer is D.**

Often the clinical response to therapies like azacitidine is after four to six cycles of therapy, so it is important to allow enough time to see efficacy from these drugs. Azacitidine is a DNA demethylating agent that is able to be administered by either intravenous or subcutaneous routes. It is very unstable and needs to be administered quickly after reconstitution.

Answer 11.12.   **The answer is C.**

Mesna bladder protection is required for all patients receiving ifosfamide and for those patients receiving high doses of cyclophosphamide. It works by providing a free sulfhydryl group that conjugates with the toxic metabolite (acrolein) of ifosfamide and cyclophosphamide. The dosing of mesna should be equal to 60% of the total dose of ifosfamide or cyclophosphamide.

Answer 11.13.   **The answer is B.**

Oxaliplatin is associated with significant acute neuropathy that is exacerbated by cold and delayed peripheral neuropathy. It has been demonstrated in colon cancer that infusions of calcium and magnesium prior to and after oxaliplatin infusions can lessen the incidence and severity of the delayed peripheral neuropathy. Cisplatin is associated with a much higher rate of ototoxicity than carboplatin. Cisplatin should also be avoided in patients with renal insufficiency, while oxaliplatin is well tolerated in patients with mild-to-moderate renal insufficiency.

Answer 11.14.   **The answer is C.**

The binding of oblimersen (an antisense oligodeoxyribonucleotide) to its target mRNA forms an mRNA–DNA complex. This elicits the activity of RNase H that cleaves the mRNA strand coding for the Bcl-2 protein from the mRNA–DNA complex. This leads to decreased transcription of Bcl-2.

Answer 11.15.   **The answer is A.**

Bortezomib is FDA approved for use in combination with melphalan and prednisone for front-line therapy of multiple myeloma. The drug is given on days 1, 4, 8, 11, of a 3-week cycle. The drug is also approved for use as a single agent for patients with relapsed multiple myeloma.

Answer 11.16.   **The answer is D.**

At low concentrations (0.2 to 1 mcM), the azacytosine nucleosides show dose-dependent reversal of DNA methylation and induction of terminal differentiation. As concentrations are increased; however, induction of cell apoptosis and DNA damage become the prominent cytotoxic effects.

Answer 11.17.   **The answer is B.**

Preclinical studies have shown that combining PARP inhibitors with anti-cancer treatment modalities that result in DNA instability (e.g., radiation therapy and platinum chemotherapy agents) potentiates their cytotoxicity. In the presence of BRCA mutations, PARP inhibitors cause impaired homologous recombination, loss of repair mechanisms, and cell death. PARP inhibition has also been implicated in decreased production of hypoxia-inducible factor-1 function that may contribute to cancer cell death.

Answer 11.18.   **The answer is C.**

Pulmonary toxicities are a relatively rare event in patients taking everolimus, occurring in less than 1% of patients. Dry skin with an acneiform rash is one of the most common side effects of everolimus therapy seen in up to 18% of patients. Deep vein thrombosis has been reported in 1% to 10% of patients taking everolimus, but no recommendations exist for prophylactic anticoagulation. Rates of endocrine and other metabolic adverse events (including hypercholesterolemia, hypertriglyceridemia, and hyperglycemia) with everolimus have been as high as 90%.

Answer 11.19.   **The answer is D.**

Asparaginase has been shown to antagonize the cytotoxic antimetabolite activity of methotrexate when administered either concurrently with or immediately before the drug. The proposed mechanism is via decreased methotrexate polyglutamation leading to lower levels of unbound intracellular drug. It is recommended, therefore, that the two drugs be given sequentially at least 24 hours apart.

Answer 11.20.   **The answer is C.**

The biologic effects seen with interferons are associated with interactions with both the innate and adaptive immune systems. Anorexia and weight loss are commonly seen with higher dose regimens, such as those used for malignant melanoma. While not studied extensively, no clinically significant drug–drug interactions have been proven for interferons to date.

Answer 11.21.   **The answer is A.**

High-dose interferon therapy can cause acute elevations in serum transaminases. This toxicity may result in fatal hepatic failure. Dose reductions have been recommended in the setting of transaminitis that have allowed for safe continued administration of the drug.

Answer 11.22.   **The answer is B.**

Delayed, prolonged, and severe cytopenias have been reported with ibritumomab therapy. It is recommended that therapy not be administered to patients with greater than or equal to 25% lymphoma marrow involvement or to patients with prior stem cell mobilization failure.

Answer 11.23.   **The answer is C.**

Doses of IL-2 should be withheld or interrupted for toxicities; doses should not be reduced. It is recommended that treatment be withheld for patients with moderate-to-severe lethargy or somnolence, as continued treatment may result in coma. Retreatment with subsequent doses of IL-2 is contraindicated in patients with repetitive or refractory seizures.

Answer 11.24.   **The answer is D.**

Bevacizumab was the first angiogenesis inhibitor to be approved by the FDA for cancer treatment following a phase III trial showing a survival benefit. Drugs that only exhibit antiangiogenic properties are known as exclusive inhibitors. Drugs such as vorinostat, celecoxib, and bortezomib all inhibit angiogenesis as a secondary function and thus are known as inclusive inhibitors. Proangiogenic factors include, but are not limited to, vascular endothelial growth factor, platelet-derived growth factor, placental growth factor, and transforming growth factor-β.

Answer 11.25.   **The answer is B.**

The National Comprehensive Cancer Network breast cancer guidelines recommend the use of single-agent aromatase inhibitor therapy for 5 years as adjuvant endocrine therapy for postmenopausal patients. The use of tamoxifen alone for 5 years is limited to those who decline or have a contraindication to aromatase inhibitors. LHRH agonists should not be used in postmenopausal patients. The antiandrogen bicalutamide is not used to treat breast cancer.

CHAPTER 12 CANCER PREVENTION

DANIEL MORGENSZTERN • VORACHART AUETHAVEKIAT

DIRECTIONS   Each of the numbered items below is followed by lettered answers. Select the ONE lettered answer that is BEST in each case unless instructed otherwise.

QUESTIONS

Question 12.1.   Which of the following statements regarding nicotine replacement therapy (NRT) is TRUE:

A.   All commercially available forms of NRT are equally effective treatments of smoking cessation.
B.   NRTs do not compromise postsurgical wound healing.
C.   A and B
D.   None of the above

Question 12.2.   What is the estimated prevalence of smokers among US adults?

A.   10%
B.   15%
C.   20%
D.   25%

Question 12.3.   Which of the following may be classified as nonsmoker?

A.   An 82-year-old man who smoked for 10 years and quit 50 years ago.
B.   A 25-year-old woman who never smoked cigarettes.
C.   A 38-year-old man who smoked approximately 75 cigarettes in his lifetime.
D.   B and C.

Question 12.4.   What is the best measurement for nicotine dependence?

A.   Number of cigarettes smoked per day
B.   Age of smoking initiation
C.   Time from waking up to the first cigarette smoking
D.   All the above

Corresponding chapters in *Cancer: Principles & Practice of Oncology,* Ninth Edition: 50 (Preventive Cancer Vaccines), 51 (Tobacco Dependence and Its Treatment), 52 (Role of Surgery in Cancer Prevention), 53 (Principles of Cancer Risk Reduction Intervention), 54 (Retinoids, Carotenoids, and Other Micronutrients in Cancer Prevention), and 55 (Drugs and Nutritional Extracts for Cancer Risk Reduction (Chemoprevention)).

Question 12.5.   What is the mechanism of action for bupropion?

    A. Increase synaptic concentration of norepinephrine
    B. α2β4 partial agonist and antagonist
    C. Blockade of the dopamine reuptake
    D. None of the above

Question 12.6.   Which of the following neoplasias is NOT an intraepithelial marker for invasive cancer?

    A. Colorectal adenoma
    B. Junctional nevus
    C. Actinic keratosis
    D. Bronchial dysplasia

Question 12.7.   In clinical trials, systemic retinoids and beta-carotene were shown to reduce cancer incidence in this group of high-risk individuals:

    A. Skin cancer in patients with xeroderma pigmentosum
    B. Lung cancer in heavy smokers
    C. Cervical cancer in patients with cervical dysplasia
    D. Colorectal cancer in patients with adenoma

Question 12.8.   Which of the statements is/are TRUE regarding nonsteroidal anti-inflammatory drugs (NSAIDs) in the prevention of colorectal cancer?

    A. Chemopreventive effects of low-dose aspirin on colorectal cancer development were demonstrated in clinical trials, and its overall benefits outweigh the risks in adults at average risks of developing colorectal cancer.
    B. High-dose sulindac prevents the development of new polyps, although it does not cause the regression of established polyps.
    C. In randomized trials, both rofecoxib and celecoxib were shown to reduce the risk of metachronous colorectal adenomas and colorectal cancer.
    D. Considering the risks associated with these agents, screening strategy alone seems to be sufficient in average-risk adults.

Question 12.9.   The risk of which of the following toxicities is increased in patients treated with raloxifene?

    A. Endometrial cancer
    B. Vertebral fracture
    C. Venous thromboembolism
    D. Coronary artery heart disease

Question 12.10. Which of the following statements regarding *BRCA* mutations is false?

    A. The lifetime risk of ovarian cancer increases to 15% to 25% in *BRCA2* mutation carriers.

    B. The frequency of *BRCA* mutation carriers in Ashkenazi Jewish population is approximately 2.5%.

    C. *BRCA2*-associated ovarian cancer occurs at younger age compared to sporadic cases.

    D. *BRCA1* is mutated more often than *BRCA2* in women with hereditary ovarian cancer.

Question 12.11. Which of the following statements regarding familial adenomatous polyposis (FAP) is FALSE?

    A. The development of colorectal cancer is inevitable in the absence of colectomy.

    B. It is characterized by the presence of 100 or more adenomatous polyps in the colorectum.

    C. It accounts for approximately 5% of the colorectal cancer cases.

    D. It is an autosomal-dominant disorder.

Question 12.12. What is the best treatment of a patient with FAP presenting with approximately 300 colorectal polyps and 15 rectal adenomas?

    A. Observation

    B. Total proctocolectomy with permanent ileostomy (TPC)

    C. Proctocolectomy with ileal pouch-anal anastomosis (IPAA)

    D. Total colectomy with ileorectal anastomosis (IRA)

Question 12.13. Which of the following does not represent an indication for microsatellite instability (MSI) testing in patients with suspected hereditary nonpolyposis colorectal cancer (HNPCC) according to the revised Bethesda guidelines?

    A. Colorectal cancer in a patient aged less than 50 years

    B. Presence of synchronous colorectal cancer regardless of age

    C. Colorectal cancer with MSI histology regardless of age

    D. Colorectal cancer diagnosed in two or more first-degree relatives with HNPCC-related tumor regardless of age

Question 12.14. Which of the following does NOT represent an HNPCC-related tumor?

    A. Gastric cancer

    B. Carcinoma of the small bowel

    C. Pancreatic cancer

    D. Breast cancer

Question 12.15. Which of the following malignancies are associated with germ line mutations in the *RET* protooncogene?

    A. Multiple endocrine neoplasia (MEN) 2A

    B. MEN 2B

    C. Sporadic medullary thyroid carcinoma

    D. All the above

ANSWERS

Answer 12.1.   **The answer is A.**

There are no significant differences in smoking cessation rates among the several forms of NRT. Nicotine causes vasoconstriction and may be associated with compromised postsurgical wound healing.

Answer 12.2.   **The answer is C.**

Data from the 2008 National Health Interview Survey (NHIS) indicate that approximately 20% of US adults are smokers. Although there was a significant decrease in the prevalence of smoking over the last 10 years, the rate remained unchanged over the last 5 most recent NHIS surveys.

Answer 12.3.   **The answer is D.**

The standard definition of nonsmokers includes patients who smoked less than 100 cigarettes in their lifetime. In contrast, patients who smoked more than five packs of cigarettes and already quit are classified as former smokers.

Answer 12.4.   **The answer is C.**

The number of cigarettes smoked per day and age of initiation, subtracted from the current age, reflect the total dose of cigarette consumption. The best measurement of nicotine dependence is the time from waking up to the first cigarette smoking. Patients who smoke the first cigarette within 30 minutes from waking up have high level of dependence and will likely need more intensive cessation therapy.

Answer 12.5.   **The answer is C.**

Several pharmacological agents have been used for the treatment of nicotine dependence, including the partial agonist of the $\alpha2\beta4$ nicotinic acetylcholine receptor varenicline, nortriptyline that increases the synaptic concentration of norepinephrine and bupropion, which increased the level of dopamine in the brain through blockage of dopamine reuptake.

Answer 12.6.   **The answer is B.**

In chemopreventive studies, intraepithelial neoplasias could be used as surrogate end points, allowing cancer diagnosis at an early stage, identification of high-risk individuals, and reduction in the size and duration of chemoprevention trials. Colorectal adenoma, actinic keratosis, and bronchial dysplasia are neoplastic surrogates for colorectal carcinoma, squamous cell carcinoma of the skin, and lung carcinoma, respectively. Unlike dysplastic nevus, which is a premalignant pigmented skin lesion, junctional nevi are not a premalignant lesion.

Answer 12.7.   **The answer is A.**

In smokers, the Alpha-Tocopherol, Beta-Carotene Trial (ATBC) and the Carotene and Retinol Efficacy Trial (CARET) showed increased risk of lung cancer in patients receiving beta-carotene with or without retinol. Although topical all-trans retinoic acid (ATRA) might cause regression of cervical dysplasia, this effect was not seen in studies involving systemic retinoids or beta-carotene. Prospective studies found no protective effect of beta-carotene supplementation. Retinoids and beta-carotene have been studied extensively in both clinical and epidemiologic trials. Systemic retinoids were initially shown to reduce skin cancer incidence by 63% during therapy in patients with xeroderma pigmentosum. However, the protective effect was lost after discontinuing the treatment.

Answer 12.8.   **The answer is D.**

Several studies have shown protective effects from NSAIDs in patients with colorectal cancer. Although regular use of aspirin was associated with protective effects in population base studies, the benefit of low-dose aspirin was not yet clear in randomized clinical trials. The limited benefit of NSAIDS, including low-dose aspirin, in preventing colorectal cancer, does not justify their use in average-risk individuals. Sulindac, at high dose, was associated with both regression of existing polyps and prevention of new polyps in patients with FAP, but the protection was transient and incomplete. Although the cyclooxygenase-2 inhibitors rofecoxib and celecoxib were shown to reduce the risks of metachronous adenoma, the studies were terminated early because of their side effects, being unable to detect the reduction of colorectal cancer incidence. Although NSAIDs reduce the risk of colorectal adenoma and colorectal cancer, these agents are associated with significant gastrointestinal and cardiovascular toxicities, which outweigh the benefits. Therefore, the best strategy for the general population remains effective screening.

Answer 12.9.   **The answer is C.**

Raloxifene is a nonsteroidal selective estrogen receptor modulator that binds to estrogen receptor leading to estrogen agonist effects in some tissues and estrogen antagonist effects in others. Raloxifene has estrogen agonist activity in the bone but is less active than tamoxifen in the uterus. Unlike tamoxifen, raloxifene was not associated with increased risk of uterine cancer. Because of raloxifene's agonist activity in bone, it reduced the risk of vertebral fracture. Raloxifene does not increase the risk of coronary artery heart disease, but studies showed increased risk of venous thromboembolism and fatal stroke.

Answer 12.10.   **The answer is C.**

The lifetime risk of ovarian cancer increases from a baseline of 1.5% to about 15% to 25% in *BRCA2* carriers. Although *BRCA* mutations are rare in most populations, they occur in approximately 1 in 40 Ashkenazi Jews. The median age for sporadic epithelial ovarian cancer is 60 years. Among patients with hereditary ovarian cancer, *BRCA1* mutation is more common than *BRCA2*. In contrast to *BRCA1* mutants, who usually develop ovarian cancer by their mid-1940s, the median age at presentation for *BRCA2* mutants is 63 years.

Answer 12.11.   **The answer is C.**

FAP is an autosomal-dominant disorder characterized by at least 100 colorectal adenomatous polyps, and virtually all patients develop colorectal cancer in the absence of surgery. This disease, however, is uncommon, representing less than 1% of the total number of colorectal cancer cases.

Answer 12.12.   **The answer is D.**

Because of the virtually universal risk of developing cancer by the age of 40 years in the absence of therapy, patients with FAP should undergo surgery, with the timing depending on the extent of disease. Among the surgical options, TPC is rarely used and most patients will be treated with IRA or IPAA. One of the main factors in deciding whether to remove the rectum is the risk of rectal cancer. Therefore, IRA may be considered in patients with less than 1000 colorectal polyps and less than 20 rectal adenomas. In contrast, patients with a higher number of rectal adenomas, adenomas larger than 3 cm, or severe dysplasia should undergo proctectomy in addition to colectomy, through IPAA.

Answer 12.13.   **The answer is C.**

The revised Bethesda criteria are used to identify individuals and families at high risk for HNPCC, where the MSI testing is indicated. The five criteria include (a) colorectal cancer in a patient aged less than 50 years, (b) presence of synchronous or metachronous HNPCC cancer regardless of age, (c) colorectal cancer with MSI histology in patients aged less than 60 years, (d) colorectal cancer diagnosed in one or more first-degree relatives with an HNPCC-related tumor with one of the cancers being diagnosed at age less than 50 years old, and (e) colorectal cancer diagnosed in two or more first-degree or second-degree relatives with HNPCC-related tumor regardless of age. Therefore, answer C is incorrect because only patients aged less than 60 years with MSI histology should be screened. MSI histology includes the presence of tumor-infiltrating lymphocytes, Crohn's-like lymphocytic reaction, signet ring differentiation, and medullary growth pattern.

Answer 12.14.   **The answer is D.**

HNPCC is associated with several extracolonic malignancies, including endometrial cancer, ovarian cancer, urothelial tumors, biliary and pancreatic cancers, carcinomas of the small bowel, and brain tumors. Breast cancer, although commonly associated with multiple familiary disorders, is not considered one of the HNPCC-related tumors.

Answer 12.15.   **The answer is D.**

MEN 2A, MEN 2B, familial medullary thyroid carcinoma and sporadic medullary carcinoma are associated with germ line mutations in the *RET* protooncogene.

CHAPTER 13 CANCER SCREENING

MEGAN E. WREN

DIRECTIONS   Each of the numbered items below is followed by lettered answers. Select the ONE lettered answer that is BEST in each case unless instructed otherwise.

QUESTIONS

Question 13.1.   Studies of screening for cancer are subject to several types of bias. If screening detects a cancer earlier (before it becomes symptomatic), but treatment has no effect on the course of the disease, then the subject will seem to live longer, than if he or she had presented symptomatically. (That is, the cancer is known for a longer period of time, but the time of death is not altered.) This type of bias is known as:

A. Lead-time bias
B. Length bias
C. Volunteer bias
D. Overdiagnosis bias

Question 13.2.   A healthy 13-year-old girl received a vaccine against human papilloma virus (HPV). This is an example of:

A. Primary prevention
B. Secondary prevention
C. Tertiary prevention
D. Case finding

Question 13.3.   A healthy 48-year-old woman went to see her primary care physician because she found a breast lump. The work-up found a 1-cm invasive ductal carcinoma. This is an example of:

A. Primary prevention
B. Secondary prevention
C. Tertiary prevention
D. Case finding

Corresponding Chapters in *Cancer: Principles & Practice of Oncology,* Ninth Edition: 56 (Principles of Cancer Screening), 57 (Early Detection Using Proteomics), 58 (Screening for Gastrointestinal Cancers), 59 (Screening for Gynecologic Cancers), 60 (Screening for Breast Cancer), 61 (Screening for Prostate Cancer), and 62 (Screening for Lung Cancer).

Question 13.4.   A healthy 85-year-old man was found to have an elevated prostate-specific antigen (PSA) level. He had no urologic symptoms. Evaluation and biopsy revealed a localized prostate cancer with a low Gleason score. This is an example of:

A. Primary prevention
B. Secondary prevention
C. Tertiary prevention
D. Case finding

Question 13.5.   Which of the following statements regarding the risk of developing esophageal cancer is true?

A. Chronic gastroesophageal reflux disease increases the risk for esophageal cancer.
B. Surveillance with upper endoscopy reduces the risk of esophageal cancer.
C. Aggressive antireflux therapy for patients with Barrett's esophagus reduces the risk of esophageal cancer.
D. Patients with Plummer-Vinson syndrome do not have increased risk for esophageal cancer.

Question 13.6.   A new screening test for ovarian cancer was developed. It was tested in a tertiary care academic medical center in a group of women with breast cancer (BRCA) mutations and was found to have a sensitivity of 70%, specificity of 90%, and positive predictive value (PPV) of 10%. If a woman in the study population is found to have a positive (abnormal) test result, how would you interpret it?

A. There is a 30% chance that this represents a false-positive result.
B. There is a 10% chance that this represents a false-positive result.
C. There is a 9 in 10 chance that this represents a false-positive result.
D. You can be 90% sure that your patient has the disease.

Question 13.7.   If the use of this test (from Question 13.7) is expanded to the general population, it is expected that:

A. The test sensitivity will be lower.
B. The test specificity will be lower.
C. The PPV will be lower.
D. The test specificity will be higher.

Question 13.8.   Which one or more of the following screening tests for colorectal cancer have been proven effective in randomized controlled trials?

A. Fecal occult blood testing
B. Flexible sigmoidoscopy
C. Air-contrast barium enema
D. Colonoscopy

Question 13.9. More frequent screening for colorectal cancer is recommended in all of the following situations, EXCEPT:

A. Patients with one second-degree relative with colorectal cancer
B. Gene carriers for familial adenomatous polyposis
C. Gene carrier for hereditary nonpolyposis colon cancer
D. Patients with ulcerative colitis

Question 13.10. Almost all cervical cancers are associated with infection by sexually transmitted HPV. Of the following statements about HPV infection in young women (in their teens and 20s), which one is INCORRECT?

A. HPV infection is common in young, sexually active women.
B. HPV infection is often transient in young women.
C. In young women, most cases of low-grade squamous intraepithelial lesion (LSIL) will regress without treatment.
D. HPV infection and LSIL are the earliest stages in the development of cervical cancer and require aggressive treatment.

Question 13.11. Regarding population screening for ovarian cancer, which of the following tests have been proven effective? Choose one or more:

A. Annual pelvic examination
B. Annual measurement of serum CA 125
C. Two-stage screening: annual CA 125 then transvaginal ultrasound if elevated CA 125
D. None of the above

Question 13.12. The United States Preventive Services Task Force, the American College of Obstetricians and Gynecologists, and the American College of Physicians agree on which one of the following recommendations for ovarian cancer screening?

A. Annual pelvic examination for women ages 20 to 70 years
B. No population-based screening is recommended.
C. Transvaginal ultrasound every 5 years
D. Annual serum CA 125 measurement

Question 13.13. Women are at increased risk of breast cancer if they have:

A. Lobular carcinoma in situ (LCIS)
B. Atypical ductal hyperplasia (ADH)
C. A history of mantle radiation for Hodgkin's lymphoma
D. All of the above

Question 13.14.   **For women who have had a hysterectomy, which one of the following is the most appropriate practice for screening for cervical cancer with PAP smears?**

   A. PAP smears should be performed every 1 to 3 years indefinitely.

   B. PAP smears should be performed every 1 to 3 years until age 65 years.

   C. Women who have a history of cervical cancer can discontinue screening after a total abdominal hysterectomy.

   D. Women who have had a total hysterectomy for benign conditions no longer need PAP smears.

Question 13.15.   **Which statement regarding screening for breast cancer is true?**

   A. Latina women are at a lower risk for developing aggressive breast cancer than the general population.

   B. The monthly breast self-examination (BSE) is a crucial component of breast cancer screening programs.

   C. The BSE has been shown to be ineffective for breast cancer screening.

   D. Older women are more likely to develop triple negative disease.

Question 13.16.   **Which of the following statements regarding prostate cancer screening is true?**

   A. PSA levels do not change with age.

   B. African-American men are at increased risk for prostate cancer.

   C. Annual PSA level testing is recommended for men of 55 to 74 years.

   D. PSA levels are unaffected by benign prostate diseases.

Question 13.17.   **All of the following statements regarding cancer screening tests are true, EXCEPT:**

   A. Lead-time bias could affect the effectiveness of screening tests.

   B. Randomized controlled trials are necessary to evaluate the effectiveness of screening tests.

   C. Improvement in overall survival is an appropriate end point for trials on cancer screening tests.

   D. Risk models could help identify the patients to be screened.

ANSWERS

Answer 13.1.   **The answer is A.**

Lead-time bias is the interval between the diagnosis of disease at screening and when it would have been detected because of the development of symptoms. Length bias is the overrepresentation among screen-detected cases of those with a long preclinical period (thus, less rapidly fatal), leading to the incorrect conclusion that screening was beneficial. Volunteers who choose to participate in screening programs are likely to be different from the general population in ways that affect survival. They may be more compliant or may have healthier habits. Conversely, they may volunteer because they think they are at higher risk for disease.

Answer 13.2.   **The answer is A.**

Primary prevention refers to the prevention of disease, such as the removal of colon polyps to prevent the development of colon cancer. Secondary prevention refers to the identification of disease at an early asymptomatic stage through screening. Case finding occurs when a patient with symptomatic disease presents to a physician for evaluation.

Answer 13.3.   **The answer is D.**

Primary prevention refers to the prevention of disease, such as the removal of colon polyps to prevent the development of colon cancer. Secondary prevention refers to the identification of disease at an early asymptomatic stage through screening. Case finding occurs when a patient with symptomatic disease presents to a physician for evaluation.

Answer 13.4.   **The answer is B.**

Primary prevention refers to the prevention of disease, such as the removal of colon polyps to prevent the development of colon cancer. Secondary prevention refers to the identification of disease at an early asymptomatic stage through screening. Case finding occurs when a patient with symptomatic disease presents to a physician for evaluation.

Answer 13.5.   **The answer is A.**

Chronic gastroesophageal reflux disease is associated with increased risk for esophageal cancer. Plummer-Vinson syndrome is associated with increased risk of squamous cell carcinoma of the esophagus. Screening upper endoscopy or aggressive antireflux therapy for Barrett's esophagus has not been shown to decrease the risk for esophageal cancer.

Answer 13.6.   **The answer is C.**

The sensitivity of a test reflects its ability to detect a known disease, and the specificity reflects the ability of a test to give a normal result when the disease is known to be absent. From the point of view of the clinician, the presence or absence of a disease is unknown, and the pertinent question is the accuracy of the test result. The PPV or PV+ is an estimate of the accuracy of the test in predicting the presence of disease; the negative predictive value (NPV or PV−) is an estimate of the accuracy of the test in predicting the absence of disease. The PPV represents the proportion of all positive tests that are true positives: TP/(TP+FP). A PPV of 10% means that 10% of positive test results are true positives, so 90% are false positives.

Answer 13.7.   **The answer is C.**

The sensitivity and specificity are characteristics of the test itself and are not affected by the population characteristics. On the other hand, the PPV and NPV values are influenced by the disease prevalence in the population being tested.

Answer 13.8.   **The answer is A.**

Fecal occult blood testing and flexible sigmoidoscopy have been proven effective in randomized controlled trials. For the other screening modalities, the only published data are from observational and case-control studies. There are ongoing randomized controlled trials of colonoscopy, but no data are yet available.

Answer 13.9.   **The answer is A.**

Patients with a second-degree relative diagnosed with colon cancer are not at increased risk for developing colorectal cancer. The screening recommendations for this group are same as that for the general population.

Answer 13.10.   **The answer is D.**

HPV infection is common in young, sexually active women but is often transient. Up to 70% of high-risk HPV infections will resolve spontaneously. Similarly, up to 90% of LSILs will regress without treatment. Concerns have been raised that screening young women could lead to overdiagnosis, aggressive treatment, and unnecessary harm from ablative surgical procedures.

Answer 13.11.   **The answer is D.**

No screening strategies have been shown to be effective for screening for ovarian cancer for several reasons. Ovarian cancer has a low prevalence in the population, thus lowering the PPVs of any tests. CA 125 has limited sensitivity (it misses many early-stage cancers) and limited specificity (many false positives). Transvaginal ultrasound has inadequate specificity.

Answer 13.12.   **The answer is B.**

The United States Preventive Services Task Force, the American College of Obstetricians and Gynecologists, and the American College of Physicians all discourage routine screening for ovarian cancer in the general population. The currently available screening tests do not have adequate sensitivity and specificity, especially considering the relatively low prevalence in the population.

Answer 13.13.   **The answer is D.**

LCIS is associated with an annual risk of developing breast cancer of up to 1% per year. Screening with mammography and physical examination can reduce breast cancer mortality in women with LCIS to the same level as that of the general population. ADH or ductal atypia increases cancer risk four- to fivefold, or even higher in women with a family history of breast cancer or those with ADH at ages less than 30 years. A personal history of mantle radiation (especially between the ages of 10 and 30 years) has also been shown to elevate breast cancer risk. Cases of breast cancer have been reported as early as 8 years after treatment, so screening of these women as early as 8 years posttreatment has been recommended.

Answer 13.14.   **The answer is D.**

Women without a cervix are not at risk for cervical cancer unless there was a history of cervical cancer (then PAP smears are for follow-up of the cancer, not for screening). Vaginal cuff smears are unnecessary; they have an extremely low likelihood of detecting vaginal dysplasia, and the false-positive rate is high.

Answer 13.15.   **The answer is C.**

Large trials of careful BSE instruction have failed to show any mortality benefit, so BSE is no longer a standard component of breast cancer screening programs (the American Cancer Society lists BSE as an option). Latina and African-American women are at higher risk for developing triple negative disease. Older women have higher risk for developing breast cancer but they are less likely than younger women to develop triple negative disease.

Answer 13.16.   **The answer is B.**

Aging and noncancerous diseases of the prostate are associated with rising PSA levels. African-American men and men with family history of prostate cancer in a nonelderly relative are at higher risk for prostate cancer than the general population.

Answer 13.17.   **The answer is C.**

The studies to evaluate the effectiveness of screening test are susceptible to several issues that includes lead-time bias, length-time bias and overdiagnosis bias. Therefore, an improvement in survival is not an appropriate end point of cancer screening trials. Mortality rates are a more appropriate end point for these trials. Risk modeling techniques can identify patients at high risk for developing cancer and are therefore candidates for screening trials.

CHAPTER 14 GENETIC COUNSELING

JENNIFER IVANOVICH

DIRECTIONS Each of the numbered items below is followed by lettered answers. Select the ONE lettered answer that is BEST in each case unless instructed otherwise.

QUESTIONS

Refer to the following pedigree for Questions 14.1 to 14.4.

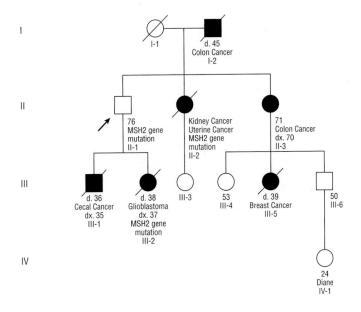

Corresponding Chapter in *Cancer: Principles & Practice of Oncology*, Ninth Edition: 63 (Genetic Counseling).

149

Question 14.1.   The family depicted has hereditary nonpolyposis colon cancer (HNPCC) syndrome. This syndrome is characterized by a high risk to develop colon and endometrial cancer and an increased risk to develop various other tumor types. Before her death, individual III-2 had genetic testing of the *MLH1* and *MSH2* genes, and an *MSH2* gene mutation was identified. Specifically, the mutation is c.942 + 3A > T. MLH1, and *MSH2* gene mutations account for 80% to 90% of families with HNPCC. Individual II-1, depicted with the arrow, has not been diagnosed with cancer. He has undergone frequent colonoscopy screening. He has also had genetic testing and was found to carry the family *MSH2* gene mutation. The finding that individual II-1 has not been diagnosed with cancer can be explained by which of the following concepts?

A.   Genetic testing laboratory error
B.   Clinical variability
C.   Genetic heterogeneity
D.   Reduced penetrance

Question 14.2.   Assuming individual II-3 has the family *MSH2* gene mutation, what is the calculated probability Diane (individual IV-1) has inherited the *MSH2* gene mutation?

A.   0%
B.   12.5%
C.   25%
D.   50%

Question 14.3.   Diane (individual IV-1) is 24 years of age. She approaches her primary care physician about her medical management, given her family history of HNPCC syndrome. She has a healthy body weight and does not smoke. Both her paternal grandmother (II-3) and her father (III-6) refuse to have genetic testing. In addition to her annual PAP smear, which of the following cancer screening is most appropriate for Diane?

A.   Colonoscopy screening to begin at 50 years of age
B.   Sigmoidoscopy screening to begin by 25 years of age
C.   Colonoscopy screening to begin by 25 years of age
D.   Colonoscopy and mammography screening to begin by 25 years of age

Question 14.4.   Diane (individual IV-1) decides to pursue genetic testing to aid in her medical management. She states that her father will not undergo genetic testing. What specific genetic test should be ordered?

A.   Full sequencing of the *MSH2* gene
B.   Full sequencing of the *MSH2* and *MLH1* genes
C.   Site-specific targeted mutation analysis of the *MSH2* gene
D.   Deletion analysis using multiplex ligation-dependent probe amplification

Question 14.5.   Which of the following factors suggest that a family may have hereditary cancer?

    A. Young age at diagnosis
    B. Bilateral cancer in an affected family member
    C. Multiple affected generations
    D. All of the above

Refer to the following pedigree for Questions 14.6 to 14.8.

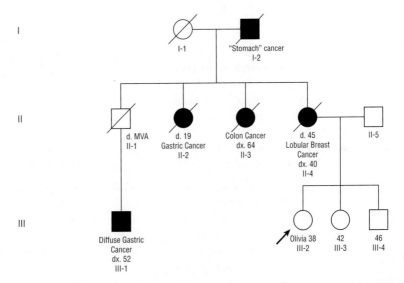

Olivia is a 38-year-old healthy woman who presents to her primary care physician concerned about her family history of cancer. She has no chronic health concerns. Both her mother's and father's family are of Ashkenazi Jewish ancestry. Olivia pursues an evaluation with a clinical geneticist for assessment and genetic testing.

Question 14.6.   The clinical geneticist diagnoses the family with which cancer predisposition syndrome?

    A. HNPCC syndrome
    B. Hereditary breast cancer 1 (BRCA1) syndrome
    C. Li-Fraumeni syndrome
    D. Hereditary BRCA2 syndrome
    E. None of the above

Question 14.7.   Which of the following features is NOT consistent with hereditary cancer in the family depicted?

    A. Multiple affected family members
    B. Lobular breast cancer and diffuse gastric cancer pathology
    C. Ashkenazi Jewish heritage
    D. Affected family member diagnosed at a young age

Question 14.8.   Which of the following statements regarding prophylactic oophorectomy is true?

A. Prophylactic bilateral salpingo-oophorectomy (BSO) is the most effective therapy to reduce the risk of ovarian cancer in women with *BRCA1* or *BRCA2* gene mutation.

B. BSO in *BRCA1* or *BRCA2* gene mutation carriers is indicated at age 30.

C. BSO in *BRCA1* or *BRCA2* gene mutation carriers has no effect on the risk of developing breast cancer.

D. All the above.

Question 14.9.   Jennifer is a 38-year-old woman who was diagnosed with stage IIA ductal carcinoma at 30 years of age. She undergoes direct genetic testing of the *BRCA1* and *BRCA2* genes and is found to have a *BRCA2* gene variant. Specifically the variant is Q713L (2366A > T), which results in the substitution of leucine for glutamine at amino acid 713 of the BRCA2 protein. The functional significance is unknown. Jennifer's sister, Angela, is 40 years of age and has no personal history of cancer. Which is the most appropriate genetic testing approach for Angela?

A. Genetic testing is recommended for Angela because it will clarify her breast cancer risk.

B. Genetic testing is not recommended for Angela because it will not clarify her breast cancer risk.

C. Genetic testing is recommended for Angela because it will help clarify Jennifer's genetic test results.

D. A and C.

Question 14.10.   Which of the following statements regarding BRCA is NOT TRUE?

A. The majority of *BRCA* 2 gene mutation carriers who develop breast cancer have estrogen-receptor positive tumors.

B. *BRCA1* and *BRCA2* gene mutation carriers are at increased risk for developing second contralateral or ipsilateral breast tumors.

C. Treatment with tamoxifen does not decrease the risk of contralateral breast cancer in women with *BRCA2* gene mutations.

D. Prophylactic bilateral mastectomy decreases the risk of breast cancer in more than 90% of high-risk women with *BRCA1* or *BRCA2* gene mutation.

Refer to the following pedigree for Questions 14.11 and 14.12.

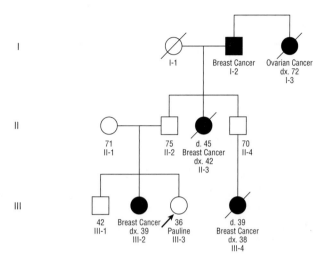

Question 14.11. Pauline, depicted by the arrow, is a healthy 36-year-old woman who presents to her gynecologist concerned about her breast cancer risk. She requests genetic testing. No other family member has undergone genetic testing. The gynecologist orders *BRCA1* and *BRCA2* gene testing. No mutation is identified. Which of the following statements is the correct interpretation of Pauline's testing?

A. Pauline's test result is a true negative.
B. Pauline's test result is an unknown variant.
C. Pauline's test result is uninformative.
D. Pauline's test result is positive.

Question 14.12. Pauline's sister, individual III-2, is currently undergoing neoadjuvant chemotherapy for an aggressive ductal carcinoma of the breast. She is not interested in pursuing genetic testing at this time given the demands of her treatment. What breast health screening recommendations do you make for Pauline given her negative genetic testing?

A. Mammography beginning at age 40 years
B. Mammography and breast ultrasound beginning at age 40 years
C. Mammography and breast ultrasound beginning now
D. Mammography and breast MRI beginning now

Question 14.13. Which of the following malignancies does not have a significant increase in incidence among patients with Lynch syndrome?

A. Colon cancer
B. Cervical cancer
C. Ovarian cancer
D. Endometrial cancer

Question 14.14.   A 28-year-old woman with bilateral ductal cancer presents to the medical oncologist for assessment and treatment. Her medical history is notable for intussusception at 6 years of age. On her physical examination, the medicine resident notices small blue/black hyperpigmented macules on her lips, buccal mucosa, and fingertips. What is her syndrome diagnosis?

A. Hereditary BRCA1 syndrome
B. Hereditary BRCA2 syndrome
C. Li-Fraumeni syndrome
D. Peutz-Jeghers syndrome
E. Cowden syndrome

ANSWERS

Answer 14.1.   **The answer is D.**

Penetrance may be defined as the proportion of individuals with a mutant genotype who show any manifestation of the given disorder. A disorder that is expressed in less than 100% of individuals with the mutant genotype is said to have reduced penetrance. For example, if only 60% of individuals with the genotype express clinical features, the disease is considered to be 60% penetrant. Expression in hereditary cancer syndromes occurs when an individual is diagnosed with one of the associated malignancies or associated benign lesions. Almost all cancer syndromes show reduced penetrance. This concept is important to understand because many families believe that if a family member has not developed a specific cancer, he/she cannot pass on the gene mutation to a child.

Answer 14.2.   **The answer is C.**

HNPCC syndrome is an autosomal-dominant disease. Calculation of Diane's probability to have inherited the gene mutation is based on straightforward autosomal-dominant inheritance. By assuming that individual II-3 has the *MSH2* gene mutation, the calculated probability Diane's father (III-6) has inherited the mutation is 50%. The probability Diane has inherited it from her father is 50%. Thus, Diane's calculated probability to have inherited the *MSH2* gene mutation is 25% (50% × 50%). Most hereditary cancer syndromes identified to date are inherited in an autosomal-dominant manner with reduced penetrance. In a clinical setting, it would be important not to assume that individual II-3 has the mutation. Although she has been diagnosed with colon cancer, the cardinal feature of HNPCC syndrome, individuals may be diagnosed with an associated cancer type and not have the causal gene mutation. That is, an individual may develop a sporadic cancer that does not result from the underlying family gene mutation. If individual II-3 does not have the *MSH2* gene mutation, her sporadic colon cancer would be a phenocopy, a mimic of the syndrome phenotype. II-3's daughter, who died of breast cancer at 39 years of age, does not provide any insight as to whether II-3 has the gene mutation. Breast cancer has been reported in some families with HNPCC; however, an association in larger studies has not consistently been demonstrated.

Answer 14.3.   **The answer is C.**

HNPCC syndrome is associated with a 70% to 80% lifetime risk for colon cancer and a 20% to 60% risk for endometrial cancer. There are also increased risks for gastric (intestinal type), ovarian, urinary tract, and central nervous system tumors, with the level of risk varying for each cancer type. Colonoscopy screening is recommended to begin by 20 to 25 years of age or 10 years before the youngest age of cancer diagnosis and repeated every 1 to 2 years. Sigmoidoscopy is not recommended because of the predominance of right-sided colon cancers.

Approximately two-thirds of all colon cancers in HNPCC occur in the ascending colon. Consensus recommendations also include endometrial cancer surveillance with transvaginal ultrasound and endometrial biopsy; however, the efficacy of this screening regimen is unknown. Although Diane's (IV-1) paternal aunt (III-5) died of breast cancer at a young age, there are insufficient data to prove breast cancer is one of the associated cancers in HNPCC syndrome. As such, intensified mammography screening is not warranted. Intensified surveillance recommendations are available for many hereditary cancer syndromes. Limited data exist to prove the efficacy of these screening protocols. However, until larger data sets are developed, consensus recommendations are issued to help guide clinicians in the care of high-risk families.

Answer 14.4.   **The answer is C.**

The *MSH2* gene mutation, c.942 + 3A > T, identified in an affected family member, results in an A > T change at the third nucleotide of the splice-donor site of intron 5 and causes an in-frame deletion of exon 5. The mutation can be detected using sequencing.

As such, site-specific sequencing, also known as targeted mutation analysis, is the only test that is needed. Full sequencing of the *MSH2* gene is unnecessary and may result in excess cost to the individual pursuing genetic testing. Approximately 20% of *MSH2* gene mutations are large deletions or gene rearrangements. These mutations cannot be detected using sequencing. Southern blot analysis and multiplex ligation-dependent probe amplification are techniques used to detect large deletions. A working knowledge of the types of mutations that have been described for a given gene, as well as an understanding of the limitations of the techniques used by a given laboratory, is crucial in overseeing the clinical genetic testing of a family.

Diane (IV-1) has the right to pursue clinical genetic testing to aid in her medical management. If her testing is positive for the *MSH2* gene mutation, then her father and paternal grandmother may gain information they have previously chosen not to obtain. In advance of ordering the testing, it is crucial to discuss if and how Diane is going to communicate her test results with her family and their potential reactions. By facilitating this discussion, the clinician is acknowledging some of the psychosocial implications associated with hereditary disease and providing anticipatory guidance as to how Diane may address potential reactions from her family.

Answer 14.5.   **The answer is D.**

Several factors warrant genetic counseling for hereditary cancer syndrome including young age at diagnosis, bilateral cancer in an affected family member, and multiple affected generations.

Answer 14.6.   **The answer is E.**

The family cancer history meets the diagnostic criteria for the hereditary diffuse gastric cancer syndrome. HDGC is an autosomal-dominant, highly penetrant cancer predisposition syndrome that results from mutations in the E-cadherin gene (CDH1). This syndrome is associated with a 70% cumulative lifetime risk for diffuse gastric cancer, an adenocarcinoma that causes thickening of the gastric wall (linitis plastica) without a distinct mass. There is also a 40% lifetime risk for lobular breast cancer. The youngest reported case of gastric cancer is 14 years with a median age at diagnosis of 38 years. Intensified surveillance with upper endoscopy and breast mammography with MRI is recommended. Prophylactic gastrectomy may also be considered given the limitation in detecting diffuse lesions. Precancerous lesions have been detected in a small series of "prophylactic" gastrectomy specimens.

It is a challenge for healthcare providers to stay well informed of their own medical discipline, let alone to maintain a working knowledge of the advances for other specialties and rare syndromes. Working collaboratively with a clinical geneticist and genetic counselor may help to facilitate the identification of families with hereditary cancer. Although these syndromes may be considered "rare," they often go unrecognized and the opportunity for positive medical intervention for a family is lost. The first step in the identification of hereditary cancer begins with a thorough collection and evaluation of the family cancer history. Detailed reviews of many hereditary cancer syndromes can be found at http://www.genetests.org

Answer 14.7.   **The answer is C.**

Most hereditary cancer syndromes identified to date are characterized by their highly penetrant, autosomal-dominant (AD) inheritance. As such, the features of hereditary cancer are the same as other highly penetrant AD diseases. The characteristics include young age of onset, multiple primary cancers in one individual, multiple affected family members in at least two generations, diverse cancer types that are part of a known cancer syndrome, and specific pathology known to be associated with a given syndrome. A family's ethnic and religious background is important to consider. As with any genetic disease, the frequency of cancer predisposition gene mutations may vary among ethnic groups. Knowing a family's ethnic background may provide a helpful clue in deciding to pursue a given diagnosis over another. In the family presented, the Ashkenazi Jewish ancestry was not a feature or clue to their diagnosis. Although *BRCA1* and *BRCA2* gene mutations occur more commonly among Jewish families, E-cadherin gene mutations do not. In contrast, the pathology of the breast and gastric cancers proved invaluable in the syndrome identification of this family. The HDGC syndrome is associated with lobular breast cancer and diffuse gastric cancer. Consider whether the family had reported only a history of breast and gastric cancer with no specific pathology details. The differential diagnoses would have expanded to include BRCA1 and BRCA2 cancer syndromes and HNPCC syndrome. Knowing the histopathologic features allowed for a direct diagnosis to be made in this family. The use of tumor pathology to identify hereditary disease is quickly evolving.

Answer 14.8.   **The answer is A.**

BSO in BRCA carriers is the most effective procedure to reduce the risk of ovarian cancer and is generally recommended upon completion of child-bearing. BSO also decreases the risk of subsequent breast cancer.

Answer 14.9.   **The answer is B.**

Missense variants result in the substitution of one amino acid for another. These variants occur frequently in the *BRCA1* and *BRCA2* genes. The functional significance cannot be determined with gene sequencing alone. Functional analysis of the BRCA1 and BRCA2 proteins is not available. Angela has a 50% probability to have the *BRCA2* gene variant, but because the functional significance is unknown, testing Angela does not provide any clinically relevant information for her. Furthermore, because Angela has not been diagnosed with cancer, genetic analysis does not provide any new information to clarify Jennifer's test results. If Angela had been diagnosed with early-onset breast cancer, then analysis for the *BRCA2* gene variant would have been offered for research purposes only to help determine whether the variant is tracking with disease in the family.

For this family, genetic testing did not provide any new information to facilitate their medical decision making. Individuals with these types of gene variants are often left intellectually and emotionally frustrated by the testing. Imagine deciding to pursue expensive genetic testing with the intention of using the results to guide your personal and family medical care only to learn the testing provides no clear answer. As clinical genetic testing quickly becomes available following gene discovery, clinicians must contend with the identification of variants of unknown functional significance. The development of functional, rather than descriptive, testing will help to address this challenging clinical issue. Until such techniques are developed, it is important to inform individuals of the possibility of identifying these types of variants of unknown before the initiation of genetic testing.

Answer 14.10.   **The answer is C.**

Breast cancer in BRCA2 carriers is usually ER positive and these patients are at risk of developing second primaries, with the risk decreasing to less than 10% after prophylactic bilateral mastectomy. Treatment with tamoxifen decreases the risk of contralateral breast cancer in BRCA2 carriers.

Answer 14.11.   **The answer is C.**

Pauline's testing is uninformative because the underlying genetic basis for cancer predisposition has not yet been identified in her family. When possible, genetic testing should always begin with an affected family member. In essence, when evaluating a family with genetic disease, testing should begin with the person who expresses features of the inherited condition. In the case of hereditary cancer syndromes, expression is defined as a person who is diagnosed with one of the associated malignancies or benign lesions. If Pauline's sister undergoes clinical *BRCA1* and *BRCA2* genetic testing, then these results may change the interpretation of Pauline's testing. For example, if Pauline's sister's testing is positive for a mutation, then Pauline's testing would be interpreted as a true negative. If Pauline's sister's testing is negative, then Pauline's testing was of no clinical value because the basis for disease remains unknown. Without prior knowledge of the family's gene mutation, Pauline's negative testing may have provided a false and dangerous sense of security.

Answer 14.12.   **The answer is D.**

The underlying genetic basis for cancer predisposition remains unknown. Even though Pauline had negative genetic testing, it is not known whether she inherited the disease causing gene mutation. As such, Pauline, and her paternal family members, should continue to be considered at high risk and followed accordingly. The clinician must return to the family cancer history to determine her medical follow-up. The family history is consistent with the clinical diagnosis of either the hereditary BRCA1 or BRCA2 syndrome. Pauline should follow the same recommendations as families with a confirmed diagnosis of one of these syndromes, until genetic testing proves informative for her family. Intensified surveillance with mammography and breast MRI screening, beginning by 25 years of age, is recommended. In studies of individuals with an increased breast cancer risk, the combination of mammography and breast MRI proved to be more effective in identifying abnormal breast lesions than mammography alone. The combination of mammography and breast ultrasound for women with an increased breast cancer risk is still under investigation.

In a 1997 study published by Giradello and colleagues in the *New England Journal of Medicine,* approximately one-third of all ordering physicians misinterpreted the results of *APC* gene testing. The majority of errors arose as physicians misinterpreted a negative test result when the genetic basis for disease had not previously been established in a given family. Ongoing genetics education is needed for practitioners who assume the genetics care and testing of families with hereditary disease.

Answer 14.13.   **The answer is B.**

HNPCC (also known as Lynch syndrome) is primarily associated with a high risk for colon and endometrial cancer and an increased risk for other tumors including ovary, stomach, small intestine, hepatobiliary tract, urinary tract, brain, and skin. Cervical cancer is not one of the known associated cancer types. The life time risk for colon cancer is estimated to range from 60–80% and for uterine cancer as high as 60% lifetime risk.

Answer 14.14.   **The answer is D.**

Peutz-Jeghers syndrome is characterized by the association of hyperpigmented macules, increased cancer risk, and gastrointestinal polyposis. Blue/black macules may be found around the mouth, buccal mucosa, nostrils, eyes, and fingertips. These lesions may fade over time. Hamartomatous polyps (Peutz-Jeghers type) most commonly occur in the small bowel but can also develop in the colon or the stomach. Recurrent obstruction and intussusception may occur. Individuals with Peutz-Jeghers syndrome are at increased risk for various tumors, including breast, colorectal, ovarian, gastric, and pancreatic cancers. Affected females are also at increased risk for adenoma malignum of the cervix and a benign ovarian tumor, sex cord tumors with annular tubules (SCTAT). Peutz-Jeghers syndrome results from mutations in the *STK11* gene found on chromosome 19. The Peutz-Jeghers syndrome serves as an example of the importance of a detailed physical examination, in combination with the family cancer history, to identify individuals with a hereditary cancer syndrome. Other physical features that provide important diagnostic clues include the mucosal neuromas of the lips and tongue in the multiple endocrine neoplasia syndrome type 2B, trichilemmomas or papillomatous lesions in the Cowden syndrome, and sebaceous adenomas in the Muir-Torre syndrome.

CHAPTER 15 ADVANCES IN DIAGNOSTICS AND INTERVENTION

SANJEEV BHALLA • CYLEN JAVIDAN-NEJAD

DIRECTIONS   Each of the numbered items below is followed by lettered answers. Select the ONE lettered answer that is BEST in each case unless instructed otherwise.

QUESTIONS

Question 15.1.   Which of the following statements regarding the use of tumor markers in colorectal cancer is TRUE?

A. Patients with KRAS mutations in codons 12 or 13 should not receive anti-EGFR antibody therapy.
B. CEA is recommended as a screening for colorectal cancer.
C. CEA has limited utility in the surveillance of resected colorectal cancer.
D. Microsatellite instability (MSI) predicts efficacy of adjuvant chemotherapy in colorectal cancer.

Question 15.2.   Tissue expression of CDX2 is characteristic of which malignancy?

A. Ovarian cancer
B. Lung cancer
C. Colon cancer
D. None of the above

Question 15.3.   Patient with deficiency in UDP glucuronosyltransferase 1A1 (*UGT1A1*) have increased risk for toxicity from which chemotherapy drug?

A. Irinotecan
B. 5-Fluorouracil
C. Capecitabine
D. B and C

Corresponding Chapters in *Cancer: Principles & Practice of Oncology*, Ninth Edition: 64 (Vascular Access and Specialized Techniques), 65 (Interventional Radiology), 66 (Functional Imaging), 67 (Molecular Imaging), 68 (Photodynamic Therapy), and 69 (Biomarkers).

Question 15.4.   **Which of the following statements regarding catheter complications is NOT true?**

A. Infection is the most common cause of catheter loss.
B. Tunneled catheters with externalized hubs are less likely to develop infection than implanted subcutaneous devices.
C. The most common pathogen in catheter-associated bacteremia is a coagulase-negative staphylococci.
D. Catheter salvage is possible with several weeks of antibiotics.

Question 15.5.   **Which of the following is an indication for infected catheter removal?**

A. Inability to clear the infection with antibiotic therapy.
B. Continued signs and symptoms of bacteremia.
C. Recurrent infection after completion of a full course of antibiotics.
D. All the above.

Question 15.6.   **Regarding percutaneous ablation of pulmonary tumors, which is NOT true?**

A. Currently reserved for patients whose operative risk is too high.
B. Performed under conscious sedation.
C. Efficacy is based on size and location of the lesion.
D. Most common complication is pulmonary hemorrhage.

Question 15.7.   **Regarding percutaneous abdominal and pelvic biopsies, which is NOT true?**

A. Pneumothorax is a well-known potential complication of adrenal biopsies.
B. Liver biopsies may need a core biopsy to distinguish well-differentiated neoplasms from benign lesions.
C. Fewer complications are sustained from crossing the transverse colon than the inferior vena cava (IVC) when performing pancreatic biopsies.
D. Pelvic percutaneous biopsies are the preferred technique when ovarian cancer leads the differential diagnosis.
E. Pelvic sarcomas often require core biopsies.

Question 15.8.   **Regarding percutaneous gastrostomy tubes, which is NOT true?**

A. Requires less sedation than endoscopy-placed feeding tube.
B. May be placed for feeding or decompression.
C. Contraindicated in patients with prior gastrectomy.
D. Contraindicated in patients with ascites.
E. If in place more than 4 weeks, no imaging guidance is required to reinsert the tube if it falls out.

Question 15.9.   Regarding percutaneous nephrostomy, which is NOT true?

    A. Treatment of pyonephrosis
    B. Useful for diverting urine proximally from a genitourinary fistula
    C. Requires preprocedural antibiotics
    D. Requires CT guidance to access the kidneys

Question 15.10.   Regarding biliary procedures, which is NOT true?

    A. High strictures are usually treated by interventional radiology, and low strictures are usually treated by gastroenterology.
    B. The right biliary system is more likely to have isolated dilated segments from a central mass.
    C. Biliary dilatation is the major indication for intervention.
    D. Pruritus can be cured by draining just one segment.
    E. Cholangitis may require multiple catheters to cure sepsis.

Question 15.11.   Regarding percutaneous transhepatic biliary drainage, which is NOT true?

    A. Preprocedural antibiotics are required.
    B. Drainage is usually via a two-staged procedure: external drainage then internal drainage.
    C. High biliary outputs warrant nutritional replenishment.
    D. Contrast is usually used.
    E. Liver function usually takes weeks to return to normal.

Question 15.12.   Regarding percutaneous cholecystostomy, which is NOT true?

    A. May be a diagnostic tool in unexplained sepsis.
    B. May be a therapeutic tool in acute cholecystitis.
    C. A transhepatic approach is preferred.
    D. Distension of the gallbladder during cholecystography is avoided in the acute setting.
    E. It usually avoids a future cholecystectomy.

Question 15.13.   Regarding malignant pleural effusions, which is TRUE?

    A. Surgical pleurodesis offers a higher success rate in their management than chemical pleurodesis.
    B. Usually transudates from tumor obstruction
    C. Usually asymptomatic
    D. Thoracentesis is the definitive treatment.
    E. Large-bore tubes are better than small-bore catheters in their management.

Question 15.14. **Regarding superior vena cava (SVC) obstruction, which is NOT true?**

   A. Occlusion is a common consequence of thoracic malignancy.
   B. Collateral vessels predispose to hemorrhage and require embolization.
   C. Radiographic occlusion may be asymptomatic.
   D. Angioplasty with stenting is better than radiation therapy for immediate symptomatic relief.
   E. Recurrent obstruction may be treated with thrombolysis, balloon angioplasty, or repeat stenting.

Question 15.15. **Which is NOT an indication for an inferior vena cava (IVC) filter?**

   A. History of recurrent gastrointestinal hemorrhage
   B. Recurrent venous thrombus despite anticoagulation
   C. Propagating lower-extremity thrombus
   D. Eccentric mural thrombus in IVC
   E. Planned surgery

Question 15.16. **Regarding IVC filters, which is TRUE?**

   A. Femoral approach is preferred for their deployment.
   B. Symptomatic caval thrombosis is a fairly rare complication.
   C. It is permanent.
   D. Jugular approach requires the patient to lie flat for 6 hours.
   E. There is no role for inferior vena cavogram before deployment.

Question 15.17. **With respect to recurrent ascites, which is NOT true?**

   A. Transjugular intrahepatic portosystemic shunt (TIPS) has been used to control ascites from portal hypertension.
   B. TIPS is contraindicated in patients with hepatic encephalopathy.
   C. Peritoneovenous shunting is an effective method of dealing with malignant ascites.
   D. TIPS is more beneficial in dealing with ascites from portal hypertension than medical management alone.
   E. Large-volume paracentesis is an effective method for obtaining symptomatic relief from malignant ascites.

Question 15.18. **Regarding percutaneous abscess drainage, which is TRUE?**

   A. Urinomas are readily distinguished from abscesses with routine imaging.
   B. Transbowel approach is an acceptable route of drainage.
   C. Bilomas do not require drainage because they are sterile.
   D. Pancreatic leaks may be suspected because of high amylase.
   E. Small bowel leaks require surgical intervention.

Question 15.19.   **Regarding concepts of hepatic embolization, which is NOT true?**

    A. Coils provide an effective hepatic embolization technique.

    B. The hepatic artery provides greater blood supply to hepatic tumors than the portal vein.

    C. Hypervascular lesions are more sensitive to ischemia than hypovascular lesions.

    D. For neuroendocrine tumors, therapy is often aimed at symptomatic relief.

    E. Postembolization symptoms are often self-limited.

Question 15.20.   **Regarding transarterial chemoembolization for patients with hepatocellular carcinoma, which of the following is NOT an absolute contraindication?**

    A. Child-Pugh C cirrhosis

    B. Total bilirubin of 5 mg/dL

    C. Mild encephalopathy

    D. Poor performance status

    E. radiofrequency ablation (RFA) AND alcohol injection ablation (PEI) are usually reserved for larger tumors (>7cm)

Question 15.21.   **Regarding the variety of imaging modalities, which is NOT true?**

    A. Bone magnetic resonance imaging (MRI) has essentially replaced radiography for the evaluation of osseous lesions.

    B. Sonography may be used for the evaluation of chest lesions.

    C. Multidetector computed tomography (MDCT) has resulted in improved temporal resolution in cross-sectional imaging.

    D. MRI has the advantage of functional analysis.

    E. Both MDCT and MRI allow for high-quality multiplanar imaging.

Question 15.22.   **Regarding nuclear medicine studies, which is TRUE?**

    A. Increased number of images results in increased radiation dose.

    B. Bone scintigraphy is a good screening for bone metastases from prostate cancer when the prostate-specific antigen (PSA) is less than 5.

    C. Sentinel node mapping is of no value in the staging of melanoma.

    D. Positron emission tomography (PET)/CT relies on spiral CT for its attenuation correction.

    E. Single-photon emission computed tomography relies on injection of fluorodeoxyglucose (FDG) for diagnosis.

Question 15.23.   Regarding therapeutic response assessment, which is TRUE?

    A. There are three categories of response: complete response, partial response, and disease progression.

    B. Response Evaluation Criteria in Solid Tumors (RECIST) rely on bidirectional measurements.

    C. Partial response represents less than 25% reduction in the sum of the tumor cross-products.

    D. One shortcoming of the RECIST is the lack of inclusion of bone marrow involvement by neoplasm.

    E. There is no role in using perfusion techniques to assess tumor response.

Question 15.24.   Regarding brain neoplasms, which is TRUE?

    A. Cross-sectional imaging is a highly specific way to distinguish recurrent tumor from radiation change.

    B. MRI with contrast is superior to CT for the evaluation of sellar lesions.

    C. CT plays no role in the presurgical evaluation when high-quality MRI is used.

    D. Because of high spatial resolution, MRI does not require contrast to detect cerebral lesions.

    E. Functional MRI is a great way to look at the behavior of small nodules and avoid overstaging a patient.

Question 15.25.   Regarding head and neck cancers, which is TRUE?

    A. MRI is favored over CT when the lesion is in the upper aerodigestive tract near the skull base.

    B. Neck CT with intravenous contrast is better than endoscopy in the evaluation of small mucosal lesions of the aerodigestive tract.

    C. There is no role for PET/CT in head and neck cancers because intravenous contrast material is not used.

    D. CT does not delineate bone involvement in paranasal sinus tumors.

Question 15.26.   Regarding lung cancer, which is TRUE?

    A. Chest radiography screening results in improved mortality.

    B. CT screening further improves mortality because smaller lesions are detected.

    C. MDCT can accurately predict chest wall or mediastinal invasion in greater than 95% of patients.

    D. MRI is useful in the evaluation of superior sulcus tumors.

    E. PET/CT obviates the need for any additional imaging in the staging of clinically suspected metastatic non-small cell lung cancer.

Question 15.27.   **Regarding lung cancer treatment planning, which is TRUE?**

   A. Adrenal lesion biopsy is no longer needed in the era of MRI and MDCT.
   B. Routine imaging of the brain and bone in the absence of clinical suspicion of metastases is unwarranted.
   C. CT of the chest requires intravenous contrast to exclude adrenal metastases.
   D. Liver should be imaged in its entirety on an initial staging CT because of the high incidence of liver metastases.

Question 15.28.   **Regarding lymphoma, which is TRUE?**

   A. Lymphangiography remains a highly sensitive and specific way to evaluate portal and mesenteric lymphadenopathy.
   B. CT is an effective way to evaluate bone marrow involvement.
   C. Routine MRI is equally as sensitive as CT for detection of lymphadenopathy in the chest, abdomen, or pelvis.
   D. Gallium scintigraphy is better than PET in the detection of lymphadenopathy from lymphoma.
   E. The added sensitivity of PET is its ability to adequately characterize bone marrow involvement by lymphoma.

Question 15.29.   **Regarding breast cancer, which is TRUE?**

   A. Annual screening mammography should begin at age 50 years.
   B. There is no role for early screening in high-risk patients.
   C. Calcium is an indication of benign disease.
   D. Final assessment on mammography is based on likelihood of malignancy.
   E. Percutaneous biopsy of a potential cancer is contraindicated for fear of seeding the needle tract.

Question 15.30.   **Regarding nonmammographic breast imaging, which is TRUE?**

   A. Sonography is not useful for the evaluation of dense breasts.
   B. To distinguish cysts from solid masses, sonography should be used as a first-line tool.
   C. Because of breast geometry, sonography cannot be used for needle biopsy guidance.
   D. MRI is limited because of the inability to have MRI-guided biopsies.

Question 15.31.   **Regarding breast cancer staging, which is NOT true?**

   A. Lymphoscintigraphy is useful for the staging of large breast cancers (>5 cm).
   B. Disease greater than one quadrant is known as multicentric disease.
   C. More than one focus of disease in the same quadrant is known as multifocal disease.
   D. Sonography is limited in the detection of depicting carcinoma in situ.
   E. MRI is useful in the detection of infiltrating lobular cancer.

Question 15.32.   **Regarding breast MRI, which is TRUE?**

    A. Not useful in the postoperative breast.
    B. More specific than sensitive in neoplasm detection.
    C. Intravenous contrast is not needed.
    D. Obviates need for biopsy.
    E. Impact on mortality has yet to be determined.

Question 15.33.   **Regarding colorectal cancer, which is TRUE?**

    A. CT colography is limited by reliance on intravenous contrast.
    B. Transrectal ultrasound (TRUS) is a useful way of evaluating the entire colon.
    C. MDCT is an accurate way to evaluate the bowel wall tumor extension.
    D. MRI is better than CT in the evaluation of distant metastasis.
    E. MRI is a more sensitive way to assess localized disease extension than MDCT.

Question 15.34.   **Regarding gynecologic malignancies, which is TRUE?**

    A. Transabdominal ultrasound is the first step in staging endometrial cancer.
    B. CT is limited in the assessment of localized extension of cervical cancer.
    C. MRI is more sensitive than MDCT for detecting myometrial invasion of cervical cancer.
    D. MRI is much better than MDCT in detecting lymphadenopathy from gynecologic malignancies.

Question 15.35.   **Regarding cervical cancer, which is TRUE?**

    A. Ultrasound is a highly effective way to stage cervical cancer.
    B. MRI is a more effective technique for evaluating parametrial invasion than CT.
    C. CT is an effective staging tool for localized disease.
    D. No role for PET in the staging of cervical cancer.

Question 15.36.   **Regarding ovarian cancer, which is NOT true?**

    A. Ultrasound is an effective method for distinguishing ovarian from uterine lesions.
    B. MRI is superior to ultrasound in determining whether an adnexal lesion is malignant.
    C. CT and MRI are better than ultrasound for the detection of peritoneal disease.
    D. MRI is better than CT for detection of lymphadenopathy from ovarian cancer.

Question 15.37.   **Regarding prostate cancer, which is TRUE?**

    A. Imaging is key in its early detection.

    B. MDCT is a useful way to localize a biopsy site.

    C. CT is not useful for the detection of distant nodal disease.

    D. The role of MRI is to determine whether the cancer is confined to the prostate.

    E. The main role of MR spectroscopy is to determine whether a prostate nodule is malignant.

ANSWERS

Answer 15.1.   **The answer is A.**

Patients with KRAS mutation in codons 12 or 13 have low probability of achieving benefit from anti-EGFR antibodies and should not receive these drugs. CEA is not recommended in the screening of colorectal cancer but is valuable in the postsurgical surveillance and for monitoring metastatic disease during systemic therapy. MSI is not recommended to determine the prognosis or efficacy from adjuvant chemotherapy.

Answer 15.2.   **The answer is C.**

The presence of tissue CDX2 suggests the diagnosis of colon cancer.

Answer 15.3.   **The answer is A.**

Patients with *UGTA1A* deficiency are unable to metabolize irinotecan with increased risk for significant toxicity. The risk of toxicity from 5-fluorouracil or capecitabine is increased in patients with dihydropyrimidine dehydrogenase deficiency.

Answer 15.4.   **The answer is B.**

Infection is significantly more common in tunneled catheters with externalized hubs than in implanted subcutaneous devices.

Answer 15.5.   **The answer is D.**

Inability to clear the infection with antibiotic therapy, continued bacteremia, and recurrent infection after treatment completion are all indications for catheter removal.

Answer 15.6.   **The answer is D.**

Percutaneous thermal ablation of lung cancer is a relatively new technique that uses CT guidance to place a probe within a lung neoplasm. This probe is then used to deliver targeted thermal therapy. Studies are under way to determine how this technique compares with more well-established therapies. The procedure is performed under conscious sedation and can usually be completed within 1 hour. Efficacy is predominantly based on the volume of the lesion and the location. Accessible lesions less than 3 cm are likely to completely respond. Complications include hemorrhage, infection, and pneumothorax. The first two are unusual if sterile technique is used and any coagulopathy is corrected before beginning. Pneumothorax may be seen in 25% to 40% of patients undergoing ablation.

Answer 15.7.   **The answer is C.**

As with lung biopsies, preprocedural imaging is important in determining the route of approach and type of needles to be used for percutaneous abdominal and pelvic biopsies. Certain organs, because of their most common locations, are associated with certain complications. The adrenal gland is one such organ. Because of its cranial location in the retroperitoneum, percutaneous biopsy may lead to pneumothorax. The pancreas is another such organ. It is often surrounded by bowel, precluding an unobstructed approach to a pancreatic mass. In such cases, a transcaval approach is preferred. The differential diagnosis from any preprocedural imaging will also dictate biopsy technique. Although liver masses may represent well-differentiated neoplasm (e.g., fibrolamellar HCC), core biopsies are required to distinguish them from normal liver or benign lesions, such as focal nodular hyperplasia. Core biopsies are also valuable in diagnosing histology or retroperitoneal and pelvic masses that may be sarcomas. When ovarian cancer heads the differential diagnosis, alternatives to percutaneous biopsy should be sought. High risk of tract and peritoneal seeding make an open procedure the favored route of tissue sampling.

Answer 15.8.   **The answer is D.**

Percutaneous gastrostomy (also known as g-tube) is an alternative to an endoscopically placed gastrostomy tube that has gained acceptance as a method of providing nutrition or gastric decompression. It can be placed quickly with less sedation than required for its endoscopic counterpart. Percutaneous placement can be via a pull technique, where the catheter is advanced into the stomach and a snare is used to retrieve it through the skin, or in a push technique, where the catheter is pushed externally into the stomach via a tract that is serially dilated. The former method may allow for larger catheters to be placed, but the latter method may result in less seeding of the tract in aerodigestive malignancies. Contraindications to the percutaneous technique include uncorrectable coagulopathy, gastric varices, and previous gastrectomy. Ascites may hinder endoscopic placement because of the increased distance of stomach to skin and therefore decreased effectiveness of gastric transillumination. It is not a contraindication for percutaneous placement. The presence of ascites may require gastropexy, whereby the stomach is affixed to the abdominal wall. When gastropexy has been performed or after a tract has been established (usually after 4 weeks of a gastrostomy tube in place), catheter replacement may be performed without image guidance.

Answer 15.9.   **The answer is D.**

Percutaneous nephrostomy (referred to informally as a "perc" or "PCN") is a way of percutaneously draining a kidney that is usually hydronephrotic. Preprocedural imaging is key to identifying the site of obstruction and relevant information regarding the collecting system. It is performed as a way to treat an infected, hydronephrotic kidney (pyonephrosis), divert urine away from a fistula, or preserve renal function if the obstruction is temporary or treatable. Percutaneous nephrostomies are usually performed from a posterior or flank approach with fluoroscopic or ultrasound guidance and do not require CT guidance. Preprocedural antibiotics are used that target skin organisms to prevent infection from the procedure itself. Postprocedural antibiotics depend on the quality of the urine aspirated at the time of the procedure.

Answer 15.10.   **The answer is C.**

Hepatobiliary drainage is one of the main procedures in most interventional radiology suites today. Bile duct obstructions can be divided into high and low obstructions, an important distinction because the former are usually referred to interventional radiologists and the latter are usually treated endoscopically by gastroenterologists. Dilation of isolated segments or isolated bile ducts occur when the duct is obstructed and no longer is communicating with the other ducts. These, too, usually fall to interventional radiologists for treatment. Because the right duct is shorter than the left, isolated right segmental biliary dilatation is more common than isolated left segments from a central mass. Percutaneous drains can only drain a portion of the liver, but that may be all that is required to cure pruritus. For an infected biliary tree (cholangitis), multiple catheters may be required to cure sepsis. Because catheters may be in place for a long time and the remainder of a terminally ill patient's life, percutaneous drainage should be reserved for patients who are symptomatic or in whom clear benefit will be obtained. Biliary dilatation on its own is not an indication for drainage.

Answer 15.11.   **The answer is E.**

Patients who are scheduled to undergo percutaneous biliary drainage receive prophylactic antibiotics targeting skin flora to avoid infection from the procedure. First, percutaneous transhepatic cholangiography is performed to provide information about the biliary tree. This step provides invaluable information regarding the nature of an obstruction. Drainage is usually done as a two-step procedure. First, an external drain is used to cross a level of obstruction. If the patient can tolerate this catheter with side holes proximal and distal to the obstruction without any external drainage, the catheter is converted to an internal one. When external outputs are high, oral replenishment of electrolytes may be required. In a majority of patients, drainage can result in rapid recovery of hepatic function with decrease in liver enzymes and bilirubin.

Answer 15.12.   **The answer is E.**

Percutaneous cholecystostomy is a safe procedure in the treatment of acute cholecystitis (calculus or acalculous) in patients who are unable to undergo cholecystectomy. Because of its few complications, percutaneous cholecystostomy can be a useful diagnostic tool in patients with sepsis of unknown cause. Ultrasound or CT is used for needle guidance. A transhepatic route is usually preferred to minimize intraperitoneal leakage and subsequent bile peritonitis. Although cholecystography can be a useful diagnostic tool, distension of the gallbladder in the acute setting is avoided to prevent rupture. In a majority of patients, the catheter will be left in place until the patient's condition improves, the tract is established (2 to 4 weeks), and the tube can be removed. In others, the tube will be left in place until the time of definitive treatment, which is usually a cholecystectomy. In certain high-risk patients, percutaneous stone removal can be performed via the cholecystostomy. Recurrent disease may be found in up to 50% of these patients within 5 years. This conservative approach is often reserved for patients with limited life expectancy. Most patients will undergo a future cholecystectomy after the acute illness has resolved because of the high incidence of recurrence of cholecystitis.

Answer 15.13.   **The answer is A.**

Malignant pleural effusions are a common cause of chest pain, dyspnea, and cough in patients with metastatic cancer, usually breast carcinoma, lung carcinoma, and lymphoma. These effusions are usually symptomatic and exudative. Thoracentesis will result in immediate relief of symptoms, but the majority of these effusions will recur. Definitive treatment requires tube drainage at first, which may be better accomplished via image guidance so that the tube rests in the location of the majority of the fluid. This is particularly true when the amount of fluid is small or the effusion is loculated. Although surgical teaching suggests large-bore catheters are required for successful drainage, recent data suggest that smaller bore catheters are equally as effective and may be associated with less pain and restriction of mobility. A majority of patients will not be adequately treated with chest tube drainage alone. In these patients, pleurodesis is performed to give better long-term results. Mechanical pleurodesis can be performed at surgery (usually video-assisted thoracoscopic surgery) and offers a slightly higher success rate than chemical pleurodesis (which relies on a sclerosing agent such as talc, doxycycline, or bleomycin). Although hospital stays are shorter with surgical pleurodesis, chemical pleurodesis is less invasive and expensive, and has a lower morbidity. Another approach currently under investigation is the use of a long-term tunneled chest tube drainage catheter. Drainage can be performed in an outpatient setting. In this group, mechanical pleurodesis may be achieved in up to 50% of patients in 30 days.

Answer 15.14.   **The answer is B.**

SVC obstruction is a fairly common consequence of thoracic malignancy, usually lung cancer. Radiographic SVC occlusion is often asymptomatic secondary to collateral formation throughout the mediastinum with diversion of blood to the azygous or IVC systems. These patients do not warrant any treatment. In others, no collateral vessels have formed, resulting in symptoms of head and neck swelling, headache, and mental status changes. In these symptomatic patients, radiation may be beneficial when the tumors are radiosensitive. This form of therapy usually works but may require therapy over weeks with symptomatic relief over days. An alternative therapy is balloon angioplasty with stent deployment. This technique (if the obstruction can be crossed intravascularly) results in immediate symptomatic relief. Recurrent symptoms may follow stent deployment and are usually related to tumor overgrowth, neointimal hyperplasia, and rarely stent migration. Recurrent occlusion may be treated with thrombolysis, angioplasty, or repeat stenting.

Answer 15.15.   **The answer is D.**

The incidence of pulmonary embolism in cancer is three times that in the general population. The first-line treatment of pulmonary embolism or deep venous thrombosis is systemic anticoagulation. In patients in whom anticoagulation is contraindicated (brain metastases, gastrointestinal hemorrhage), an IVC interruption filter should be considered. An IVC filter is also warranted when a deep venous thrombus continues to propagate or emboli continue to be observed despite anticoagulation or if surgery is planned. Free-floating clots within the IVC or a deep vein is also another relative indication for a filter because these types of thrombi tend to embolize. Eccentric, mural thrombi are usually chronic and less likely to embolize. Their presence alone would initially warrant systemic anticoagulation.

Answer 15.16. **The answer is B.**

IVC filters can be deployed by a femoral or jugular approach. The latter is preferred because of a decreased chance of dislodging a clot in a deep femoral vein or the IVC, the ability to place a simultaneous venous line if needed, and the ability of the patient to sit upright in bed after the procedure. A femoral approach requires the patient to lie flat in bed for 4 hours after the procedure, which is less comfortable. The predeployment cavogram is important in excluding any congenital anomalies or IVC thrombus that may alter the site of deployment. Therefore, intravenous contrast is usually used for IVC filter placement. Complications of IVC filter placement are fairly uncommon and include symptomatic IVC thrombosis. Recent work suggests that this may be seen in less than 3% of patients with IVC filters. A retrievable filter was recently approved for use in the United States. This filter can be left in place, however, if the need for it persists.

Answer 15.17. **The answer is C.**

Ascites is a common association with malignancy, from either malignant peritoneal deposits or end-stage liver disease. In the latter group, refractory ascites may be managed by a portal vein bypass in the form of a percutaneous shunt known as a TIPS. In this procedure, a stent is placed in the liver from the portal vein to the hepatic vein. Portal pressures are reduced and ascites resolves. Although TIPS has gained in its use in patients with portal hypertension, certain patients are not TIPS candidates: Those with congestive heart failure and preexisting hepatic encephalopathy, because the TIPS can exacerbate these underlying conditions. TIPS has been shown to be superior to medical therapy alone in patients with ascites. In patients with malignant ascites, large-volume paracentesis is the most common means of managing their condition. Although this technique allows for immediate, symptomatic relief, it is rarely definitive, and repeat treatments with all their associated risks are often required. Long-term catheters have been used with some degree of success. Another alternative is a peritoneovenous shunt (e.g., a Denver shunt). Their role in the management of malignant ascites remains unclear.

Answer 15.18. **The answer is D.**

Percutaneous techniques have dramatically changed the way postoperative abdominal fluid collections are managed. A majority can be drained without the need for reoperation. Postoperative leaks may result from urine leaks, bile leaks, bowel leaks, pancreatic leaks, or lymphatic obstruction. These may warrant drainage if infection is suspected, leak is suspected, mass effect is symptomatic, or the fluid requires further characterization. Cross-sectional imaging has made tremendous strides with recent advances in CT but does not always allow for adequate characterization of fluid collections with standard protocols. An example is a urinoma, which may be overlooked unless delayed images are obtained, and small bowel leaks, which may be confused with ascites if oral contrast is not administered. Bilomas can be another confusing fluid collection, which may be suspected in patients with a history of hepatobiliary surgery. Because of communication with the bowel via the bile ducts, these fluid collections can lead to peritonitis and should be drained. Pancreatic leaks should be suspected when the amylase is elevated (three to five times serum levels).

Answer 15.19.   **The answer is A.**

Hepatic tumor embolotherapy is a promising tool for the treatment of hepatic lesions. This therapy relies on the increased reliance of tumors on hepatic arterial perfusion compared with normal liver. The result is that various agents can be used intraarterially to cause in situ tumor death. Hypervascular tumors are known to be sensitive to ischemia, which has given rise to hepatic particle embolization with very small particles. Because of their larger size, coils are not used for hepatic embolotherapy. In patients with hepatocellular carcinoma (HCC), the goal of embolization is to prolong survival. In patients with neuroendocrine tumor, the control of symptoms is the more common end point. When tumors are bulky, pain control may be the main goal of treatment. Occasionally, postembolization syndrome may be witnessed and is marked by pain, fever, nausea, and vomiting; its course is usually self-limited.

Answer 15.20.   **The answer is C.**

The main contraindications for transarterial chemoembolization are Child-Pugh C cirrhosis, uncorrectable bleeding diathesis, ECOG performance status 3, total bilirubin greater than 4 mg/dL, and significant encephalopathy.

Answer 15.21.   **The answer is A.**

Recent years have seen great advances in anatomic imaging. Among these is faster scanning techniques with MRI and faster CT. The advent of MDCT has resulted in improved temporal resolution and the ability to scan a targeted region in many phases of enhancement. The improved spatial resolution of MDCT has resulted in improved reconstructions in both coronal and sagittal plains. Although acquired axially, these images can rival MRI in their depiction of complex nonaxial anatomy. MRI remains superior to CT in its ability to create functional images (spectroscopy, perfusion, and cine images). Ultrasound also has seen dramatic improvements with better probes and more sophisticated techniques of scanning (tissue harmonics, extended field of view). Although not traditionally used for thoracic imaging because of the air interface with normal lung, sonography may be useful for needle guidance in thoracentesis and peripheral lung lesion biopsy. Occasionally, a mass can be characterized by sonography by use of color Doppler. With all of the recent advances, it would be tempting to discount the role of conventional radiography. One area in which plain films are still of great value is bone radiography. The high spatial resolution of bone films allows for lesion characterization that is complementary to MRI. At Washington University, no bone MRI is interpreted without a comparison radiograph. Lack of a comparison bone film may result in benign disease being confused with malignancy.

Answer 15.22.   **The answer is D.**

Nuclear medicine studies are a form of molecular imaging that have been around for a while but continue to occupy an important role in staging and diagnosis. This has become even more true in the era of PET and PET/CT. Nuclear medicine studies rely on the administration of biologically active material (usually injected). Images are then obtained to document the biodistribution of the material. Although resolution of the images is somewhat limited, when viewed in conjunction with anatomic imaging, the studies can be enormously powerful. Because radioactivity is with the agent that is administered, radiation dose is completely independent of the number of images obtained, unlike CT, which increases the radiation dose with increased number of images. Bone scintigraphy represents one of the older techniques in which a tracer is injected that is taken up by osteoblasts. Tumors with a predisposition to osseous metastases are well imaged by this technique. However, it is very sensitive but not very specific, because any process resulting in increased bone turnover will result in increased tracer uptake. As a result, bone scintigraphy should be reserved for instances in which there is a reasonable likelihood of osseous metastasis. For example, in prostate cancer, a bone scan is recommended when serum PSA levels are greater than 10. Another technique that has been in use for a few years is sentinel node mapping. In this technique, radiotracer is injected into a tumor and the lymph node drainage pattern is mapped. The first or sentinel node that is seen can then be biopsied. This technique is useful when lymph node drainage patterns are unpredictable, such as melanoma or breast cancer. A recent major advance in nuclear medicine has been the increased use of PET in the diagnosis and staging of various tumors. PET relies on the injection of a radiotracer (currently, usually FDG), which is taken up by metabolically active tissues. These tissues may represent infection, inflammation, or neoplasm. When combined with CT (PET/CT), this has become a powerful tool in neoplasm detection and characterization. A major pitfall of anatomic imaging is that it relies on an abnormal mass or abnormal size of a normal structure before pathology is appreciated. PET/CT allows for normal-sized structures (e.g., lymph nodes) with disease to be imaged before they become enlarged. This has been helpful in accurately staging many different types of tumors. The advantage of using a simultaneous CT for attenuation correction is that areas of increased uptake can be more accurately localized. Another major advantage is that by using spiral CT for the transmission scan for attenuation correction, the entire process has become faster, which has resulted in improved patient satisfaction and throughput.

Answer 15.23.   **The answer is D.**

A major role of imaging in oncology is to determine the effect of therapy on the clinical behavior of a tumor. To that end, a new study may show complete response to therapy, partial response (defined as >50% reduction in the sum of tumor cross products), and stability or progression (defined as 25% increase in the sum of one or more of the tumor deposits). In 1994, an attempt was made to create a more reliable method of assessing tumor response. These principles were published as the RECIST guidelines. These RECIST principles relied on the same four categories of tumor response assessment and used unidimensional measurements to quantify tumor size. RECIST also more strictly defined disease progression. Major criticism of RECIST rests on the lack of universal application of one measurement to all tumors, which may vary in shape, and the lack of inclusion of bone or marrow involvement. Newer techniques may make measurement less important in assessing tumor response to therapy. These include PET, where altered FDG metabolism may be seen as a sign of response, and rapid perfusion techniques that may measure altered tissue perfusion, which may be another early sign of tissue response.

Answer 15.24.   **The answer is B.**

Neuroimaging continues to be on the forefront of modern anatomic imaging. MRI with contrast has become the standard method for detecting and characterizing intracerebral masses. It is very helpful in diagnosing and planning surgery for brain masses, especially those near the brain stem, posterior fossa, pituitary region, and cerebellopontine angle. CT is limited in these regions secondary to beam hardening from adjacent bone. Although spatial resolution of MRI is higher than CT, intravenous contrast is still used. It can be helpful in the detection of small lesions and meningeal lesions. CT with contrast is usually reserved for patients unable to undergo MRI or in some cases in which it may help in refining a differential diagnosis by showing calcium or osseous destruction. Both techniques are limited in their ability to differentiate between tumor recurrence and radiation change. Newer techniques have recently been developed that may allow for improved performance in the MRI detection and characterization of brain lesions and in the presurgical planning. These include MR spectroscopy, perfusion, and diffusion-weighted imaging. Spectroscopy, which relies on noninvasive measurements of brain tumor metabolites, is useful in guiding biopsy. It is limited, however, in small lesions (<2 cm) and in those adjacent to bone, fat, or cerebrospinal fluid.

Answer 15.25.   **The answer is A.**

Head and neck cancers can be challenging to detect on imaging. Usually, CT or MRI is reserved once a lesion is detected by endoscopy. Endoscopy is far better than imaging for the detection of small mucosal lesions.

The role of imaging is to evaluate any extension of disease. Both CT with contrast and MRI with contrast are used for staging of head and neck cancers. The preference seems to vary by institution. For upper aerodigestive malignancies, MRI is the favored technique because of fewer artifacts from the skull base. PET/CT has become a valuable tool in the staging of head and neck cancer. Although CT with intravenous contrast is usually used initially, PET/CT with FDG but no intravenous contrast allows for a nice complement. This is particularly true in the postoperative neck, which can be confusing on routine CT or MRI. CT is usually favored when early cortical base erosion is suspected or if invasion of the orbital walls or paranasal sinus walls is the clinical question.

Answer 15.26.   **The answer is D.**

Lung cancer is the most common cancer in both men and women, and its incidence is increasing. Screening, therefore, has been a topic of a great deal of discussion. Unfortunately, studies have not demonstrated any improvement in mortality from chest radiograph screening, although lesions were detected at more favorable stages. Studies are currently under way to determine whether CT with its ability to detect smaller lesions will be any better. It is still too early to tell whether detecting smaller lesions will affect mortality from this dreaded disease. Another role of imaging lung cancer is in the staging of disease. Despite improvements in spatial resolution, CT is still limited in its ability to detect chest wall and mediastinal invasion. MRI has shown greater promise in the evaluation of tumor extension because of its improved multiplanar capability and soft-tissue resolution. This is particularly true in the superior sulcus or lung apex where MRI can delineate tumor involvement of the subclavian vessels and brachial plexus better than CT. PET/CT is also useful in the staging of lung cancer. It is better than CT alone in the detection of mediastinal lymphadenopathy and sensitive for adrenal and bone metastases. Because of its high sensitivity, PET/CT may overstage patients with non-small cell lung cancer. Because of the high glucose uptake of normal brain, PET/CT with FDG is limited for the evaluation of brain metastases. If these are suspected clinically, further imaging with MRI may be indicated.

Answer 15.27.   **The answer is B.**

Adrenal glands represent the most common site of abdominal metastases from lung cancer. For this reason, a routine chest CT should include the adrenal glands. Most adrenal nodules in patients with lung cancer will be adrenal adenomas. Because of their high lipid content, many (but not all) will be low attenuating on noncontrast CT examinations. If intravenous contrast is given, adenomas will enhance and may not be distinguishable from metastases. Many adrenal adenomas will show signal dropout on opposed phase gradient recalled echo imaging. PET may also be helpful in adrenal imaging in that metastases should have increased uptake when they are larger than 1 cm. Because of false positives with CT, PET, and MRI, any patient with isolated suspected adrenal metastasis should be biopsied to prevent false overstaging. Routine imaging of the brain, liver, and bone is not warranted in patients with lung cancer unless suspected metastasis has a clinical basis because likelihood of disease is low.

Answer 15.28. **The answer is C.**

Lymphoma is a fairly common neoplasm that has seen dramatic change in its imaging in the era of cross-sectional imaging. In the past, lymphangiography was used for evaluation of paraaortic lymphadenopathy, but its role in lymphoma imaging has been replaced by CT, MRI, and PET. CT is an efficient way to evaluate nodal and solid-organ involvement by lymphoma but is limited in the evaluation of bone marrow involvement. MRI is equally as effective as CT in the evaluation of nodal and solid-organ involvement. MRI tends to take longer, is more expensive, and often is performed in patients unable to undergo CT or who cannot receive intravenous iodinated contrast. MRI is also useful in depicting bone marrow involvement. PET is highly accurate in the staging of lymphoma and with CT fusion is better than gallium scintigraphy for the staging of lymphoma. PET is limited in evaluating bone marrow involvement by lymphoma because increased uptake can be seen diffusely in reactive bone marrow, especially after chemotherapy and marrow-stimulating drugs.

Answer 15.29. **The answer is D.**

Mammography remains the standard of care for breast cancer screening. Annual screening is recommended beginning at 40 years. High-risk patients (those with personal or strong family history of breast cancer) should consult their physician regarding initiation of screening at an earlier age. In these patients, there may be a role for screening sonography or MRI. On mammography, screening is based on the detection of a spiculated mass, architectural distortion, or microcalcifications that may be indicative of in situ carcinoma. Each mammogram has a final assessment category defined by the American College of Radiology breast imaging reporting and data system lexicon based on the likelihood of malignancy (1 = normal; 5 = highly suggestive of malignancy). This standardized reporting format has gained wide acceptance and serves as a model for other screening imaging modalities. Imaging can provide guidance for biopsy of any suspicious lesion (by ultrasound, mammography, and, most recently, MRI). Unlike with ovarian cancer, there is no fear of seeding the needle tract. Percutaneous needle biopsy is faster, safer, and less expensive than surgical biopsy. Patients undergoing percutaneous needle biopsy are more likely to be treated with a single, definitive surgery than patients undergoing surgical biopsy.

Answer 15.30. **The answer is B.**

Breast sonography is an important adjunct to mammography in the detection of breast cancer. It is especially useful in patients with dense breasts but is not standard of care in breast cancer screening. It is a great first-line tool in the evaluation of a mass to determine whether it is cystic or solid and to guide intervention. It is faster and cheaper than breast MRI. The role of MRI of the breast is currently under study. Until recently, the role of MRI in screening has been limited because of the inability to biopsy lesions that were not palpable and only seen on MRI. MRI-compatible biopsy devices have recently been developed. Studies are under way to determine the makeup of these mammographically occult, sonographically occult, and nonpalpable lesions.

Answer 15.31.   **The answer is A.**

Understanding breast cancer staging and potential therapy requires one to realize that more than one focus of breast cancer in one quadrant (multifocal disease) may warrant a wider excision and that disease in more than one quadrant (multicentric disease) may warrant mastectomy. Sonography is useful in depicting axillary adenopathy, which also affects staging, but sonography is limited in depicting carcinoma in situ. MRI is sensitive in evaluating ipsilateral and contralateral breasts in women with cancer. It is particularly useful in depicting invasive lobular carcinoma and finding an occult primary tumor in patients presenting with axillary lymphadenopathy. Nuclear medicine techniques may also be used for breast cancer staging. PET may play a role in depicting metastases and showing tumor response to therapy. Lymphoscintigraphy also has become useful for lesions less than 5 cm and in some centers is considered the standard of care. For larger lesions, the results of lymphoscintigraphy may not be reliable for sentinel node mapping.

Answer 15.32.   **The answer is E.**

As useful as breast MRI may be on a case-by-case basis, its impact on breast cancer mortality has yet to be determined. MRI is a sensitive technique that is not as specific; consequently, biopsy of detected lesions may be needed. For this reason, MRI-compatible biopsy instruments have been devised. MRI is still expensive and requires intravenous contrast for dynamic enhancement. In the postoperative breast, however, MRI can be useful in separating recurrent tumor from postoperative change.

Answer 15.33.   **The answer is E.**

Colorectal cancer is the most common gastrointestinal malignancy. As a result, many studies have been performed to determine an effective way of screening for this malignancy. MDCT has recently allowed for the propagation of CT colography, which shows early promise. This technique is relatively noninvasive and does not require intravenous contrast. In the initial staging of colorectal cancer, CT, MRI, and TRUS are all commonly used. TRUS allows for clear visualization of the layers of the bowel wall and can allow for accurate depiction of tumor penetration. TRUS does not allow for visualization of the entire colon. CT is best used for assessing metastases and lymphadenopathy. Even MDCT does not allow for differentiation of the layers of the bowel wall. MRI, because of its better soft-tissue resolution, is superior to CT for localized staging. High-resolution sequences may allow for clearer depiction of extension into adjacent fat and organs. CT and MRI have similar sensitivity and specificity for assessing nodal involvement.

Answer 15.34.   **The answer is C.**

Imaging in endometrial and cervical cancer is usually performed after a diagnosis is clinically made. The main role of imaging is to determine the depth of myometrial invasion, endocervical tumor extension and lymphadenopathy with endometrial cancer, and the extent of parametrial extension and lymphadenopathy with cervical cancer. Imaging is also performed to evaluate for distant metastases. MRI is better than CT in delineating localized invasion of both tumors. CT is limited in depicting the extent of myometrial invasion from endometrial carcinoma and the extent of parametrial invasion from cervical cancer. MRI is approximately equal to CT in delineating lymphadenopathy from gynecologic malignancy. Although transabdominal sonography is often used to investigate the pelvis, it should not be routinely performed in endometrial cancer staging. Even transvaginal ultrasound is limited because of its limited field of view and lack of soft-tissue resolution.

Answer 15.35.   **The answer is B.**

Imaging in cervical cancer is usually performed after a positive biopsy or PAP smear. The main role of imaging is to determine the extent of parametrial extension and lymphadenopathy. MRI is better than CT in delineating localized invasion. CT is limited in depicting the extent of parametrial invasion from cervical cancer. MRI is slightly better than CT in delineating lymphadenopathy from cervical cancer. Although transabdominal sonography is often used to investigate the pelvis, it should not be routinely performed in cervical cancer staging. Even transvaginal ultrasound is limited because of its limited field of view and lack of soft-tissue resolution.

Answer 15.36.   **The answer is D.**

Imaging in adnexal masses is aimed at delineating the origin of the mass (ovarian or uterine), whether a mass is malignant, and whether distant metastases are present. Ultrasound is effective at identifying the location of an adnexal tumor (bowel, ovarian, or uterine) and in distinguishing benign from malignant disease. When ultrasound is inconclusive, CT or MRI may be used. MRI is more accurate in separating malignant from benign ovarian pathology. Staging accuracy for MRI equals that of CT. Both are thought to be slightly more accurate than ultrasound, especially in the evaluation of peritoneal disease. CT is slightly better than MRI for the evaluation of lymphadenopathy. Both are equal in their depiction of hepatic metastases.

Answer 15.37.   **The answer is D.**

Digital rectal examination and serum PSA are effective means of screening for prostate cancer. Imaging plays no role in prostate cancer detection. It is useful (usually by ultrasound) for guiding biopsy. CT does not allow adequate soft tissue resolution for cancer detection in an abnormal prostate. It is useful, however, for detection of metastases. MRI, especially with an endorectal coil, provides high-quality imaging of the zones of the prostate. Its role is to determine whether the cancer is confined to the prostate. Spectroscopy is a relatively new technique that may improve tumor localization and detection of extracapsular spread. The role of spectroscopy is not in the characterization of a prostate nodule.

CHAPTER 16 DESIGN AND ANALYSIS OF CLINICAL TRIALS

FENG GAO • KATHRYN TRINKAUS

DIRECTIONS   Each of the numbered items below is followed by lettered answers. Select the ONE lettered answer that is BEST in each case unless instructed otherwise.

QUESTIONS

Question 16.1.   Which of the following is NOT true concerning a clinical trial?

A. The sample size of a clinical trial is fixed and determined before the trial begins.

B. Clinical trials are prospectively planned experiments involving human subjects.

C. A well-chosen control group provides a baseline against which to measure effects of experimental treatment.

D. Clinical trials test a clearly stated hypothesis using a predefined analysis plan.

Question 16.2.   Phase I trials on cytotoxic agents are designed to determine a dose that is appropriate for use in Phase II trials. Which of the following statements is TRUE of Phase I trials?

A. Phase I trials involve the first use of a drug, device, or procedure in humans in a new disease setting or a new combination of therapies.

B. Patients for Phase I trials are usually not chosen on the basis of their likelihood of having a favorable response to the experimental treatment.

C. Phase I trials do not require statistical justification because the sample sizes are usually small.

D. A and B.

Question 16.3.   Which of the following regarding the conventional $3 + 3$ Phase I designs is NOT true?

A. Participants are often those with end-stage disease whose treatment options have been exhausted.

B. Dose levels are usually prespecified and based on a modified Fibonacci series.

C. Cohorts of three to six patients are treated at each dose level, and the initial dose is chosen to cause little or no toxicity.

D. The optimal dose recommended for Phase II is chosen using a dose-toxicity curve generated from a statistical model fitted to the full data.

Corresponding Chapter in *Cancer: Principles & Practice of Oncology*, Ninth Edition: 70 (Design and Analysis of Clinical Trials).

Question 16.4.   Traditional Phase I trials are designed to determine a dose that is appropriate for use in Phase II trials. Which of the following statements on traditional Phase I trials are NOT true?

A. Some patients may receive subtherapeutic doses of the treatment drug.
B. A prolonged period of time may be required to complete the trial.
C. Dose escalation in the individual patient is allowed.
D. Information regarding cumulative toxicity from the study drug may be limited.

Question 16.5.   A drug, device, or other treatment may be considered for Phase II testing when:

A. The maximum tolerable dose is known but there is genuine doubt about efficacy, and patients with the condition of interest and a likely favorable outcome can be recruited as study participants.
B. A standard treatment exists for comparison.
C. Accrual is rapid enough to allow recruitment of 20 to 30 patients.
D. An appropriate control group can be recruited at the same time as the experimental group.

Question 16.6.   All of the following statements regarding Phase II trial are correct, EXCEPT:

A. Phase II trials are traditionally performed in patients with the same tumor type.
B. Two-stage designs allow for early elimination of ineffective drugs.
C. Patient eligibility should not be restricted by biomarker testing.
D. Phase II trials can help develop predictive biomarker assays for the study drug.

Question 16.7.   Phase II trials of a single agent are designed to determine whether the experimental drug has any antitumor activity against a given type of tumor, and the antitumor effect is often measured as an objective response based on tumor shrinkage. However, such a trial is not appropriate for the question of patient welfare because:

A. The welfare of patients with cancer is often measured by survival or symptom control, but there is no necessary relationship between such beneficial end points and tumor response.
B. Survival is inherently a comparative end point that should be assessed in a prognostically comparable set of patients. Unfortunately, Phase II trials are often conducted without concurrent controls.
C. Comparing the survival times of responders and nonresponders is not a valid means of showing a treatment is beneficial to patients because responders may have more favorable prognostic factors than nonresponders.
D. All of the above.

Question 16.8.   Patients in a Phase II trial are often recruited in a two-stage manner that allows a potential early stopping, thus saving patients from unnecessary exposure to inactive agents. Which of the following is NOT true of a two-stage design?

A. The optimal two-stage design minimizes the average sample size and thus optimizes the protection of patients given an inactive agent.

B. Simon's two-stage designs are often applied in Phase II trials on molecularly targeted drugs and therapeutic cancer vaccines.

C. The minimax design minimizes the total sample size. Compared with the optimal design, the minimax design usually enrolls more patients in the first stage and fewer patients in total sample size.

D. With $p0 = 0.10$, $p1 = 0.25$, a type I error of 0.05, and 80% power, for example, a Simon's minimax design will enroll 22 patients in the first stage. If three or more responses are observed, 18 more patients will be enrolled in the second stage. If eight or more responses are observed at the end of study, it will be concluded that the treatment shows preliminary evidence of efficacy.

Question 16.9.   Unlike cytotoxic agents that work by killing tumor cells, cytostatic agents work via biologic effects that modify the environment of tumor growth; that is, inhibition of a molecular target. Which of the following is NOT true regarding early-phase trials on cytostatic agents such as molecularly targeted drugs and cancer therapeutic vaccines?

A. Because cytostatic agents usually have a good safety profile, Phase I trials on such drugs are often designed to identify a biologically active dose rather than maximum tolerated dose.

B. Because therapeutic cancer vaccines work via stimulation of tumor-reactive T cells, heavily treated patients with end-stage disease are less likely to benefit from a cancer vaccine.

C. The response rate based on tumor shrinkage is the best primary end point measuring treatment efficacy in Phase II trials on cytostatic agents.

D. Because of the low toxicity profiles in cytostatic agents, factorial designs and randomized studies have appealing features and are used to evaluate multiple drugs in a single trial.

Question 16.10.   Which of the following best describes Simon's Phase 2.5 design on molecularly targeted drugs and cancer therapeutic vaccines?

A. The design compares progression-free survival times of the same patient from the current trial with his/her previous trial.

B. The design first treats all eligible patients with two to four courses of the experimental drugs. Patients are then evaluated, and the experimental drug is either continued or discontinued, depending on their response to the initial treatment.

C. The design is similar to a Phase III trial except that it allows a relatively large type I (false positive) error and targets for a relatively large difference, thus requiring fewer patients.

D. The design will compare time to progression of patients in the study with a prospectively identified and prognostically comparable historical control.

Question 16.11.   **Which of the following is NOT true of Phase III trials?**

A. The primary end points should be demonstrably related to patient benefit.
B. Eligibility criteria should be broad to enhance generalizability of results.
C. Conditions of treatment should be suited to community patient care.
D. A quality-of-life measure should be included to measure benefit to patients.

Question 16.12.   **Which of the following is TRUE of randomized treatment assignment?**

A. Trial participants are a representative sample of patients with the disease of interest.
B. Randomization may fail to balance unknown prognostic factors in small studies.
C. Randomization is unnecessary if controls can be matched closely enough to trial participants.
D. Randomization is effective only if patients and treating physicians are unaware of treatment assignment for the duration of the study.

Question 16.13.   **Randomization is generally NOT necessary in which of the following scenarios?**

A. Study of patients with a disease that will uniformly and rapidly progress to an end-stage.
B. Phase III trial
C. Screening study on multiple cytostatic agents, such as molecularly targeted drugs or cancer therapeutic vaccines
D. Phase II trial on cytotoxic agents using time to progression as the primary efficacy end point

Question 16.14.   **Which of the following is NOT true of power and hypothesis testing in clinical trials?**

A. Statistical power mainly depends on the anticipated size of treatment effect. Trials designed to detect a small effect will demand large sample sizes.
B. Statistical power is also heavily influenced by the prespecified type I error (probability of erroneously claiming a "positive" result), and a two-sided type I error of 0.05 has been widely accepted, especially in Phase III trials.
C. Because a confidence interval provides information about the size and direction of treatment effect, it is more informative than significance testing, especially for "negative" trials.
D. Because data from small randomized trials can be pooled for meta-analysis, the calculation of sample size for a randomized clinical trial is no longer as critical as it was.

Question 16.15.   Which of the following is NOT true for therapeutic equivalence (or non-inferiority) trials?

A. Therapeutic equivalence trials are designed to test similarity, as measured by a clinical end point, between the experimental drugs and the standard treatment.

B. Because it is impossible to prove equivalence in true sense, in practice therapeutic equivalence will be accepted if the difference in efficacy is within a prespecified level (δ).

C. The traditional superiority trials cannot be used to prove equivalence because a "negative" finding may be simply due to inadequate sample size.

D. A trial designed to demonstrate therapeutic equivalence requires fewer patients because it usually allows a relatively large type I error.

Question 16.16.   Therapeutic equivalence trials often express results as an estimate of difference between two treatments with a 95% confidence interval. Which of the following statements about the 95% confidence interval is NOT correct?

A. The confidence interval is a range of values consistent with the observed difference, given the precision with which the trial can measure that difference.

B. The trial estimates that in 5 of 100 cases the true difference will fall outside the 95% confidence interval.

C. It is unlikely that the true difference is smaller than the lower limit or larger than the upper limit of the confidence interval.

D. If the confidence interval includes 0, then the trial has shown that the two treatments do not differ.

Question 16.17.   Which one of the following describing the pros and cons of Bayesian methods in planning clinical trials is NOT true?

A. In the traditional statistical (frequentist) methods, the treatment effect is regarded as a fixed but unknown parameter, and the likelihood of the parameter is described using a probability derived from observed frequencies in a defined distribution. In contrast, a Bayesian statistical method assumes that the treatment effect itself is a random quantity drawn from a prior distribution.

B. Bayesian methods are widely applied in planning Phase III trials.

C. Because Bayesian methods can incorporate information from preclinical studies and sources outside of the trial, many designs for Phase I and II trials have been developed within a Bayesian framework.

D. The prior distribution of parameters heavily influences the meaningfulness and interpretation of Bayesian-based clinical trials.

Question 16.18.   The intention-to-treat analysis is considered the primary analysis of data from a clinical trial. Which of the following describes an intention-to-treat analysis?

    A. An ineligible patient is not included in an intention-to-treat analysis because the study treatment is not appropriate for that patient.

    B. All patients who give consent and are randomized are included in the intention-to-treat analysis in the study arm to which they were randomized.

    C. Data from patients who are ineligible or who die or withdraw from the study before completion should be analyzed separately from data from eligible patients who complete the trial.

    D. Lack of compliance can distort the results from patients who fail to complete the trial, so these data should be dropped from an intention-to-treat analysis.

Question 16.19.   An interim analysis is any assessment of data performed during patient enrollment or follow-up period of a trial. Which of the following is NOT true for planning clinical trials with interim analyses?

    A. Multiple looks at outcome data over the course of a trial will alter type I and II errors. Unless they are included in the design, multiple looks will cause the operating characteristics of the trial to deviate from the planned values.

    B. Various group-sequential designs have been proposed to guide the statistical significance testing of a fixed number of interim analyses that are usually specified from the outset.

    C. The method of stochastic curtailment is designed to calculate conditional power (the projected probability of rejecting the null hypothesis at the end of study), conditional on the accumulated information, and to stop the trial if the conditional power is small (e.g., 0.2). In such a "futility" analysis, the number of interim analyses does not need to be fixed in advance.

    D. A data-safety committee is usually put in charge of the interpretation of interim analyses. The committee also includes the study leaders to notify the patients and medical community in a timely manner.

Question 16.20.   One of the most important features that makes survival data different from other kinds of data is the presence of censoring. That is, the actual survival times for some patients cannot be observed during study. Which of the following is NOT true for the analysis of survival data?

A. Survival (or disease-free survival) curves provide a superior tool for summarizing survival data.

B. Two methods are most frequently used for the estimation of survival curves. The life table method requires relatively large sample size, and the Kaplan-Meier product limit method is appropriate for any sample size.

C. Traditional summary statistics, such as means and standard deviations, can provide a sufficient summary for survival data without censoring.

D. The statistical power of clinical trials using survival as a primary end point will be mainly determined by the actual number of events (i.e., death or progression) rather than the total number of patients.

Question 16.21.   An important assumption in the analysis of survival data is noninformative censoring. That is, censoring is not related to the outcome of interest. For a clinical trial with cancer-specific survival as the primary end point, which of the following patients is more likely to suffer from informative censoring?

A. Alive at the time of study closeout

B. Withdrawal from the trial because of disease progression

C. Died of accident

D. Moving out of the region

Question 16.22.   All of the following are characteristics of Phase 0 trials EXCEPT:

A. Requires an assay for measuring the pharmacodynamic end point.

B. Patients receive multiple doses of the experimental drug.

C. Identifies whether the experimental drug has an inhibitory effect against its specified molecular target.

D. Drug doses used in these trials are not expected to cause toxicity.

Question 16.23.   All of the following statements regarding clinical trials are true EXCEPT:

A. Response rate is the most commonly utilized end point in Phase II trials.

B. More than 25% of current clinical trials select patients based on biomarker testing.

C. Universities are listed as the primary sponsor for the majority of clinical trials.

D. None of the above.

Answer 16.7.   **The answer is D.**

There is no biologically inherent relationship between response and survival. For example, a meta-analysis on randomized clinical trials by Torri et al. showed that a large improvement in response rate only corresponded to a minor increase in survival. In addition, survival end points are comparative in nature and require taking the distribution of potential prognostic factors into consideration.

Answer 16.8.   **The answer is B.**

Trials of cytostatic agents often choose time to progression as the primary end points. When testing cytotoxic agents, the use of Simon's two-stage designs is limited to situations where outcome assessment can be made shortly after patients are treated. These designs usually are not practical for end points requiring a long period of follow-up.

Answer 16.9.   **The answer is C.**

Cytostatic agents, such as antiangiogenesis factors, growth modulators, or cancer vaccines, usually selectively work on molecular targets to modulate tumor environment. They may prolong patient survival without causing tumor shrinkage. Therefore, time to progression is often used as the primary end point for such trials.

Answer 16.10.   **The answer is C.**

Option A represents a design that used growth modulation index for the assessment of efficacy, option B describes a randomized discontinuation design, and option D is frequently used for trials on the combination of cytotoxic agents. Simon's Phase 2.5 designs are similar to Phase III trials except that they allow a relatively large type I error and are able to identify only a relatively large difference.

Answer 16.11.   **The answer is D.**

Validated quality-of-life instruments are useful parts of Phase III trials, especially if they are directly related to areas of concern to patients. Many areas of patient benefit (e.g., longer survival, lower risk of relapse, accessibility, or lower cost) may not be readily measured by these instruments.

Answer 16.12.   **The answer is B.**

A random sample helps to provide a fair, unbiased comparison of the treatments within the population of patients from whom participants are recruited, although this population may not be representative of all patients with the disease. Randomization may not result in equal, or nearly equal, numbers of patients with a particular characteristic in each treatment group, but it does distribute biasing characteristics according to a known probability distribution so that they do not obscure identification of treatment effects, if any, by statistical tests. Matching is not a substitute for randomization; in fact, matching too closely can mask real treatment effects. Blinding of participants or treating physicians to treatment assignment can reduce bias introduced in the process of treatment, whereas randomization reduces bias in patient selection. Randomized assignment to treatment can be used with or without blinding.

Answer 16.13.   **The answer is A.**

Randomization is not necessary for patients with a disease that will uniformly and rapidly progress to an end-stage. In such a setting of homogeneity, a historical control usually is sufficient.

Answer 16.14.   **The answer is D.**

It is true that meta-analysis can combine the results of small randomized studies and may address questions that cannot be answered by any individual study alone. However, by no means can meta-analyses replace carefully designed and adequately powered randomized trials. This is because different trials can be heterogeneous in terms of diagnostic and staging procedures, supportive care, and methods of patient evaluation and follow-up. Such heterogeneity may obscure small-to-moderate therapeutic effects and undermine the ground for any pooled analyses.

Answer 16.15.   **The answer is D.**

This claim may be true for bioequivalence studies but not for therapeutic equivalence trials. In the former, for example, the objective is to show biological equivalence of two proprietary preparations of a drug, and a relatively large type I error or large tolerable difference (δ) is acceptable. For trials targeting equivalence in therapeutic effect (e.g., mortality rate), however, usually a much smaller δ is of interest, and this will require a very large sample size.

Answer 16.16.   **The answer is D.**

The trial has shown that 0 is a plausible value for the difference but not that the difference equals zero.

Answer 16.17.   **The answer is B.**

Because Bayesian methods can incorporate information from preclinical studies and sources outside of the trial, they are appealing in planning Phase I and II trials. In these trials, information regarding the experimental treatment is sparse, and study design is based on various (usually subjective) assumptions. However, Phase III trials intend to provide reliable and objective guidance for decision making in a given disease, so the subjective nature of prior distributions in Bayesian methods limits their popularity in planning Phase III trials.

Answer 16.18.   **The answer is B.**

Omitting patients who die or withdraw without completing the study is a serious source of bias, as is dropping patients for noncompliance or deviation from protocol. These may be patients for whom the treatment does not work or has serious adverse consequences. There is no sound way to identify and eliminate this bias in the context of the trial, so the intention-to-treat analysis includes all consenting, randomized patients in the study arm to which they were randomized.

Answer 16.19.   **The answer is D.**

For Phase III trials, it is mandatory to have an independent data-safety committee that has the power to recommend termination of the study based on safety concerns, outstanding benefit, or futility. Because the study leaders have a conflict of interest with respect to the decision to continue the study, they are not part of the committee.

Answer 16.20.   **The answer is C.**

Even if survival data have no censoring, a survival curve still provides a better approach for data summary because it takes the length of follow-up time into consideration. In addition, survival times are usually skewed to the right, and the conventional means and standard deviations may not be adequate for data description.

Answer 16.21.   **The answer is B.**

For this study, noninformative censoring means that the probability distributions of cancer-specific survival are similar for both censored and noncensored patients. However, patients who have experienced disease progression are more likely to have a poor prognosis.

Answer 16.22.   **The answer is B.**

Phase 0 trials are first in human trials that help eliminate ineffective and toxic drugs at a very early stage of clinical development. A small sample of patients receive a onetime low dose of the study drug at which it is not expected to cause toxic adverse effects. These trials provide preliminary pharmacokinetic and pharmcodynamic information that enable the go/no-go decisions on further evaluation of the study drug. These studies do require the prior development of an assay to measure the pharmaco-dynamic end point for the study drug.

Answer 16.23.   **The answer is B.**

In a 2009 review of the ClinicalTrials.gov website, response rate was the most frequent (37%) end point in Phase II clinical trials. Universities were listed as the sponsor for 45% of all clinical trials. Only 7% of all clinical trials utilized biomarker testing for patient selection.

Answer 16.24.   **The answer is B.**

Meta-analysis allows for combining and summarizing the results from several therapeutic trials. To achieve meaningful results and avoid bias, meta-analysis includes only randomized clinical trials including unpublished studies. Studies are not restricted to any particular geographic region. Furthermore, access to individual patient data and collaboration of the individual study investigators is required for meta-analysis.

CHAPTER 17 CANCER OF THE HEAD AND NECK

DAVID I. KUPERMAN

DIRECTIONS   Each of the numbered items below is followed by lettered answers. Select the ONE lettered answer that is BEST in each case unless instructed otherwise.

QUESTIONS

Question 17.1.   In the progressive development of squamous cell cancer of the head and neck (SCCHN), which of the following is the latest event?

A. Loss of 9p
B. Loss of 3p
C. Loss of 17p
D. Loss of 11q

Question 17.2.   Which of the following statements about the epidermal growth factor receptor (EGFR) in SCCHN is FALSE?

A. EGFR overexpression can be equally and effectively targeted with erlotinib or cetuximab in SCCHN.
B. Activated EGFR signaling results in cell growth and division.
C. EGFR overexpression enhances tumor angiogenesis.
D. High EGFR expression is associated with resistance to radiation therapy.

Question 17.3.   Which of the following are the risk factors for SCCHN?

A. Tobacco use
B. Alcohol use
C. Fanconi's anemia
D. All of the above

Question 17.4.   All of the following are characteristics of human papilloma virus (HPV) positive SCCHN, EXCEPT:

A. Most patients are never smokers.
B. Survival outcomes are better than in patients with tobacco smoking-associated SCCHN.
C. Chemotherapy response is unrelated to HPV status.
D. HPV causes nonkeratinizing tumors.

Corresponding Chapters in *Cancer: Principles & Practice of Oncology,* Ninth Edition: 71 (Molecular Biology of Head and Neck Cancers), 72 (Treatment of Head and Neck Cancer) and 73 (Rehabilitation after Treatment of Head and Neck Cancer).

Question 17.5.   A 56-year-old man presents to his primary care physician with a 3-month history of right ear pain and two masses on the right side of his neck. On examination, he is found to have a 3-cm right tonsil mass and two separate right-sided lymph nodes below the sternocleidomastoid. One lymph node is 2 cm, and the other is 1 cm in diameter. He has a fine-needle aspiration (FNA) of one of the neck lymph nodes, and it is consistent with a squamous cell carcinoma. A neck and chest computed tomography (CT) shows no additional lymphadenopathy or distant metastasis. What is the stage of his disease?

   A. Stage II
   B. Stage III
   C. Stage IVA
   D. Stage IVC

Question 17.6.   Which of the following statements is TRUE?

   A. Only classic radical neck dissections should be performed for the management of SCCHN.
   B. Complications from neck dissections include hematoma; seroma; lymphedema; wound infections and dehiscence; damage to the VII, X, XI, and XII cranial nerves; carotid exposure; and carotid rupture.
   C. In a surgically treated tumor without radiographic evidence of lymph node metastasis, an elective neck dissection should only be performed if the risk of occult metastasis to the neck is greater than 50%.
   D. For patients who have had a neck dissection for SCCHN, there is no benefit from postoperative radiation.

Question 17.7.   Which of the following statements is TRUE?

   A. The combination of cisplatin and 5FU has been clearly shown to improve survival over single-agent methotrexate in the treatment of metastatic SCCHN.
   B. Cetuximab has no activity in metastatic or recurrent SCCHN.
   C. The combination of cisplatin and 5FU has a higher response rate than single-agent methotrexate in the treatment of metastatic SCCHN.
   D. Higher doses of chemotherapy have led to improved survival.

Question 17.8.   A 66-year-old man presents to his otolaryngologist with a 4-cm left floor of mouth squamous cell cancer. He has a left-sided 3-cm lymph node felt on examination and seen on CT. Magnetic resonance imaging (MRI) shows that the primary tumor is invading into the mandible. He has no evidence of distant metastasis on CT of his chest. What is the most appropriate primary therapy for this patient?

   A. Surgery
   B. Radiation
   C. Chemoradiation

Question 17.9.   A 54-year-old woman recently had a resection of a squamous cell cancer of the supraglottis with bilateral neck dissections. The pathology shows a T2 lesion, which was completely excised with negative margins but perivascular and perineural invasion. There are 2 of 28 positive lymph nodes with extracapsular extension on the right and no positive lymph nodes. What is the most appropriate primary therapy for this patient?

A. Observation
B. Radiation
C. Chemoradiation

Question 17.10.   All of the following are true regarding the addition of cetuximab to definitive radiation in patients with SCCHN, EXCEPT:

A. Results in improved survival compared to radiation alone.
B. Concurrent cetuximab has been proven to be equally effective to concurrent cisplatin with radiation.
C. Addition of cetuximab results in increased incidence of acne and infusion reactions.
D. No significant difference in the incidence of mucositis between patients receiving radiation alone or concurrent radiation and cetuximab.

Question 17.11.   Which of the following statements is FALSE?

A. Radiation therapy alone for locally advanced squamous cell cancer of the larynx has a lower overall survival than concurrent chemoradiation.
B. Concurrent chemoradiation allows for better local control than radiation alone for squamous cell cancer of the larynx.
C. A total laryngectomy may not be necessary for the treatment of laryngeal cancer.
D. Large-volume laryngeal tumors are best treated with surgery.

Question 17.12.   True or False: There is an overall survival benefit from adjuvant chemotherapy after resection of a squamous cell cancer of the larynx.

A. True
B. False

Question 17.13.   Which of the following statements is FALSE?

A. The three subtypes of nasopharyngeal carcinoma are World Health Organization (WHO) type I, squamous cell carcinoma; WHO type II, nonkeratinizing carcinoma; and WHO type III, undifferentiated carcinoma or lymphoepithelioma.
B. Most nasopharyngeal carcinomas are treated with surgery.
C. Common presenting symptoms of nasopharyngeal carcinomas include painless upper neck mass, nasal stuffiness, facial pain, and headache.
D. The majority of nasopharyngeal carcinomas are metastatic to neck lymph nodes at presentation.

Question 17.14. A 56-year-old woman presents to her primary care physician with left-sided facial swelling and facial drooping. The patient has weakness of the lower portion of her facial nerve and a palpable parotid mass. A biopsy is performed showing a high-grade mucoepidermoid carcinoma. There are no palpable neck lymph nodes. What is the best treatment for this patient?

A. Radiation
B. Chemoradiation
C. Surgery
D. Surgery followed by adjuvant radiation

Question 17.15. Which of the following statements is FALSE?

A. Treatment of head and neck cancer requires a multidisciplinary team, including medical oncologists, otorhinolaryngologists, radiation oncologists, nurses, speech therapists, nutritionists, and social workers.
B. Once the patient is able to get nutrition via a G-tube, there is no benefit from having the patient continue to swallow during radiation.
C. Intensity-modulated radiation therapy (IMRT) can decrease xerostomia in patients treated with radiation for head and neck cancer.
D. The severity of the side effects of radiation depends on the radiation field, the radiation dose, and the concomitant chemotherapy agents.

Question 17.16. All of the following statements are true regarding second primaries in patients with SCCHN, EXCEPT:

A. Low dose isotretinoin is ineffective in preventing second primaries.
B. Never smokers with resected SCCHN have a lower incidence of second primaries.
C. Treatment with α-tocopherol decreases the incidence of second primary cancers.
D. Treatment with β-carotene decreases the incidence of second primary cancers.

Question 17.17. Which of the following statements regarding induction chemotherapy in the treatment of SCCHN is NOT true?

A. Treatment with concurrent chemoradiation with cisplatin resulted in improved overall survival compared to induction cisplatin and 5FU followed by radiation therapy
B. Addition of docetaxel to cisplatin and 5FU was associated with superior overall survival when compared to cisplatin and 5FU alone in the TAX 324 trial.
C. Induction chemotherapy has the potential for organ preservation.
D. Patients with unresectable SCCHN are candidates for induction chemotherapy followed by concurrent chemoradiation.

ANSWERS

Answer 17.1.   **The answer is D.**

Dr. Sriranski has proposed a molecular progression model of the development of SCCHN based on analysis of the 10 most common allelic changes found in these malignancies. The earliest events appear to be the loss of 9p and 3p given that these are found in preinvasive lesions. This is to be followed soon afterward by the loss of 17p. The loss of 11q, 13q, 14q, and p53 mutation is not typically found in preinvasive lesions and, therefore, must be a later event.

Answer 17.2.   **The answer is A.**

EGFR plays a key role in the development of SCCHN. There is often a moderate increase in the number of copies of this gene. EGFR overexpression leads to activation of multiple signaling pathways that lead to cell growth and resistance to apoptosis. Evidence suggests that EGFR overexpression can lead to an increase in vascular endothelial growth factor production, leading to angiogenesis. Analysis of EGFR expression in archived tumor tissue from a prospective clinical trial suggests that EGFR overexpression is associated with resistance to radiation therapy. Even though erlotinib is a small molecule inhibitor of the EGFR tyrosine kinase domain, it has not been shown so far to be effective in the treatment of SCCHN while cetuximab has shown a survival benefit when given concurrently with radiation for locally advanced or used as a part of treatment for distantly metastatic disease.

Answer 17.3.   **The answer is D.**

Several risk factors for the development of SCCHN have been identified. The two most important are tobacco and alcohol use. They seem to be synergistic. Other risk factors include occupational exposure to chemicals and irritants, such as aromatic hydrocarbons and wood dust, and viruses, such as HPV and EBV. In addition, patients with Fanconi's anemia are at increased risk.

Answer 17.4.   **The answer is C.**

It has been recognized recently that HPV is the primary cause of many squamous cell cancers of the oropharynx. HPV DNA can be found in approximately 50% of tonsil and base of tongue tumors. These tumors are often described as having a basal cell-like appearance and are frequently nonkeratinizing. These tumors are more commonly found in never smokers. In general, these tumors carry a better prognosis than other tumors of the head and neck. The overall survival and disease-free survival are improved, and the risk of second primaries is lower compared with non–HPV-associated tumors. Patients with HPV-associated SCCHN have better response to chemotherapy than patient s with tobacco-smoking-associated SCCHN.

Answer 17.5.   **The answer is C.**

The patient has a tonsil mass that is between 2 and 4 cm. This makes his primary tumor T2. He has multiple ipsilateral regional lymph nodes with the largest lymph node being smaller than 6 cm, which is N2b disease. His tumor shows no evidence of distant metastasis. The patient's disease is T2N2bM0, which is stage IVA.

Answer 17.6.   **The answer is B.**

Control of neck disease is very important in the management of SCCHN. Both surgery and radiation can be used. When a tumor is treated surgically, a neck dissection is recommended even in a clinically negative neck if the risk of occult metastasis exceeds 10% to 15%. Modified neck dissections that can preserve structures such as cranial nerve XI, internal jugular vein, and sternocleidomastoid can often be performed without compromise of disease control. Patients with positive neck lymph nodes clearly have a benefit from postoperative radiation if multiple lymph nodes are involved or N3 disease and sometimes chemoradiation depending on the pathologic findings. Complications from neck dissections include hematoma; seroma; lymphedema; wound infections and dehiscence; damage to the VII, X, XI, and XII cranial nerves; carotid exposure; and carotid rupture.

Answer 17.7.   **The answer is C.**

The treatment of metastatic squamous cell cancer is challenging. Many cytotoxic chemotherapeutic agents including cisplatin, carboplatin, 5FU, taxanes, ifosfamide, and methotrexate have activity against metastatic SCCHN. Combinations of conventional cytotoxic chemotherapy and higher doses of chemotherapy have a higher response rate but have not shown a clear survival benefit over single agent cytotoxic chemotherapy. The anti-EGFR antibody cetuximab has shown significant activity against SCCHN. Recently in the EXTREME trial, the addition of cetuximab to conventional cytotoxic chemotherapy showed a survival benefit.

Answer 17.8.   **The answer is A.**

This patient has a stage IVA (T4aN1M0) squamous cell cancer of the oral cavity. The therapy that is most effective in this situation is surgery. Radiation and chemoradiation as primary therapy will be of little utility here, particularly with invasion of the mandible. He will most likely require radiation or chemoradiation after surgery depending on the findings.

Answer 17.9.   **The answer is C.**

After gross tumor resection, adjuvant therapy with radiation or chemoradiation is recommended for locally advanced SCCHN. The decision on what adjuvant therapy is to be recommended is based on operative findings. Major risk factors for local recurrence are positive margins or lymph node disease with extracapsular extension. Minor risk factors include primary tumors that are T3 or T4, N2, or N3 disease, perineural invasion, and vascular embolism. If the patient has any major risk factor or two or more minor risk factors, adjuvant chemoradiation is recommended. If the patient has a minor risk factor, adjuvant radiation is recommended. If the patient has no adverse risk factors, observation is recommended.

Answer 17.10.   **The answer is B.**

Cetuximab is an EGFR antibody that has been used to treat SCCHN. It has been used alone or combined with chemotherapy for treatment of metastatic disease, as well as with radiation, to treat locally advanced SCCHN. In a multicenter, randomized phase III trial comparing chemoradiation with cetuximab with radiation alone for SCCHN of the oropharynx, larynx, and hypopharynx, cetuximab improved both local control and overall survival. In patients receiving cetuximab with radiation, there was increased incidence of acne and infusion reactions but no difference in the incidence of mucositis. However, concurrent cetuximab with radiation has not been compared with cisplatin and radiation.

Answer 17.11.   **The answer is D.**

The treatment of larynx cancers has changed significantly over the last 20 years. The traditional approach to locally advanced tumors of the larynx was a total laryngectomy often followed by adjuvant radiation. With improvements in surgical techniques and chemoradiation, it is often possible to preserve the larynx. For low-volume disease, a hemilaryngectomy can be performed saving the voice. Nonsurgical treatments can also be good options. Both radiation alone and concurrent chemoradiation for locally advanced tumors of the larynx have equal chance of cure. Concurrent chemoradiation, however, gives the best local control; therefore, it is the standard of care. Unfortunately, large-volume tumors of the larynx may not be curable by chemoradiation or larynx-preserving surgery and should be treated with a total laryngectomy.

Answer 17.12.   **The answer is B.**

Adjuvant chemotherapy has been tested in several trials to improve the survival of patients with SCCHN. Unfortunately, it has not been shown to improve survival. Currently, adjuvant chemotherapy is only used in the treatment of locally advanced nasopharyngeal cancer. Even its benefit is unclear.

Answer 17.13.   **The answer is B.**

Nasopharyngeal carcinomas are unusual in the United States but are much more common in China and Southeast Asia. On the basis of pathology, there are three subtypes of nasopharyngeal carcinoma: WHO type I, squamous cell carcinoma; WHO type II, nonkeratinizing carcinoma; and WHO type III, undifferentiated carcinoma or lymphoepithelioma. The WHO type III is associated with EBV. These tumors typically present with a painless upper neck mass, nasal stuffiness, facial pain, and headache. Cranial nerve involvement occurs in approximately 25% of the patients.

Cranial nerves II, III, IV, V, and VI can be affected by the tumor extending into the cavernous sinus. Lateral pharyngeal space extension of the tumor affects cranial nerves IX through XII. Approximately 80% to 90% of the patients have neck lymph node involvement at presentation with half of the patients having bilateral neck disease. These tumors are almost exclusively treated with radiation because it is very difficult to obtain a complete resection. For more locally advanced tumors (node positive or T3–4N0), chemoradiation with concurrent cisplatin followed by adjuvant cisplatin–5FU is used.

Answer 17.14.   **The answer is D.**

The treatment of choice for both benign and malignant tumors is primarily surgical. Inoperable malignancies are treated by radiation therapy with occasional success. Radiation therapy is given postoperatively for nearly all high-grade lesions. Radiation therapy is advised for low-grade malignant lesions that are recurrent and those with positive margins or narrow margins on the facial nerve. Postoperative radiation therapy is advised for selected benign mixed tumors when there is microscopic residual disease after operation and for nearly all patients after surgery for recurrent disease.

Answer 17.15.   **The answer is B.**

The treatment of head and neck cancer requires a multidisciplinary approach. This is because the treatment will often require several different modalities (e.g., surgery followed by chemoradiation) to support the patient through treatment and recovery from the side effects. Radiation to the head and neck has many short- and long-term toxicities. Short-term side effects include severe mucositis with pain and inability to swallow and burns. The long-term effects include xerostomia, dental caries, and fibrosis resulting in trismus and difficulty swallowing. The degree of toxicity from radiation varies from patient to patient and depends on the dose of radiation, the radiation port, the radiation technique, and whether chemotherapy is used concurrently. IMRT is a radiation technique that allows varying doses of radiation to be given to different parts of a radiation field. This allows a parotid gland to be spared resulting in less long-term xerostomia. To decrease the risk of long-term swallowing dysfunction, patients should be strongly encouraged to continue to swallow to exercise the pharyngeal muscles even if they are receiving the majority of nutrition via a G-tube.

Answer 17.16.   **The answer is C.**

Prospective trials on secondary chemoprevention with isotretinoin and α-tocopherol have shown no significant benefit in preventing second primary cancers in patients with resected SCCHN. Tobacco smoking status is an important risk factor for the development of second primaries and never smokers have lower risk for second primaries compared to former and current smokers.

Answer 17.17.   The answer is A.

Induction chemotherapy followed by definitive radiation has the potential to treat unresectable tumors and increase organ preservation rates. In a phase III trial of patients with glottis and supraglottic SCC, there was no significant survival difference between induction chemotherapy followed by definitive radiation versus concurrent chemoradiation. However, there was a statistically significant organ preservation advantage with the concurrent chemoradiation approach. The addition of docetaxel improved overall survival in the TAX 324 trial.

CHAPTER 18 CANCER OF THE LUNG

SAIAMA N. WAQAR

DIRECTIONS   Each of the numbered items below is followed by lettered answers. Select the ONE lettered answer that is BEST in each case unless instructed otherwise.

QUESTIONS

Question 18.1.   Which of the following statements is INCORRECT regarding epidermal growth factor receptor (EGFR) mutations in lung cancer?

   A. EGFR mutations are observed in approximately 80% of non-small cell lung cancers (NSCLCs).
   B. Mutations which predict response to EGFR–tyrosine kinase inhibitors include exon 19 deletion and a point mutation (L858R) in exon 21.
   C. The L858R mutation renders EGFR constitutively active.
   D. EGFR mutations are seen more frequently in tumors from patients who are nonsmokers, in women, and in Asian populations.

Question 18.2.   Which of the following statements is/are CORRECT regarding molecular abnormalities observed in lung cancer?

   A. Chromosomal translocations have not been seen in NSCLC.
   B. C-Kit expression is seen in most NSCLCs.
   C. Chromosome 3p allele loss is one the most common events in lung cancer pathogenesis.
   D. All of the above.

Question 18.3.   A 55-year-old man with a 30 pack-year history of smoking, presents to the emergency room with shortness of breath. Chest radiograph demonstrates a right upper lobe opacity. Computed tomography scan reveals a 3.5-cm spiculated mass in the peripheral right upper lobe, which is suspicious for malignancy, without any hilar or mediastinal lymphadenopathy. What is the next best step in management?

   A. Bronchoscopy and biopsy of the mass
   B. CT-guided biopsy of the mass
   C. Brain MRI
   D. Refer to thoracic surgeon for resection.

Corresponding Chapters in *Cancer: Principles & Practice of Oncology*, Ninth Edition: 74 (Molecular Biology of Lung Cancer), 75 (Non–Small Cell Lung Cancer), and 76 (Small Cell and Neuroendocrine Tumors of the Lung).

Question 18.4.   A 65-year-old man with a 40 pack-year history of smoking, presents to the emergency room with shortness of breath. Chest radiograph demonstrates a left lower lobe mass and left pleural effusion. CT reveals a 3-cm left lower lobe mass, left hilar fullness, and a moderate left pleural effusion. Biopsy of the mass and thoracentesis are both positive for adenocarcinoma. Staging studies do not reveal any distant metastases. Which of the following is the next best step in his management?

A. Referral to a thoracic surgeon
B. Radiation to the chest
C. Concurrent chemotherapy and radiation
D. Platinum-based doublet therapy

Question 18.5.   A 66-year-old man, with a 30 pack-year history of smoking, presents to your office for consultation regarding chemotherapy options for metastatic NSCLC, squamous histology. He has no significant medical problems and his performance status (PS) is 1. Laboratory studies reveal normal blood counts, liver enzymes, and kidney function. Which of the following treatment regimens would you recommend?

A. Cisplatin and pemetrexed
B. Carboplatin, paclitaxel, and bevacizumab
C. Carboplatin and paclitaxel
D. Carboplatin and erlotinib

Question 18.6.   A 55-year-old Asian woman, who is a never smoker, completed four cycles of front-line carboplatin and paclitaxel, for metastatic NSCLC. Imaging studies done after completion of therapy show stable disease. She is very active, and has continued to work as a nurse throughout her treatment. Her PS is 0 and she has tolerated the treatment well, other than grade I neuropathy. Her tumor EGFR status is wild type. She wants "the best treatment possible" and desires further treatment. What would you recommend?

A. Treatment break, erlotinib at the time of disease progression
B. Stopping carboplatin, continuing paclitaxel till disease progression
C. Continuing carboplatin and paclitaxel for four additional cycles
D. Pemetrexed maintenance therapy

Question 18.7.   Which of the following statements is INCORRECT regarding the role of prophylactic cranial irradiation (PCI) in lung cancer?

A. PCI reduces the incidence of brain metastases in limited-stage and extensive-stage small cell lung cancer (SCLC).
B. PCI improves survival in patients with extensive-stage SCLC, who respond to front-line chemotherapy.
C. PCI improves survival in patients with early-stage NSCLC.
D. Patients who receive PCI therapy have long-term cognitive defects.

Question 18.8.   A 58-year-old man, with a 40 pack-year history of smoking is referred to you by a radiation oncologist for management of limited-stage SCLC. What treatment would you recommend?

A. Cisplatin and etoposide chemotherapy
B. Cisplatin and etoposide chemotherapy with concurrent thoracic radiation
C. Cisplatin and etoposide chemotherapy, followed by PCI if response to chemotherapy
D. Cisplatin and etoposide chemotherapy with concurrent thoracic radiation, followed by PCI if response to treatment

Question 18.9.   Which of the following statements is/are correct regarding the role of adjuvant chemotherapy after resection for NSCLC?

A. Adjuvant chemotherapy does not appear to benefit patients with stage IA disease.
B. Adjuvant chemotherapy benefits patients with node-positive disease.
C. Adjuvant chemotherapy may benefit patients with stage IB disease, who have primary tumors larger than 4 cm in size.
D. All of the above.

Question 18.10.   Which of the following statements is correct regarding pulmonary carcinoid tumors?

A. Patients usually present with carcinoid syndrome.
B. Surgery has a curative potential for resectable localized tumors.
C. Adjuvant chemotherapy is the standard of care following complete surgical resection.
D. Most pulmonary carcinoids are atypical carcinoids.

Question 18.11.   Which of the following is INCORRECT regarding erlotinib for the treatment of advanced NSCLC?

A. Patients with L858R mutations respond better than those with exon 19 deletions.
B. Resistance to erlotinib therapy occurs through acquisition of T790M mutation in EGFR.
C. MET amplification in tumors can lead to resistance to erlotinib therapy.
D. Presence of erlotinib-induced skin rash correlates with response to therapy.

Question 18.12.   A 60-year-old man with a 45 pack-year history of smoking, presents with central chest pain. Chest x-ray reveals a right upper lobe mass. CT scan of the chest demonstrates a 4-cm right upper lobe lung mass, with right hilar and multiple ipsilateral enlarged mediastinal lymph nodes. Bronchoscopy and biopsy of the mass reveals NSCLC. PET scan demonstrates increased FDG-uptake in the lung mass, right hilar and mediastinal lymph nodes, but no other site of metastatic disease. CT of the abdomen and brain MRI are within normal limits. Mediastinoscopy and biopsy reveals NSCLC. His cancer is staged as T2a N2 M0, stage IIIB NSCLC. His PS is 1, and he is otherwise in good health. Which of the following is the best management for this patient?

A. Definitive radiation to the chest
B. Radiation to the chest, followed by platinum-based chemotherapy
C. Concurrent radiation to the chest and platinum-based chemotherapy
D. Platinum-based chemotherapy

Question 18.13.   Which of the following statements is INCORRECT regarding large cell neuroendocrine tumors (LCNEC)?

A. Paraneoplastic syndromes are commonly associated with LNEC.
B. Like SCLC, LCNEC have an aggressive natural history and propensity to metastasize.
C. LCNEC are treated in the same manner as NSCLC, with the same treatment algorithm, stage for stage.
D. LCNEC are less chemosensitive than SCLC.

Question 18.14.   A 45-year-old Asian woman, who is a never smoker, presents to your office for consultation regarding systemic therapy for metastatic adeno-carcinoma of the lung. Her tumor has activating EGFR mutation and she inquires regarding the use of erlotinib in the first-line setting. Which of the following statements is INCORRECT regarding the use of EGFR TKIs in previously untreated patients with NSCLC?

A. In patients with activating EGFR mutations, initial therapy with an EGFR inhibitor results in longer time to progression compared with chemotherapy.
B. In patients with activating EGFR mutations, initial therapy with either an EGFR TKI or with chemotherapy results in similar over-all survival.
C. Front-line EGFR TKIs are less effective than chemotherapy in patients with unknown EGFR status, or wild-type EGFR.
D. Erlotinib should be combined with chemotherapy in patients with activating EGFR mutation-positive tumors.

Question 18.15.   A 65-year-old Caucasian man, who is a never smoker, presents to your office for consultation regarding therapy for metastatic adenocarcinoma of the lung. He was initially treated with cisplatin and pemetrexed, but developed progressive disease. EGFR mutational analysis on his tumor revealed exon 19 deletion, and he received second-line erlotinib therapy. Despite initial response, he had disease progression 10 months later. The patient is now inquiring about EML4–ALK testing. Which of the following is INCORRECT regarding ALK testing for NSCLC?

A. The frequency of EML4–ALK translocations in never smokers is 4%.

B. EGFR mutations and ALK rearrangements are for the most part mutually exclusive.

C. The gold standard for diagnosing ALK-positive NSCLC is the ALK Dual Color break-apart probe.

D. Most tumors with EML4–ALK translocations are adenocarcinomas.

Question 18.16.   A 65-year-old man, who is a former smoker presents for consultation regarding management of unresectable stage IIIB adenocarcinoma of the lung. He has a PS of 0 and adequate blood counts, hepatic and renal function. Which of the following would you recommend?

A. Concurrent definitive cisplatin and etoposide therapy, no consolidation therapy, no PCI

B. Concurrent definitive cisplatin and etoposide therapy, consolidation docetaxel therapy, no PCI

C. Concurrent definitive cisplatin and etoposide therapy, consolidation gefitinib therapy, no PCI

D. Concurrent definitive cisplatin and etoposide therapy, consolidation gefitinib therapy, followed by PCI

Question 18.17.   A 48-year-old man, presents to your office for consultation regarding management of newly diagnosed extensive-stage SCLC. He has a PS of 0 and adequate blood counts, hepatic and renal function. Which of the following would be a reasonable first-line treatment option for him?

A. Cisplatin and irinotecan

B. Cisplatin and etoposide

C. Cisplatin and topotecan

D. Cisplatin, paclitaxel, and etoposide

ANSWERS

Answer 18.1.   **The answer is A.**

EGFR overexpression is seen in 80% of lung cancers. However, EGFR mutations occur in only 10% of NSCLCs, though these mutations are found more frequently in Asian populations (40%), women, and never smokers. EGFR mutations predict response to EGFR–tyrosine kinase inhibitors. The most common mutations observed are an in-frame deletion in exon 19 and a point mutation in exon 21 (L858R). These mutations result in prolonged EGFR activation and downstream signaling.

Answer 18.2.   **The answer is C.**

Chromosome 3p allele loss is one of the most common events in the pathogenesis of lung cancer, and is an early event. It occurs in 90% of SCLCs and 80% of NSCLCs. HER2/neu is expressed in over a third of NSCLCs, especially in adenocarcinoma. EML4–ALK translocations occur in 3% to 5% of NSCLCs. Like EGFR mutations, these also are enriched in never smokers. EML4–ALK translocations and EGFR mutations occur in a mutually exclusive manner; tumors with EGFR mutations do not have EML4–ALK translocations and vice versa.

Answer 18.3.   **The answer is B.**

The right upper lobe mass is suspicious for malignancy, however, a tissue diagnosis is needed. Since the location of the mass is peripheral, the best way to approach it would be through CT-guided biopsy, rather than bronchoscopy and biopsy. Once a diagnosis of lung cancer is established, staging studies, such as CT of the abdomen, MRI of the brain, PET, or bone scan may be performed. If the diagnosis is NSCLC, and there is no evidence of distant metastases on staging studies, then he should be referred to a thoracic surgeon for discussion regarding surgical interventions.

Answer 18.4.   **The answer is D.**

The seventh edition of the TNM staging system includes several changes to the T descriptors including the addition of size cutoffs, of 2, 3, 5, and 7 cm, subdivision of T1 into T1a and T1b, and of T2 into T2a and T2b, downstaging of separate tumor nodules in the same lobe as the primary tumor from T4 to T3, downstaging of separate tumor nodules in a different ipsilateral lobe as the primary tumor from M1 to T4, and reclassification of malignant pleural nodules, pleural effusions and pericardial effusions as M1 disease. He has stage IV disease due to the presence of malignant pleural effusion and should receive treatment with platinum-based doublet chemotherapy for metastatic disease. Surgery would be appropriate only for early-stage disease, while chemoradiation would be the way to treat locally advanced, stage III disease, in patients with good PS and no significant weight loss.

Answer 18.5.   **The answer is C.**

Cisplatin, pemetrexed and carboplatin, paclitaxel, bevacizumab are possible treatment options to consider for patients with advanced NSCLC with non-squamous histology. For patients with squamous histology, carboplatin and paclitaxel is a reasonable treatment regimen. The addition of erlotinib to chemotherapy does not appear to improve survival, compared to chemotherapy alone, in patients with advanced NSCLC.

Answer 18.6.   **The answer is D.**

Several randomized studies have demonstrated that there is no survival advantage to continuing platinum doublet therapy beyond four to six cycles. If patients experience significant toxicities following upfront therapy, delaying further treatment till disease progression is a reasonable option. Agents used in the second-line setting for the treatment of NSCLC include docetaxel, erlotinib, and pemetrexed. Patients whose tumors have an activating mutation in the EGFR–tyrosine kinase domain, have the most durable benefit from erlotinib. Maintenance chemotherapy is an option for patients with good PS and stable disease following front-line chemotherapy, who do not experience significant treatment-related toxicities. Maintenance chemotherapy (either pemetrexed or erlotinib) has been shown to improve overall survival in patients with NSCLC. Pemetrexed maintenance would be an appropriate option for her.

Answer 18.7.   **The answer is C.**

PCI reduces the incidence of brain metastases in patients with both limited-stage and extensive-stage SCLC, and improves survival in patients with limited-stage SCLC. Patients with extensive-stage SCLC, who respond well to initial front-line therapy also benefit from PCI. However, PCI does not have a role in the management of patients with early-stage NSCLC. Long-term cognitive decline is a side effect of PCI.

Answer 18.8.   **The answer is D.**

In a patient with limited-stage SCLC, the optimal treatment would comprise cisplatin and etoposide chemotherapy, concurrent with thoracic radiation. If the tumor responds to chemotherapy, PCI should follow, once primary treatment is complete.

Answer 18.9.   **The answer is D.**

Adjuvant platinum-based chemotherapy has been shown to improve survival in patients with stage II and III NSCLC who undergo surgical resection. Patients with stage I disease do not benefit from chemotherapy, and a subset analysis of the JBR-10 study suggested that patients with tumor size greater than 4 cm may benefit from adjuvant chemotherapy.

Answer 18.10.   **The answer is B.**

Patients with pulmonary carcinoid rarely present with the carcinoid syndrome (2%). Approximately 30% of patients are asymptomatic at presentation. Ninety percentage of pulmonary carcinoids are typical, while 10% are atypical carcinoids. Surgery is the primary treatment for carcinoid tumors. There is no role for adjuvant chemotherapy, following complete resection for carcinoid tumors.

Answer 18.11.   **The answer is A.**

Erlotinib is a small molecule EGFR–tyrosine kinase inhibitor. Though it is approved in the second-line setting for treatment of NSCLC, its benefit appears to be mainly in patients with activating mutations in the tyrosine kinase domain of EGFR (exon 19 deletion or exon 21 point mutation L858R). Patients with exon 19 deletion respond better to erlotinib, than patients with L858R mutations. The presence of dermatologic toxicity from erlotinib therapy correlates with response to treatment. Resistance to erlotinib therapy is mediated through two main mechanisms: acquisition of a second mutation in EGFR (T790M), or through MET oncogene amplification.

Answer 18.12.   **The answer is C.**

This patient has locally advanced NSCLC. Chemotherapy in addition to radiation has been shown to improve survival over radiation alone, and concurrent chemotherapy and radiation has been demonstrated to be superior to sequential therapy. Chemotherapy alone would be indicated for palliation of metastatic disease and is not appropriate in this setting. Concurrent chemotherapy and radiation would provide the best chance for cure.

Answer 18.13.   **The answer is A.**

LNEC accounts for 3% of surgically resected lung cancers. They are diagnosed based on the following criteria: neuroendocrine morphology with rosette-like structures, high mitotic rate, NSCLC features, such as large cell size, low nuclear/cytoplasmic ratio, nucleoli, or vesicular chromatin and finally, neuroendocrine differentiation by immunohistochemistry. They are not associated with paraneoplastic syndromes or ectopic hormone secretion. They have an aggressive natural history, though are less chemosensitive than SCLCs. They are managed according to the same treatment algorithm as NSCLC, stage for stage, though they carry a worse prognosis.

Answer 18.14.   **The answer is D.**

In patients with EGFR mutations, initial therapy with an EGFR TKI results in longer time to progression compared with chemotherapy, though overall survival is similar in both groups. Though EGFR TKI therapy does not confer a survival benefit in the first-line setting, most patients prefer oral therapy, and the toxicities of EGFR TKI therapy (diarrhea and acneform rash) compare more favorably than conventional chemotherapy. However, first-line EGFR TKI therapy in patients with EGFR wild-type tumors, or tumors with unknown EGFR status is less efficacious than chemotherapy. Both erlotinib and gefitinib have been studied in combination with chemotherapy in the first-line setting and do not result in improved response rates, progression-free survival or overall survival.

Answer 18.15.   **The answer is A.**

The frequency of EML4–ALK translocations in unselected patients is 4%, though is as high as 22% in patients who are never smokers. Most tumors with EML4–ALK translocations are adenocarcinomas. EGFR mutations and ALK rearrangements are for the most part mutually exclusive. The gold standard for diagnosing ALK-positive NSCLC is the ALK Dual Color break-apart probe.

Answer 18.16.   **The answer is A.**

The standard of care for locally advanced unresectable NSCLC is concurrent definitive chemoradiation with cisplatin and etoposide. The role of consolidation docetaxel was investigated in a phase III study conducted by the Hoosier Oncology Group (HOG), and was not found to improve survival over concurrent chemoradiation without consolidation therapy, and increases toxicity. The Southwest Oncology Group (SWOG) conducted another study in which patients who completed chemoradiation and did not experience progressive disease, were randomized to receive gefitinib or placebo. The gefitinib arm had a shorter survival than the placebo arm. Prophylactic cranial radiation decreases the incidence of brain metastases in patients with stage III disease, but does not improve overall survival in these patients. At present there is no sufficient evidence to recommend PCI in patients with stage III disease.

Answer 18.17.   **The answer is B.**

The standard treatment for patients with extensive stage SCLC is combination chemotherapy. Historically, alkylating agent-based regimens were used, though the standard of care has evolved into the use of a platinum agent and etoposide. Cisplatin and irinotecan combination does not confer increased response rates or survival benefit over the use of cisplatin and etoposide, and is associated with increased rates of grade 3 or 4 diarrhea, while cisplatin and etoposide is associated with increased myelosuppression. Carboplatin is commonly substituted for cisplatin, due to better toxicity profile and similar efficacy. The addition of a third agent (paclitaxel or ifosfamide) results in increased toxicities without clear survival benefit. Topotecan is used in patients with relapsed/refractory disease.

GREGORY P. KALEMKERIAN

CHAPTER 19 NEOPLASMS OF
THE MEDIASTINUM

DIRECTIONS   Each of the numbered items below is followed by lettered answers. Select the ONE lettered answer that is BEST in each case unless instructed otherwise.

QUESTIONS

Question 19.1.   A 51-year-old woman presents with dull anterior chest pain. She is a lifelong nonsmoker. Her medical history is significant for Hashimoto's thyroiditis, for which she has been taking levothyroxine for 1 year. Examination is unremarkable. Laboratory studies show normal blood counts, lactate dehydrogenase (LDH), α-fetoprotein, and beta-human chorionic gonadotropin (β-hCG). Chest radiograph reveals clear lung fields with a retrosternal density. Computed tomography (CT) scan shows a 4-cm, smooth, anterior mediastinal mass. What is the most likely diagnosis?

A. Small cell lung cancer
B. Pericardial cyst
C. Nonseminomatous germ cell tumor (NSGCT)
D. Thymoma

Question 19.2.   A 5-year-old boy has been experiencing left upper back pain that radiates around his left chest wall for 2 months. Examination reveals a healthy-appearing boy with no spinal or chest wall deformity, tenderness or masses. He is neurologically intact. A chest radiograph suggests a left paravertebral mass adjacent to T5. A magnetic resonance imaging (MRI) scan shows a 2-cm, smooth, fusiform mass abutting the left T5–6 neural foramen without bony erosion. What is the most likely diagnosis?

A. Non-Hodgkin's lymphoma
B. Neurogenic tumor
C. Thymoma
D. Mediastinal germ cell tumor

Corresponding Chapter in *Cancer: Principles & Practice of Oncology*, Ninth Edition: 77 (Neoplasms of the Mediastinum).

Question 19.3.   Which of the following imaging modalities provides the most accurate assessment of the invasiveness of a posterior mediastinal mass?

    A. Posteroanterior (PA) and lateral chest radiograph
    B. Intravenous contrast-enhanced CT scan
    C. Transesophageal ultrasonography
    D. Positron emission tomography (PET)

Question 19.4.   A 36-year-old woman presents with an anterior mediastinal mass that was identified incidentally on a chest radiograph done as part of an employment examination. She is asymptomatic and a lifelong nonsmoker, with no significant medical history. Examination is unremarkable. CT scan shows a 3-cm, smooth, anterior mediastinal mass without local invasion. Resection of the mass reveals an encapsulated, lymphocyte-rich thymoma (World Health Organization [WHO] type B1) with no capsular invasion. She recovers from surgery without complications. What is the most appropriate next step in the management of this patient?

    A. Clinical surveillance
    B. Adjuvant radiotherapy alone
    C. Adjuvant chemotherapy alone
    D. Adjuvant chemotherapy plus radiotherapy

Question 19.5.   A 48-year-old man presents with progressive fatigue and dyspnea on exertion over the past 6 months. He is a former smoker, and his medical history is significant for well-controlled hypertension. Examination reveals tachycardia with a regular rhythm, mild tachypnea, and conjunctival and mucosal pallor. Stool is guaiac negative. Laboratory studies show hemoglobin of 5.5 g/dL, hematocrit of 17%, white blood cell count of 6800/μL, platelet count of 343,000/μL, and normal electrolytes, renal function, and liver function test results. A chest radiograph reveals superior mediastinal widening. CT scan shows a large, irregular, anterior mediastinal mass. Bone marrow aspiration and biopsy show profound erythrocytic hypoplasia with no dysplasia and normal granulocytic and megakaryocytic maturation with no clonal lymphoid proliferation. Serum LDH, α-fetoprotein, and β-hCG are normal. He is transfused with packed red blood cells, and his hemoglobin increases to 10.4 g/dL. Resection of the mass reveals a cortical thymoma (WHO type B2) with microscopic invasion of the capsule and negative surgical margins. He recovers without complications, and his hemoglobin is 11.5 g/dL 4 weeks after surgery. What is the most appropriate next step in the management of this patient?

    A. Clinical surveillance
    B. Adjuvant radiotherapy alone
    C. Adjuvant chemotherapy alone
    D. Adjuvant chemotherapy plus radiotherapy

Question 19.6.   Which of the following paraneoplastic syndromes are associated with thymoma?

  A. Myasthenia gravis and pure red cell aplasia
  B. Eaton–Lambert myasthenic syndrome and hypogammaglobulinemia
  C. Polymyositis and hypothyroidism
  D. All of the above

Question 19.7.   A 62-year-old man presents with substernal chest pain. Cardiac evaluation is negative. CT angiogram shows no aortic dissection, but does reveal an irregular, anterior mediastinal mass abutting the upper lobe of the left lung. PET scan shows a fluorodeoxyglucose (FDG)-avid anterior mediastinal mass without evidence of metastases. Resection of the mass with en bloc wedge resection of the left upper lobe shows high-grade thymic carcinoma (WHO type C) with invasion into the pericardium and the left upper lobe. The surgical margins are positive on microscopic examination. He recovers from surgery without complications. What is the most appropriate next step in the management of this patient?

  A. Clinical surveillance
  B. Adjuvant radiotherapy alone
  C. Adjuvant chemotherapy alone
  D. Adjuvant chemotherapy plus radiotherapy

Question 19.8.   A previously healthy 38-year-old man presents with facial and bilateral upper-extremity edema that has progressed over the past 2 weeks. Examination reveals moderate facial, cervical, and bilateral upper-extremity edema with facial plethora and prominent anterior chest wall vasculature. He is tachycardic, but his heart sounds are regular and his lungs are clear. There is no lower-extremity edema. CT scan of the chest shows a large anterior mediastinal mass encasing the superior vena cava, displacing the aortic arch and trachea, and invading the pericardium and upper lobe of the left lung. The superior vena cava is compressed and there are numerous dilated, intrathoracic collateral vessels. An experienced thoracic surgeon deems that the lesion is primarily unresectable. Mediastinotomy with biopsy of the mass reveals well-differentiated thymic carcinoma (WHO type B3). PET scan shows a large FDG-avid mediastinal mass with no evidence of metastatic disease. What is the most appropriate management of this patient?

  A. Palliative radiotherapy followed by chemotherapy
  B. Definitive radiotherapy with concurrent chemotherapy
  C. Neoadjuvant chemotherapy followed by surgical resection and postoperative radiotherapy
  D. Palliative chemotherapy alone

Question 19.9.   Which of the following histologic features is associated with an unfavorable outcome in patients with thymic carcinoma?

    A.   Lobular growth pattern
    B.   Well-differentiated squamous cell carcinoma
    C.   Low mitotic activity
    D.   Clear cell carcinoma

Question 19.10.   A 24-year-old man with multiple endocrine neoplasia type 1 (MEN I) has undergone two resections for pancreatic islet cell carcinoma metastatic to regional lymph nodes. He is asymptomatic. Examination shows well-healed abdominal scars. Surveillance CT scan identifies a new 3-cm, smooth, anterior mediastinal mass. Serum LDH, α-fetoprotein, and β-hCG are normal. Testicular ultrasonography is unremarkable. Which of the following is the most likely diagnosis?

    A.   Thymolipoma
    B.   Thymoma
    C.   Thymic carcinoid
    D.   Metastatic islet cell tumor

Question 19.11.   A 24-year-old man presents with anterior chest discomfort and cough of 3 weeks duration. Examination is unremarkable. Chest radiograph shows widening of the superior mediastinum. CT scan shows a 6-cm anterior mediastinal mass encasing the trachea and great vessels and three 1-cm pulmonary nodules. CT scan of the abdomen and pelvis and a testicular ultrasound examination are normal. Laboratory studies reveal a hemoglobin of 11.4 with normal white blood cell count and platelet count, LDH of 880 IU/L (normal, 120–240 IU/L), α-fetoprotein of 1800 ng/mL (normal, <8 ng/mL), and β-hCG of 1.2 mIU/mL (normal, <5 mIU/mL). What is the most likely diagnosis?

    A.   Hodgkin's lymphoma
    B.   Benign teratoma
    C.   Nonseminomatous germ cell tumor (NSGCT)
    D.   Seminoma

Question 19.12.   Which of the following statements regarding mediastinal germ cell tumors is correct?

    A.   The incidence of malignant mediastinal germ cell tumors is the same in men and women.
    B.   Seminoma is the most common mediastinal germ cell tumor.
    C.   An elevated serum α-fetoprotein level in a patient with biopsy-proven seminoma indicates the presence of a NSGCT component.
    D.   Mediastinal NSGCTs are associated with better overall survival than testicular NSGCTs.

Question 19.13.   A 39-year-old woman presents with a cough and dyspnea that have progressed over the past 4 months. She is now dyspneic on walking less than 100 feet. Examination shows an anxious woman with a pulse of 110 beats/min, a respiratory rate of 24 breaths/min, and mild stridor. Lungs are otherwise clear to auscultation, and heart sounds are regular. Chest radiograph shows a large anterior mediastinal mass with narrowing of the mid-trachea. CT scan shows a 10-cm, highly heterogeneous anterior mediastinal mass with foci of dense calcification that compresses the trachea and superior vena cava without obstruction. Laboratory studies reveal normal blood counts, chemistries, LDH, carcinoembryonic antigen (CEA), α-fetoprotein, and β-hCG. She undergoes complete resection of the mass, which is adherent to the trachea, superior vena cava, left pleura, and pericardium without gross invasion. Pathologic evaluation reveals a multicystic mass with foci of mature gland formation, respiratory epithelium, cartilage, and bone. There is no invasion into adjacent structures, and surgical margins are negative. What is the most appropriate management of this patient?

A. Clinical surveillance
B. Adjuvant radiotherapy
C. Cisplatin plus etoposide × four cycles
D. Doxorubicin plus ifosfamide × six cycles

Question 19.14.   A 23-year-old man presents with hoarseness, cough, and anterior chest pain. He has a 30 pack-year smoking history. Examination is normal. Chest radiograph shows a large left mediastinal mass and clear lung fields. CT scan of the chest shows a 5-cm irregular left paratracheal mass. CT scan of the abdomen is normal. Serum CEA, β-hCG, and α-fetoprotein are normal. Bronchoscopy reveals extrinsic compression of the left mainstem bronchus without an endobronchial lesion. Left mediastinotomy with biopsy of the anterior mediastinal mass reveals a poorly differentiated malignant neoplasm that is immunohistochemically negative for leukocyte common antigen, vimentin, S100, TTF1, and chromogranin, but positive for low molecular weight cytokeratin. Genetic studies reveal no B- or T-cell rearrangements, and karyotypic analysis shows aneuploidy with an isochromosome 12p. Which of the following is the most appropriate therapy for this patient?

A. Cisplatin plus etoposide
B. Cisplatin, etoposide, and bleomycin
C. Concurrent chemotherapy and radiation therapy
D. Cyclophosphamide, doxorubicin, vincristine, and prednisone

Question 19.15.   A previously healthy 32-year-old man presents with fatigue and vague chest discomfort. A chest radiograph shows a widened mediastinum, and the CT scan confirms a large anterior mediastinal mass with focal areas of hemorrhage that fills the substernal space and invades into the upper lobe of the left lung. Laboratory studies show LDH of 850 IU/L (normal, 120–240 IU/L), α-fetoprotein of 8700 ng/mL (normal, <8 ng/mL), and β-hCG of 220 mIU/mL (normal, <5 mIU/mL). Biopsy confirms embryonal carcinoma with elements of choriocarcinoma. After four cycles of cisplatin, etoposide, and bleomycin, a CT scan shows marked shrinkage of the mediastinal mass, now measuring 3 cm in maximal diameter. One month after completion of therapy, LDH is 150 IU/L, α-fetoprotein is 5.0 ng/mL, and β-hCG 2.4 is mIU/mL. Which of the following is the most appropriate management of this patient?

A. Clinical surveillance
B. Cisplatin, ifosfamide, and vinblastine (VIP)
C. Two additional cycles of cisplatin, etoposide, and bleomycin
D. Resection of the residual mediastinal mass

Question 19.16.   A 22-year-old man has a retrosternal mass identified on a chest radiograph done during his enlistment into military service. He is an asymptomatic nonsmoker with no significant medical history. CT scan shows a 2.5-cm smooth anterior mediastinal mass without local invasion. Serum LDH, β-hCG, and α-fetoprotein are normal. Testicular ultrasound is normal. He refuses primary surgical resection, and a percutaneous core biopsy shows pure seminoma. Which of the following is the most appropriate management of this patient?

A. Surgical resection
B. Radiotherapy
C. Cisplatin, etoposide, and bleomycin
D. Cisplatin plus etoposide followed by surgical resection

Question 19.17.   An increased incidence of hematologic malignancies, such as acute megakaryocytic leukemia, has been reported with which of the following mediastinal tumors?

A. Seminoma
B. NSGCT
C. Malignant schwannoma
D. Thymic carcinoid

Question 19.18.   A 33-year-old man presents with chest tightness and shortness of breath. A chest radiograph shows a large mediastinal mass. CT scan shows a 9-cm lobulated anterior mediastinal mass invading the left lung and the pericardium with a small pericardial effusion, a 3-cm right paratracheal lymph node, and a 5-cm subcarinal lymph node. Echocardiogram shows no tamponade. Serum LDH is 440 IU/L (normal, 120–240 IU/L), but α-fetoprotein and β-hCG are normal. Testicular ultrasound is normal. Bronchoscopic core biopsy of the subcarinal mass reveals seminoma. Which of the following is the most appropriate management of this patient?

A. Carboplatin plus etoposide
B. Radiotherapy
C. Surgical resection
D. Cisplatin, etoposide, and bleomycin

Question 19.19.   A previously healthy 52-year-old man presents with hoarseness and vague chest discomfort. A chest radiograph shows a widened mediastinum, and a CT scan confirms a large anterior mediastinal mass encasing the trachea and abutting the superior vena cava, left pleura, and superior pericardium. Serum α-fetoprotein is normal, but β-hCG is 10 mIU/mL (normal, <5 mIU/mL). Biopsy shows seminoma. He is treated with cisplatin, etoposide, and bleomycin. CT scan after treatment shows marked shrinkage of the mediastinal mass, now measuring 2 cm in maximal diameter. β-hCG is now 1.2 mIU/mL. Which of the following is the most appropriate management of this patient?

A. Clinical surveillance
B. Cisplatin, ifosfamide, and vinblastine (VIP)
C. Resection of the residual mediastinal mass
D. Involved-field radiotherapy

Question 19.20.   A 17-year-old boy is evaluated for cough and fatigue. Physical exam is notable for scant facial, pubic and axillary hair, breast enlargement, and small testes. His serum testosterone level is low, but serum follicle-stimulating hormone (FSH) and luteinizing hormone (LH) levels are mildly elevated. Karyotypic analysis reveals 47XXY. Chest radiograph reveals an anterior mediastinal mass. CT scan of the chest shows a lobulated, 5.2-cm anterior mediastinal mass with areas of hemorrhage and necrosis. What is the most likely diagnosis?

A. Lymphoblastic lymphoma
B. Thymoma
C. NSGCT
D. Seminoma

ANSWERS

Answer 19.1.   **The answer is D.**

This middle-aged woman has an anterior mediastinal mass that appears localized on radiologic imaging. Thymomas are the most common tumors arising in the anterior mediastinum. They occur in patients of all ages, and approximately one-half of patients are symptomatic because of compression of mediastinal structures (e.g., pain, cough, superior vena cava syndrome) or associated paraneoplastic syndromes. Paraneoplastic syndromes can be identified in up to 70% of patients with thymoma but are uncommon in patients with thymic carcinoma. Myasthenia gravis is the most common paraneoplastic syndrome associated with thymoma, although a wide variety of other syndromes, primarily caused by autoimmune dysregulation, have been reported. Small cell lung cancer typically presents with a central lung mass and bulky mediastinal lymphadenopathy, and nearly all patients have a history of tobacco use. Pericardial cysts occur primarily in the middle mediastinum and, in adults, are usually asymptomatic. NSGCTs occur predominantly in young men, and 80% to 85% are associated with elevations of α-fetoprotein and/or β-hCG.

Answer 19.2.   **The answer is B.**

This child presents with radicular pain and a noninvasive posterior mediastinal mass arising from the paravertebral sulcus. Thoracic neurogenic tumors occur most commonly in the posterior mediastinum and account for 75% of tumors in this location. They are predominantly seen in children, in whom they are frequently malignant, and in young adults, in whom they are usually benign. In children, neurogenic tumors account for nearly half of all mediastinal neoplasms. Histologic subtypes of thoracic neurogenic tumors include neurofibroma, neurilemmoma, neurosarcoma, ganglioneuroma, paraganglioma, and neuroblastoma. Because thoracic neurogenic tumors arise in the paravertebral sulcus, they frequently cause pain and a variety of neurologic symptoms, including spinal cord compression, paresthesia, Horner's syndrome, and muscular atrophy. Surgical resection is the primary treatment option for all thoracic neurogenic tumors if it can be accomplished with acceptable risk. Observation is an option for asymptomatic patients with benign tumors who are poor candidates for surgery. Thymomas are found predominantly in the anterior mediastinum, although ectopic thymic tissue can rarely result in tumors in other mediastinal compartments. Mediastinal germ cell tumors are uncommon in young children and nearly always arise in the anterior mediastinum. Lymphomas account for 26% of mediastinal tumors in adults, but only 9% in children, and are mainly noted in the anterior mediastinum.

Answer 19.3.   **The answer is C.**

Transesophageal ultrasonography provides the best assessment of the invasiveness of a posterior mediastinal mass, while the other modalities have limited utility for this indication. Posteroanterior (PA) and lateral chest radiographs can define the general location, size and density of a mediastinal mass. Intravenous contrast-enhanced CT scan is the best imaging modality for accurately defining whether the lesion is solid or cystic, detecting fat and calcium, and determining the relationship of the mass to surrounding structures. PET scan is useful for assessing mediastinal lymphoma, but its role in the evaluation of other mediastinal masses continues to be evaluated.

Answer 19.4.   **The answer is A.**

This woman has undergone complete resection of a noninvasive, low-grade thymoma. Several histologic classification schemes and staging systems have been developed for thymic neoplasms. The WHO histologic classification is most commonly used and includes both thymomas (types A, AB, B1, and B2) and thymic carcinomas (types B3 and C) with varying degrees of pathologic atypia and aggressiveness. The most commonly used staging system was derived by Masaoka: stage I, no microscopic capsular invasion (noninvasive); stage II, microscopic capsular invasion or gross invasion into perithymic fat; stage III, gross invasion into adjacent organs; stage IVa, pleural or pericardial dissemination; and stage IVb, lymphogenous or hematogenous metastases. Complete resection of Masaoka stage I low-grade thymoma is associated with 5- and 10-year survival rates of 90% to 100% and 70% to 80%, respectively. Neither adjuvant radiotherapy nor chemotherapy has been shown to benefit patients who have undergone complete resection of Masaoka stage I, or noninvasive, thymoma.

Answer 19.5.   **The answer is B.**

This middle-aged man presents with anemia and a mediastinal mass that is found to be a microscopically invasive, low-grade thymoma. The presence of capsular invasion is an adverse prognostic factor for patients with completely resected thymoma, leading to a classification of Masaoka stage II. Studies have suggested a survival advantage for adjuvant radiotherapy after complete resection in patients with invasion into the capsule (stage II) or adjacent organs (stage III). The role of adjuvant chemotherapy in such patients remains unclear. Pure red cell aplasia occurs in 5% of patients with thymoma and is believed to be caused by autoimmune dysregulation. Conversely, 30% to 50% of patients with pure red cell aplasia have an associated thymoma. Bone marrow examination shows marked reduction or absence of erythroid precursors. Approximately 30% of patients also have a reduction in megakaryocytes or leukocyte precursors. Thymectomy induces remission of pure red cell aplasia in only 40% of patients.

Answer 19.6.   **The answer is D.**

Many paraneoplastic syndromes are associated with thymoma, including autoimmune disorders (polymyositis, systemic lupus erythematosus, Sjogren's syndrome, Hashimoto's thyroiditis, and scleroderma), endocrine disorders (Addison's disease, hypothyroidism, and panhypopituitarism), neuromuscular syndromes (myasthenia gravis, Eaton–Lambert myasthenic syndrome, and myotonic dystrophy), hematologic disorders (pure red cell aplasia, hypogammaglobinemia, T-cell deficiency syndrome, and amegakaryocytic thrombocytopenia) and miscellaneous disorders (hypertrophic pulmonary osteoarthropathy, nephrotic syndrome and paraneoplastic pemphigus).

Answer 19.7.   **The answer is D.**

This man presents after incomplete surgical resection of a high-grade thymic carcinoma. Thymic carcinoma is a rare, aggressive malignancy that is frequently locally advanced or metastatic at diagnosis. The many histologic subtypes of thymic carcinoma generally fall into two clinically relevant categories: low grade or well differentiated (WHO type B3) and high grade (WHO type C). Low-grade thymic carcinomas can have a relatively indolent course leading to reported median survivals of 25 months to over 6 years. However, the median survival of patients with high-grade thymic carcinoma is only 11 to 15 months. Although the rarity of thymic carcinoma precludes evidence-based treatment guidelines, most patients undergo multimodality therapy because of the locally invasive nature of the disease. Adjuvant chemotherapy plus radiotherapy is recommended for patients with thymic carcinoma with either grossly (R2) or microscopically (R1) positive surgical margins. Clinical surveillance is recommended only for patients with no evidence of capsular invasion, and adjuvant radiotherapy alone is recommended for those with capsular invasion after complete surgical resection (R0). Recommendations are similar for patients with thymoma after R0 and R2 resections, except that adjuvant radiotherapy alone is usually used after R1 resection. Further surgical resection and adjuvant chemotherapy alone are not generally indicated for thymic tumors.

Answer 19.8.   **The answer is C.**

This young man presents with symptoms of superior vena cava syndrome caused by a locally advanced, primarily unresectable thymic carcinoma. Symptoms caused by compression or invasion of mediastinal structures, including anterior chest pain, cough, dyspnea, and superior vena cava syndrome, occur in up to 70% of patients with thymic carcinoma, whereas paraneoplastic syndromes are rare. Because completeness of resection is one of the most important predictors of outcome, multimodality therapy should be recommended for all patients with thymic neoplasms, both thymoma and thymic carcinoma, whose tumors are judged to be primarily unresectable because of the extent of local invasion. The most commonly studied approach includes neoadjuvant cisplatin-based chemotherapy followed by surgical resection and postoperative radiotherapy. Cumulative results reveal that neoadjuvant chemotherapy results in an objective response rate of 89% and a complete response rate of 31%. These studies included patients with both thymoma and thymic carcinoma. Long-term survival remains the goal of therapy for patients with locally advanced disease, with one trial noting a 7-year disease-free survival rate of 83% after trimodality therapy. Therefore, purely palliative approaches are only justifiable in patients whose performance status or comorbidities preclude potentially curative combined modality therapy. Although there are some data supporting the use of definitive chemotherapy plus radiotherapy without surgical resection, further studies are needed to define the utility of this approach.

Answer 19.9.   **The answer is D.**

In patients with thymic carcinoma, improved survival has been correlated with the following histologic features: negative margins/complete resection, encapsulated tumors, lobular growth pattern, low mitotic activity, and low histologic grade. Low-grade tumors include well-differentiated squamous cell carcinoma, well-differentiated mucoepidermoid carcinoma and basaloid carcinoma. High-grade thymic tumors include small cell carcinoma, poorly differentiated lymphoepithelioma-like carcinoma, sarcomatoid carcinoma, anaplastic carcinoma, and clear cell carcinoma.

Answer 19.10.   **The answer is C.**

This young man with MEN I presented with a localized anterior mediastinal mass. Thymic carcinoid is a rare tumor that is associated with MEN I. Thymic carcinoids can produce adrenocorticotropic hormone (ACTH), leading to Cushing's syndrome, but rarely cause classical, serotonin-induced carcinoid syndrome. The primary treatment is complete surgical resection, which results in a 5-year survival rate of 60%, although late recurrences and mortality are not uncommon. Adjuvant radiotherapy is reserved for patients with incomplete resections, and the role of chemotherapy is unclear. Thymolipomas are rare, benign tumors that occur mainly in young adults and consist of mature thymic and adipose tissue. Although they are noninvasive, thymolipomas can grow to a large size and cause symptoms resulting from compression of mediastinal structures. Complete resection is curative. Thymoma is not associated with any of the MEN syndromes. Malignant islet cell tumors tend to recur locally in the pancreatic bed or to metastasize to the peritoneum, regional lymph nodes, and liver.

Answer 19.11.   **The answer is C.**

This young man presents with an anterior mediastinal mass and an elevated α-fetoprotein (AFP) that is pathognomonic for an NSGCT. Germ cell tumors account for 10% to 12% of all mediastinal tumors in adults and 6% in children and usually arise in the anterior mediastinum. Approximately 10% of germ cell tumors originate in extragonadal sites, with 50% to 70% of these arising in the mediastinum. Serum tumor markers, namely, LDH, AFP, and β-hCG, are helpful in the diagnosis and management of germ cell tumors. Benign teratomas, the most common mediastinal germ cell tumors (60% to 70%), are not associated with significant tumor marker elevations. Pure seminoma can cause modest elevations of β-hCG, but not AFP. AFP is produced by yolk sac elements, and in the setting of a mediastinal mass, an elevated serum AFP level is pathognomonic of NSGCT. Although lymphoma is commonly associated with elevations of LDH, AFP is not affected.

Answer 19.12.   **The answer is C.**

Although benign teratomas occur with equal frequency in men and women, approximately 85% of malignant mediastinal germ cell tumors occur in men. Primary pure seminoma accounts for only 35% of malignant mediastinal germ cell tumors. Patients with pure seminoma may have modest elevations of serum β-HCG, but an elevated serum α-fetoprotein level indicates the presence of an NSGCT component, even in a patient with biopsy-proven seminoma. Mediastinal NSGCTs carry a poorer prognosis than testicular NSGCTs. All patients with mediastinal NSGCT are considered poor-risk per the International Germ Cell Consensus Classification, with 85% to 95% having distant metastases at presentation. The overall 5-year survival rate of patients with mediastinal NSGCT is about 50%.

Answer 19.13.   **The answer is A.**

This woman has undergone complete resection of a tumor with radiologic and histologic characteristics of a benign, noninvasive teratoma. Benign teratoma is the most common mediastinal germ cell tumor. Unlike malignant germ cell tumors, benign teratomas, also known as dermoid cysts, occur with equal incidence in both men and women, primarily affecting patients between 20 and 40 years of age. Benign teratomas frequently present as large anterior mediastinal masses with normal serum tumor markers that cause symptoms resulting from compression of mediastinal structures. Although they may be adherent to adjacent structures, they are typically noninvasive. Histologically, both benign and malignant teratomas contain elements from all three germ cell layers: ectoderm (skin, hair, sweat glands, teeth); mesoderm (fat, muscle, bone, cartilage); and endoderm (bronchial or intestinal epithelium). Malignant teratomas, in which one or more of these elements have an invasive or metastatic phenotype, are aggressive tumors that usually have a poor response to therapy and are associated with an unfavorable prognosis. In contrast, surgical resection of benign teratoma results in excellent long-term survival rates with a low risk of recurrence. Neither adjuvant radiotherapy nor chemotherapy is indicated in the management of patients with benign teratoma.

Answer 19.14.   **The answer is B.**

This young man presents with a mediastinal poorly differentiated carcinoma of unknown primary site that is clinically and molecularly consistent with an extragonadal germ cell tumor. Poorly differentiated carcinoma arising in the midline structures of a young man is highly suggestive of an unrecognized extragonadal germ cell tumor, even in the face of normal tumor markers. In this patient, immunohistochemical analysis is suggestive of carcinoma with positive cytokeratin and argues against lymphoma (common leukocyte antigen), neuroendocrine tumor (chromogranin), sarcoma (vimentin), lung cancer (TTF1), and melanoma (S100). Genetic analysis can frequently be useful in clarifying histogenesis in such situations. Isochromosome 12p (i[12p]) is pathognomonic of germ cell tumors and can be found in approximately 30% of patients in this setting. A long-term survival rate of 16% has been reported for patients with midline poorly differentiated carcinoma of unknown primary site treated with cisplatin-based chemotherapy appropriate for NSGCT. The presence of i(12p) has been favorably associated with response and survival. Because the International Germ Cell Cancer Collaborative Group considers mediastinal NSGCT a "poor-risk" tumor, appropriate treatment should consist of cisplatin, etoposide, and bleomycin for four cycles. Therapy aimed at good-risk NSGCT (answer A), stage III NSCLC (answer C), or lymphoma (answer D) would not be appropriate.

Answer 19.15.   **The answer is D.**

This young man had an excellent response to initial chemotherapy for mediastinal NSGCT with normalization of tumor markers and a small residual mediastinal mass. Mediastinal NSGSTs commonly arise in the anterior compartment, and most patients are symptomatic at diagnosis. Elevations of β-hCG and α-fetoprotein are found in 30% to 50% and 60% to 80% of patients, respectively. NSGCTs frequently consist of a mixture of histologic subtypes, including choriocarcinoma, embryonal carcinoma, endodermal sinus (yolk sac) elements, and teratoma. Primary treatment of mediastinal NSGCTs is cisplatin, etoposide, and bleomycin, as per the guidelines for poor-risk nonseminomatous testicular cancer, which yields a complete response rate of 40% to 64% and a long-term survival rate of 45%. Surgical resection is recommended for patients with residual masses after completion of initial chemotherapy and normalization of tumor markers. If viable NSGCT elements are identified in the resected specimen, then two further cycles of cisplatin-based therapy are indicated. If the residual mass reveals only mature teratoma or necrosis, then clinical surveillance without further treatment is indicated. The role of surgical resection in patients with incomplete tumor marker responses has not been clearly defined, but such patients would typically proceed to salvage chemotherapy with a regimen such as VIP.

Answer 19.16.   **The answer is B.**

This young man presents with a localized mediastinal seminoma. Pure mediastinal seminoma is a rare disease, accounting for 35% of malignant mediastinal germ cell tumors and occurring mainly in men 20 to 40 years of age. Despite their slow growth rate, mediastinal seminomas tend to present as large tumors that cause symptoms resulting from compression of mediastinal structures. Serum β-hCG and LDH levels may be modestly elevated in patients with pure seminoma, but an elevated α-fetoprotein level would be indicative of a nonseminomatous germ cell component. Radiotherapy is the treatment of choice for localized mediastinal seminoma, yielding long-term survival rates of 60% to 80%. The total radiation dose should be in excess of 45 Gy, and the field should include the mediastinum and bilateral supraclavicular fossae. Although surgery followed by adjuvant therapy also yields high long-term survival rates, resection is not generally indicated in the management of mediastinal seminoma. Because of the exquisite sensitivity of seminoma to radiotherapy, the relatively low rates of recurrence after radiotherapy and the high cure rates associated with salvage chemotherapy, systemic treatment is not recommended for patients with localized disease.

Answer 19.17.   **The answer is B.**

A number of hematologic malignancies have been reported in association with mediastinal NSGCT, including acute megakaryocytic leukemia, acute myeloid leukemia, erythroleukemia, malignant histiocytosis, and myelodysplastic syndromes. These may be diagnosed either before or at the same time as the NSGCT. Solid tumors may also occur at an increased frequency in patients with mediastinal germ cell tumors. In addition, mediastinal NSGCTs have a propensity to develop malignant non-germ cell components, such as adenocarcinoma, squamous cell carcinoma, and sarcoma.

Answer 19.18.   **The answer is D.**

This man presents with locally advanced mediastinal seminoma that invades adjacent structures and involves regional lymph nodes. More than half of patients with mediastinal seminoma will have metastases at diagnosis, primarily to the intrathoracic lymph nodes, lung, or bone. Patients with locally advanced disease are usually treated with cisplatin-based chemotherapy with or without radiotherapy, whereas those with distant disease are treated with chemotherapy alone. Cisplatin-based treatment has been reported to result in an objective response rate that approaches 95% and a complete response rate of up to 85%, with a long-term disease-free survival rate of 80% to 85%. Carboplatin-based therapy is known to be inferior to cisplatin-based regimens. For patients with bulky, locally advanced mediastinal seminoma, the large radiation fields required to encompass all disease can result in excessive pulmonary or cardiac toxicity. In addition, despite high rates of local control, 20% to 40% of patients with locally advanced disease who are treated with radiotherapy alone will develop distant metastases, leading to the recommendation for primary systemic chemotherapy in such patients. Surgery is not indicated in the primary treatment of mediastinal seminoma.

Answer 19.19.   **The answer is A.**

This man has had an excellent response to initial chemotherapy for locally advanced mediastinal seminoma with normalization of β-HCG and a small residual mediastinal mass. The optimal management of patients with a residual mass on radiographic follow-up after treatment with initial chemotherapy or radiotherapy for seminoma remains controversial. Most studies have demonstrated that viable seminoma is rare in resected residual masses, and that 85% to 90% of such specimens consist entirely of scar tissue. Other studies have shown that up to 25% of residual masses more than 3 cm in size after initial chemotherapy contain viable seminoma. Nevertheless, resection of a residual mass is currently not recommended unless the mass enlarges during clinical surveillance. Similarly, the addition of radiotherapy after chemotherapy has not been shown to be of significant benefit. Salvage chemotherapy with a regimen such as VIP, with or without aggressive local therapy, is indicated for recurrent disease.

Answer 19.20.   **The answer is C.**

This young man presents with symptoms of mediastinal compression and physical signs of Klinefelter's syndrome. Karyotypic analyses of mediastinal germ cell tumors have revealed the 47XXY pattern of Klinefelter's syndrome in up to 20% of patients. Klinefelter's syndrome is also associated with male breast cancer and rare cases of seminoma have been reported, but it has not been associated with an increased risk of thymic tumors or non-Hodgkin's lymphoma.

 # CHAPTER 20 CANCER OF THE GASTROINTESTINAL TRACT

RENUKA V. IYER • RAVI CHHATRALA

RENUKA V. IYER • RAVI CHHATRALA

SECTION 1 ESOPHAGUS AND STOMACH

DIRECTIONS   Each of the numbered items below is followed by lettered answers. Select the ONE lettered answer that is BEST in each case unless instructed otherwise.

QUESTIONS

Question 20.1.1. **Which of the following statements about the incidence of esophageal cancer is TRUE?**

  A. Esophageal cancer is relatively uncommon in the United States, and the lifetime risk of being diagnosed with the disease is less than 1%.
  B. Incidence rates among white men continue to increase and now exceed 8 per 100,000 person-years, and reflect the marked increase in the incidence of adenocarcinoma of the esophagus of more than 400% in the past 2 decades.
  C. Although the incidence of adenocarcinoma in white women (2 per 100,000) is lower than that in white men, rates of adenocarcinoma have increased in women by more than 300% during the past 20 years.
  D. Only A and B.
  E. All of the above.

Question 20.1.2. **All of the following are risk factors for the development of squamous cell cancer of the esophagus, EXCEPT:**

  A. Plummer–Vinson syndrome
  B. Gastroesophageal reflux disease
  C. Achalasia
  D. Tylosis

Corresponding Chapters in *Cancer: Principles & Practice of Oncology,* Ninth Edition: 78 (Molecular Biology of the Esophagus and Stomach), 79 (Cancer of the Esophagus), 80 (Cancer of the Stomach).

Question 20.1.3. Which of the following statements about Barrett's esophagus is TRUE?

A. The prevalence of Barrett's esophagus in the general population undergoing endoscopy is approximately 5%.

B. Both medical and antireflux therapies are associated with reduced risk of developing esophageal cancer.

C. Patients with low-grade dysplasia should undergo surveillance annual endoscopy.

D. Patients with Barrett's esophagus have a 5- to 10-fold higher risk of developing esophageal carcinoma compared to the normal population.

Question 20.1.4. Which of the following statements about the role of trastuzumab in the treatment of gastroesophageal cancers is FALSE?

A. The percentage of patients with overexpression of HER2 by FISH or immunohistochemistry is approximately 10%.

B. The addition of trastuzumab to cisplatin-based chemotherapy has been shown to improve response rates compared to chemotherapy alone.

C. The addition of trastuzumab to cisplatin-based chemotherapy has been shown to improve overall survival rates compared to chemotherapy alone.

D. None of the above.

Question 20.1.5. A 22-year-old woman is diagnosed with metastatic gastric cancer, with diffuse involvement of the stomach and linitis plastica. Her father died of the same cancer at age 42 years. Her mother is concerned about familial gastric cancer and is asking for information about hereditary gastric cancer and appropriate screening for her other children. Which of the following would be the most appropriate recommendation to this family?

A. Hereditary gastric cancer is rare and unlikely. She may just have some environmental exposures or DNA mismatch repair gene mutations that cannot be screened for.

B. She may very well have hereditary early-onset diffuse gastric cancer, but no surveillance or workup is recommended because this has yet to be confirmed in larger studies.

C. E-cadherin mutation testing should be considered here, and, in fact, prophylactic gastrectomy should be considered strongly for her siblings if a germ line E-cadherin mutation is confirmed and mucosal abnormality can be documented by endoscopic examination of the stomach.

D. E-cadherin mutation testing should be considered, and, in fact, prophylactic gastrectomy should be considered strongly for her siblings if a germ line E-cadherin mutation is confirmed even if no mucosal abnormalities are seen by endoscopic examination of the stomach.

Question 20.1.6. Which of the following statements is TRUE about molecular genetic alterations in gastric cancer?

A. Many sporadic diffuse gastric cancers display altered E-cadherin, a transmembrane, calcium-dependent adhesion molecule important in epithelial cell homophilic and heterophilic interactions.

B. The p53 tumor suppressor gene is consistently altered in most gastric cancers.

C. Microsatellite instability has been found in 13% to 44% of sporadic gastric carcinomas.

D. All of the above.

Question 20.1.7. A 72-year-old man diagnosed with squamous cancer of the esophagus has questions regarding the benefit of chemoradiation plus surgery for his locally advanced cancer. He would like to know about the natural history of his disease and the expected benefit of combined modality therapy. Which of the following statements best describes the likely outcome/prognosis of his cancer?

A. In patients with cancers of the upper and middle thirds of the esophagus, which are predominately squamous cell carcinomas, distant recurrence predominates over locoregional recurrence.

B. Preoperative radiotherapy and chemoradiotherapy may reduce the rate of locoregional recurrence but have no obvious effect on the rate of distant metastases.

C. Two recent prospective randomized trials evaluating chemoradiotherapy alone or chemoradiotherapy followed by surgery in squamous cancer indicate that improvement in local control with the addition of surgery also resulted in improved survival.

D. Concurrent administration of chemotherapy and radiotherapy provides better local control than radiotherapy alone, and the administration of chemotherapy has been shown in follow-up studies to reduce systemic recurrence.

Question 20.1.8. Which of the following statements about the role of fluorodeoxyglucose positron emission tomography (FDG-PET) use in the diagnosis and management of esophageal cancers is TRUE?

A. In the detection of distant metastases, FDG-PET is superior to computed tomography (CT), with sensitivity, specificity, and accuracy all in the range of 80% to 90%.

B. PET in combination with CT (PET/CT fusion or hybrid FDG-PET/CT) further improves specificity and accuracy of noninvasive staging.

C. FDG-PET seems to have value in evaluating response to chemotherapy and radiotherapy.

D. All of the above.

Question 20.1.9.   A 58-year-old Caucasian man with a long-standing history of alcohol abuse and 40 pack-year smoking history is evaluated by his primary care physician for symptoms of acid reflux. He is placed on a trial of proton pump inhibitor with partial relief of symptoms. He undergoes an upper endoscopy, and salmon pink color mucosa extending in a tongue-like fashion is identified at the gastroesophageal junction, extending 8 cm in length. Biopsy results reveal Barrett's esophagus with high-grade dysplasia and a 1.5-cm focus of submucosal adenocarcinoma. Staging PET/CT scan is negative for metastatic disease. The patient has neoadjuvant chemoradiation followed by esophagogastrectomy, and pathology is consistent with a residual 0.8-cm area of moderately differentiated adenocarcinoma extending into the muscularis, with no lymphovascular invasion or lymph node involvement with tumor. The patient is here for follow-up today 6 weeks postoperatively. He feels well and states he is thinking of returning to work. What are your recommendations?

A. Baseline postoperative restaging scan and annual radiographic surveillance, 3-month history, and physical examination
B. Adjuvant chemotherapy with cisplatin + 5-fluorouracil (5FU)
C. Adjuvant chemoradiation therapy with cisplatin + 5FU
D. Follow-up in 4 months with complete blood count (CBC) and comprehensive metabolic panel (CMP)

Question 20.1.10.   In the case described in Question 9, what is the pathologic stage of the patient?

A. T1N0M0 stage I
B. T2N0M0 stage IIA
C. T3N0M0 stage IIB
D. T3N0M0 stage III

Question 20.1.11.   Which of the following statements regarding the use of capecitabine and oxaliplatin in patients with advanced carcinoma of the esophagus or stomach is FALSE?

A. Capecitabine and oxaliplatin are non-inferior to infusional 5FU and cisplatin, respectively.
B. Oxaliplatin was associated with higher incidence of neutropenia compared to cisplatin.
C. The median survival for EOX (epirubicin, oxaliplatin, and capecitabine) is superior to ECF (epirubicin, cisplatin, and 5FU).
D. None of the above.

Question 20.1.12. In the United States, preoperative chemoradiation for locally advanced esophageal cancer followed by esophagectomy is commonly used as evidence suggests that this approach offers a survival advantage over surgery alone. Which of the following statements about the benefits of neoadjuvant chemoradiation are TRUE?

A. In approximately two-thirds of patients, disease is downstaged.

B. A survival advantage exists for patients experiencing downstaging to pathologically confirmed complete response or minimal residual disease status.

C. Locoregional control is improved, whereas distant failure is frequent and is the major cause of death.

D. All of the above.

Question 20.1.13. A 67-year-old man with dysphagia to solids and a 20-lb weight loss presents for evaluation and workup. Endoscopy reveals a 4-cm-long stricture from 28 to 32 cm, and biopsy confirms moderately differentiated squamous cell cancer, likely with regional nodal involvement noted on PET scan. The patient has long-standing diabetes mellitus, hypertension, and peripheral vascular disease and is not thought to be a good surgical candidate. The best treatment approach would be:

A. Photodynamic therapy followed by salvage chemoradiation

B. Chemoradiation with cisplatin, 5FU, and 64.8 Gy of radiation to tumor and involved nodal regions, including 5-cm margins above and below the tumor

C. Chemoradiation with cisplatin, 5FU, and 50.4 Gy of radiation to tumor, including the nodes involved

D. Radiation alone because he is unlikely to tolerate any kind of chemotherapy.

Question 20.1.14. A 57-year-old Caucasian woman with long-standing reflux symptoms presented with hematemesis to a local emergency department. Endoscopy revealed a distal esophageal malignant ulcer with involvement of the gastroesophageal (GE) junction and 5 cm of the gastric cardia. Biopsy revealed intestinal metaplasia at the GE junction and confirmed a diagnosis of adenocarcinoma. CT shows thickened distal esophagus and proximal stomach, hiatal hernia, and enlarged celiac nodes. Which statement most accurately describes her cancer?

A. She has a Siewert type I cancer: adenocarcinoma of the distal esophagus, which usually arises from an area with specialized intestinal metaplasia of the esophagus (i.e., Barrett's esophagus) and may infiltrate the esophagogastric junction from above.

B. She has a Siewert type II cancer: adenocarcinoma of the cardia, which arises from the epithelium of the cardia or from short segments with intestinal metaplasia at the esophagogastric junction.

C. She has a Siewert type III cancer: adenocarcinoma of the subcardial stomach, which may infiltrate the esophagogastric junction or distal esophagus from below.

Question 20.1.15. A 65-year-old woman underwent a D2 subtotal gastrectomy for a T3N1 moderately differentiated gastric cancer at a community hospital. On recovery from the operation, 9 weeks later, she was offered adjuvant fluoropyrimidine-based chemoradiation. Which of the following statements about adjuvant therapy for completely resected gastric cancer is TRUE?

A. Comparable local control can be achieved with optimal surgery that includes D2 lymph node dissection, and if this can be confirmed by a second pathology review, she does not need additional therapy.

B. Adjuvant chemotherapy alone based on data from the MAGIC trial is indicated because she has had adequate surgery. Radiation will not add any further improvement in local control.

C. The recommendation is based on results of the Intergroup study where D2 dissections were performed in only 10% of patients; thus, this may not be the best approach for this patient.

D. Adjuvant 5FU-based chemoradiation with 45 Gy radiotherapy has been shown to have a major advantage in survival, disease-free survival, and local–regional control compared with surgery alone, with much of the advantage in terms of improved local and regional control.

Question 20.1.16. A 79-year-old African American man presents with advanced gastric cancer, peritoneal carcinomatosis, and malnutrition. Parenteral nutrition is initiated, and his performance status is slowly improving. He is now able to perform activities of daily living and has gained 8 lbs. His daughter would like to know what your recommendations are at this point. Your response would be:

A. His survival with best supportive care alone is likely to be approximately 3 months. Now that he is strong enough to tolerate the side effects of chemotherapy, he could have a prolonged survival and better quality of life if he opts for chemotherapy.

B. His survival with best supportive care alone is likely to be 3 months; chemotherapy may improve his quality of life.

C. With chemotherapy, an improvement in survival is expected in patients with a performance status of 0 or 1, essentially only those who are fit and relatively asymptomatic from their cancer.

D. Intraperitoneal chemotherapy may be better in this case for better delivery of chemotherapy in the peritoneal cavity because it would avoid the toxicities of systemic therapy.

Question 20.1.17. All of the following are thought to be protective against the development of adenocarcinoma of the esophagus, EXCEPT:

A. Smoking cessation
B. Consumption of raw fruits and vegetables
C. Aspirin use
D. H. pylori infection

Question 20.1.18. Which of the following statements about the molecular biology of esophageal cancer is/are TRUE?

    A. EGFR overexpression correlates with poor prognosis including poor response to chemotherapy.

    B. Presence of p53 point mutation correlates with response to induction chemotherapy and predicts survival after esophagectomy.

    C. Reduced expression of E-cadherin correlates with progression from Barrett's esophagus to dysplasia and finally to adenocarcinoma.

    D. All of above.

Question 20.1.19. Which of the following statements is/are correct regarding gastric cancer?

    A. Prophylactic gastrectomy should be considered strongly in families with germ line E-cadherin mutation even without gross mucosal abnormalities on endoscopic examination of the stomach.

    B. p53 tumor suppressor gene is not involved in most gastric cancers.

    C. 'Microsatellite instability' is one of the mechanisms involved in the pathogenesis of sporadic gastric cancers.

    D. A & C.

ANSWERS

Answer 20.1.1.   **The answer is E.**

Similar trends have been noted in Western European countries. This trend of increased incidence of adenocarcinoma of the esophagus has paralleled the upward trend in rates of both GE reflux disease and obesity.

Answer 20.1.2.   **The answer is B.**

Achalasia, tylosis, characterized by hyperkeratosis of the palms and soles as well as esophageal papillomas, Plummer–Vinson syndrome, characterized by iron deficiency anemia, brittle fingernails, and esophageal webs, are all associated with the development of squamous cell carcinoma of the esophagus. Gastroesophageal reflux, however, is associated with the development of Barrett's esophagus and adenocarcinoma.

Answer 20.1.3.   **The answer is C.**

The prevalence of Barrett's esophagus in the general population undergoing endoscopy is approximately 1.5%, ranging from 1.2% to 2.3% in those without and with reflux symptoms, respectively. Although antireflux therapies are effective in reducing or even eliminating the symptoms, there is no clear evidence that either medical or surgical procedures decrease the risk of developing esophageal carcinoma. Patients with Barrett's esophagus have a 40- to 125-fold increase in the risk of developing esophageal carcinoma compared to the general population. The presence of any degree of dysplasia indicates the need for endoscopic surveillance, with annual endoscopy recommended for those with low-grade dysplasia and more frequent surveillance for those with higher grades of dysplasia.

Answer 20.1.4.   **The answer is A.**

In a recent study evaluating the role of trastuzumab in combination with chemotherapy for patients with gastroesophageal cancer, more than 3800 patients were screened for HER2 overexpression and 22.5% had HER2 overexpression. The addition of trastuzumab to cisplatin-based chemotherapy was associated with improved response rates, progression-free survival, and overall survival compared to chemotherapy alone.

Answer 20.1.5.   **The answer is D.**

Large families with an autosomal dominant, highly penetrant inherited predisposition for the development of gastric cancer are rare. However, early-onset diffuse gastric cancers have been described and linked to the E-cadherin/CDH1 locus on 16q and associated with mutations in this gene, which may be the case in this family. This seminal finding has been confirmed in other studies with gastric cancers at a relatively high (67% to 83%) penetrance rate. Thus, E-cadherin mutation testing should be considered in the appropriate clinical setting. In fact, prophylactic gastrectomy should be considered strongly in families with germ line E-cadherin mutation even without gross mucosal abnormalities on endoscopic examination of the stomach. Hereditary nonpolyposis colon cancer (HNPCC) involves germ line mutations of DNA mismatch repair genes. Gastric adenocarcinoma may be observed in families with HNPCC.

Answer 20.1.6. **The answer is D.**

A reasonably prevalent alteration is microsatellite instability, the result of changes in DNA mismatch repair genes (*PPO* Table 39.1.1). Microsatellite instability and associated alterations of the TGF-b II receptor, IGFRII, BAX, E2F-4, hMSH3, and hMSH6 genes are found in a subset of gastric carcinomas. Microsatellite instability has been found in 13% to 44% of sporadic gastric carcinomas. A high degree of microsatellite instability occurs in gastric cancers of the intestinal type, reduced involvement of lymph nodes, enhanced lymphoid infiltration, and better prognosis. This is reminiscent of colon cancers associated with HNPCC. The p53 tumor suppressor gene is consistently altered in most gastric cancers. In a study of the promoter region of p16 in gastric cancers, a significant number (41%) exhibited CpG island methylation. Many cases with hypermethylation of promoter regions displayed the phenotype with a high degree of microsatellite instability and multiple sites of methylation, including the hMLH1 promoter region. Many sporadic diffuse gastric cancers display altered E-cadherin. E-cadherin may be downregulated in gastric carcinogenesis (especially diffuse gastric adenocarcinoma) by point mutation, allelic deletion, or promoter methylation. In addition, during epithelial–mesenchymal transition, E-cadherin transcription can be silenced by transcriptional factors such as Snail and Slug.

Answer 20.1.7. **The answer is B.**

Median survival after esophagectomy for patients with localized disease is 15 to 18 months with a 5-year overall survival rate of 20% to 25%. Patterns of failure after esophagectomy suggest that both location of tumor and histologic type may influence the distribution of recurrence. In patients with cancers of the upper and middle thirds of the esophagus, which are predominately squamous cell carcinomas, locoregional recurrence predominates over distant recurrence. In patients with lesions of the lower third, where adenocarcinomas are more frequently located, distant recurrence is more common. Treatment failure patterns after definitive chemoradiotherapy without surgical resection reveal that concurrent administration of chemotherapy and radiotherapy provides better local control than radiotherapy alone, and that the administration of chemotherapy may reduce systemic recurrence; however, long-term follow-up of both randomized and nonrandomized patients treated with primary chemoradiotherapy failed to indicate a clear reduction in distant disease recurrence compared with radiation therapy alone. Although the addition of surgery further reduces local failure from 45% to 32%, it does not diminish systemic recurrence and, in fact, may enhance it by allowing patients to manifest distant disease because they do not succumb to locoregional failure. Two recent prospective randomized trials evaluating primary chemoradiotherapy alone or chemoradiotherapy followed by surgery in squamous cancer indicate that improvement in local control with the addition of surgery failed to improve survival. These patterns of relapse suggest that any further improvement in overall outcome for patients with esophageal cancer will be achieved through advances in systemic therapy.

Answer 20.1.8.   **The answer is D.**

The addition of CT to PET improves sensitivity and specificity, which translates into the detection of unsuspected metastatic disease (upstaging) in approximately 15% of patients and refutation of suspected disease (downstaging) in 10% of patients, which leads to alteration of the intended treatment plan in at least 20% of patients. Weber et al. demonstrated that decreased FDG uptake significantly correlated with pathologically confirmed response in patients treated with induction chemotherapy before esophagectomy for esophageal adenocarcinoma.

Answer 20.1.9.   **The answer is A.**

The available data for postoperative adjuvant chemotherapy suggest a possible prolongation of survival for patients who have had a potentially curative (R0) resection and have lymph node-positive (N1) disease. There are no data to indicate or suggest that administration of postoperative adjuvant chemotherapy will prolong survival for patients who have undergone a curative resection and have negative nodes (N0). Patients who have positive margins of resection should be considered for postoperative radiation. Those who have had R0 resections but have regional nodal metastases (stages IIB and III) should be enrolled in clinical trials evaluating adjuvant therapies.

Answer 20.1.10.   **The answer is B.**

Stage IIA.

Answer 20.1.11.   **The answer is B.**

A large phase III trial comparing four chemotherapy arms including epirubicin, cisplatin or oxaliplatin, and 5FU or capecitabine, showed non-inferiority for oxaliplatin compared to cisplatin and capecitabine compared to 5FU. In a planned comparison between EOX (epirubicin, oxaliplatin and capecitabine) and ECF (epirubicin, cisplatin and 5FU), the former was associated with a significant improvement in median overall survival (11.2 vs. 9.9 months).

Answer 20.1.12.   **The answer is D.**

Although two of the five randomized trials demonstrated a survival advantage for combined modality therapy, they are limited by small numbers of patients. The efficacy of preoperative combined modality treatment for patients with resectable esophageal cancer remains controversial. The accumulated experience from phase II and III trials support all of the statements listed here concerning chemoradiotherapy using cisplatin and infusional 5FU-based therapy followed by esophagectomy. Surgery seems to be an important component of treatment to eliminate persistent disease after chemoradiotherapy. Some 20% to 30% of this group will be long-term survivors. Rates of curative resection may be improved with preoperative chemoradiotherapy.

Answer 20.1.13. **The answer is C.**

The INT 0123 trial was the follow-up to RTOG 85–01. In this trial, patients with either squamous cell carcinoma or adenocarcinoma who were selected for nonsurgical treatment were randomly assigned to receive a slightly modified RTOG 85–01 combined modality regimen with 50.4 Gy of radiation versus the same chemotherapy with 64.8 Gy of radiation. It was closed early after an interim analysis showed that the high-dose arm was unlikely to have a superior survival compared with the lower dose arm. In addition, 11 treatment-related deaths occurred in the high-dose arm compared with two deaths in the standard-dose arm, with 7 of the 11 deaths occurring in patients who had received 50.4 Gy or less.

Although the crude incidence of local failure or persistence of local disease (or both) was lower in the high-dose arm than in the standard-dose arm (50% vs. 55%), as was the incidence of distant failure (9% vs. 16%), these differences did not reach statistical significance. At 2 years, the cumulative incidence of local failure was 56% for the high-dose arm versus 52% for the standard-dose arm ($p = .71$). Although retrospective data from the M. D. Anderson Cancer Center suggests a positive correlation between radiation dose and locoregional control, based on results of the INT 0123 trial, the standard dose of external-beam radiation remains 50.4 Gy.

Answer 20.1.14. **The answer is B.**

The Siewert classification has important therapeutic implications. The lymphatic drainage routes differ for type 1 versus types II and III lesions. As shown in lymphographic studies, the lymphatic pathways from the lower esophagus pass both cephalad (into the mediastinum) and caudad (toward the celiac axis). In contrast, the lymphatic drainage from the cardia and subcardial regions is toward the celiac axis, splenic hilus, and para-aortic nodes. Thus, the Siewert classification provides a practical means for choosing among surgical options. For type I tumors, esophagectomy is required, whereas types II and III tumors can be treated by transabdominal extended gastrectomy (resection of the stomach and distal intra-abdominal esophagus).

Answer 20.1.15. **The answer is D.**

The major change in the past decade in the adjuvant radiation therapy of gastric cancer comes from the results of the Gastrointestinal Intergroup trial that tested the value of adjuvant postoperative radiation therapy and chemotherapy for patients with T2 to T4 and/or node-positive gastric cancer after surgery with no evidence of residual disease. A total of 550 patients were entered in the study, with patients generally having advanced stage disease; 85% of patients had node-positive tumors and 69% of patients had T3 or T4 disease. Median overall survival in the Intergroup 116 study of observation versus postoperative chemoradiation therapy after potentially curative gastrectomy was 27 months in the surgery alone group and 36 months in the surgery plus chemoradiotherapy group. The hazard ratio for death in the surgery-alone group was 1.35 (95% confidence interval [CI], 1.09–1.66; $p = .005$). The Intergroup study has been criticized for not having good surgical quality control, with only a minimal number of nodes found in many surgical specimens and with D2 dissections having been performed in only 10% of patients. However, commentators often overlook the fact that the Intergroup protocol was a study of postoperative chemoradiation treatment for patients with completely resected high-risk gastric cancer; gastrectomy and lymph node dissection were not part of the protocol treatment because patients were evaluated for protocol eligibility only after successful recovery following gastrectomy. As such, the "surgical results" of the Intergroup trial are best viewed as a reflection of the standard practice of US surgeons and pathologists.

Answer 20.1.16.   **The answer is A.**

The results of the studies and supportive evidence from more recent trials indicate that fit patients with advanced incurable gastric cancer who can tolerate potential toxicities have a modest but real benefit in survival compared with best supportive care. The majority of studies that have evaluated intraperitoneal therapy for gastric cancer used mitomycin C, and most trials were performed in Asia. They have all examined intraperitoneal therapy in the adjuvant setting after surgery. A meta-analysis of these studies showed that the majority involved less than 100 patients per arm. A total of 552 patients had a resection alone, and 609 patients were randomized to operation plus intraperitoneal treatment. The odds ratio (OR) was in favor of postoperative intraperitoneal therapy (OR 0.51; 95% CI, 0.4 to 0.65). However, the authors thought that only a few of the studies were of high quality. They suggested that more rigorously designed trials with larger numbers of patients and greater power were necessary before definitive conclusions regarding the effectiveness of postoperative intraperitoneal treatment could be made. In summary, the use of intraperitoneal chemotherapy involving either technique is a reasonable experimental strategy, particularly until more effective systemic agents can be developed. The goal is improvement in overall survival, as well as prevention of abdominal carcinomatosis with its associated morbidities, such as recurrent bowel obstruction.

Answer 20.1.17.   **The answer is A.**

Smoking cessation does not appear to decrease the risk of adenocarcinoma of the esophagus. H. pylori infection, particularly cagA+ strains, is inversely associated with the risk of adenocarcinoma of the esophagus. H. pylori infection can result in chronic atrophic gastritis, leading to decreased acid production, and potentially reducing the development of Barrett's esophagus. Carcinogenesis in Barrett's esophagus is associated with increased expression of the enzyme cyclooxygenase-2 (COX-2). COX-2 inhibitors such as aspirin inhibit Barrett's esophagus-adenocarcinoma. Consumption of raw fruits and vegetables also exerts a protective effect.

Answer 20.1.18.   **The answer is D.**

All of these molecular mechanisms are involved in the pathogenesis of esophageal cancer.

Answer 20.1.19.   **The answer is D.**

Microsatellite instability is found in 13% to 44% of sporadic gastric carcinomas. A high degree of microsatellite instability occurs in gastric cancer of the intestinal type, reduced involvement of lymph nodes and better prognosis. p53 is consistently altered in most cases of gastric cancers.

SECTION 2   PANCREAS

RENUKA V. IYER • RAVI CHHATRALA

DIRECTIONS   Each of the numbered items below is followed by lettered answers. Select the ONE lettered answer that is BEST in each case unless instructed otherwise.

QUESTIONS

Question 20.2.1.   **Which of the following factors are not associated with an increased risk of pancreatic cancer?**

A. Cigarette smoke
B. Cirrhosis
C. High-protein diet
D. African American men

Question 20.2.2.   **Which of the following statements regarding pancreatic cancer is NOT true?**

A. At diagnosis, 31% have evidence of distant metastases.
B. Pancreatic cancer tends to occur later in life.
C. Activation of the K-ras oncogene plus inactivation of tumor suppressor genes (p53, DPC4, p16, and BRCA2) are associated with the development of pancreatic cancer.
D. Pancreatic intraepithelial neoplasms (PanINs) are intraductal proliferative epithelial lesions that are precancerous.
E. Patients with advanced pancreatic cancer may have undetectable levels of CA 19-9 if they are Lewis antigen-a or -b negative.

Corresponding Chapters in *Cancer: Principles & Practice of Oncology,* Ninth Edition: 81 (Molecular Biology of Pancreas Cancer), and 82 (Cancer of the Pancreas).

Question 20.2.3.   A 56-year-old African American man with a medical history of hypertension and type II diabetes presented to his primary care physician with a 1-month history of gradually worsening painless jaundice and a 10-lb weight loss. Computed tomography (CT) scan of the abdomen and pelvis revealed a 3.3-cm pancreatic head mass adjacent to the superior mesenteric vein with no intervening fat plan and encasing both the superior mesenteric vein and artery. The common bile duct was dilated, with a diameter of 1.8 cm, and the pancreatic body and tail were atrophied with dilatation of the pancreatic duct. Portal lymphadenopathy measuring 2 cm was present. The patient underwent endoscopic retrograde cholangiopancreatography ERCP, and a biliary stent was placed. Biopsy of the mass was consistent with moderately differentiated pancreatic adenocarcinoma. What is this patient's stage?

A.   Stage I
B.   Stage II
C.   Stage III
D.   Stage IV

Question 20.2.4.   A 67-year-old woman presents to her local emergency department with a 2-month history of right upper quadrant pain, jaundice, and 20-lb weight loss. She has no fever and chills. Standard CT of the abdomen reveals a 2.5-cm, ill-defined soft tissue density within the head of the pancreas and mild celiac axis, porta hepatis, and porta caval adenopathy, with the largest being within the celiac axis region measuring 2.0 × 1.8 cm. Endoscopic retrograde cholangiopancreatography is done, and a biliary stent is placed. Biopsy of the mass reveals poorly differentiated adenocarcinoma. CA 19-9 is 798. Which of the following should be done next for staging?

A.   Multiphase multidetector helical computerized axial tomography
B.   Magnetic resonance imaging
C.   Ultrasonography
D.   Staging laparoscopy
E.   Endoscopic ultrasonography

Question 20.2.5.   A 71-year-old Hispanic woman undergoes Whipple resection for a T3, N1, M0 pancreatic adenocarcinoma. Postoperative recovery was uneventful, and she starts adjuvant therapy 7 weeks later with gemcitabine given intravenously weekly for 2 weeks, followed by a 1-week break. In a follow-up visit after her first cycle she reports a 5-lb weight loss, nausea, decreased appetite, occasional abdominal cramping, and diarrhea. What should be done next?

A.   Increase pancreatic enzyme supplementation
B.   Admit the patient for small bowel obstruction
C.   Hold chemotherapy for 1 week and follow up on symptoms
D.   CT scan of the chest, abdomen and pelvis to rule out metastatic disease

Question 20.2.6.   Which of the following statements regarding adjuvant therapy is NOT true?

A. In patients with resected pancreatic head lesions, survival is superior with gemcitabine compared with infusional 5FU, when given after 5FU-based chemoradiation.

B. Gemcitabine when compared with observation is associated with prolonged disease-free survival and overall survival.

C. 5FU-based chemoradiation followed by chemotherapy with 5FU can also be considered for adjuvant therapy.

D. In the ESPAC-1 trial, patients who received chemotherapy did better than those who did not.

Question 20.2.7.   A 64-year-old Caucasian woman is diagnosed with locally advanced unresectable pancreatic cancer. She receives 2 months of gemcitabine, and restaging CT scan of the abdomen and pelvis shows a decrease in the size of the lesion and her CA19-9 decreases from 854 to 201. What should be done next?

A. Start 5FU-based chemoradiation

B. Continue gemcitabine chemotherapy for another 2 months, and then reassess

C. Start gemcitabine-based chemoradiation

D. Add 5FU to her chemotherapy regimen

Question 20.2.8.   A 52-year-old Asian woman is evaluated for chronic right upper quadrant abdominal pain. Workup leads to diagnosis of pancreatic adenocarcinoma with metastasis to the liver. She is extremely anxious and tearful and wants to do everything possible to prolong her life. Which of the following regimens has been shown to prolong overall survival compared with gemcitabine alone?

A. Gemcitabine and oxaliplatin

B. Gemcitabine and capecitabine

C. Gemcitabine and erlotinib

D. Gemcitabine and cisplatin and bevacizumab

E. Gemcitabine and cetuximab

Question 20.2.9.   A 45-year-old man is diagnosed with metastatic adenocarcinoma of the pancreas. Which of the following chemotherapy regimens would be appropriate first-line treatment choice in this otherwise healthy patient with normal organ function?

A. Gemcitabine

B. FOLFIRINOX (5FU+leucovorin+irinotecan+oxaliplatin)

C. 5FU with radiation

D. FOLFOX (5FU+leucovorin+oxaliplatin)

Question 20.2.10. Mutation of which tumor suppressor gene is most frequently associated with familial pancreatic cancer?

    A. BRCA2

    B. PALB2

    C. K-RAS

    D. TP53

Question 20.2.11. Which of the following statements regarding risk factors for pancreatic cancer is CORRECT?

    A. ABO blood group is associated with increased risk for pancreatic cancer.

    B. Testing for K-RAS mutations in the pancreatic juice of patients is an effective screening test for pancreatic cancer in high risk patients.

    C. Patients with hereditary nonpolyposis colorectal cancer syndrome do not have an increased risk for pancreatic cancer.

    D. Hereditary pancreatitis is not a significant risk factor for pancreatic cancer.

Question 20.2.12. A 65-year-old male was diagnosed with metastatic pancreatic cancer and received treatment with single-agent gemcitabine. However, he now has disease progression and is interested in pursuing systemic therapy. Which of the following could be considered as a second-line treatment choice?

    A. FOLFOX6

    B. Erlotinib

    C. Paclitaxel

    D. Irinotecan and raltitrexed

Question 20.2.13. Which of the following is true about pancreatic cancer?

    A. Most pancreatic cancers have mutations in KRAS, TP53, SMAD4, p16/CDKN2A.

    B. Telomere shortening is the earliest and most prevalent genetic change identified in the precursor lesions.

    C. Underexpression of TGF-β is observed in few pancreatic cancers.

    D. p16-mediated CDK inhibition is a protective mechanism against pancreatic cancer.

    E. All of above.

ANSWERS

Answer 20.2.1.   **The answer is C.**

Tobacco smoke exposure plays a significant role in the development of pancreatic adenocarcinoma. It has been estimated that tobacco smoking contributes to the development of 20% to 30% of pancreatic cancers. The strongest associations between cigarette smoking and pancreatic cancer have been observed when the smoking occurred within the previous 10 years. Smoking cessation can reduce this risk. Environmental tobacco smoke contains the same toxins, irritants, and carcinogens, such as carbon monoxide, nicotine, cyanide, ammonia, benzene, nitrosamines, vinyl chloride, arsenic, and hydrocarbons, as primary cigarette smoke. Host etiologic factors associated with an increased risk of pancreatic cancer include a history of diabetes mellitus (DM), chronic cirrhosis, pancreatitis, a high-fat/cholesterol diet, and prior cholecystectomy. Although not all studies have supported a relationship between DM and pancreatic cancer, a meta-analysis of 20 epidemiologic studies confirms that the pooled relative risk of pancreatic cancer in persons with DM for 5 years is double (relative risk, 2.0; 95% confidence interval [CI], 1.2 to 3.2) the risk of persons without DM. However, there is no association with a high-protein diet. People of African American descent experience a higher rate of pancreatic cancer than those of European ancestry in the United States, with an annual incidence of 16.7 per 100,000 versus 10.9 per 100,000, respectively. Death from pancreatic cancer is similarly elevated, with an annual rate of 14.6 per 100,000 versus 10.6 per 100,000. The diagnosis is slightly but significantly earlier in African Americans compared with Caucasians, with a median age of diagnosis of 68 and 73 years, respectively. In developed countries, the incidence and mortality rates range from 7 to 9 per 100,000 for men and 4.5 to 6 per 100,000 for women.

Answer 20.2.2.   **The answer is A.**

CA 19-9 is a clinically useful tumor marker. The epitope of this antibody is a sialylated lacto-N-fucopentaose II related to the Lewis-a blood group antigen. Limitations of CA 19-9 are that it is not specific for pancreatic cancer and has been found to be elevated in other tumor types, such as biliary tract, colon, and stomach cancers. Ten percent of patients are Lewis antigen-a or b negative and unable to synthesize this antigen, and therefore may have undetectable levels of CA 19-9, even in the setting of advanced pancreatic cancer. Cholestasis can falsely elevate serum CA 19-9 levels; therefore, in patients who present with obstructive jaundice, an elevated CA 19-9 is not specific for the presence of pancreatic malignancy. Despite these caveats, serum CA 19-9 levels seem to have prognostic utility, particularly when measured either preoperatively or postoperatively in patients with resectable pancreatic cancer. Pancreatic ductal adenocarcinoma arises from ductal epithelial cells. Neoplasia arising from these cells progresses from initial PanINs to invasive carcinomas. The evidence that these lesions are precancerous includes the observation that after segmental resection of pancreas with PanINs in the resected tissue, pancreatic cancer can develop in the pancreatic remnant. The strongest evidence that PanINs are precancerous lesions is the stepwise progression of genetic mutational events that correlates with the stepwise progression of worsening PanINs culminating in adenocarcinoma. PanIN-1 lesions show a predominance of K-ras mutations and overexpression of HER-2/neu. In PanIN-2 lesions, p16 mutations are the typical mutational event, and in PanIN-3 lesions, p53, DPC4, and BRCA2 mutations predominate. The mutational pattern of PanIN-3 lesions is equivalent to mutations found in pancreatic adenocarcinoma. These events are the basis of a current progression model for pancreatic cancer in which point mutation of K-ras and overexpression of HER-2/neu are initiating early events, p16 inactivation is an intermediate event, and p53, DPCA, BRCA2 inactivation follow just before invasion outside of the duct. Approximately 90% of all cases have p16 mutations, 75% have p53 mutations, and 55% have DPC4 mutations. It is estimated that 10% to 20% of pancreatic cancers are hereditary or have a familial link. Of patients with available data in the United States who were diagnosed with pancreatic cancer from 1996 to 2002, 8% presented with local disease, 31% presented with regional disease, and 61% had distant metastases. Therefore, the majority of patients are metastatic at diagnosis. Five-year survival from all stages of disease is 5%. Pancreatic cancer tends to occur later in life. Only 10% of patients in Europe present before the age of 50 years, whereas those aged 50 to 54 years experience an incidence of 9.8 per 100,000, and those aged 70 to 74 years experience an incidence of 57 per 100,000. The median age of diagnosis with pancreatic cancer in the United States is 72 years.

Answer 20.2.3.   **The answer is C.**

The patient has a stage III, T4N1M0 pancreatic cancer. As per the sixth edition of the American Joint Committee on Cancer staging system, this represents unresectable disease. The T-stage designation classifies T1 to T3 tumors as potentially resectable and T4 tumors as locally advanced (unresectable). Tumors with any involvement of the superior mesenteric or celiac arteries are classified as T4; however, tumors that involve the superior mesenteric, splenic, or portal veins are classified as T3 because these veins can be resected and reconstructed provided that they are patent.

Answer 20.2.4.   **The answer is A.**

Laparoscopy and multiphase CT have evolved concurrently as methods to evaluate a pancreatic mass. Both have emerged as highly effective in evaluating the tumors, but CT as a noninvasive modality supplants the use of routine laparoscopy. Currently, routine use of laparoscopy is not warranted. The cornerstone of diagnostic evaluation of a pancreatic tumor is the multiphase CT scan, coordinating intravenous contrast administration with subsequent rapid thin-cut CT through the pancreas during arterial, portal venous, and parenchymal phases of enhancement. With this type of CT, extension of the tumor to the superior mesenteric artery, celiac axis, superior mesenteric vein/portal vein complex, and contiguous structures can be clearly determined, as well as an assessment of distant metastasis. Optimally, CT imaging should precede stent placement and biopsy because of the possibility of postprocedure inflammation from the biopsy and artifact from the stent that can confound interpretation of the images. Magnetic resonance imaging has not been widely used to assess pancreatic cancer. Endoscopic ultrasound can image the primary cancer and be a means of obtaining a fine-needle aspiration of pancreatic adeno-carcinoma, but in general the procedure is noncontributory when CT scan characterizes the tumor. When a mass cannot be visualized on CT scan, sonography through the wall of the stomach or duodenum can image tumors in the body/tail and head of the pancreas, respectively. Although preoperative ultrasonography is useful in assessing tumor characteristics and resectability of pancreatic adenocarcinoma, it is particularly opera-tor dependent. It has a high sensitivity and specificity (92.3% and 72.7%, respectively) in defining superior mesenteric vein and portal vein invasion, although lower than helical CT (98% and 79%, respectively).

Answer 20.2.5.   **The answer is A.**

Malabsorption is a frequent complication seen in patients after Whipple surgery because of pancreatic enzyme insufficiency. Most patients require adjustment of the pancreatic enzyme supplement for adequate control of this symptomatology. Although small bowel obstruction and metastatic disease can be seen, the patient's clinical picture does not go along with these diagnoses. The aim during adjuvant therapy is to adminis-ter the chemotherapy with minimal delays to obtain the full benefit from therapy.

Answer 20.2.6.   **The answer is B.**

The Radiation Therapy Oncology Group (RTOG) performed a prospec-tive randomized trial (RTOG 9704) comparing gemcitabine with infu-sional 5FU as the systemic component of therapy with all patients also receiving 5FU-based chemoradiation. There was no survival difference between patients randomized to gemcitabine and those who received infusional 5FU. However, among the 380 patients with resected pancre-atic head lesions, survival was superior for patients randomized to gemc-itabine compared with those who received infusional 5FU (20.6 months vs. 15.9 months; hazard ratio [HR] for death 0.79; 95% CI, 0.63 to 0.99; $p = .033$). In CONKO-001, patients randomized to receive gem-citabine had a median disease-free survival of 13.9 months (95% CI, 11.4 to 15.3), whereas those patients who underwent surgery alone had a median disease-free survival of only 6.9 months (95% CI, 6.1 to 7.8; $p = .001$). However, there was no statistically significant difference in overall survival. 5FU-based chemoradiation followed by up to 2 years of weekly bolus 5FU was evaluated against observation alone in the GITSG trial. A preliminary analysis of survival was reported after only 43 patients had completed treatment and showed a striking survival advantage for patients receiving combined modality therapy compared with survival of patients who underwent surgery alone (median 21.0 months vs. 10.9 months, respectively; one-tailed $p = .03$). In ESPAC-1, patients receiving chemoradiation did worse (median survival of 15.9 months; HR for death 1.28; 95% CI, .99 to 1.66) than those not receiving chemoradiation (median survival of 17.9 months; $p = .05$). Conversely, patients who received chemotherapy had a median survival of 20.6 months (HR for death 0.71; 95% CI, 0.55 to 0.92) versus 15.5 months for those patients who did not receive chemotherapy, a statistically significant result ($p = .009$).

Answer 20.2.7.   **The answer is B.**

The optimal treatment of locally advanced pancreatic cancer remains controversial. Locally advanced disease is generally incurable, and all therapies have significant limitations. Gemcitabine-based chemotherapy for 2 to 4 months followed by 5FU or capecitabine-based chemoradiation is the most appropriate choice for the majority of patients with locally advanced, unresectable disease. If patients are responding to chemotherapy (objective radiographic response or CA 19-9 level decline) after 2 months and tolerating therapy well, it is reasonable to continue for 2 more months. When there is radiographic local progression, a CA 19-9 level plateau or increase, local symptomatic progression, or chemotherapy is poorly tolerated, chemoradiation should be initiated. In patients in whom distant progression has become evident during chemotherapy, a 2-week course of 30 Gy of 5FU or capecitabine-based chemoradiation should be considered only in patients with symptomatic primary tumors. The patients who have not progressed after systemic therapy are most likely to benefit from chemoradiation, and typically a 5.5-week course (50.4 Gy) of radiation therapy is appropriate with concurrent chemotherapy.

Answer 20.2.8.   **The answer is C.**

Thus far, only inhibition of epidermal growth factor receptor with erlotinib combined with gemcitabine has led to a small, but statistically significant improvement in survival compared with gemcitabine alone. In a study performed by the National Cancer Institute of Canada Clinical Trials Group, patients with advanced pancreatic cancer were randomized to receive gemcitabine alone at 1000 mg/m^2 weekly for 7 weeks, then 1 week off, followed by gemcitabine days 1, 8, 15, every 28 days, or the combination of gemcitabine with erlotinib at a dose of 100 to 150 mg orally daily. Overall survival was improved for patients randomized to receive gemcitabine and erlotinib compared with patients receiving gemcitabine alone (191 vs. 177 days, respectively; HR for death 0.82; $p = .02$).

Answer 20.2.9.   **The answer is B.**

Results from an interim analysis of phase III randomized trial reported significant improvement in overall survival for patients receiving

FOLFIRINOX compared to single-agent gemcitabine alone. Therefore, FOLFIRINOX should be considered for first-line treatment in patient with good performance status and normal serum bilirubin level. FOL-FOX has shown activity in patients with pancreatic cancer but further evaluation is required in the frontline setting. 5FU with concurrent radiation is more appropriate in patients with locally advanced disease.

Answer 20.2.10.   **The answer is A.**

BRCA2 is the most commonly mutated tumor suppressor gene in familial pancreatic cancer followed by PALB2. K-RAS is an oncogene and not a tumor suppressor gene. TP53 gene mutation is found in more than 70% of all pancreatic cancers, but there is no evidence to link this mutation with familial pancreatic cancer.

Answer 20.2.11.   **The answer is A.**

ABO blood type has been long known to be associated with increased risk for lung cancer. A recent genome wide association study identified high risk single nucleotide polymorphism for pancreatic cancer in the gene encoding for the ABO blood type. Patients with nonpolyposis colorectal cancer syndrome are at higher risk for gastrointestinal malignancies including pancreatic cancer. K-ras mutation testing has so far not proven to be effective in differentiating between pancreatic cancer and other conditions such as pancreatitis and pancreatic adenoma.

Answer 20.2.12.   **The answer is A.**

Data on second-line treatment of patients with pancreatic cancer who failed first-line gemcitabine are limited. Fluoropyrimidine (5FU or capecitabine) and oxaliplatin combination has the most evidence for treatment benefit in the second-line setting. Hence, a FOLFOX chemotherapy regimen would be an appropriate second-line option in fit patients. Single-agent erlotinib has not shown significant treatment benefit for patients with metastatic pancreatic cancer. Raltitrexed is thymidylate synthase inhibitor that is currently unavailable in the United States has shown activity in the second-line setting in combination with irinotecan or oxaliplatin.

Answer 20.2.13.   **The answer is E.**

Telomere shortening is thought to predispose to chromosome fusion (translocation) and missegregation of genetic material during the mitosis and later during tumor genesis, telomerase is reactivated. SMAD4 (DPC4) pathway mediates signals initiated on the binding of the extracellular proteins TGF-β. The underexpression of TGF-β receptors results in cellular resistance to the usual suppressive effects of the TGF-β ligand. The cyclin D oncogene complexes with CDKs and phosphorylates the retinoblastoma protein (tumor suppressive protein) that results in loss of negative regulatory effect of retinoblastoma protein.

SECTION 3   HEPATOBILIARY

RENUKA V. IYER • RAVI CHHATRALA

DIRECTIONS   Each of the numbered items below is followed by lettered answers. Select the ONE lettered answer that is BEST in each case unless instructed otherwise.

QUESTIONS

Question 20.3.1.   A 52-year-old man is found to have abnormal liver function and an elevated serum alpha-fetoprotein (AFP). Workup reveals prior hepatitis B viral (HBV) infection, but it was not previously known or treated. An ultrasound reveals a 4-cm lesion in the left hepatic lobe, and a computed tomography (CT) scan reveals no evidence of metastatic disease or vascular involvement. A needle biopsy reveals hepatocellular carcinoma (HCC). The patient undergoes successful partial hepatectomy, surgical margins are clear, and the patient recovers from surgery. Which of the following approaches should be followed?

A. Adjuvant chemotherapy with sorafenib
B. Combination chemotherapy that is doxorubicin based
C. Adjuvant radiation to surgical bed
D. None of the above

Question 20.3.2.   Which of the following criteria are useful for selection of patients appropriate for liver transplantation?

A. Patients with solitary tumors ≤5 cm, or patients with multifocal disease with ≤3 tumor nodules each ≤3 cm in size
B. Patients with Child-Pugh B or C cirrhosis
C. Tumors without evidence of macrovascular invasion and patients who are not candidates for primary liver resection
D. All of the above

Corresponding Chapters in *Cancer: Principles & Practice of Oncology,* Ninth Edition: 83 (Molecular Biology of Liver Cancer), 84 (Cancer of the Liver), 85 (Cancer of the Biliary Tree).

Question 20.3.3. Which of the following statements about staging systems for liver cancer is TRUE?

A. The Okuda system takes into account several clinical features that include tumor size (>50% of liver), ascites (positive or negative), hypoalbuminemia (<3 g/dL), and hyperbilirubinemia (>3 mg/dL).

B. The Cancer of the Liver Italian Program system uses hepatic tumor morphology and extent of liver replacement, Child-Pugh score, portal vein thrombosis, and serum AFP levels.

C. The Barcelona Clinic Liver Cancer scoring system combines assessment of tumor stage, liver function, and patient symptoms with a treatment algorithm and has been shown to correlate well with patient outcomes.

D. All of the above.

Question 20.3.4. Which of the following biochemical abnormalities is both a paraneoplastic syndrome associated with HCC, and may also be caused by end-stage liver failure?

A. Hypoglycemia

B. Erythrocytosis

C. Hypercalcemia

D. Hypercholesterolemia

Question 20.3.5. An increased risk of developing HCC is associated with all of the following, EXCEPT:

A. Wilson disease

B. Hemochromatosis

C. Alpha1-antitrypsin deficiency

D. Primary biliary cirrhosis

Question 20.3.6. Which of the following statements about screening and prevention is INCORRECT?

A. The advent of vaccination for hepatitis B has the potential to reduce HCC in endemic areas.

B. A combination of AFP and ultrasound screening is used in high-risk populations.

C. Aggressive screening programs for HCC have been shown to improve survival.

D. Detection of HCC, through surveillance of patients awaiting liver transplantation, results in increased priority for orthotopic liver transplantation.

Question 20.3.7. Which of the following is a risk factor for developing cholangiocarcinoma?

A. Primary sclerosing cholangitis

B. Clonorchis sinensis infestation

C. Chronic portal bacteremia and portal phlebitis

D. All of the above

Question 20.3.8.   A 66-year-old man is noted to have painless jaundice on a routine follow-up at his primary care physician's office. Workup reveals biliary obstruction at the hilum. Endoscopic retrograde cholangiopancreatography confirms a high-grade stricture predominantly involving the left hepatic duct; however, brushings reveal atypical cells and no malignancy. He is seen at a tertiary care center and offered surgical management, an en bloc resection of the left hepatic lobe and extrahepatic bile duct, and a complete periportal lymphadenectomy. Which of the following statements about management/natural history of hilar cholangiocarcinoma is/are TRUE?

  A. Surgical resection is associated with an operative mortality rate of 30%.
  B. Recurrences occur most commonly at the bed of resection, followed by retroperitoneal lymph nodes. Distant metastases occur in one-third of cases.
  C. Less than 10% of patients have resectable cancer at the time of diagnosis.
  D. All of the above.

Question 20.3.9.   A 70-year-old man presents to an emergency department with a history of 16-lb recent weight loss and persistent right upper quadrant pain. CT scan reveals a gall bladder stone and thickening of the anterior wall of the gall bladder. He undergoes a laparoscopic cholecystectomy. Pathology reveals a moderately differentiated 2-cm gall bladder adenocarcinoma invading the perimuscular connective tissue. Margins of resection are negative for tumor. What is the stage of this cancer?

  A. Stage IA
  B. Stage IB
  C. Stage IIA
  D. Stage IIB

Question 20.3.10.   The patient in Question 20.3.9 recovers after his surgery and receives a second opinion at a tertiary care center 5 weeks after his cholecystectomy. A follow-up CT scan 2 weeks after surgery shows mild periportal fullness. What would be the best approach at this time?

  A. Perform en bloc resection of the gallbladder, resection of segments IVb and V of the liver, and regional lymph node dissection.
  B. No further therapy is warranted; surveillance with CT scans and laboratories done every 3 months.
  C. He requires a second laparotomy to assess the extent of remaining disease to guide further therapy.
  D. Perform ultrasound-guided biopsy of the periportal nodes; if positive, then fluoropyrimidine-based chemoradiation is indicated.

Question 20.3.11. Which of the following statements about adjuvant therapy for biliary cancers is TRUE?

    A. Although there is no clear evidence from one prospective randomized trial, it appears patients treated in the adjuvant setting have a median survival of approximately 2 years.

    B. Adjuvant radiation is superior to chemotherapy alone.

    C. Adjuvant therapy can improve overall survival for patients with R0 resections.

    D. Fluoropyrimidine-based chemoradiation is standard because it is superior to radiation alone.

Question 20.3.12. Which of the following statements regarding fibrolamellar HCC is INCORRECT?

    A. Fibrolamellar HCC occurs in equal frequencies in men and women.

    B. This variant of HCC is uncommonly associated with prior cirrhosis or viral hepatitis.

    C. Lymph node metastases at the time of presentation are uncommon.

    D. Most patients with fibrolamellar HCC present in their third decade of life.

Question 20.3.13. You are consulted on a 50-year-old man with a history of chronic hepatitis B infection and Child-Pugh A cirrhosis, who presents with abdominal pain. He is otherwise in good health. CT of the abdomen reveals a cirrhotic liver with a 2.5 cm liver mass that rapidly enhances during the arterial phase of contrast administration and "washout" during the later venous phases. There is no involvement of the portal vein. AFP is 300 ng/mL. What is the next best step in his management?

    A. Insist that he should get a biopsy.

    B. Refer him to a hepatobiliary surgeon.

    C. Start him on sorafenib.

    D. Refer him to a radiation oncologist.

Question 20.3.14. Which of the following statements is NOT correct regarding hepatoblastoma?

    A. This is the most common primary cancer of the liver in children.

    B. Hepatoblastoma is a very chemosensitive tumor.

    C. Patients with this tumor have a poor outcome after liver transplantation, with a 5-year survival rate of 20%.

    D. The peak incidence of hepatoblastoma is within the first 2 years of life.

Question 20.3.15. **Which of the following statements is INCORRECT?**

A. The hepatitis B x gene product has been implicated in causing HCC.
B. NS5A protein product of hepatitis C viral (HCV) genome does not interact with p53.
C. Level of HBV replication is not inversely related to the risk of liver cancer.
D. Hepatitis B virus genotype C is associated with increased risk of HCC.

Question 20.3.16. **Which of the following statements is/are correct?**

A. 60% to 80% HCV infections become chronic in contrast to 10% HBV infections.
B. HBV genome integrates into hepatocyte DNA while HCV genome does not.
C. The average interval from HCV infection to HCC is 30 years in contrast to 40 to 50 years for HBV infection.
D. All of above.

Question 20.3.17. **Which of the following is NOT an independent predictor for the development of HCC in chronic hepatitis C infection?**

A. Thrombocytosis
B. Esophageal varices
C. Smoking
D. African American ethnicity

Question 20.3.18. **Which of the following features are characteristic of the appearance of HCC on four-phase CT?**

A. Presence of arterial hypervascularity
B. Rapid enhancement during the arterial phase of contrast administration
C. Washout during the later portal venous and delayed phase
D. All of the above

Question 20.3.19. **Which of the following individuals would not meet criteria to have surveillance for HCC?**

A. 28-year-old African American woman who is a hepatitis B carrier.
B. 47-year-old Indian woman who is hepatitis B carrier.
C. 62-year-old Hispanic male with alcoholic cirrhosis.
D. 42-year-old Chinese man who is a hepatitis B carrier.

ANSWERS

Answer 20.3.1.   **The answer is D.**

No adjuvant therapies have been shown to affect survival or delay progression thus far.

Answer 20.3.2.   **The answer is D.**

The Milan criteria for selection of patients appropriate for liver transplantation include patients with solitary tumors less than or equal to 5 cm, patients with multifocal disease with less than or equal to 3 tumor nodules each less than or equal to 3 cm in size, patients with Child-Pugh B or C cirrhosis, patients who are not candidates for primary liver resection, and patients who have tumors with no evidence of macrovascular invasion.

Answer 20.3.3.   **The answer is D.**

Multiple clinical staging systems for hepatic tumors have been described. The most widely used is the American Joint Committee on Cancer/Tumor-Node-Metastasis. A staging system based entirely on clinical grounds that incorporate the contribution of the underlying liver disease was originally developed by Okuda et al. Adverse prognostic signs are as listed. Patients with Okuda stage III (advanced), namely, with three or more positive features, have a dire prognosis because they usually cannot be curatively resected and the condition of their liver typically precludes chemotherapy. The American Association for the Study of Liver Diseases has endorsed the use of the Barcelona Clinic Liver Cancer system for staging of HCC. This has now been validated both internally and externally in several studies.

Answer 20.3.4.   **The answer is A.**

Various paraneoplastic syndromes have been described to occur in patients with hepatocellular cancer. Most of these are biochemical abnormalities without associated clinical consequences. The most important ones include hypoglycemia (also caused by end-stage liver failure), erythrocytosis, hypercalcemia, hypercholesterolemia, dysfibrinogenemia, carcinoid syndrome, increased thyroxin-binding globulin, sexual changes (gynecomastia, testicular atrophy, and precocious puberty), and porphyria cutanea tarda. Pathogenesis of hypoglycemia is unclear but may be related to production by the tumor of insulin-like growth factor I.

Answer 20.3.5.   **The answer is D.**

Primary biliary cirrhosis is associated with an increased risk of cholangiocarcinoma.

Answer 20.3.6.   **The answer is C.**

A combination of ultrasonography and serum AFP levels is used for the screening of high-risk populations for HCC. Although screening programs are in place in endemic areas of HCC and in high-risk populations, it is unclear whether screening identifies patients at an earlier stage or improves patient survival. Detection of HCC, through surveillance of patients awaiting liver transplantation, results in increased priority for orthotopic liver transplantation.

Answer 20.3.7.   **The answer is D.**

In most patients, cholangiocarcinoma is sporadic and no precipitating factor can be identified. Risk factors that have been associated with the development of cholangiocarcinoma can be divided into congenital (choledochal cysts, anomalous pancreatic-biliary tree junction), autoimmune (primary biliary cirrhosis), infectious (clonorchis sinensis and *Opisthorchis viverrini* infestation, chronic portal bacteremia, and portal phlebitis) and finally environmental exposures (thorotrast and possibly cigarette smoking).

Answer 20.3.8.   **The answer is B.**

Approximately one-third of patients presenting with the suspected diagnosis of cholangiocarcinoma will have resectable disease. Operative mortality averages approximately 8%, indicating the high-risk population that this tumor affects and the complexity of the procedure. Some 10% to 35% of patients survive 5 years after surgical resection. Recurrences occur most commonly at the bed of resection, followed by retroperitoneal lymph nodes. Distant metastases occur in one-third of cases. The most common site is the lung or mediastinum, followed by liver and peritoneum. Comparisons of outcome over time suggest improved outcome in more recent series as a result of routine inclusion of liver resection. Prognostic factors for survival include negative microscopic margin status, lymph node metastases, tumor size, tumor grade, preoperative serum albumin, hepatic resection, and postoperative sepsis.

Answer 20.3.9.   **The answer is B.**

The patient's pathology reveals a T2 NX stage IB gall bladder cancer.

Answer 20.3.10.   **The answer is A.**

Numerous studies have demonstrated that simple cholecystectomy is curative for stage I disease (T1, N0). Recent studies have suggested that the prognosis is different for pT1a and pT1b tumors after simple cholecystectomy. Invasion of the muscular layer allows access to lymphatics and vessels, providing the rationale for extended cholecystectomy in this population. When an extended cholecystectomy is performed for T2 disease, the 5-year survival has been reported to be as high as 100%, but probably falls in the range of 70% to 90% (*PPO* Table 39.8.13). Simple cholecystectomy alone is associated with a 5-year survival rate of 20% to 40.5%. Lymph node metastases are seen in 46% of patients with T2 primary tumors, providing another reason in favor of radical repeat resection after simple cholecystectomy. In series of extended cholecystectomies, the operative morbidity ranges from 5% to 46%, and the mortality ranges from 0% to 21%. The risk of resection for each patient and each type of resection needs to be weighed against the chance of benefiting from the procedure on the basis of the tumor stage.

Answer 20.3.11.   **The answer is A.**

Balachandran et al. reported on 117 patients with gallbladder cancer, of whom 80 underwent simple cholecystectomy and 37 underwent extended resections. Seventy-three patients received adjuvant chemoradiotherapy and 44 patients did not. The median survival of all 117 patients was 16 months. On multivariate analysis, the T stage and use of adjuvant therapy were the only statistically significant independent predictors of survival. Median survival was 24 months and 11 months in patients with or without adjuvant chemoradiotherapy ($p = .001$), respectively, and this difference was most pronounced for patients with T3, node-positive disease, or after a simple cholecystectomy. Ben-David et al. reported on 14 patients with gallbladder cancer treated at the University of Michigan with resection followed by radiotherapy or chemoradiotherapy. The median radiation dose was 54 Gy, and approximately half the patients received concurrent chemotherapy. The median survival was 23 months. Interestingly, there was no difference in survival between patients with R0 or R1 resection. No differences were observed in survival or pattern of failure between patients with gallbladder cancer and bile duct cancer (distal or hilar). The high risk of systemic spread and locoregional failure associated with gallbladder cancer that extends beyond the mucosa has led most cancer centers in the United States to recommend consideration of adjuvant chemotherapy and radiotherapy. For external beam radiation therapy, the target volume should include the gallbladder fossa and adjacent liver, as well as the regional nodal areas.

Answer 20.3.12.   **The answer is C.**

Fibrolamellar HCC is a rare histologic variant of HCC. Most patients present in the third decade of life, and it affects men and women equally. This variant of HCC is uncommonly associated with prior cirrhosis or viral hepatitis. In addition, a higher proportion of patients with fibrolamellar HCC have lymph node metastases at presentation, than the usual HCC.

Answer 20.3.13.   **The answer is B.**

This man has a hepatic mass within a cirrhotic liver, which is very suspicious for HCC. The radiologic features are also highly suggestive of HCC. If the mass is more than 2 cm in size with characteristic appearance of HCC on imaging, and AFP is more than 200ng/ml, biopsy is not essential for management. Patients with a high clinical suspicion for HCC who are deemed appropriate surgical candidates should be taken to surgery without a preoperative biopsy.

Answer 20.3.14.   **The answer is C.**

Hepatoblastoma is the most common primary cancer of the liver in children. The peak incidence is within the first 2 years of life. Surgical resection is the first line of therapy; however, these tumors are very chemosensitive, and neoadjuvant chemotherapy can render unresectable tumors operable. Five-year survival after liver transplantation is excellent (83%).

Answer 20.3.15.   **The answer is B.**

The NS5A protein product of HCV genome has been demonstrated to inactivate p53 by sequestration. The hepatitis B x gene product has been implicated in causing HCC because it is a transcriptional activator of various cellular genes associated with growth control. The elevated serum level of HBV DNA (a marker of higher levels of HBV replication) is associated with a higher risk of HCC. The HBV genotype C is generally thought to increase the risk of HCC because these individuals are likely to remain seropositive for hepatitis B e antigen and thus have higher serum levels of HBV DNA for a longer time.

Answer 20.3.16.   **The answer is D.**

Hepatitis B virus is a DNA virus and it may become integrated within the chromosomes of infected hepatocyte. On the other hand, hepatitis C virus is an RNA virus without a DNA intermediate form, and therefore cannot integrate into hepatocyte DNA.

Answer 20.3.17.   **The answer is A.**

Old age, black race, lower platelet count, elevated serum alkaline phosphatase, elevated AST, presence of esophageal varices, and history of smoking are the independent predictors for the development of HCC in the setting of chronic hepatitis C infection.

Answer 20.3.18.   **The answer is D.**

Presence of arterial hypervascularity, rapid enhancement during the arterial phase of contrast administration, and washout during the later portal venous and delayed phase are features characteristic of the appearance of HCC on four-phase CT.

Answer 20.3.19.   **The answer is B.**

The following groups should undergo surveillance for HCC.

Hepatitis B carrier—Asian men more than 40 years old, Asian women more than 50 years old, Africans more than 20 years old, all cirrhotic hepatitis B carriers, family history of HCC and patients with high hepatitis B virus DNA with ongoing hepatic injury.

Nonhepatitis B cirrhosis—hepatitis C, alcoholic cirrhosis, genetic hemochromatosis, and primary biliary cirrhosis

Tests that have been used for surveillance for HCC include serologic tests (measurement of serum AFP) and radiologic tests (such as ultrasonography). Although the ideal surveillance interval is not known, a surveillance interval of 6 to 12 months has been proposed based on estimates of tumor doubling time.

SECTION 4	SMALL INTESTINE AND GASTROINTESTINAL STROMAL TUMORS

BENJAMIN R. TAN, Jr.

DIRECTIONS   Each of the numbered items below is followed by lettered answers. Select the ONE lettered answer that is BEST in each case unless instructed otherwise.

QUESTIONS

Question 20.4.1. A 60-year-old previously healthy woman noted abdominal distension and discomfort for 6 months, associated with nausea and vomiting. A computed tomography (CT) scan confirms a 20 × 25-cm abdominal mass, and exploratory laparotomy demonstrated a pedunculated mass arising from the stomach. No other metastases were found. A partial gastrectomy was done, and pathology revealed a gastrointestinal stromal tumor (GIST) that strongly stains for CD117 and CD34. Fifteen mitoses were seen per high-power field (hpf). Which of the following is true regarding GISTs?

A. The most common mutation associated with GIST involves the inactivation of a tumor suppressor gene.

B. Both tumor size and mitotic index predict response to imatinib therapy.

C. Gastric GISTs are associated with relatively worse outcomes compared with small intestinal GISTs.

D. Patients with metastatic GIST tumors harboring exon 9 mutations have a better prognosis and response to imatinib compared with those with exon 11 mutation.

E. None of the above.

Question 20.4.2. After the patient in Question 20.4.1 has recovered from surgery, what would you recommend for this patient on the basis of current data?

A. Observation with serial scans

B. Imatinib 400 mg per os (PO) daily for 1 to 2 years

C. Imatinib 400 mg PO daily for 5 years

D. Sunitinib 50 mg 4 weeks on/2 weeks off therapy for 5 years

---

Corresponding Chapters in *Cancer: Principles & Practice of Oncology,* Ninth Edition: 86 (Cancer of the Small Intestine) and 87 (Gastrointestinal Stromal Tumor).

Question 20.4.3.   A 62-year-old patient with diabetes, hypertension, and chronic moderate renal insufficiency developed abdominal discomfort and early satiety. An esophagogastroduodenoscopy revealed a gastric mass measuring 6 cm, and biopsy confirmed GIST with three mitoses per hpf. A CT scan revealed at least three hepatic metastases and multiple omental lesions. His current creatinine clearance is 36 mL/min. You recommend:

A. No dose adjustment is necessary for moderate renal insufficiency, and start imatinib 400 mg PO daily.
B. A 25% dose reduction and give 300 mg PO daily
C. A 50% dose reduction and give 200 mg PO daily
D. Give sunitinib because imatinib is contraindicated for patients with moderate renal insufficiency.

Question 20.4.4.   A 52-year-old woman with metastatic gastric GIST had an initial complete response to daily imatinib 400 mg with resolution of her hepatic and peritoneal metastases after 6 months of therapy. Imatinib was continued for 18 months when her CT scan showed recurrent hepatic lesions. Imatinib was increased to 800 mg daily. However, subsequent scans revealed progressive disease. You recommend starting sunitinib for this patient. Which of the following statements is NOT true?

A. Secondary resistance to imatinib therapy may be associated with the development of secondary KIT or PDGFRA mutations.
B. Sunitinib therapy for patients with imatinib-resistant GIST improved progression-free survival compared with placebo.
C. Patients with GIST harboring exon 9 mutation have a higher response to sunitinib than those with exon 11 mutation.
D. Patients with the wild-type GIST are resistant to both imatinib and sunitinib therapy.

Question 20.4.5.   The patient in Question 20.4.4 started sunitinib 50 mg daily for 28 days followed by a 2-week break. After two cycles, repeat CT scans showed a decrease in her measurable lesions. In addition to hypopigmentation of her hair, she also noted progressive generalized fatigue. She denies any dyspnea on exertion, diarrhea, or pedal edema. Physical examination reveals an erythematous rash in her hands, clear lungs, no cardiac gallops or rubs, and no focal neurologic deficits. Pertinent laboratory tests are as follows:
   White blood cell 5.6×10^3 cells/μL
   Hemoglobin 11.8 g/dL
   Sodium 145 mmol/L
   Potassium 4.5 mmol/L
   Creatinine 0.8 mg/dL
   Total bilirubin 0.5 mg/dL
   Alkaline phosphatase 118 μ/L
   What would you order next?

A. Magnesium level
B. Magnetic resonance imaging of the brain
C. Thyroid function tests
D. 25-Hydroxycholecalciferol level

Question 20.4.6.   Familial and genetic syndromes associated with GIST include all of the following, EXCEPT:

A. Cowden syndrome
B. Familial paraganglioma
C. Carney triad
D. Neurofibromatosis

Question 20.4.7.   Conditions that predispose one to the development of small intestinal cancer are the following, EXCEPT:

A. Crohn's disease
B. Familial adenomatous polyposis
C. Celiac disease
D. Hereditary nonpolyposis colorectal cancer
E. All of the above

Question 20.4.8.   What is the most common type of small bowel malignancy?

A. Adenocarcinoma
B. Lymphoma
C. Carcinoid
D. Schwannoma

Question 20.4.9.   Which of the following is NOT a characteristic of primary intestinal mucosal-associated lymphoid tissue (MALT) lymphoma?

A. Association with Hashimoto's thyroiditis
B. The majority of patients present with stage I and II
C. Most common in men
D. Associated with the translocation $t(11;14)$

Question 20.4.10.   Which of the following statements regarding small bowel adenocarcinoma is FALSE?

A. Duodenum is the most common location.
B. Jejunal and ileal tumors are associated with worse outcomes.
C. There is a slight male predominance in men.
D. Patients with duodenal tumors are usually older than those with more distal lesions.

Question 20.4.11. The patient in Question 20.4.10 was found to have three ileal lesions. Exploratory laparotomy revealed a total of five 1 to 1.5-cm lesions in the ileum. A frozen biopsy of one of the lesions confirmed a well-differentiated neuroendocrine (carcinoid) tumor. Segmental resection of the small bowel with regional lymph node revealed two mesenteric lymph nodes involved with carcinoid. His diarrhea, flushing, and bleeding resolved after surgery. Other than obtaining baseline scans, chromogranin A level, 24-hour urine 5-HIAA, what would be the most optimal management?

A. Short-acting octreotide 150 μg three times per day
B. Octreotide LAR 30 mg once per month
C. Adjuvant chemotherapy with 5FU, streptozotocin, and doxorubicin
D. No further therapy. The patient just needs follow-up with laboratory tests ± scans every 3 months.

Question 20.4.12. Which of the following is a criterion to differentiate between primary intestinal and secondary lymphomas?

A. No superficial adenopathy
B. No evidence of splenic involvement except through direct extension of the primary tumor
C. No evidence of peripheral blood or bone marrow involvement
D. All the above

Question 20.4.13. The risk for progressive disease for a patient with small intestinal GIST measuring less than 2 cm with more than five mitoses/50 hpf is:

A. 0%
B. 4.3%
C. 24%
D. 50%
E. 85%

Question 20.4.14. A 20-year-old student presented to the emergency department with a 2-day history of right lower abdominal pain associated with fever. His abdomen was slightly distended with diffuse tenderness but without guarding or rebound tenderness. Rectal examination showed no masses and was negative for occult blood. Complete blood count showed a slightly elevated white blood cell at 11,000. CT scan showed a mass in the terminal ileum with no evidence of free peritoneal air. Colonoscopy revealed a terminal ileum mass, the biopsy of which showed sheets of monotonous round nucleated cells with abundant basophilic cytoplasm with numerous macrophages. Ki-67 index is 100%. What is your diagnosis?

A. MALT lymphoma
B. Burkitt's lymphoma
C. Peripheral T-cell lymphoma
D. Medullary carcinoma of the small intestine

ANSWERS

Answer 20.4.1.   **The answer is E.**

In the majority of malignant GISTs, a gain-of-function mutation results in the constitutive activation of the KIT proto-oncogene. Approximately 80% of GISTs harbor mutations in the KIT receptor, whereas another 5% to 7% have activating PDGFRA mutations. The most common mutation is identified in the KIT juxtamembrane domain, exon 11. Other mutations in exon 9, 13, 17, and 18 have been described. In the Intergroup US-Finland study, higher response rates and better outcomes were observed among patients with GIST with the exon 11 mutation compared with those with exon 9 mutation. Objective responses to imatinib therapy among patients with GIST with exon 11 and exon 9 mutations are approximately 70% and 40%, respectively. Patients with wild-type GIST have a response rate of approximately 30%. Median time to progression also is longer for those with exon 11 compared with other genotypes. The higher prevalence of a specific exon 9 mutation among GISTs originating in the small intestine may explain in part the observation of worse prognosis of these tumors compared with gastric GISTs. Although tumor size and mitotic index carry prognostic significance for patients with GIST, both have not been associated with response to tyrosine kinase inhibition.

Answer 20.4.2.   **The answer is B.**

Current data on adjuvant therapy for patients with resected GIST are derived from the American College of Surgeons Oncology Group studies, which demonstrated a 1-year relapse-free survival rate of 97% among patients who received imatinib at 400 mg PO daily for 1 year, compared with 83% for those who received placebo, with a hazard ratio of 0.325 (DeMatteo, J Clin Oncol. 25:18S, abstract 10079). Although no survival benefit was demonstrated, those with tumors greater than 10 cm derived the most benefit from adjuvant imatinib. A Phase II study on adjuvant imatinib in resected high-risk GIST (tumor size ≥10 cm, tumor rupture, or ≤5 peritoneal metastases) demonstrated improved overall survival compared with historical controls (DeMatteo, Proc 2008 Gastrointestinal Cancers Symposium, abstract 8). Three-year recurrence-free survival and overall survival rates were 61% and 97%, respectively. Current studies are evaluating longer duration of adjuvant therapy, but there are no data on the benefit of adjuvant therapy beyond 1 to 2 years or on the use of sunitinib in the adjuvant setting.

Answer 20.4.3.   **The answer is A.**

No dose adjustment is necessary for patients with mild-to-moderate renal dysfunction receiving imatinib therapy based on the National Cancer Institute Organ Dysfunction Working Group Study published by Gibbons et al. (Gibbons J, Egorin MJ, Ramanathan RK, et al. Phase I and pharmacokinetic study of imatinib mesylate in patients with advanced malignancies and varying degrees of renal dysfunction: a study by the

National Cancer Institute Organ Dysfunction Working Group. J Clin Oncol. 2008;26:570–576). Although there was an increase in imatinib drug exposure in patients with mild-to-moderate renal dysfunction, this was not associated with any meaningful toxicities. Doses up to 600 to 800 mg daily were tolerable for those with moderate and mild renal dysfunction, respectively. In another study by Ramanathan et al. (Gibbons J, Egorin MJ, Ramanathan RK, et al. Phase I and pharmacokinetic study of imatinib mesylate in patients with advanced malignancies and varying degrees of liver dysfunction: a study by the National Cancer Institute Organ Dysfunction Working Group. J Clin Oncol. 2008;26:563–569), patients with mild hepatic dysfunction were able to tolerate imatinib doses up to 500 mg daily. No relationship was found between imatinib pharmacokinetics and severity of hepatic dysfunction. The authors recommended that for patients with moderate or severe hepatic dysfunction, patients can be dosed at 400 mg daily with close monitoring for toxicity or to start at 300 mg daily and rapidly escalate the dose to 400 mg daily if tolerated.

Answer 20.4.4.   **The answer is D.**

Primary resistance to imatinib, manifested by continued tumor growth within the first 6 months of imatinib therapy, occurs in a minority of GISTs. Secondary resistance generally occurs after a median of 24 months of continued tyrosine kinase inhibition. Acquired mutations in KIT or PDGFRA have been implicated in the development of drug resistance to imatinib. The emergence of KIT-independent genotypes may also result in imatinib resistance. Sunitinib was approved by the Food and Drug Administration for the treatment of GIST after disease progression or intolerance to imatinib. The pivotal Phase III study demonstrated a superior time to progression of 27.3 weeks for patients treated with sunitinib compared with 6.4 weeks for patients treated with placebo. Six-month survival rates also favor sunitinib at 79.4% compared with 56.9% for placebo. With the crossover design, the advantage for survival benefit on longer follow-up diminished. A subset analysis showed improvement in response rates and outcomes for patients with GIST harboring exon 9 mutation compared with those harboring exon 11 mutations. Responses were also observed among patients with wild-type genotype.

Answer 20.4.5.   **The answer is C.**

Biochemical and clinical hypothyroidism has been associated with sunitinib therapy. Rini et al. reported an 85% rate of thyroid dysfunction associated with sunitinib use (Hypothyroidism in patients with metastatic renal cell carcinoma treated with sunitinib. J Natl Cancer Inst. 2007;99:81). Routine monitoring of thyroid function test is warranted, and thyroid hormone replacement therapy may alleviate symptoms. The precise mechanism for sunitinib-associated hypothyroidism is unclear. Destructive thyroiditis through follicular apoptosis has been postulated for sunitinib-associated thyroid dysfunction based on the observation of transient thyroid-stimulating hormone suppression and subsequent absence of visualized thyroid tissue. Other causes of fatigue associated with sunitinib include adrenal insufficiency or congestive heart failure.

Answer 20.4.6.   **The answer is A.**

Carney triad, which encompasses multifocal GIST with pulmonary chondroma and extra-adrenal paraganglioma, familial paraganglioma, and neurofibromatosis type 1 are associated with GIST. These syndromes, along with pediatric GIST, can be characterized by the wild-type KIT gene. It is unclear whether GISTs associated with these syndromes have a similar response to imatinib therapy as sporadic GIST.

Answer 20.4.7.   **The answer is E.**

All of the conditions listed are associated with increased risk for the development of cancer in the small intestine. Other conditions include AIDS, neurofibromatosis, Gardner syndrome, Peutz-Jeghers, and a history of other primary tumors, such as uterine, ovarian, prostate, thyroid, skin, and soft tissue sarcomas.

Answer 20.4.8.   **The answer is C.**

The most common tumors of the small bowel are carcinoids, followed by adenocarcinomas and lymphomas. Sarcomas are less likely and schwannomas are rare.

Answer 20.4.9.   **The answer is D.**

MALT lymphomas are most commonly seen in men, with a peak in the sixth decade. These malignancies may be associated with chronic inflammatory disorders such as Hashimoto's thyroiditis and the majority of patients present with stages I or II. The translocation $t(11;14)$ causing overexpression of cyclin D1 is characteristic of mantle cell lymphoma.

Answer 20.4.10.   **The answer is B.**

Small bowel tumors are slightly more common in men. Duodenum represents with most common location, accounting for approximately half of the cases. Compared to more distal lesions, tumors of the duodenum tend to occur in older patients and are associated with worse outcomes.

Answer 20.4.11.   **The answer is D.**

Although the patient is at high risk for developing recurrent or metastatic disease, there is currently no clear role for the use of adjuvant octreotide therapy or chemotherapy. Close follow-up is necessary, and if tumor markers are elevated, repeat CT or octreotide scans may be done to determine metastatic disease.

Answer 20.4.12.   **The answer is D.**

The main criteria to distinguish between primary intestinal lymphomas and secondary involvement include no superficial palpable lymphadenopathy, no mediastinal adenopathy, no evidence of peripheral blood or bone marrow involvement, no involvement of the liver or spleen unless by direct extension of the primary tumor, and disease confined to the affected small bowel and regional draining mesenteric lymph nodes.

Answer 20.4.13.   **The answer is D.**

GISTs arising from the small intestine appear to have a more malignant behavior at a smaller size compared with those found in the stomach or in the colon. For small tumors less than 2 cm, those with more than 5 mitoses per 50 hpf have a 0% risk of progression according to one study, whereas those with more than 5 mitoses per 50 hpf have a 50% risk for progression. GISTs larger than 10 cm with more than 10 mitoses per 50 hpf have a 90% risk of progression.

Answer 20.4.14.   **The answer is B.**

This patient has Burkitt's lymphoma arising from the terminal ileum presenting with appendicitis-like symptoms. This type of lymphoma accounts for less than 5% of all lymphomas in the small intestine. A "starry-eyed" pattern interspersed throughout monomorphic cells with abundant basophilic cytoplasm is characteristic and related to numerous macrophages with ingested apoptotic tumors within. A high proliferative index is also characteristic. Treatment consists primarily of aggressive chemotherapy.

SECTION 5 ▏ COLORECTAL AND ANAL CANCERS

BENJAMIN R. TAN, Jr.

DIRECTIONS   Each of the numbered items below is followed by lettered answers. Select the ONE lettered answer that is BEST in each case unless instructed otherwise.

QUESTIONS

Question 20.5.1.   A 30-year-old multigravid woman presents with a large abdominal mass associated with abdominal pain. She underwent a total proctocolectomy for colon cancer secondary to familial adenomatous polyposis (FAP) 4 years ago. She received adjuvant chemotherapy for node-positive disease. A recent esophagogastric endoscopy revealed only a tubulovillous adenoma in the duodenum. A computed tomography (CT) scan revealed a 10-cm mass filling the pelvis. Biopsy confirmed desmoid tumor. A TRUE statement regarding desmoids tumors is:

A. Desmoid tumors represent the second most common cause of death for patients with FAP.
B. Desmoid tumors are uniformly aggressive and locally invasive.
C. Adjuvant radiation is recommended.
D. Adjuvant chemotherapy is recommended.

Corresponding Chapters in *Cancer: Principles & Practice of Oncology,* Ninth Edition: 88 (Molecular Biology of Colorectal Cancer), 89 (Cancer of the Colon), 90 (Cancer of the Rectum), and 91 (Cancer of the Anal Region).

Question 20.5.2.   A 55-year-old woman underwent a right hemicolectomy for a cecal mass 15 years ago. Four years later, she was found to have a hepatic flexure adenocarcinoma and a total colectomy was performed. Four years ago, she presented with postmenopausal bleeding and was found to have endometrial adenocarcinoma. She also had multiple skin malignancies, including sebaceous adenomas and keratoacanthomas. One year ago, she underwent a Whipple procedure for a duodenal adenocarcinoma invading into the pancreas. She has three siblings and a paternal uncle with colorectal cancer all diagnosed in their late 30s. What is the most probable PRIMARY genetic explanation for her inherited colorectal cancer syndrome?

A. Chromosomal instability characterized by the deletion or mutation of a tumor suppressor gene
B. Chromosomal instability characterized by activation of an oncogene
C. Microsatellite instability (MSI) caused by germ line mutations in a DNA mismatch repair (MMR) gene
D. MSI caused by epigenetic changes associated with hypermethylation in CpG islands

Question 20.5.3.   Other than genetic counseling, which test would you order to confirm the diagnosis?

A. p53 mutation and loss of heterozygosity of chromosome 18q
B. APC mutation, including the I1307K allele
C. MSI testing and methylation of CpG islands
D. MSI test and MMR gene mutation including MLH1, MSH2, MSH6

Question 20.5.4.   The patient in Question 20.5.3 had a positive test result. What screening tests and surveillance program would you recommend to her three daughters aged 24, 22, and 20 years?

A. Colonoscopy now and repeat every 1 to 2 years and transvaginal ultrasound for her daughters starting by age 30 to 35 years
B. Colonoscopy for all and transvaginal ultrasound for her daughters starting at age 30 to 35 years
C. Colonoscopy now and repeat every 1 to 2 years with transvaginal ultrasound at age 30 to 35 years only for her children confirmed to have the same genetic mutation as the patient; colonoscopy at age 40 to 50 years for those with no mutation
D. Colonoscopy and transvaginal ultrasound at age 30 to 35 years only for those confirmed with the same mutation as the patient; colonoscopy by age 40 to 50 years for those with no mutation

Question 20.5.5.   Which gene is associated with hereditary nonpolyposis colorectal cancer (HNPCC)?

A. APC
B. MYH
C. STK11
D. MSH2

Question 20.5.6.   A 65-year-old woman presented with intermittent constipation and diarrhea associated with abdominal cramping. A colonoscopy revealed a near-obstructing mass, and biopsy revealed a villoglandular polyp. She underwent an exploratory laparotomy and resection of a 5 × 5-cm circumferential necrotic and fungating mass. Pathology revealed a moderately differentiated adenocarcinoma invading into the pericolonic fat with 2 of 30 positive lymph nodes. Margins were negative. CT scan showed no evidence of metastatic disease. After recovery from her surgery, based on current evidence, you would recommend:

   A.   5FU with leucovorin × 6 months
   B.   Capecitabine × 6 months
   C.   Irinotecan with 5FU (FOLFIRI) × 6 months
   D.   Oxaliplatin with 5FU (FOLFOX) × 6 months
   E.   Oxaliplatin with 5FU (FOLFOX) and bevacizumab × 6 months

Question 20.5.7.   One week after the first dose of chemotherapy, the patient in Question 20.5.6 developed a fever at 102°F associated with chills. She also developed diarrhea, mucositis, confusion, and ataxia. Repeat complete blood count showed a white blood cell count of 0.5×103 cells/μL with an absolute neutrophil count of 100, hemoglobin of 11.7 g/dL, band platelet count of 42,000. Which one of the following pharmacogenetic conditions would best explain her clinical course?

   A.   The patient is homozygous for the thymidylate synthase (TYMS) *3/*3 polymorphism.
   B.   The patient is homozygous for UGT1A1 *28 polymorphism.
   C.   The patient is heterozygous for the IVS14 + 1 G > A DPYD*2A mutation.
   D.   The patient is heterozygous for the ERCC2 Lys751Gln polymorphism.

Question 20.5.8.   A 62-year-old engineer was diagnosed with metastatic cecal adenocarcinoma with lung and liver metastases. He was initially treated with oxaliplatin plus infusional 5FU (FOLFOX6) and bevacizumab. After four cycles (2 months), his CT scan showed progressive disease. You discussed irinotecan 180 mg/m² every 2 weeks plus weekly cetuximab based on the results of the EPIC study. A test for UGT1A1 polymorphism was done, and results revealed him to be homozygous for UGT1A1 *28/*28. Which of the following statements is TRUE?

   A.   Patients homozygous for the UGT1A1 *28 polymorphism glucuronidate SN38 more efficiently than those with the wild-type *1 genotype.
   B.   Patients homozygous for the UGT1A1 *28 polymorphism glucuronidate SN38 less efficiently than those with the wild-type *1 genotype.
   C.   Patients homozygous for UGT1A1 *28 polymorphism are at greater risk for severe neutropenia with irinotecan compared with those with the wild-type *1 genotype.
   D.   A and C are true.
   E.   B and C are true.

Question 20.5.9.   A 52-year-old teacher presents with a 2-month history of rectal bleeding. A rectal examination revealed a palpable mass 6 cm from the anal verge. Subsequent colonoscopy confirmed a friable, tethered mass biopsy that showed moderately differentiated adenocarcinoma. Transrectal ultrasound revealed a T3 N1 cancer. CT scans of the chest, abdomen, and pelvis revealed no metastatic sites. Which of the following treatment strategies would you recommend?

A. Abdominoperineal resection (APR) with a total mesorectal excision (TME) followed by adjuvant chemoradiation
B. APR with TME followed by chemotherapy alone
C. Short-course 5-day neoadjuvant radiation (25 Gy) followed by APR with TME
D. Prolonged-course neoadjuvant 5FU-based chemoradiation followed by APR with TME and adjuvant chemotherapy

Question 20.5.10.   Which of the following appropriately staged patients with rectal cancer would be the BEST candidate for transanal excision?

A. A 48-year-old woman with a 2.5-cm T1 moderately differentiated rectal adenocarcinoma 4 cm from the anal verge.
B. A 65-year-old man with a 4.5-cm T2 well-differentiated circumferential rectal mass 6 cm from the anal verge.
C. A 30-year-old man with a 2-cm well-differentiated T1 mucinous adenocarcinoma 12 cm from the anal verge.
D. A 52-year-old woman with a 3-cm well-differentiated T1N1 adenocarcinoma 5 cm from the anal verge.
E. None of the above.

Question 20.5.11.   For the patient you have selected for transanal resection in Question 20.5.10, pathological review of the excised specimen showed no lymphovascular invasion and all margins were negative. Which of the following options would you recommend?

A. No further therapy
B. Short-course (25 Gy/5 fractions) radiation
C. Intracavitary radiation
D. Adjuvant chemotherapy without radiation
E. Adjuvant chemotherapy with radiation

Question 20.5.12.   The following are true statements regarding MYH-associated polyposis, EXCEPT:

A. Inheritance is autosomal dominant.
B. Clinical features of MYH-related polyposis are similar to FAP.
C. The MYH-gene is a base-excision repair gene.
D. A deficiency in MYH leads to accumulation of somatic mutations in the APC gene.

Question 20.5.13. A 49-year-old woman noted rectal bleeding for 2 months. She denied any pain, diarrhea, constipation, or weight loss. A colonoscopy was done that revealed a 2-cm low-lying mass 1 cm from the anal verge. A transrectal ultrasound revealed no lymph nodes. Biopsy confirmed basaloid squamous cell carcinoma. CT scans of the abdomen and pelvis did not reveal any metastatic disease. The BEST curative treatment option for this patient is:

A. APR
B. Short-course (25 Gy/5 fractions) radiation followed by APR
C. Neoadjuvant chemoradiation with 5FU followed by APR
D. Chemoradiation alone with 5FU and mitomycin

Question 20.5.14. A 58-year-old man presented with a 6-month history of anorexia, fatigue, and a vague right-sided abdominal discomfort. His physical examination was unremarkable except for mild pallor. Initial laboratory test revealed a hemoglobin level of 10.7 g/dL with a mean corpuscular volume of 73. He also had mildly elevated alkaline phosphatase and hepatic transaminases. Colonoscopy revealed a nonobstructing transverse colon mass. Biopsy demonstrated moderately differentiated adenocarcinoma. CT scan revealed a 3-cm lesion in the left lobe of the liver and two other lesions measuring 1.5 to 2 cm in the right lobe of the liver. Positron emission tomography revealed uptake in the transverse colon and all three known hepatic lesions. Among the following options, what would be the best option for this patient based on current studies?

A. Curative-intent resection of the transverse colon primary and all three hepatic lesions followed by active surveillance
B. Palliative-intent frontline chemotherapy with bevacizumab for metastatic colon cancer until progression, followed by palliative second-line chemotherapy
C. Curative-intent resection of the transverse colon primary and all three hepatic lesions with chemotherapy
D. Curative-intent resection of the transverse colon primary and all three hepatic lesions with radiotherapy

Question 20.5.15. Which of the following statements regarding colorectal cancer is correct?

A. Tumors with MSI may be resistant to treatment with 5FU.
B. Patients with DNA repair defects have poor outcomes with systemic therapy.
C. High levels of MSI are reported in less than 10% of all colorectal cancers.
D. MSI is the result of chromosomal instability.

Question 20.5.16. Which genetic change is associated with resistance to treatment with cetuximab?

A. K-RAS mutation
B. EGFR over expression
C. K-RAS wild type
D. MLH1 inactivation

Question 20.5.17. **All of the following statements regarding systemic therapy for metastatic colorectal cancer is true, EXCEPT:**

    A. Treatment with FOLFOX and panitumumab results in improved progression-free survival compared to FOLFOX alone in patients with KRAS wild type.

    B. Both FOLFOX and FOLFIRI have similar treatment efficacy in the first-line setting.

    C. Treatment with combination chemotherapy regimens leads to superior outcomes than single-agent chemotherapy in the first-line setting.

    D. Arterial thrombotic events and bowel perforation are serious risk factors associated with bevacizumab.

ANSWERS

Answer 20.5.1.   **The answer is A.**

Desmoid disease is second only to colorectal cancer as a common cause of death among patients with FAP. There is heterogeneity in the clinical presentation of desmoid tumors from asymptomatic abdominal mass to bowel or ureteral obstruction. Sporadic desmoid tumors also occur. Retrospective studies have not confirmed the role of adjuvant radiation or chemotherapy for desmoid tumors. For unresectable tumors, chemotherapy, hormonal therapy, and targeted agents such as imatinib have been reported in literature as possible palliative options.

Answer 20.5.2.   **The answer is C.**

This patient meets the Amsterdam criteria for HNPCC with at least three affected relatives in at least two successive-generation relatives and one first-degree relative diagnosed with colorectal cancer before age 50 years. Unlike FAP, which is characterized by chromosomal instability caused by mutations in the APC tumor suppressor gene, HNPCC is characterized by MSI caused by mutations in the DNA MMR genes. HNPCC is the most common hereditary syndrome predisposing one to colorectal cancers. It accounts for approximately 2% to 3% of all colorectal cancer cases. The lifetime risk for developing colon cancer among patients with HNPCC approaches 80%. HNPCC is also associated with other malignancies, including endometrial, gastric, ampullary, biliary, and urinary tract cancers. This patient has Muir-Torre syndrome characterized by multiple colon cancers and multiple cutaneous neoplasia, including sebaceous adenomas.

Answer 20.5.3.   **The answer is D.**

HNPCC can be confirmed by the demonstration of the MSI-H phenotype and germ line mutation in any of the DNA MMR genes, such as MLH1 on chromosome 3p, MSH2 on chromosome 2p, MSH6 on chromosome 2p, PMS1 on 2q, and PMS2 on 7q. Germ line mutations involving MSH2 and MLH1 genes account for more than 60% of the known mutations present in patients with HNPCC. The National Comprehensive Cancer Network guidelines recommend the use of tumor screening with MSI and lack of expression of MMR protein expression by immunohistochemistry initially, followed by MMR mutation testing, although proceeding directly to MMR mutation testing is also acceptable. A negative MMR mutation test result does not rule out Lynch syndrome or HNPCC.

Answer 20.5.4.   **The answer is C.**

Once a germ line MMR mutation is identified in a patient, genetic counseling and testing of at-risk family members are essential. The patient's three daughters, along with all her first-degree relatives, have a 50% probability of being a carrier of the mutant gene. In general, for family members who do not carry the known mutation, there is no need for intensive surveillance, and routine colorectal screening according to national guidelines is recommended. For family members who carry the germ line MMR mutation, the National Comprehensive Cancer Network recommends colonoscopies every 1 to 2 years beginning at age 20 to 25 years or 5 to 10 years younger than the earliest age of diagnosis in the family, whichever comes first. For women with the MMR mutation, screening for endometrial cancer with transvaginal ultrasound with or without CA 125 for ovarian cancer screening is recommended by age 30 to 35 years. Women who have completed childbearing could opt for prophylactic hysterectomy and bilateral salpingo-oophorectomy to reduce their risks for developing endometrial and ovarian cancers.

Answer 20.5.5.   **The answer is D.**

Germ line mutations in the MMR genes MSH2, MLH1, and MSH6 account for 90% of all patients with HNPCC. APC gene mutation is commonly associated with FAP. MYH-associated polyposis is a rare inherited syndrome with increased for colorectal cancer.

Answer 20.5.6.   **The answer is D.**

The standard adjuvant therapy for patients with stage III colon cancer is oxaliplatin with 5FU based on the MOSAIC and the NSABP-C07 studies. Recent updates of the MOSAIC study demonstrated a significant improvement in 6-year overall survival among patients with stage III colorectal cancer treated with FOLFOX compared with those treated with infusional 5FU/LV. Irinotecan-based regimens are not recommended for adjuvant therapy for patients with stage III according to the negative results of three large randomized studies. Current studies on adding bevacizumab and cetuximab to oxaliplatin regimens are ongoing.

Answer 20.5.7.   **The answer is C.**

More than 80% of the administered dose of 5FU is eliminated via the dihydropyrimidine dehydrogenase (DPD) enzyme. Patients with DPD deficiency are at high risk for 5FU toxicities, such as severe neutropenia, neutropenic fever, diarrhea, mucositis, cerebellar ataxia, neurotoxicity, and even death. The most common mutation associated with DPD deficiency is the IVS14 + 1 G > A, DPYD*2A mutation. Complete DPD deficiency has been reported in patients homozygous for this allele, whereas partial DPD deficiency occurs in patients heterozygous for this allele. More than 40 other mutations and polymorphism have been identified in the DPD gene, although the functional significance of these polymorphisms is not clear. Moreover, instances of low DPD activity have been reported in patients without any identified DPD mutation or polymorphism. The TSER *3/*3 genotype is associated with higher levels of thymidine synthase and lower tumor response to 5FU therapy. Although it is possible that this patient is homozygous for the UGT1A1*28 gene resulting in severe neutropenia and diarrhea, the constellation of the patient's symptoms, including cerebellar ataxia and mucositis, is more consistent with 5FU-related toxicities. Furthermore, irinotecan therapy would not have been given to this patient with stage III colon cancer.

Answer 20.5.8.   **The answer is E.**

SN-38 is the active metabolite of irinotecan and is 100- to 1000-fold more potent than irinotecan as a topoisomerase I inhibitor. Glucuronidation is the principal elimination pathway for SN-38. UDP-glucuronosyltransferase 1 family polypeptide A1 mediates this glucuronidation of irinotecan encoded by the UGT1A1 gene. Patients who are homozygous for the UGT1A1*28 allele glucuronidate SN-38 less efficiently than patients who have one or two wild-type alleles; therefore, homozygous patients are exposed to higher plasma concentrations of SN-38 and are thus at a greater risk for severe neutropenia.

Answer 20.5.9.   **The answer is D.**

The results of the German Rectal Cancer Study published by Sauer et al. confirmed the benefit of neoadjuvant prolonged course RT with 5FU-based chemotherapy for patients with T3+/N0-2 rectal cancer. Although overall survival was similar for patients treated with neoadjuvant chemoradiotherapy compared with those treated with postoperative chemoradiotherapy, local recurrence rates and toxicities are more favorable with neoadjuvant chemoradiotherapy.

Answer 20.5.10.   **The answer is A.**

Transanal excision should only be considered for select patients with early-stage rectal cancer with the following characteristics: small rectal cancers less than 3 cm; well to moderately differentiated T1 tumors within 8 cm from the anal verge and limited to less than 30% of the rectal circumference with no evidence of nodal metastases. Only patient A meets all of these criteria.

Answer 20.5.11.   **The answer is A.**

After transanal resection of appropriately selected patients with early-stage rectal cancer, no further therapy is recommended.

Answer 20.5.12.   **The answer is A.**

MYH-associated polyposis is an autosomal-recessive disease affecting the MYH gene, a base-excision repair gene. A deficiency in MYH leads to somatic, not germ line, mutations in the APC gene. Thus, clinical features of patients with MYH-associated polyposis are similar to FAP.

Answer 20.5.13.   **The answer is D.**

The standard therapy for early localized squamous carcinoma of the anus is chemoradiation with 5FU and mitomycin. This is associated with excellent cure rates. Salvage APR is reserved for recurrent anal cancer.

Answer 20.5.14.   **The answer is C.**

This patient is potentially curable with an aggressive multidisciplinary approach. Resection of all tumor sites with close surveillance certainly is an option for this patient. However, the results of the recently published study, EORTC 40983, showed an improvement in progression-free survival for patients treated with perioperative chemotherapy with resection. Historically, cure rates of up to 35% have been observed even in patients with metastatic disease, as long as all tumor sites are resected. Thus, palliative chemotherapy would not be the best option for this patient. There is currently no role for radiotherapy for this patient.

Answer 20.5.15.   **The answer is A.**

Over 80% of all colorectal tumors show evidence of chromosomal instability characterized by loss of heterozygosity at multiple tumor suppressor loci including 5q, 17p, and 18q. The other 15% to 20% of sporadic colorectal tumors are characterized by MSI and in many cases the MSI is due to silencing of the MMR gene MLH1 by hypermethylation. Patients with MSI usually are more responsive to chemotherapy and have better outcomes. However, they appear to be resistant to treatment with 5FU.

Answer 20.5.16.   **The answer is A.**

Patients with colorectal cancer who test positive for the KRAS mutation are resistant to treatment with cetuximab. In addition, BRAF V600E mutation is also associated with resistance to cetuximab.

Answer 20.5.17.   **The answer is C.**

Sequential single-agent therapies were compared to combination chemotherapy regimens including FOLFOX and FOLFIRI in two randomized phase III trials. Even though the overall median survival was better with combination regimens, the difference was not statistically significant. Therefore, not all patients with metastatic unresectable colorectal cancer are candidates for combination chemotherapy. Adding panitumumab to FOLFOX was shown to improve progression-free survival in patients with metastatic colorectal cancer whose tumors tested positive for the wild-type KRAS gene. FOLFOX and FOLFIRI are both equally effective in the first-line setting. Bowel perforation and thromboembolic events are well known but rare toxicities seen in patients treated with bevacizumab.

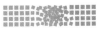

CHAPTER 21 GENITOURINARY CANCER

WALTER M. STADLER

DIRECTIONS   Each of the numbered items below is followed by lettered answers. Select the ONE lettered answer that is BEST in each case unless instructed otherwise.

QUESTIONS

Question 21.1.   Activating mutations in which of the following genes is seen in patients with hereditary papillary renal cell carcinoma?

    A. VHL
    B. MET
    C. FLCN
    D. SDHB

Question 21.2.   A 56-year-old moderately obese woman with a medical history of chronic hypertension well controlled on a thiazide diuretic presents to the emergency department with a 1-day history of abdominal pain, diarrhea, nausea, and fever. General physical examination is significant only for some mild abdominal tenderness; negative stool guaiac; a white blood cell count of 14.2/μL; hemoglobin of 14.5 g/dL; a normal platelet count; normal electrolytes, amylase, lipase, and transaminases; and a creatinine of 0.9 mg/dL. Workup includes an abdominal computed tomography (CT) scan, which is remarkable for a 1.5-cm enhancing left renal mass in the left lower pole that is interpreted by the radiologist as a "probable renal cell carcinoma" without evidence of other metastases. The patient undergoes a laparoscopic partial nephrectomy. There are no postoperative complications, and she is back to work 3 weeks later. Postoperative creatinine is 1.3, and pathology reveals a 2.5-cm renal cell carcinoma, granular cell type, that is confined to the renal parenchyma. No lymph nodes were recovered. The next appropriate step is:

    A. Open retroperitoneal lymph node dissection
    B. Adjuvant sunitinib
    C. Adjuvant local radiotherapy
    D. Submission of pathology specimen for second review

Corresponding Chapters in *Cancer: Principles & Practice of Oncology,* Ninth Edition: 92 (Molecular Biology of Kidney Cancer), 93 (Cancer of the Kidney), 94 (Molecular Biology of Bladder Cancer), 95 (Cancer of the Bladder, Ureter, and Renal Pelvis), 96 (Molecular Biology of Prostate Cancer), 97 (Cancer of the Prostate), 98 (Cancer of the Urethra and Penis).

Question 21.3.   A 55-year-old woman undergoes partial nephrectomy for clear cell carcinoma of the kidney, Fuhrman grade IV. The patient does well for 10 years, at which time she develops a pathologic intratrochanteric fracture of her left hip. CT scanning of the chest, abdomen, pelvis, and brain and bone scan reveals no other sites of disease. The MOST appropriate next step is:

A. Radiation alone
B. High-dose interleukin-2 alone
C. Orthopedic resection of the tumor with reconstruction followed by radiation
D. Temsirolimus

Questions   A 76-year-old man with chronic obstructive pulmonary disorder
21.4.–21.5.   and diabetes mellitus presents with back pain and confusion. Workup reveals extensive metastatic disease in the lungs, bones, and liver and a 6-cm tumor in the kidney. There is no evidence of cord compression. Laboratory studies reveal a calcium of 11.5 mg/dL and a creatinine of 2.0 mg/dL. After hydration and zoledronate, his calcium normalizes, hemoglobin is 9.5, creatinine decreases to 1.7, and Eastern Cooperative Oncology Group performance status is 2.

Question 21.4.   The poor-risk features present in this patient include all, EXCEPT:

A. His age of >75 years
B. Hypercalcemia
C. Performance status of 2
D. Anemia

Question 21.5.   The LEAST appropriate therapy in this case is:

A. Interferon-α
B. Temsirolimus
C. Sunitinib
D. Sorafenib

Question 21.6.   A 25-year-old Caucasian man without a medical history presents with hematuria. Workup reveals bilateral renal cysts, at least one of them suspicious for malignancy. Family history is significant for a pheochromocytoma in his father and a pancreatic islet cell tumor and early death from kidney cancer in a paternal aunt. The MOST likely familial cancer syndrome is:

A. Von Hippel-Lindau disease
B. Birt-Hogg-Dube syndrome
C. Hereditary papillary renal cancer
D. Hereditary leiomyomatosis and renal cancer

Question 21.7.   Which of the following statements about the VHL gene is INCORRECT?

A. It is mutated or altered in >60% of spontaneous clear cell carcinomas of the kidney.
B. It is critical for the normal oxygen sensing and response system in all cells.
C. It is part of a ubiquitin ligase complex.
D. Expression is regulated by vascular endothelial growth factor.

Question 21.8.   Inactivation or alteration in which of the following tumor suppressor genes is implicated in the pathogenesis of invasive bladder cancer?

A. TP53
B. RB1
C. PTEN
D. All of the above

Question 21.9.   The patient is taken to the operating room, where an examination under general anesthesia reveals a mobile bladder. Resection of the papillary lesion reveals grade III urothelial papillary carcinoma, and multiple biopsies of the erythematous areas of the bladder all reveal diffuse carcinoma in situ. Muscle is present in the pathologic specimens, and there is no evidence for invasive tumor. The appropriate therapy is:

A. Intravesical Bacillus Calmette–Guérin (BCG) vaccine
B. Intravesical cyclophosphamide
C. Radiation
D. Cystectomy

Question 21.10.   The patient receives definitive treatment, as well as with a follow-up maintenance program; however, 4 months after initiating the maintenance BCG program, the urologist notes multiple recurrent papillary lesions. Repeat biopsy reveals urothelial cancer invasive into muscle. CT scans of the chest, abdomen, and pelvis are unremarkable, creatinine remains normal at 1.2 mg/dL, and his performance status is excellent. Appropriate therapy at this point is:

A. Reinduction with intravesical BCG
B. Intravesical chemotherapy with mitomycin-C
C. Partial cystectomy
D. Cisplatin-based multiagent chemotherapy

Question 21.11.   Which of the following is the most common molecular abnormality seen in patients with prostate cancer?

A. KRAS mutation
B. BRAF mutation
C. p53 mutation
D. Chromosomal translocations involving TMPRSS2

Question 21.12. All of the following are risk factors for cancer of the male urethra, EXCEPT?

   A. HPV-16
   B. Chronic urethritis
   C. Urethral stricture
   D. Caucasian race

Questions 21.13.–21.14. A 62-year-old woman is newly diagnosed with muscle-invasive bladder cancer. She quit smoking 10 years ago, had a non-ST-elevated myocardial infarction 4 years ago, underwent coronary artery bypass surgery and has had no residual cardiac symptoms, takes only a beta-blocker and a thiazide for hypertension, and has normal laboratory test results, including a creatinine of 0.9. Cystoscopic biopsy revealed a muscle-invasive bladder cancer without associated carcinoma in situ (Tcis), and CT of the chest, abdomen, and pelvis is unremarkable.

Question 21.13. Which of the following statements about radical cystectomy is MOST correct?

   A. An orthotopic neobladder is less effective in women than in men.
   B. An abdominal wall diversion will require a urostomy bag.
   C. An orthotopic neobladder will require the patient to be willing and able to perform self-catheterization.
   D. Metabolic acidosis is not a significant problem with continent diversions.

Question 21.14. Which of the following statements about combined radiation and chemotherapy is MOST correct?

   A. Toxicity profile and tolerability of combined radiation and chemotherapy are significantly better than that of radical cystectomy.
   B. Long-term cancer outcome is similar to cystectomy.
   C. It is preferred over cystectomy because of her cardiac history.
   D. It will obviate the need for cystectomy.

Question 21.15. Which of the following is CORRECT about neoadjuvant chemotherapy?

   A. Three cycles of methotrexate, vinblastine, doxorubicin, and cisplatin before cystectomy are a standard of care.
   B. Gemcitabine/carboplatin should be considered to decrease the risk of renal failure with cystectomy.
   C. It increases the risk of surgical complications of cystectomy.
   D. It should always be used with an organ preservation approach but is optional if cystectomy is chosen.

Question 21.16. Which of the following statements about the molecular pathogenesis of urothelial cancer of the bladder is INCORRECT?

A. Chromosome 9 deletions are common and occur on both the short and long arms.

B. p53 mutations are associated with carcinoma in situ and aggressive disease.

C. pRb alterations are observed and correlate with poor prognosis.

D. Activating FGFR3 mutations are most common in metastatic lesions.

Question 21.17. A 71-year-old man without significant medical history presents with hematuria and flank pain. CT scan reveals a mass at the pelvic-ureteral junction with associated hydronephrosis, but no associated lymphadenopathy. Cystoscopy and ureteroscopy reveal an obstructing mass at the pelvic-ureteral junction, and cytology is diagnostic for a urothelial cancer. Which of the following is the MOST appropriate therapy?

A. Open nephroureterectomy and bladder cuff resection

B. Open radical nephrectomy with retroperitoneal lymph node dissection

C. Laparoscopic radical nephrectomy without retroperitoneal lymph node dissection

D. Definitive radiation and combined chemotherapy

Question 21.18. A 51-year-old man with a strong family history of prostate cancer, a normal digital rectal examination, no significant comorbid medical problems, and a PSA of 2.9 seeks advice on prostate cancer prevention. He is sexually active in a monogamous relationship and denies any urinary or rectal symptoms. The following are all true, EXCEPT:

A. Finasteride has been shown to decrease his risk of developing prostate cancer.

B. Taking supplemental vitamin E has been shown to decrease his risk of developing prostate cancer.

C. Taking finasteride will decrease the PSA.

D. 8q24 polymorphisms have been identified as risk alleles in patients such as this.

Questions 21.19.–21.20. A 71-year-old white man with a history of hypertension, hyperlipidemia, coronary artery disease, and prior angioplasty with stent placement, but no prior myocardial infarction, is noted to have a increase in his PSA from 3.0 to 3.9 ng/mL and then to 4.6 ng/mL over 19 months. He is a semiretired accountant, swims actively three times per week, and helps care for his mildly demented 95-year-old father. General physical examination is unremarkable; a rectal examination reveals a mildly enlarged prostate gland without any palpable nodules.

Question 21.19.   The MOST correct statement about this case is:

A. Biopsy should be discussed because the PSA increase is >0.75 ng/mL/yr.
B. Biopsy should not be discussed because PSA is normal for his age.
C. Biopsy should not be discussed because his expected survival makes treatment not worthwhile, even if prostate cancer is discovered.
D. Biopsy should be discussed because the PSA is >4 ng/mL.
E. The free-to-total PSA ratio will determine the need for biopsy.

Question 21.20.   Biopsy reveals Gleason 8 prostate cancer in six of six cores. CT scan of the abdomen and pelvis and bone scan are unremarkable. The MOST appropriate therapy is:

A. Radical retropubic prostatectomy
B. Three-dimensional conformal radiotherapy with concomitant androgen ablation
C. Interstitial radiotherapy with 125I
D. All of the above

Question 21.21.   After discussion with a radiation oncologist and a urologist, the patient elects to undergo combined androgen ablation and external beam radiation therapy. The androgen ablation is administered before the radiation therapy and continued for 3 months thereafter. Radiotherapy is complicated only by a mild diarrhea that resolves once the radiation therapy is complete. The PSA nadirs at 1.2 ng/mL; however, 9 months after his last dose of the luteinizing hormone-releasing hormone (LHRH) agonist, the PSA increases to 2.4 ng/mL and then to 3.6 ng/mL 1 month later. Testosterone level is normal at 350 ng/mL. The MOST appropriate next therapeutic and/or diagnostic maneuver is:

A. Perform MRI of the pelvis to assess for local recurrence
B. Reinitiate androgen ablation
C. Refer the patient to a urologist for salvage prostatectomy
D. Initiate docetaxel-based chemotherapy

Question 21.22.   The patient is treated with an LHRH agonist along with the antiandrogen bicalutamide. PSA declines to 0.8 ng/mL, but after 10 months, the PSA begins to slowly increase to a value of 3.7. He continues to feel well and has minimal urinary symptoms, no bone pain, and no weight loss. The MOST appropriate therapy at this point is:

A. Docetaxel-based chemotherapy
B. Discontinuing the antiandrogen bicalutamide
C. Hospice care
D. Radionuclide therapy with strontium-98 (Metastron)

Question 21.23.   Infestation with which of the following parasites is a risk factor for developing bladder cancer?

    A. *Clonorchis sinensis*
    B. *Opisthorchis viverrini*
    C. *Schistosoma haematobium*
    D. None of the above

Question 21.24–21.25.   51-year-old black male executive with no medical history undergoes a routine PSA screening evaluation and is found to have a PSA of 5.5 ng/mL. Biopsy reveals a Gleason 3 + 3 prostate cancer in two of six biopsy cores. After discussion with a radiation oncologist and urologist, he elects to receive treatment with a radical retropubic prostatectomy.

Question 21.24.   Which of the following statements about the surgery is TRUE?

    A. Robotic laparoscopic prostatectomy is associated with a lower incidence of impotence than open retropubic prostatectomy.
    B. The incidence of impotence under the assumption that a bilateral nerve sparing procedure can be performed is <10%.
    C. Problems with incontinence persist in approximately 20% of patients.
    D. Surgical experience has only a minimal impact on the positive margin rate.

Question 21.25.   Surgical pathology confirms a Gleason score 6 tumor in both lobes of the prostate. There is a focal surgical positive margin. There is no evidence of seminal vesicle or lymph node invasion. His postoperative PSA is undetectable, and he has good continence. The MOST appropriate next step is:

    A. Adjuvant radiotherapy
    B. Repeat surgical exploration with possible reexcision of the prostatic bed
    C. Pelvic CT scan
    D. Prostascint scan

Question 21.26.   The patient maintains an undetectable PSA until 8 years later (at the age of 59 years), recurrent biochemical disease is noted. After appropriate discussion, androgen ablation with an LHRH agonist alone is initiated, and the PSA once again becomes undetectable. The patient maintains an undetectable PSA while on androgen ablation for 3 years, when he develops sudden mid-back pain after lifting his grandson. There are no associated neurologic signs or symptoms. Bone scan shows marked uptake at the T8 vertebra, and PSA remains undetectable. The MOST appropriate therapeutic or diagnostic maneuver is:

    A. Immediate radiotherapy to T8
    B. Therapy with ketoconazole, 400 mg three times daily with hydrocortisone replacement
    C. Spinal MRI to rule out cord compression
    D. Bone densitometry to assess for osteoporosis

Question 21.27.   A 75-year-old man with diabetes, hypertension, and coronary artery disease who is receiving atorvastatin, glyburide, and an angiotensin-converting enzyme inhibitor is under surveillance after external beam radiotherapy for a Gleason 3 + 3 prostate cancer that was diagnosed and treated 10 years earlier when he was found to have a PSA of 4.3 on routine screening. His PSA level, which had been 0.2 ng/mL, has increased to 0.3, 0.35, and then 0.40 over the period of 18 months. The MOST appropriate therapy at this time is:

    A. Androgen ablation with an LHRH agonist
    B. Continued active surveillance
    C. High-intensity focused ultrasound to his prostate
    D. High-dose (150 mg) bicalutamide

Question 21.28.   A 65-year-old man has been receiving combined androgen ablation with leuprolide and bicalutamide for 4 years for biochemical recurrence after radical prostatectomy. His PSA has increased from an undetectable nadir to 1.1 ng/mL on serial measurement over the period of 6 months. The PSA continues to increase 2 months after discontinuation of bicalutamide to 1.5, with serum testosterone of 10 ng/mL. Bone scan and CT of the abdomen/pelvis do not reveal any metastatic disease, and he remains asymptomatic. Treatment options include all the following, EXCEPT:

    A. Active surveillance
    B. Docetaxel-based chemotherapy
    C. Thalidomide
    D. High-dose ketoconazole

Question 21.29.   All the following statements about prostate cancer epidemiology are correct, EXCEPT:

    A. There is a marked difference in mortality from prostate cancer in different parts of the world.
    B. The difference in mortality between African Americans and Caucasian Americans can be completely explained by socioeconomic factors.
    C. Epidemiologic studies suggest a dietary or lifestyle component to prostate cancer development.
    D. There is molecular confirmation for genetic risk factors for prostate cancer.

Question 21.30.   The following statements about prostate cancer biology are all correct, EXCEPT:

    A. GSTπ loss is common in prostate intraepithelial neoplasia (PIN).
    B. TMPRSS2 translocations juxtapose an androgen-responsive gene promoter with a transcription factor.
    C. PTEN loss is as common in PIN as in more advanced cancer.
    D. NKX3.1 has been postulated to be a gatekeeper tumor suppressor.

Question 21.31.   Which of the following statements about the androgen receptor is MOST correct?

   A.   The majority of its activity in prostate cancer is due to its cytoplasmic effects.
   B.   Upregulation of androgen receptor expression has been linked to prostate cancer development.
   C.   Castration leads to complete inactivation of all androgen receptor-mediated pathways.
   D.   Castrate-resistant prostate cancer is associated with upregulation of androgen receptor expression.

Question 21.32.   A 63-year-old uncircumcised man without any significant medical history presents to his physician with an inability to retract the foreskin. Examination reveals phimosis, with an underlying painless ulcerated mass of 1×2 cm. A 2.5-cm hard node is palpated in the left inguinal region. Biopsy of the penile lesion reveals squamous cell cancer. In addition to wide surgical resection of the primary lesion, other appropriate therapeutic and/or diagnostic maneuvers at this time include:

   A.   Four-week course of a broad-spectrum antibiotic
   B.   Left inguinal lymph node dissection
   C.   Bilateral inguinal radiotherapy
   D.   Taxane-based chemotherapy

ANSWERS

Answer 21.1.   **The answer is B.**

Hereditary papillary renal cell carcinoma is an autosomal-dominant hereditary cancer syndrome characterized by mutations in the MET protooncogene, which encodes the hepatocyte growth factor/scatter factor receptor tyrosine kinase. Although MET overexpression has been demonstrated in a number of epithelial cancers, HRPC is the first cancer syndrome for which germ line MET mutations have been identified. Individuals with this syndrome are at risk for developing multifocal, bilateral papillary type 1 kidney cancer in their fifth and sixth decades of life, with age-dependent penetrance of 67% by 60 years of age.

Answer 21.2.   **The answer is D.**

Renal cell cancer is currently divided into clear cell and nonclear cell subtypes. The nonclear cell subtypes have been further divided into papillary, chromophobe, and collecting duct tumors. Several renal cancers cannot be accurately subtyped, often because of poor histologic differentiation such that the originating subtype cannot be easily recognized. Such tumors are often classified as "sarcomatoid." Granular cell carcinoma has been used in the past but is not currently an accepted pathologic classification. Thus, a second opinion and pathologic review should be requested. The risk of recurrence in this case is low, and adjuvant sunitinib has not been shown to decrease the risk of recurrence. Patients who do have recurrence after nephrectomy almost always recur systemically, and thus additional local radiotherapy is not indicated. Likewise, the role of extensive lymph node dissection is highly controversial and generally not recommended. In any case, formal retroperitoneal lymph node dissection as is carried out in testes cancer would certainly not be standard in patients with localized renal cell carcinoma.

Answer 21.3.   **The answer is C.**

Patients with renal cancer can develop recurrent disease more than 5 years after initial definitive therapy. Development of a single metastatic site is not unusual. Patients with a single site of metastatic disease and a long interval between initial diagnosis and recurrent metastatic disease typically have a good prognosis. Thus, aggressive surgical resection including orthopedic stabilization is indicated. Because orthopedic surgery such as this often leaves microscopic tumors behind in the surgical field, additional radiotherapy to the site is appropriate. Radiation alone is insufficient to completely eradicate metastatic renal cancer and does not repair the underlying structural bony abnormality. High-dose interleukin-2 is approved for metastatic renal cancer but is less effective than aggressive local surgery for complete eradication of disease when possible. Temsirolimus improves survival in patients with poor prognosis metastatic disease, which does not apply here. In addition, it is not curative.

Answer 21.4.   **The answer is A.**

Several prognostic factors have been identified that can help explain the highly heterogeneous natural history of metastatic renal cancer. Hypercalcemia, poor performance status, and anemia are significant prognostic factors in most studies. Age, in and of itself, is not a prognostic factor.

Answer 21.5.   **The answer is A.**

Of the choices, phase III data supportive of a survival benefit in a patient with poor prognosis such as this are available only for temsirolimus. The available data suggest that sunitinib or sorafenib could be considered. However, data suggest that interferon is not effective in patients with poor prognosis, and phase III data show that sunitinib is more effective than interferon for metastatic disease in patients with a good and intermediate prognosis.

Answer 21.6.   **The answer is A.**

Von Hippel-Lindau disease, caused by mutation of the VHL gene, is an autosomal-dominant cancer syndrome characterized by multiple renal cysts, early onset and multiple renal tumors, retinal angiomas and central nervous system hemangioblastomas, pheochromocytomas, and pancreatic islet cell tumors. The Birt-Hogg-Dube syndrome, caused by mutations of the BHD gene, is characterized by early onset chromophobe cancers, benign hair follicle tumors (fibrofolliculomas), and pulmonary cysts. Hereditary papillary renal cancer, caused by mutations of the MET gene, is characterized by multiple type I papillary cancers. The hereditary leiomyomatosis and renal cancer syndrome, caused by mutation of the fumarate hydratase gene, is characterized by cutaneous and uterine leiomyomas and aggressive type II papillary cancers.

Answer 21.7.   **The answer is D.**

VHL is part of the normal oxygen sensing and response system in all cells and is mutated or altered in greater than 60% of sporadic clear cell carcinomas of the kidney. Under normoxic conditions, VHL is part of a multiprotein complex that recognizes the hydroxylated HIF transcription factor, acts as a ubiquitin ligase, and thus targets it for proteasomal degradation. Under hypoxic conditions, HIF is not hydroxylated, not targeted to VHL and thus not degraded leading to upregulation of multiple genes critical for the hypoxic response including vascular endothelial growth factor. The VHL gene is expressed constitutively.

Answer 21.8.   **The answer is D.**

The tumor suppressor genes TP53, RB1 CDKN2A, and PTEN are implicated in the pathogenesis of invasive bladder cancer.

Answer 21.9.   **The answer is A.**

Indications for intravesical therapy are multiple recurrent Ta lesions, especially if they are high grade, or Tcis. It is critical that the pathologic specimen in patients diagnosed with superficial bladder cancer contains muscle to determine whether there is an non-invasive component. Most, but not all, studies have suggested that intravesical BCG is more effective than intravesical chemotherapy. Although other chemotherapeutic agents are being investigated, cyclophosphamide needs to be activated to 4-hydroxy-cyclosphosphamide in the liver to act as an alkylating agent, and thus bladder instillation of the parent compound is not expected to be effective. Radiation or cystectomy, although potentially useful for invasive carcinoma or refractory bladder cancer, is not appropriate as initial therapy in this patient.

Answer 21.10.   **The answer is D.**

Patients with muscle-invasive bladder cancer require definitive local therapy. Additional intravesical therapy is inappropriate. Partial cystectomies are only rarely indicated and should be performed in only a very highly select group, which does not include patients with a history of Tcis or patients with multiple tumors. The standard definitive therapy for bladder cancer is cystectomy. Multiagent cisplatin-based neoadjuvant chemotherapy improves survival for patients with invasive urothelial bladder cancer and is considered a standard of care.

Answer 21.11.   **The answer is D.**

Chromosomal translocations fusing the TMPRSS2 androgen-responsive gene to various ETS family transcription factors, of which ERG is the most common, occur in approximately 60% of patients. Prostate cancer is characterized by a relatively low rate of mutations in KRAS, BRAF, and p53, unlike most other tumors.

Answer 21.12.   **The answer is D.**

Risk factors for male urethral cancers include HPV-16, chronic irritation, and infection. The incidence of urethral cancer in men with urethral strictures ranges from 24% to 76%. No racial predisposition has been noted for urethral cancers.

Answer 21.13.   **The answer is C.**

There are several options for urinary diversion after cystectomy, and no clear evidence has emerged that any is more or less desirable or effective based on patient gender. Diversion to the abdominal wall with a urostomy can be performed as a conduit, requiring a urine collection device, or as a continent diversion, requiring regular catheterization. Metabolic complications, including metabolic acidosis, can occur with both conduits and continent diversions. Complications of orthotopic continent diversions, or neobladders, include intermittent urethral obstruction and frequent requirement for intermittent or temporary self-catheterization.

Answer 21.14.   **The answer is B.**

Organ preservation with combined radiation and chemotherapy has been investigated in numerous trials, and long-term outcomes are similar to those observed in cystectomy series. The therapy is, however, an aggressive and potentially toxic approach in which approximately 30% of patients will require cystectomy for incomplete response. It is thus not more tolerable than cystectomy. The patient's cardiac history does not preclude major surgery, and in fact willingness to accept a cystectomy has been an inclusion criterion for most organ preservation trials.

Answer 21.15.   **The answer is A.**

Randomized studies have demonstrated that cisplatin-based combination chemotherapy provides a survival advantage. The largest phase III studies used methotrexate, vinblastine, doxorubicin, and cisplatin or a similar regimen in which the doxorubicin was eliminated (MVC). The strongest data supporting neoadjuvant chemotherapy are in the surgical setting, with no survival advantage demonstrated in modest-sized trials using combined chemotherapy and radiation for primary tumor treatment. The randomized data further demonstrate that there is no increase in surgical morbidity or complications after neoadjuvant chemotherapy. There are no data on the neoadjuvant use of carboplatin-based regimens, and data in the metastatic setting strongly suggest that carboplatin is an inferior agent in comparison with cisplatin for this disease.

Answer 21.16.   **The answer is D.**

Chromosome 9 deletions are the most common alteration in urothelial carcinoma of the bladder, appear to be critical for the initiation of bladder cancer, and occur on both the long and short arms. Alterations of both p53 and pRb are most common in invasive disease and are markers of poor prognosis. Activating mutations of FGFR3 are common in papillary noninvasive cancers but are actually unusual in more invasive lesions.

Answer 21.17.   **The answer is A.**

The standard definitive treatment for renal pelvis urothelial cancers is radical nephroureterectomy with resection of the bladder cuff at the ureteral insertion site. Radical nephrectomy without ureter resection is inappropriate because of the high incidence of undiagnosed or recurrent disease in the ureter. Definitive radiotherapy would also be inappropriate because this would be expected to lead to kidney necrosis.

Answer 21.18.   **The answer is B.**

The Prostate Cancer Prevention Trial randomized patients with normal rectal examination and PSA less than 3.0 ng/dL to finasteride or placebo, and required an end-of-treatment biopsy because of the decrease in PSA observed with 5-α reductase inhibitor therapy. It demonstrated an overall decrease in the incidence of prostate cancer but an increase in the number of high-risk prostate cancers. Single nucleotide polymorphisms on 8q24 have been identified as risk alleles for prostate cancer in multiple independent studies. Although dietary studies have suggested that vitamin E correlates with a decreased incidence of prostate cancer, early data from the phase III intervention study (SELECT) of selenium and vitamin E to prevent prostate cancer demonstrates that vitamin E use is actually associated with an increased risk of developing prostate cancer (JAMA 2011;306:1549).

Answer 21.19.   **The answer is A.**

The decision to screen for and diagnose prostate cancer always needs to be accompanied by a discussion between the physician and the patient regarding risks and benefits of screening. To this end, it should be recognized that the median survival of an average 70-year-old man without significant comorbidities is more than 10 years, and that such a patient could benefit from the treatment of localized disease. Nonetheless, there is a risk of treating disease that will never become clinically significant within the patient's lifetime. It also needs to be recalled that the sensitivity and specificity of all PSA-based screening methods are limited, and there are no absolute "normal" criteria. Therefore, no single test can determine the absolute need for a biopsy. Predictors of cancer on biopsy include PSA greater than 4.0 ng/mL, PSA greater than age-adjusted PSA norms (based on normal increasing PSA with age), free-to-total PSA ratio, and PSA velocity. Of these, and in this case, the rapid increase in the PSA is most predictive of malignancy, and this is also predictive of aggressive disease.

Answer 21.20.   **The answer is D.**

On the basis of the high Gleason score, the aforementioned rapid PSA doubling time, and the tumor in all cores, this patient is at a high risk for locally advanced disease and systemic recurrence. As such, staging CT scan and bone scan are reasonable, although not generally necessary in patients with lower-risk disease. Because of the presence of high-risk features and the general good health of the patient, watchful waiting is probably not an appropriate option in this case. Radiotherapy, with external beam radiotherapy or interstitial brachytherapy, or surgical prostatectomy is equally appropriate for patients with clinically localized disease. The choice is dependent on a discussion of expected risks and benefits.

Answer 21.21.   **The answer is B.**

Rapidly increasing PSA before diagnosis, high Gleason score, PSA nadir of greater than 1.0 after radiotherapy, short interval between definitive local therapy and biochemical recurrence, and rapid PSA increase once recurrence is identified are all associated with a poor prognosis. The probability of locally recurrent disease alone is extremely low, and there is not much value to pelvic MRI for assessing local recurrence. Despite the poor prognosis, the role of chemotherapy in patients whose testosterone axis is intact is controversial. Although timing of androgen ablation is not clearly defined, some retrospective data suggest that "early" ablation in high-risk patients such as this provides a long-term survival advantage over "later" ablation.

Answer 21.22.   **The answer is B.**

Approximately 10% to 15% of patients receiving treatment with an antiandrogen will experience an antiandrogen withdrawal response. Although the majority of these responses are of brief duration, it is obviously the easiest therapeutic maneuver. Docetaxel-based chemotherapy leads to improved survival in castrate-resistant prostate cancer, which is generally defined as a progressive disease after androgen ablation, an antiandrogen, and antiandrogen withdrawal. Radioactive nuclides are occasionally useful for the palliation of diffuse bone pain but have not been shown to have an impact on survival.

Answer 21.23.   **The answer is C.**

Over 90% of bladder cancers in Western countries are urothelial carcinomas. In areas where the parasite *Schistosoma haematobium* is endemic, squamous cell bladder carcinomas are more common. *Opisthorchis viverrini* and *Clonorchis sinensis* are associated with cholangiocarcinoma, and not bladder cancer.

Answer 21.24.   **The answer is C.**

Although robotic laparoscopic prostatectomy has been touted as a less-invasive and potentially more effective approach, there is no reliable evidence that the risk of long-term complications, including impotence, is different than that observed in patients undergoing an open procedure with an experienced surgeon. In both groups, the incidence of impotence is at least 25%, even in young men with good erectile function before surgery. The risk of incontinence, when assessed by anonymized, validated quality of life instruments, is on the order of 20%. One of the most important variables for both pathologic outcome and complications is the surgeon's experience.

Answer 21.25.   **The answer is A.**

Adjuvant radiotherapy has been shown to decrease the risk of recurrence in patients with T3 disease. However, overall survival and clinical metastases-free survival have not been affected by this approach. Some have thus argued for close monitoring and salvage radiotherapy on biochemical recurrence in patients such as this. Imaging tests have not been shown to be helpful in identifying patients most likely to benefit from adjuvant therapy, and surgical reexploration is not indicated either.

Answer 21.26.   **The answer is D.**

Patients on long-term androgen ablation are at high risk for the development of osteoporosis and its complications, and an osteoporotic fracture must be considered in this patient before initiating any therapy for progressive metastatic disease. If progressive disease were to be diagnosed, ketoconazole is not an unreasonable second-line hormonal therapy, but the addition of an antiandrogen would likely be more appropriate. In the absence of neurologic signs or symptoms, an MRI is not necessary.

Answer 21.27.   **The answer is B.**

Patients with a slowly increasing PSA after definitive local therapy may have a very long natural history, with only a minority of patients having cancer-related mortality within 10 years. Androgen ablation, especially in elderly patients, is associated with osteoporosis, muscle loss, and changes in lipid metabolism that may have significant impact on cardiovascular comorbidities. High-intensity focused ultrasound for treatment of possible localized recurrence is still investigational. Single-agent antiandrogen therapy is not approved and may lead to higher mortality in patients such as this.

Answer 21.28.   **The answer is C.**

This patient meets all the criteria for castrate-resistant prostate cancer, and the only therapy demonstrated to improve survival is docetaxel-based chemotherapy. Nevertheless, there remains controversy regarding the timing of such therapy in otherwise asymptomatic men. Active surveillance is thus reasonable. High-dose ketoconazole has been demonstrated to lead to PSA decreases in up to 30% of men in this situation in several studies. Although thalidomide has been investigated, it has minimal activity as a single agent and is not indicated.

Answer 21.29.   **The answer is B.**

Multiple studies confirm marked differences in prostate cancer incidence and mortality between various countries that are not explainable by any kind of ascertainment bias. Changes in incidence and mortality in populations migrating from a country with a low incidence to a country with a high incidence strongly suggest that there are significant dietary or lifestyle contributors to prostate cancer development. There is now also confirmation of a genetic risk component because genetic polymorphisms, including several on 8q24, have been found to be closely associated with prostate cancer. In fact, the large difference in prostate cancer mortality between African Americans and Caucasian Americans cannot be explained by socioeconomic factors alone.

Answer 21.30.   **The answer is C.**

NKX3.1 transcription factor inactivation can be detected in the earliest identifiable PIN lesions. In contrast, PTEN loss is far more common in advanced disease. GSTπ is also commonly seen at all disease stages, including PIN. Translocation of the androgen-responsive gene promoter from TMPRSS2 to ETS family transcription factors is common in early tumors, but not in PIN.

Answer 21.31.   **The answer is D.**

Although the androgen receptor does have cytoplasmic effects, some of which may be important to prostate cancer oncogenesis, the majority of its effects occur in the nucleus where it modifies expression of genes with an androgen-responsive promoter. Upregulation of androgen receptor expression has been reported to be both necessary and sufficient for the castrate-resistant state, which is likely an adaptation to prolonged exposure to a low androgen environment. Such upregulation is not generally observed de novo and has not been linked to the development of prostate cancer. Castration dramatically lowers testosterone, but the levels of other androgenic steroids are sufficient to cause partial activation of androgen receptor-mediated pathways.

Answer 21.32.   **The answer is A.**

Penile carcinoma is a rare malignancy that presents most commonly with phimosis in an uncircumcised patient. Metastatic spread of penile carcinoma is via superficial inguinal lymphatics, followed by deep inguinal lymphatics, and then to the pelvic lymphatics. Systemic metastatic disease almost never develops in the absence of pelvic lymphadenopathy. Therefore, surgery and occasionally radiotherapy form the cornerstone of treatment for lymph node-positive patients; however, half of the patients with clinically palpable nodes will have inflammatory lesions only. Thus, a course of antibiotics before any further therapy is indicated. If the nodes persist after a course of antibiotics, biopsy and surgical dissection are indicated. Management of patients with clinical N0 is more controversial, with some authors recommending immediate lymph node dissection and others recommending a watchful waiting approach. Pathologic risk factors as assessed in the primary lesion may assist in decision making. Lymphangiography before a course of antibiotics is generally not considered helpful.

CHAPTER 22 CANCER OF THE TESTIS

SAIAMA WAQAR • DANIEL MORGENSZTERN • BRUCE ROTH

DIRECTIONS Each of the numbered items below is followed by lettered answers. Select the ONE lettered answer that is BEST in each case unless instructed otherwise.

QUESTIONS

Question 22.1. Which germ cell tumor is associated with widespread hematogenous metastases and high levels of human chorionic gonadotropin (HCG)?

A. Pure choriocarcinoma
B. Yolk sac tumor
C. Embryonal carcinoma
D. Seminoma

Question 22.2. Which of the following is associated with primary nonseminomatous mediastinal germ cell tumors?

A. Human immunodeficiency virus (HIV)
B. Klinefelter syndrome
C. Diethylstilbestrol exposure
D. None of the above

Question 22.3. Which of the following is a risk factor for central nervous system involvement in patients with testicular cancer?

A. Large volume pulmonary metastases
B. Pure choriocarcinoma histology
C. HCG >100,000
D. All of the above

Question 22.4. Which immunohistochemical markers are commonly expressed in patients with seminoma?

A. CD117
B. Placental alkaline phosphatase (PLAP)
C. None of the above
D. A and B

Corresponding Chapter in *Cancer: Principles & Practice of Oncology*, Ninth Edition: 99 (Cancer of the Testis).

Question 22.5. Which of the following statements is incorrect regarding the epidemiology and risk factors for germ cell malignancies?

    A. Orchiopexy eliminates the risk of developing testicular cancer in patients with cryptorchidism.

    B. Contralateral primaries arise in 1% to 2% of patients.

    C. Germ cell tumors are the most common malignancy seen in men between the ages of 15 and 34.

    D. HIV infection is a risk factor for developing germ cell tumors.

Question 22.6. Which of the following characterizes a pathological stage T3 testicular germ cell tumor?

    A. Invasion of the tunica vaginalis

    B. Invasion of the tunica albuginea

    C. Invasion of the spermatic cord

    D. None of the above

Question 22.7. Which of the following is NOT recommended after orchiectomy for patients with stage I seminoma?

    A. Radiation

    B. Retroperitoneal lymph node dissection (RPLND)

    C. Observation

    D. None of the above

Question 22.8. Which of the following are TRUE regarding patients with stage I seminoma?

    A. The relapse rate without radiation therapy is between 15% and 20%.

    B. The median time to relapse is 20 months.

    C. Approximately 10% of relapses occur 5 years after orchiectomy.

    D. All the above.

Question 22.9. Which of the following is a reasonable treatment option after orchiectomy for patients with stage IA nonseminomatous germ cell tumors (NSGCTs)?

    A. Observation

    B. Radiation

    C. Full bilateral RPLND with suprahilar dissection

    D. All the above

Question 22.10. Which of the following is an acceptable treatment regimen for a patient with good risk advanced germ cell tumor?

    A. Three cycles of bleomycin, etoposide, and carboplatin

    B. Three cycles of bleomycin, etoposide, and cisplatin (BEP)

    C. Three cycles of etoposide and cisplatin (EP)

    D. All of the above

Question 22.11.   Which of the following defines a seminoma with poor prognosis?

    A. Mediastinal primary site
    B. Brain metastases
    C. A and B
    D. None of the above

Question 22.12.   Which of the following may be present in patients with intermediate-risk nonseminoma?

    A. Alpha-fetoprotein (AFP) of 20,000 ng/mL
    B. HCG of 35,000 mIU/mL
    C. Primary mediastinal site
    D. None of the above

Question 22.13.   Which of the following patients has good-risk metastatic seminomatous germ cell tumor?

    A. A 23-year-old man with testicular seminoma, elevated AFP and hepatic metastases.
    B. A 38-year-old man with testicular seminoma, elevated AFP and pulmonary metastases.
    C. A 19-year-old man with primary mediastinal seminoma, normal AFP and hepatic metastases.
    D. A 28-year-old man with primary mediastinal seminoma, normal AFP and pulmonary metastases.

Question 22.14.   What is the standard chemotherapy regimen for patients with poor-risk germ cell tumors?

    A. Three cycles of BEP
    B. Four cycles of EP
    C. Four cycles of BEP
    D. A or B

Question 22.15.   Which of the following treatments have shown improved survival compared with BEP in patients with poor-risk germ cell tumors in a randomized phase III trial?

    A. Four cycles of etoposide, ifosfamide, and cisplatin (VIP)
    B. Two cycles of BEP followed by high-dose chemotherapy and stem cell support
    C. A and B
    D. None of the above

Question 22.16.   What is the best treatment for a patient with poor-risk germ cell tumor and compromised pulmonary function?

    A. Four cycles of EP
    B. Four cycles of VIP
    C. Three cycles of BEP
    D. Four cycles of bleomycin, vincristine, and cisplatin (BOP)

Question 22.17.   Which factor is a predictor for poor outcomes after salvage chemotherapy in germ cell tumors?

    A. Primary retroperitoneal site
    B. Primary mediastinal site
    C. Complete response to initial therapy
    D. A and B

ANSWERS

Answer 22.1.   **The answer is A.**

Metastases from testicular cancer usually follow the lymphatic drainage, reaching the retroperitoneal lymph nodes in a predictable way. This is the case for seminomas and almost all subtypes of nonseminomas. The main exception is pure choriocarcinoma, which is rare and associated with widespread hematogenous metastases. Choriocarcinomas are, by definition, composed of both cytotrophoblasts and syncytiotrophoblasts. Because HCG is produced by syncytiotrophoblasts, pure choriocarcinomas may be associated with high levels of this serum marker.

Answer 22.2.   **The answer is B.**

There is no established association between the use of diethylstilbestrol and the development of germ cell tumors. Although testicular cancer has been reported in patients with HIV, there is little evidence to support its increased incidence in this population. Klinefelter syndrome is diagnosed by a 47, XXY karyotype and is characterized by testicular atrophy, eunuchoid habitus, and gynecomastia. These patients are at increased risk for the development of mediastinal NSGCTs, but not seminomas.

Answer 22.3.   **The answer is D.**

Risk factors for central nervous system involvement in patients with testicular cancer include pure choriocarcinoma histology, HCG >100,000 and large volume pulmonary metastases.

Answer 22.4.   **The answer is D.**

Virtually all seminomas express CD117 (c-kit) and PLAP.

Answer 22.5.   **The answer is A.**

Orchiopexy does not eliminate the risk of developing germ cell tumors in patients with cryptorchidism. HIV infection is a risk factor for developing germ cell tumors. Contralateral primaries arise in 1% to 2% of patients. Germ cell tumors are the most common malignancy seen in men between the ages of 15 and 34.

Answer 22.6.   **The answer is C.**

According to the sixth edition of the American Joint Committee on Cancer staging handbook, invasion of the tunica albuginea and vaginalis characterizes pathological stages T1 and T2, respectively. Pathological stage T3 is defined by the invasion of the spermatic cord.

Answer 22.7.   **The answer is B.**

After resection of the primary testicular cancer, the standard treatment for patients with stage I seminoma is radiation therapy. Because of the low risk of relapse and the high probability of cure with treatment of relapsed disease, observation after orchiectomy remains an alternative option. RPLND is usually not recommended in the management of patients with seminoma.

Answer 22.8.   **The answer is D.**

After orchiectomy, the probability of relapse for patients with seminoma under surveillance is between 15% and 20%. The relapse, however, is typically 12 to 15 months longer than for nonseminomatous tumors, with the relapse rate after 2 and 5 years approximately 30% and 5%, respectively.

Answer 22.9.   **The answer is A.**

Historically, patients with clinical stage I disease were treated with a retroperitoneal lymph node dissection, and 30% of patients were found to have occult retroperitoneal disease. This rate may be dependent on the pathological stage, ranging from 15% in patients with T1 (stage IA) to 50% in patients with stage T2 or higher (stage IB). However, since chemotherapy is highly effective for treating recurrent disease, observation is a reasonable treatment option, with chemotherapy in case of recurrence. Radiation therapy has no role in the management of stage I NSGCTs as they are not very radiosensitive. Virtually all patients who undergo full bilateral RPLND have retrograde ejaculation; however, nerve-sparing RPLND has eliminated this complication.

Answer 22.10.   **The answer is B.**

In patients with advanced good-risk germ cell tumors, acceptable chemotherapy regimens include three cycles of BEP, or four cycles of EP. Carboplatin should not be substituted for cisplatin in patients with testicular cancer.

Answer 22.11.   **The answer is D.**

Although either mediastinal primary site or brain metastases define poor-risk nonseminomas, the poor-risk category is not applicable for seminomas. Furthermore, whereas the presence of nonpulmonary visceral metastases, such as brain metastases, classifies seminomas as intermediate risk, primary mediastinal seminomas remain in the good-risk category.

Answer 22.12.   **The answer is B.**

Patients with intermediate-risk nonseminomas should have AFP between 1000 and 10,000 ng/mL, HCG between 5000 and 50,000 mIU/mL, LDH between 1.5 and 10 times the upper normal limit, primary site gonadal or retroperitoneal, and no visceral metastases other than pulmonary.

Answer 22.13.   **The answer is D.**

The International Germ Cell Cancer Collaborative Group (IGCCCG) staging system stratifies patients with seminoma into two categories: good risk or intermediate risk, based on the following: primary site of tumor, pulmonary versus nonpulmonary metastases and AFP level. Patients are classified as good risk if they have a seminoma of any primary site, pulmonary only visceral metastases and normal AFP level. Patients are classified as intermediate risk if they have a seminoma of any primary site, nonpulmonary visceral metastases and normal AFP level. Elevated AFP levels are inconsistent with diagnosis of seminoma and patients should be treated for NSGCT, even if pathology fails to identify an NSGCT component.

Answer 22.14.   **The answer is C.**

Options A and B are commonly used in patients with good-risk tumors with equivalent efficacy. In patients with high-risk disease, however, the standard approach consists of four cycles of BEP.

Answer 22.15.   **The answer is D.**

VIP has similar results compared with BEP and may be offered to patients with contraindications to BEP. In a large US trial comparing four cycles of BEP with two cycles of BEP followed by high-dose chemotherapy and stem cell support, the latter showed no significant survival benefit.

Answer 22.16.   **The answer is B.**

Although significant pulmonary toxicity from bleomycin is rare, it may be fatal. Because the predictive ability of pulmonary function tests such as vital capacity and diffusion capacity of carbon monoxide is not proven, this agent is typically avoided in patients with pre-existing pulmonary compromise. Therefore, BEP and BOP should, if possible, not be used. Four cycles of EP are equivalent to three cycles of BEP in patients with good-risk germ cell tumors, but inferior to four cycles of BEP. The best option in this patient is four cycles of VIP.

Answer 22.17.   **The answer is B.**

Patients who fail to respond or relapse after first-line chemotherapy with BEP represent a heterogeneous population with a wide range of cure rates after salvage chemotherapy. The 3-year survival is approximately 35% in patients with primary tumors of the testicle or retroperitoneum and those who achieved a complete response to first-line chemotherapy. In contrast, the probability of cure from conventional therapy is less than 10% in patients with less than complete response to initial chemotherapy or relapsed mediastinal tumors.

CHAPTER 23 GYNECOLOGIC CANCERS

DAVID G. MUTCH

DIRECTIONS   Each of the numbered items below is followed by lettered answers. Select the ONE lettered answer that is BEST in each case unless instructed otherwise.

QUESTIONS

Question 23.1.1.   A 35-year-old premenopausal woman of Ashkenazi Jewish ancestry presents to you because her 60-year-old paternal aunt was recently diagnosed with ovarian cancer, and she is concerned about her own risk for ovarian cancer. She has no siblings, and there is no other family history of cancer. She has two living children and is in good health, and her pelvic examination is unremarkable. You should advise her that:

A. Ovarian cancer cannot be inherited through the paternal side, and she does not need any particular screening.

B. A single second-degree relative with cancer at age more than 50 years does not confer a significantly increased risk for her.

C. She should visit a genetic counselor.

D. Annual transvaginal ultrasound and CA-125 screening can reduce her risk of mortality.

E. She should have a prophylactic total abdominal hysterectomy/bilateral salpingo-oophorectomy (TAH/BSO) if/when she does not want to have any more children.

Corresponding Chapter in *Cancer: Principles & Practice of Oncology*, Ninth Edition: 104 (Ovarian Cancer, Fallopian Tube Carcinoma, and Peritoneal Carcinoma).

Question 23.1.2. A 35-year-old woman presents to you for recommendations regarding therapy of her newly diagnosed mucinous ovarian cancer. This was a 5-cm, grade 1, left-sided mass that was incidentally found at the time of surgery for endometriosis as part of an infertility workup. The ovary was removed, and the operative note states that there was no evidence of tumor on the external surface of the ovary or elsewhere in the abdomen, but full surgical staging was not performed. A postoperative computed tomography (CT) scan of the abdomen and the pelvis is unremarkable, and CA-125 is within normal limits. Pelvic examination is unremarkable. The patient would like to have children but does not want to compromise her survival. You should advise her that:

A. She is unlikely to have any residual cancer or a recurrence, and further surgery or chemotherapy is not needed.

B. She should have a positron emission tomography (PET) scan, and if there is no uptake, she does not need further surgery or chemotherapy.

C. Because her CT scan and CA-125 are normal, she is unlikely to have any residual disease, and further surgery is not needed; however, because the mucinous subtype of ovarian cancer has a very poor prognosis, she will require three to six cycles of carboplatin/paclitaxel chemotherapy.

D. She should have complete surgical staging, if possible, via laparoscopy, with the option of preserving her uterus and contralateral ovary if there is no further evidence of tumor; if no further tumor is found, she would have a >90% chance of 5-year survival, and chemotherapy would not be required.

E. She should have complete surgical staging, including TAH/BSO; if no further disease is found, she will need only three cycles of carboplatin/paclitaxel chemotherapy, but if there is disease outside the ovary, she will need six cycles.

Question 23.1.3. CA-125 is most useful in what aspect of ovarian cancer management?

A. Screening
B. Diagnosis
C. Monitoring treatment
D. Equally useful in all of the above

Question 23.1.4. Which of the following increases the risk of a woman developing ovarian cancer?

A. Use of oral contraceptives for >5 consecutive years
B. Nulliparity
C. Breastfeeding
D. Tubal ligation

Question 23.1.5.   All of the following statements regarding the molecular genetics of ovarian cancer are true, EXCEPT:

A. TP53 mutation is the most common mutation in patients with ovarian carcinoma.
B. BAX overexpression is associated with better prognosis.
C. Vascular endothelial growth factor (VEGF) expression is associated with better prognosis.
D. PTEN mutations are more common in endometrioid or mucinous tumors.

Question 23.1.6.   A 50-year-old woman presents with a pelvic mass. She is found to have a tumor of low malignant potential. She undergoes a TAH/BSO and staging. She has no gross disease but has positive washings on final pathology and one positive lymph node, making her disease stage IIIC. What is the most appropriate therapy postoperatively?

A. Intraperitoneal cisplatin and intravenous (IV) taxane
B. IV platinum and a taxane
C. Hormonal therapy with tamoxifen or an aromatase inhibitor
D. No further therapy

Question 23.1.7.   A 50-year-old woman was diagnosed with stage III ovarian cancer and underwent primary resection followed by chemotherapy. She is asymptomatic but has elevated CA-125. Imaging studies do not identify recurrent disease. Which of the following is the best treatment option?

A. Hormonal therapy
B. Platinum-based chemotherapy
C. Single agent doxorubicin
D. Single agent paclitaxel

Question 23.1.8.   All of the following are founder mutations associated with individuals of Ashkenazi descent, EXCEPT:

A. 185delAG
B. 5382insC
C. 617delT
D. 619delT

Question 23.1.9.   A patient of Jewish heritage who has breast cancer, but no family history of breast or ovarian cancer, has what chance of having a BRCA1 or BRCA2 mutation?

A. 5%
B. 10%
C. 40%
D. 90%

Question 23.1.10. Oral contraceptive use for ≥5 years is associated with what percentage decrease in the incidence of ovarian cancer?

    A. 5%
    B. 10%
    C. 20%
    D. 50%
    E. 80%

Question 23.1.11. A 25-year-old woman has her left ovary removed because of an ovarian mass. The final pathology shows that this is a moderately differentiated papillary serous cancer. There was no other evidence of disease in the abdominal cavity. What is the likelihood that this patient has a positive pelvic or para-aortic lymph node metastasis?

    A. 5%
    B. 15%
    C. 30%
    D. 50%

Question 23.1.12. Patients with high-risk early ovarian cancer should generally be treated:

    A. By observation
    B. With platinum-based chemotherapy
    C. With whole abdominal radiation therapy
    D. B or C

Question 23.1.13. A 55-year-old woman who has just achieved a complete clinical remission (normal CT scan, pelvic examination, and CA-125) after six cycles of chemotherapy for stage IIIC optimally debulked serous ovarian cancer presents to you for a second opinion regarding her prognosis and treatment options at this point. She is in excellent general health and tolerated chemotherapy well except for some numbness in her fingers and toes, which caused her treating oncologist to switch her treatment from paclitaxel/carboplatin to docetaxel/carboplatin after cycle three. You should advise her that:

    A. The risk of eventual relapse for an optimally debulked patient with a complete clinical remission is approximately 30%; no therapy is proven to be of any further survival benefit at this point.
    B. She should have second-look surgery; if residual disease is found, she should have four to six cycles of intraperitoneal platinum-based therapy because this can improve survival in patients with platinum-sensitive, minimal residual disease.
    C. She should have a PET scan; if residual disease is found, she should have four to six cycles of a non–cross-resistant drug, such as topotecan.
    D. Her risk of eventual relapse is approximately 70%; she should be offered consolidation therapy with paclitaxel 175 mg/m^2 every 3 weeks for 12 months with the expectation of a 30% improvement in survival.
    E. Her risk of relapse is approximately 70%; no therapy is proven to be of any survival benefit at this point.

Question 23.1.14. Which of the following statement(s) is/are TRUE about granulosa cell tumors of the ovary?

    A. They usually occur in premenopausal women.

    B. They are usually stage III/IV.

    C. Survival of patients with stage I disease is generally good, but they may relapse later.

    D. Survival of patients with stage III/IV disease is poor, and they should consider chemotherapy.

    E. They may be associated with endometrial cancer.

    F. C, D, and E.

Question 23.1.15. Which of the following statements is TRUE about germ cell tumors of the ovary?

    A. They occur more often in younger women.

    B. They are usually stage III/IV.

    C. Appropriate therapy includes TAH/BSO/full surgical staging and chemotherapy regimens similar to those used in male testicular cancer.

    D. Survival of patients with stage III/IV disease is poor.

    E. The chemotherapy will usually result in infertility.

Question 23.1.16. A 51-year-old woman presents to you for recommendations regarding the treatment of her recurrent ovarian cancer. She was optimally debulked for stage IIIC serous ovarian carcinoma and completed six cycles of carboplatin/paclitaxel 36 months ago with a clinical complete remission. She now has recurrent ascites, which is histologically positive for tumor compatible with her original primary. CT scan shows peritoneal carcinomatosis and a pelvic mass. You should advise her that:

    A. Prognosis of recurrent ovarian cancer is poor; she may get short-term benefit from chemotherapy, but hospice is a reasonable option.

    B. Tamoxifen has a 40% chance of shrinking her disease.

    C. She has a very high likelihood of disease shrinkage and symptom palliation with further platinum-based chemotherapy.

    D. She has a chance of cure with autologous stem cell transplant.

    E. Liver metastases and liver failure will probably be her ultimate cause of death.

Question 23.1.17. All of the following statements regarding ovarian cancer are true, EXCEPT:

    A. Endometrioid variants are sometimes associated with endometriosis.

    B. Mucinous tumor types are resistant to chemotherapy.

    C. Clear cell variant is associated with hypocalcemia.

    D. Immunostains on ovarian cancers are typically cytokeratin 7 positive and cytokeratin 20 negative.

Question 23.1.18. A 45-year-old woman has undergone surgical resection followed by adjuvant chemotherapy for her stage IIIC ovarian cancer. She is now in complete remission and is interested in further treatment to reduce the risk of recurrent disease. Which of the following would you recommend?

A. Maintenance treatment with single agent paclitaxel for 12 months.
B. Clinical surveillance.
C. Maintenance treatment with single agent topotecan.
D. Maintenance treatment with bevacizumab.

ANSWERS

Answer 23.1.1.   **The answer is C.**

This woman should be referred for genetic counseling and possible genetic testing. Some 40% to 60% of patients of Jewish descent who have epithelial ovarian cancer carry one of the three founder BRCA1 or BRCA2 mutations (irrespective of family history). These, like other BRCA mutations, are inherited in an autosomal dominant manner, through either the paternal or maternal side. If this woman carries a BRCA1 mutation, her lifetime risk of ovarian cancer is 20% to 60%, and her risk of breast cancer is even higher. Although transvaginal ultrasound and CA-125 screening are generally recommended for mutation carriers who have their ovaries in place, there is no good evidence that such screening will decrease mortality. Oral contraceptives have been suggested to decrease the risk of ovarian cancer by up to 50%. Removal of the ovaries likely confers the best method for reducing the risk of ovarian cancer; it remains controversial whether the uterus should be removed as well.

Answer 23.1.2.   **The answer is D.**

Understaging is common, particularly when the preoperative diagnosis is that of a benign process. Earlier laparoscopic surgical staging series suggested that up to 30% to 40% of patients thought to have FIGO stage I or II disease actually had disease in the upper abdomen. The incidence of extraovarian spread will be lower with a grade 1 tumor. Nonetheless, complete surgical staging, if possible, is advised in this case, because the recommendation for a stage IA grade 1 mucinous tumor is no chemotherapy. Although some data have suggested that advanced-stage mucinous tumors may respond less well to chemotherapy than serous tumors, a low-grade early-stage mucinous tumor does not have a poor prognosis. However, chemotherapy would be recommended in the case of any extraovarian spread. In the hands of an experienced surgeon, laparoscopic staging, including omentectomy and para-aortic lymph node examination, is an option. Preservation of the uterus and contralateral ovary is reasonable if no further disease is found at the time of staging. CA-125 is frequently normal in women with mucinous ovarian tumors, even when of advanced stage. A PET scan will not detect microscopic disease, may not be positive in low-grade malignancies, and is not likely to be helpful.

Answer 23.1.3.   **The answer is C.**

CA-125 is not useful for screening because early-stage ovarian cancer has an elevated CA-125 approximately 50% of the time. Furthermore, the positive predictive value of an elevated CA-125 is very low because many things cause an elevated CA-125 and the prevalence of the disease is quite low. It is not particularly useful in the diagnosis of ovarian cancer for the above reasons. It is useful in monitoring treatment.

Answer 23.1.4.   **The answer is B.**

Anything that decreases ovulation decreases the risk of ovarian cancer. Thus, oral contraceptives, multiparity, and breastfeeding decrease the likelihood that an individual will develop ovarian cancer. Several population-based studies show that tubal ligation decreases the likelihood of developing ovarian cancer.

Answer 23.1.5.   **The answer is C.**

p53 is mutated in approximately 50% of patients with ovarian cancer. VEGF is often overexpressed and is associated with poor prognosis. BAX is a pro-apoptotic gene and overexpression of the BAX gene is associated with increased responsiveness to chemotherapy and better prognosis. Mutations involving the KRAS and PTEN mutation are more common in mucinous or endometrioid tumors.

Answer 23.1.6.   **The answer is D.**

There are no data that suggest any adjuvant therapy will improve the survival in patients with tumors of low malignant potential.

Answer 23.1.7.   **The answer is A.**

Elevated CA-125 indicates disease recurrence and in patients who are asymptomatic with no other objective evidence of disease recurrence, the appropriate treatment would be hormonal therapy. Chemotherapy is considered when patients have symptomatic disease or there is objective evidence for disease recurrence.

Answer 23.1.8.   **The answer is D.**

The majority of inherited disease in the Jewish population is due to one of the three founder mutations in BRCA1 and BRCA2.

Answer 23.1.9.   **The answer is C.**

Answer 23.1.10.   **The answer is D.**

There are several published studies, at least two of which are referenced in the corresponding chapter (Chapter 42), that report this benefit.

Answer 23.1.11.   **The answer is B.**

Answer 23.1.12.   **The answer is B.**

There are several studies that address this issue. Most data suggest that platinum/taxane-based therapy is superior to others.

Answer 23.1.13.   **The answer is E.**

Although the majority (almost 80%) of patients with advanced-stage (III–IV) ovarian cancer will achieve a clinically complete remission with taxane/platinum combination therapy, approximately 70% will ultimately relapse from a clinical complete remission. Even patients with a surgically confirmed complete remission (negative second look) have an eventual relapse rate of approximately 50%. Although patients with optimally debulked stage III disease are a relatively favorable subgroup, those optimally debulked patients who have a larger presurgical tumor burden (IIIC) fare worse than those with a lesser presurgical tumor burden (IIIA). One randomized trial has demonstrated that maintenance paclitaxel improved progression-free survival of women with a clinical complete response (66% with optimal stage III disease) from 21 to 28 months in a randomized trial, and this option should be discussed with this patient. However, no survival benefit was observed at the time the trial was ended and the randomization code was broken, and there is a significant incidence of neuropathy. No data exist on PET scans in this situation, and consolidation topotecan has shown no benefit in two randomized trials. Although intraperitoneal therapy is a theoretically attractive option, cisplatin, the most widely used drug, carries a significant risk of neurotoxicity, and there are no data showing any survival benefit to its use in the setting of minimal residual disease.

Answer 23.1.14.   **The answer is F.**

Sex cord–stromal tumors (of which granulosa cell tumors are the most common subtype) comprise only approximately 5% of all ovarian neoplasms. The peak incidence is in women aged more than 50 years, although a significant proportion occurs in premenopausal women. Granulosa cell tumors may secrete estrogen and be associated with endometrial hyperplasia and endometrial carcinoma. The majority is diagnosed in stage I, and these patients have 10-year survivals of 75% to 95%. However, late relapses may be observed. Patients with advanced-stage disease fare more poorly. Although the rarity of the tumor precludes randomized trial data, most such patients will be offered chemotherapy, traditionally with bleomycin, etoposide, cisplatin (BEP), or other regimens used in germ cell tumors.

Answer 23.1.15.   **The answer is A.**

Germ cell tumors almost always occur in young women, with a peak incidence in their early 20s. Some 60% to 70% are stage I at diagnosis. With the use of platinum-based chemotherapy regimens similar to those used for men with testicular cancer, even patients with an advanced stage have a good prognosis. Because most of these tumors occur in young women, often before they have had children, and because the type of chemotherapy used will not cause infertility in most young female patients, the surgical approach is critical; in many patients, the contralateral ovary and uterus can and should be spared.

Answer 23.1.16.   **The answer is C.**

Recurrent ovarian cancer is not generally curable with transplant or any other modality, but patients whose disease recurs with a disease-free interval of more than 1 year have more than a 50% chance of responding to platinum-based combination therapy and should usually be offered chemotherapy. Secondary debulking surgery may also be of benefit. Hormonal therapy in ovarian cancer generally produces response rates of only 10% to 15% and is usually reserved for patients who cannot tolerate other therapy. It has also been recommended as the initial salvage therapy in patients who have an increasing CA-125 as their only manifestation of recurrent disease.

Answer 23.1.17.   **The answer is C.**

Clear cell histology is commonly associated with hypercalcemia. The other statements are true.

Answer 23.1.18.   **The answer is B.**

Current evidence does not support maintenance chemotherapy with paclitaxel or topotecan after adjuvant chemotherapy for patients with advanced disease. The role of maintenance bevacizumab is being investigated in ongoing clinical trials.

SECTION 2 NONOVARIAN
MATTHEW A. POWELL

DIRECTIONS   Each of the numbered items below is followed by lettered answers. Select the ONE lettered answer that is BEST in each case unless instructed otherwise.

QUESTIONS

Question 23.2.1.   **Type I endometrial cancers have all the following features, EXCEPT:**

A. Most of these cancers have serous or clear cell histology.
B. Type I endometrial cancers account for 80% of endometrial cancers.
C. They appear to arise via a progression pathway.
D. The precursor lesion is atypical hyperplasia.

Question 23.2.2.   **Type II endometrial cancers have which of the following features?**

A. The precursor lesion is atypical hyperplasia.
B. The majority of tumors are slow-growing.
C. These cancers are unrelated to estrogen exposure.
D. All of the above.

Corresponding Chapters in *Cancer: Principles & Practice of Oncology,* Ninth Edition: 100 (Molecular Biology of Gynecologic Cancers), 101 (Cancer of the Cervix, Vagina, and Vulva), 102 (Cancers of the Uterine Body) and 103 (Gestational Trophoblastic Neoplasms).

Question 23.2.3.   Genetic changes commonly seen in type I endometrial cancers include:

A.   KRAS mutation
B.   PTEN mutation
C.   β-catenin mutation
D.   All of the above

Question 23.2.4.   All of the following genetic changes are characteristic of type II endometrial cancers, EXCEPT:

A.   Microsatellite instability (MSI)
B.   HER2/neu amplification
C.   BCL2 overexpression
D.   p53 mutations

Question 23.2.5.   Risk factors for endometrial cancer include all of the following, EXCEPT:

A.   Increasing age
B.   Black race
C.   Family history of endometrial cancer
D.   Prior pelvic radiotherapy

Question 23.2.6.   The majority of cervical, vaginal, and vulvar cancers appear to have a common cause and are usually caused by:

A.   Increased exposure to exogenous estrogen
B.   Chronic bacterial and parasitic infections
C.   Multiple prior herpes simplex virus (HSV) infections
D.   Human papillomavirus (HPV) infection with high-risk types

Question 23.2.7.   In patients with gestational trophoblastic disease (GTD) with a complete mole, molecular features include all of the following, EXCEPT:

A.   Mutations in p53 have not been reported.
B.   Most are diploid with duplication of a haploid paternal genome.
C.   Predominance of maternal chromosomes is common.
D.   Several genes, including CMYC, ERBB2, CFMS, and BCL2, have been implicated in the pathogenesis of complete moles.

Question 23.2.8.   A 39-year-old married woman is seeing you in the office after recently having a cervical biopsy that demonstrated cervical cancer. She has no prior medical problems other than anemia and one prior uncomplicated child birth. You tell her all of the following epidemiologic factors are true, EXCEPT:

A.   During the past 80 years, death rates from cervical cancer have decreased primarily because of the adoption of routine screening programs with PAP smears.
B.   Cervical cancer is the second leading cause of cancer deaths for women aged 20 to 39 years in the United States.
C.   HSV is thought to be the causative agent for the majority of patients.
D.   The incidence of cervical cancer is 30% and 100% higher in Black and Hispanic women, respectively, compared with Whites in the United States.

Question 23.2.9. She asks about prevention and treatment of HPV infections, and you advise her:

    A. The viral infections are rare, and promiscuity has caused her cancer.

    B. Treatments for HPV infections with antiviral therapy are effective if taken within 4 days of exposure.

    C. An HPV vaccine has recently been approved by the Food and Drug Administration (FDA) to help prevent infection from the most common HPV types.

    D. An HPV vaccine has recently been FDA approved, and she should receive the vaccine now to help treat her cancer.

Question 23.2.10. You counsel her about HPV and human immunodeficiency virus (HIV). After extensive discussion, you decide to proceed with testing for HIV with all of the following justifications, EXCEPT:

    A. HIV immunosuppression is correlated with an increased risk of cervical HPV infections.

    B. Patients with HIV appear to have a faster rate of progression to high-grade dysplasia (cervical intraepithelial neoplasia [CIN]).

    C. Antiretroviral therapy to manage HIV has demonstrated direct activity against HPV.

    D. Cervical cancers in HIV-positive women may be more aggressive than in HIV-negative women.

Question 23.2.11. She has done extensive reading about cervical cancer and asks you about factors that are associated with metastatic disease. You advise her the following are associated with extracervical disease, EXCEPT:

    A. Tumor size

    B. Presence of microinvasion

    C. Depth of invasion

    D. Presence of lymph-vascular space invasion

Question 23.2.12. If her initial biopsy returned with invasive squamous cell carcinoma with 2 mm of invasion and no lymphovascular space involvement (LVSI), you recommend that:

    A. She be referred back to her gynecologist for a simple hysterectomy.

    B. She be referred to the radiation oncologist for consideration of radiation therapy with possible chemotherapy.

    C. You begin therapy with cisplatin 40 mg/m^2 weekly for six cycles.

    D. She undergo cervical conization.

Question 23.2.13. The patient has a 3-cm visible tumor found on her cervix that is biopsied and is frankly invasive squamous cell carcinoma. She has several questions regarding staging of her cancer. You advise the following, EXCEPT:

A. Staging for cervical cancer is clinical, involving pelvic examination.

B. If enlarged lymph nodes are seen on her computed tomography (CT) scan, her cancer would be staged appropriately as at least stage III.

C. If hydronephrosis is demonstrated on her CT scan, her cancer would be staged appropriately as at least stage III.

D. Positron emission tomography (PET) scanning appears to be the most sensitive noninvasive method of detecting nodal involvement.

Question 23.2.14. The patient's 3-cm visible tumor appears confined to the cervix and is staged appropriately as stage IB1. Which of the following therapies is most appropriate?

A. Radiation and chemotherapy with weekly cisplatin dosed at 40 mg/m^2

B. Simple hysterectomy with removal of fallopian tubes and ovaries

C. Radiation therapy or radical hysterectomy with lymphadenectomy

D. Brachytherapy radiation with a dose of 75 Gy

Question 23.2.15. A 40-year-old woman is diagnosed with invasive cervical cancer. She has a 5-cm cervical tumor with parametrial involvement, and evidence of hydronephrosis on imaging. Her cancer is staged appropriately as stage IIIB. You elect to treat her with combined chemotherapy and radiation. Which of the following is INCORRECT regarding the treatment of locoregionally advanced cervical cancer?

A. Several randomized trials involving patients with locally advanced cervical cancer have demonstrated a benefit to the addition of chemotherapy to standard radiation therapy.

B. Carboplatin appears to be the most appropriate agent to combine with radiation therapy for cervical cancer, and this should be followed by hysterectomy.

C. 5FU with cisplatin is an acceptable regimen to combine with radiation therapy and has demonstrated improved survival.

D. Weekly cisplatin with radiation therapy appears as active as other regimen with manageable toxicity.

Question 23.2.16. After receiving definitive concurrent chemoradiotherapy for her stage IIIB cervical cancer, she develops a recurrence in the cervix, 18 months from the completion of therapy. Imaging studies suggest no extrapelvic disease. You recommend the following:

A. Referral back to the radiation oncologist for consideration of further radiation

B. Chemotherapy with combined cisplatin and topotecan

C. Chemotherapy with combined cisplatin and paclitaxel

D. Referral for consideration of further surgery

Question 23.2.17. A 67-year-old woman presents for evaluation of a cancer found in the vagina. Before any examination or evaluation, you review with her that all of the following are true, EXCEPT:

A. Prior in utero exposure to the synthetic estrogen diethylstilbestrol (DES) places a woman at an increased risk for development of vaginal clear cell adenocarcinoma.
B. Most cancers found in the vagina are actually metastases or direct extensions from other gynecologic tumors.
C. Vaginal squamous cell carcinoma is thought to be unrelated to the HPV.
D. Staging for primary vaginal cancers is similar to cervical cancer and is clinical.

Question 23.2.18. This patient is found to have had a prior hysterectomy for mild dysplasia and benign indications. Her apparent primary vaginal cancer extends to the subvaginal tissues and is appropriately staged as a stage II cancer. You recommend:

A. Referral for total radical vaginectomy
B. Chemotherapy with a cisplatin-based regimen
C. Referral for radiation therapy
D. Local excision followed by close observation

Question 23.2.19. Which of the following statements is INCORRECT regarding invasive vulvar cancer?

A. There are two distinct types of invasive squamous vulvar cancer.
B. HPV-associated vulvar cancer tends to occur in younger women (age <55 years) and is associated with prior cervical precancerous abnormalities.
C. Melanoma of the vulva is caused by exposure to HPV.
D. Non–HPV-associated invasive squamous vulvar cancer is associated with lichen sclerosis.

Question 23.2.20. A 55-year-old patient with a history of abnormal PAP smears presents for evaluation of a 3-cm vulvar mass. It is located 1 cm lateral to the clitoris on the right and has an ulcerated appearance. She states she noticed it 2 years ago and has tried many different ointments to help control the itching and irritation. This was recently biopsied to reveal invasive squamous cell carcinoma. What treatment would you recommend?

A. Neoadjuvant chemoradiation followed by local resection
B. Concurrent chemoradiation
C. Radical vulvectomy with bilateral inguinal (groin) lymphadenectomy
D. Local resection followed by radiation and/or chemotherapy

Question 23.2.21. Which of the following histologic features does not predict the outcome for a patient with vulvar cancer?

    A. Presence of lymphovascular invasion
    B. Tumor grade
    C. Depth of invasion and tumor thickness
    D. Number of positive lymph nodes

Question 23.2.22. Her final pathology reveals a 3.3-cm invasive squamous cell carcinoma with two involved (positive) lymph nodes in the right inguinal/femoral lymph node dissection of 12 removed. The contralateral node dissection was negative. Margins around the primary tumor were negative and greater than 1 cm. Her appropriate International Federation of Obstetrician & Gynecologist (FIGO) and TNM stage are:

    A. IVA and T2N1M0
    B. II and T2N2M0
    C. III and T3N1M0
    D. III and T2N1M0

Question 23.2.23. The most appropriate therapy for this patient after she recovers from surgery is:

    A. Close observation
    B. Chemotherapy with cisplatin plus 5FU
    C. Referral for consideration of radiation therapy
    D. Exploration with dissection of the pelvic lymph nodes

Question 23.2.24. Unfortunately, despite the use of adjuvant therapy, this patient's cancer recurs locally on the vulva, and a 2-cm recurrence is documented. You advise which of the following:

    A. Repeat resection
    B. Chemotherapy with bleomycin
    C. Best supportive care
    D. Chemotherapy with cisplatin plus 5FU

Question 23.2.25. A 62-year-old woman has been diagnosed with a uterine corpus (body) cancer. You have not received her records for review, but she is seen in your office for consultation and asks many general questions. You tell her all of the following are true, EXCEPT:

    A. Approximately 90% of these cancers arise from the endometrial lining and are typically managed with hysterectomy and staging.
    B. Most of these cancers are caused by exogenous estrogen use.
    C. Uterine sarcomas are less common than endometrial cancers and represent approximately 10% of corpus cancers.
    D. Endometrial cancer typically presents at an early stage with patients having abnormal uterine bleeding.

Question 23.2.26. This patient's records arrive in the office, and the pathology verifies the diagnosis of a grade 2 endometrioid-type endometrial cancer from an office endometrial biopsy. She asks what has caused her cancer to develop. You tell her all of the following are considered to be independent risk factors for the development of endometrial cancer, EXCEPT:

    A. Obesity
    B. Diabetes mellitus
    C. Premature ovarian failure with early menopause
    D. Presence of an estrogen-producing tumor

Question 23.2.27. For this patient with an office biopsy demonstrating grade 2 endometrioid endometrial cancer who is of apparent good heath with no other medical comorbidities, you recommend:

    A. Further evaluation with CT scan and PET scan to evaluate for metastatic disease
    B. A formal dilation and curettage (D&C) to obtain a more accurate pathologic diagnosis
    C. Hysterectomy with removal of the tubes and ovaries with consideration of pelvic and para-aortic lymphadenectomy
    D. Referral for radiation therapy with possible chemoradiation

Question 23.2.28. During the patient's initial visit, she reports her mother was diagnosed with endometrial cancer at age 42 years, her maternal aunt with colon cancer at age 51 years, and her sister with endometrial cancer at age 38 years. You are concerned her cancer may be hereditary. You advise that:

    A. She undergo colon assessment if she is not up to date with age-appropriate screening and consider counseling and possible testing for hereditary nonpolyposis colorectal cancer (Lynch II syndrome).
    B. She undergo breast MRI and be tested for BRCA1 and BRCA2.
    C. Colon and endometrial cancers are common, and no further evaluation is necessary at this time.
    D. The maternal side of her family very likely has familial adenomatous polyposis and should be further evaluated.

Question 23.2.29. The patient undergoes hysterectomy with full staging, including pelvic washing for cytology, removal of both tubes and ovaries; pelvic and para-aortic lymph nodes are removed. She is noted to have cancer involving three pelvic lymph nodes. Her stage is designated:

    A. IC
    B. IIC
    C. IIIC
    D. IVA

Question 23.2.30. For this patient with three positive pelvic lymph nodes and a grade 2 endometrioid endometrial cancer, you recognize adjuvant therapy is controversial but ultimately recommend:

A. Hormone therapy with a progestational agent
B. Referral for pelvic radiation therapy
C. Chemotherapy with combined paclitaxel, cisplatin, and doxorubicin
D. Combination of radiation and chemotherapy

Question 23.2.31. The patient completes your recommended adjuvant therapy. Unfortunately, 18 months later she returns to your office with CT evidence of liver and lung recurrent cancer that is biopsy proven. All of the following are correct regarding recurrent endometrial cancer, EXCEPT:

A. Recurrence typically occurs within 3 years of the original diagnosis.
B. Approximately 50% of patients are symptomatic at the time of recurrence.
C. Serum CA-125 may be a useful surveillance marker for patients at high risk for recurrence.
D. Isolated vaginal recurrence is rare in patients, and cure is only by ultra-radical surgery.

Question 23.2.32. The most active (improved disease-free and overall survival) chemotherapy regimen as determined in randomized clinical trials in women with advanced or recurrent endometrial cancer with measurable disease is:

A. Doxorubicin plus paclitaxel
B. Cisplatin/doxorubicin
C. Cisplatin/doxorubicin/paclitaxel
D. Ifosfamide plus paclitaxel

Question 23.2.33. The following are true regarding uterine sarcomas, EXCEPT:

A. Represent approximately 10% of uterine corpus cancers.
B. The malignant mixed mullerian tumor is also known as uterine carcinosarcoma.
C. All different types of uterine sarcoma are treated similarly with resection followed by radiation therapy.
D. Uterine leiomyosarcoma is more chemoresponsive than most other types of sarcomas.

Question 23.2.34. A 17-year-old female patient presents to your office with pelvic ultrasound suggesting intrauterine gestational trophoblastic neoplasia (GTN). The most common of the distinct clinicopathologic entities of GTN is:

A. Complete hydatidiform mole
B. Partial hydatidiform mole
C. Choriocarcinoma
D. Placental site trophoblastic tumor

Question 23.2.35. This patient has a beta-human chorionic gonadotropin (hCG) of 122,300 and undergoes therapy with a suction D&C. Final pathology confirms the diagnosis of complete hydatidiform mole. The patient is followed with the following:

   A. CT scan every 3 months
   B. Ultrasound of the pelvis every 3 months
   C. Pelvic examination with PAP smear every 6 weeks
   D. Beta-hCG weekly

Question 23.2.36. This patient goes on to develop evidence of persistent GTN. You are concerned she may have "phantom" hCG. All of the following are correct regarding "phantom" hCG, EXCEPT:

   A. False-positive hCG test results are caused by the presence of het-erophile antibodies.
   B. False-positive hCG results have caused inappropriate therapies to be performed, including surgery and chemotherapy.
   C. Phantom hCG is no longer a problem with modern testing equipment.
   D. A urinary beta-hCG assay should be performed.

Question 23.2.37. After a complete metastatic workup, the patient is determined to have low-risk disease. You recommend the following chemotherapy:

   A. Etoposide
   B. Vincristine
   C. Methotrexate
   D. Cyclophosphamide

ANSWERS

Answer 23.2.1.   **The answer is A.**

Type I endometrial cancers account for 80% of endometrial cancers. The precursor lesion is atypical hyperplasia and these tumors are usually superficial and low grade. Type I endometrial cancers have endometrioid histology, and these cancers are related to prior estrogen exposure. They demonstrate a large number of genetic changes, and appear to arise via a progression pathway.

Answer 23.2.2.   **The answer is C.**

Type II endometrial cancers have serous or clear cell histology. Most tumors are aggressive and progress rapidly. They are not associated with estrogen exposure. The usual precursor lesion is endometrial intraepithelial neoplasia.

Answer 23.2.3.   **The answer is D.**

Genetic changes that are characteristic of type I endometrial cancer include KRAS, PTEN and β-catenin mutations and MSI.

Answer 23.2.4.   **The answer is A.**

MSI is seen in type I endometrial cancers. Genetic changes characteristic of type II endometrial cancers include p53 mutations and HER2/neu and BCL2 amplification/overexpression.

Answer 23.2.5.   **The answer is B.**

Risk factors for endometrial cancer include increasing age, white race, obesity, family history of endometrial cancer, prior pelvic radiation, diabetes mellitus, gallbladder disease, estrogen replacement, estrogen-producing tumors, early menarche and late menopause.

Answer 23.2.6.   **The answer is D.**

Infection with high-risk HPV appears to be the common cause for these cancers.

Answer 23.2.7.   **The answer is C.**

Complete moles have a predominance of paternal chromosomes.

Answer 23.2.8.   **The answer is C.**

Cervical cancer is caused by exposure to high-risk strains of HPV. The presence of HPV DNA has been identified in more than 99% of cervical carcinomas. The epidemiologic information presented is correct. The increased incidence of cervical cancer in Blacks and Hispanics in the United States is thought to be secondary to barriers in screening because of the lack of insurance, low income, and cultural differences.

Answer 23.2.9.   **The answer is C.**

HPV infections are not rare, and although promiscuity is more common for women with cervical cancer, it is certainly not required. There is no currently effective antiviral therapy that is active against HPV. Treatments of the precancerous and cancerous changes that develop from HPV are usually indicated, but the virus can still be often detected even after therapy. An HPV vaccine has recently been FDA approved as a preventative vaccine. It appears that primarily those patients who are naive to the virus benefit from vaccination. Young women between the ages of 9 and 26 years are currently approved for vaccination. Ideally, vaccination should occur before the onset of sexual activity.

Answer 23.2.10.   **The answer is C.**

All of the factors are correct except that current antiretroviral therapy has not demonstrated benefit against HPV.

Answer 23.2.11.   **The answer is B.**

The incidence of nodal (extracervical) involvement is directly correlated with tumor stage, size, histology, depth of invasion, and lymphovascular space invasion. For patients with stage I disease treated with radical hysterectomy, 15% to 20% and 1% to 5% of pelvic and para-aortic lymph nodes, respectively, will be involved. Cervical cancer usually follows an orderly pattern of spread from the cervix to the pelvic nodes, then to the common iliacs, and finally to the para-aortic lymph nodes before systemic spread. Distant metastatic sites can occur, and the most common are lung, extrapelvic lymph nodes, liver, and bone.

Answer 23.2.12.   **The answer is D.**

Microinvasive carcinoma of the cervix is often a source of confusion and mismanagement for patients with cervical cancer. Patient with stage IA1 cancers have been safely managed with conization only or simple hysterectomy. These patients typically are not treated with radiation and chemotherapy. The difficulty and confusion that arise result from practitioners attempting to make the diagnosis from small biopsies. To make the diagnosis, the patient should have less than 3 mm of invasion and no more than 7 mm of lateral spread, along with negative margins. LVSI remains controversial, but typically if present, patients should be treated as if they have frankly invasive disease. Thus, if superficial invasion is seen on a small biopsy and there is no visible tumor on the cervix, the patient should typically be evaluated with cervical conization before definitive therapy to properly stage the patient and allow for the most appropriate therapy.

Answer 23.2.13.   **The answer is B.**

Staging of cervical cancer is clinical, which is based on careful clinical examination and routine radiographic studies (e.g., chest radiograph, intravenous pyelogram, lower gastrointestinal) and procedures (cystoscopy, proctoscopy). Because cervical cancer is primarily a disease of the developing world, staging procedures have been kept simple to allow consistency staging throughout the world. Specific technology, such as CT and PET, is often used for treatment planning in the United States but should not be the basis for changing the stage.

Answer 23.2.14.   **The answer is C.**

For patients with small stage IB1 tumors, either radiation or radical hysterectomy with lymphadenectomy is appropriate. Factors such as patient preference, anesthetic, and surgical risks should be considered. Surgical treatment tends to be preferred for young women with small tumors because it permits preservation of the ovaries and likely better vaginal function. Radiation invariably leads to menopause with loss of ovarian hormone production and possible vaginal stenosis. Simple hysterectomy would be considered inadequate therapy for this size and stage of cancer. Chemoradiotherapy would typically be indicated for patients with more advanced cancers. Brachytherapy alone would also be inadequate because the patient is at risk for nodal involvement, and external beam therapy would also be indicated to treat the nodal area at risk.

Answer 23.2.15.   **The answer is B.**

Several randomized trials have demonstrated a benefit to the addition of chemotherapy, to standard radiation therapy, for treating women with locoregionally advanced cervical cancer. Based on these trials, regimens that are commonly used in practice include 5FU with cisplatin and concurrent radiation, and weekly cisplatin with radiation. None of the combined chemotherapy and radiation trials included the use of carboplatin. Hysterectomy following radiation and chemotherapy is no longer considered routine.

Answer 23.2.16.   **The answer is D.**

This patient has developed an apparently isolated central pelvic recurrence after combined chemoradiotherapy. Her only real curative option is surgery and will likely require pelvic exenteration. Patients typically receive the maximum tolerated dose of radiation during their primary therapy, and further meaningful doses of radiation are usually not possible. Chemotherapy is typically palliative in nature only. Recent randomized trials have suggested improved survival with combination chemotherapy over single-agent cisplatin, but this remains palliative.

Answer 23.2.17.   **The answer is C.**

All of the statements are correct except that vaginal cancers are thought to be related to HPV in at least 60% to 65% of cases. DES is a synthetic estrogen previously given to women during pregnancy primarily in women with a history of miscarriage or premature birth. First reported in 1971, an association between DES exposure in utero and clear cell vaginal cancer was made. Few cases of cancer in DES-exposed women have been reported in those aged more than 40 years, and these women continued to be followed closely. If a cancer in the vagina is in contact with the cervix or the vulva, then it is not classified as a vaginal cancer and the primary is consider either the cervix or the vulva, respectively. Staging for primary vaginal cancer is clinical, similar to cervical cancer.

Answer 23.2.18.   **The answer is C.**

Stage II vaginal cancer involves the subvaginal tissues and is typically not amendable to local resection without injury to the bladder or rectum. The most appropriate therapy is radiation, likely with both brachytherapy and external beam radiotherapy to treat the regional nodal areas. Chemotherapy is not indicated for primary therapy. Extrapolating from randomized studies in patients with cervical cancer, one could consider combination chemoradiotherapy for patients with vaginal cancer.

Answer 23.2.19.   **The answer is C.**

Vulvar melanoma is not thought to be related to HPV infection. There does appear to be two types of invasive squamous vulvar cancers. HPV-related cancers typically occur in younger women and can be multifocal and associated with vulvar-intraepithelial neoplasia (VIN), whereas non-HPV cancers occur in older women and are often associated with chronic vulvar inflammation or lichen sclerosis.

Answer 23.2.20.   **The answer is C.**

Although all options are used to treat patients with invasive vulvar cancer, the apparent best option is typically radical vulvectomy with inguinal lymphadenectomy. Staging is then determined on the basis of the surgical findings, which also dictate adjuvant therapy. Typically, neoadjuvant and definitive chemoradiation are often necessary with very large cancers involving the urethra or anus and can help achieve organ preservation, but would not be typically used with a 3-cm tumor.

Answer 23.2.21.   **The answer is B.**

Tumor grade has been inconsistent and has not typically been found to be an independent risk factor. LVSI is a very strong predictor of positive inguinal lymph nodes. Depth of invasion, tumor diameter, and tumor thickness are all directly related to lymph node involvement and the patient's ultimate survival.

Answer 23.2.22.   **The answer is D.**

Staging for carcinomas of the vulva has been established by the FIGO. In 1983, FIGO initially adopted a clinical TNM staging system. The reliability of clinical assessment of regional lymph node status was found to be poor. In 1988, FIGO adopted a surgical staging system, and this was updated in 1994 to include an additional substage for minimally invasive cancers (IA). Typically, both TNM and FIGO stages are provided.

Answer 23.2.23.   **The answer is C.**

Radiation is indicated for patients with more than one positive lymph node and should be considered with any positive lymph nodes or if resection margins are positive and further resection is not possible. Chemotherapy has not been demonstrated to be of benefit in the adjuvant setting. A randomized trial evaluating the role of pelvic lymphadenectomy for patients with positive groin lymph nodes was completed, suggesting there is no role for routine pelvic lymphadenectomy for these patients. Pelvic radiation therapy should be delivered to patients with positive groin lymph nodes.

Answer 23.2.24.   **The answer is A.**

Local recurrence of vulvar cancer is not uncommon. These patients can often be successfully managed with repeat resection. Large surgical defects from further resections in the vulva can be managed with the use of flaps and skin grafting. Chemotherapy is usually of limited efficacy and not needed if the lesion is resectable. Radical surgical resection, including pelvic exenterations, has been used successfully for large recurrent cancers.

Answer 23.2.25.   **The answer is B.**

Exogenous estrogen use appears to cause a minority of endometrial cancers. In the past, when estrogens were given frequently to women without progestins to protect the endometrial lining, this was a more frequent cause of endometrial cancer. The majority (90%) of uterine corpus cancers arise from the endometrium with sarcomas representing less than 10% of cases. Abnormal uterine bleeding typically leads to early presentation and evaluation of patients with endometrial cancer.

Answer 23.2.26.   **The answer is C.**

Risk factors for the development of endometrial cancer are typically related to chronic estrogenic stimulation. Estrogen therapy, obesity, early age of menarche, late age of menopause, anovulation, and estrogen-producing tumors have all been associated with the development of endometrial cancers. Interestingly, diabetes mellitus imparts an increased relative risk of 3, even when controlling for other known factors.

Answer 23.2.27.   **The answer is C.**

Hysterectomy, whether performed through a large open incision, laparoscopically, or vaginally, is indicated. Ovarian preservation has been performed in rare circumstances but is typically discouraged. Preoperative imaging, beyond a chest radiograph for patients with disease apparently confined to the uterus on clinical examination, is rarely helpful. Thus, CT, MRI, and PET scans are not typically recommended as a preoperative evaluation for these patients. The office endometrial biopsy is sufficiently accurate in this setting, and a D&C would not offer any further benefit to the preoperative evaluation. Radiation can be used as primary therapy for the treatment of endometrial cancer but is typically reserved for patients with severe medical comorbidities in whom surgery is thought to be too high a risk. These patients will still typically require general anesthesia to allow for brachytherapy implantation into the uterine fundus.

Answer 23.2.28.   **The answer is A.**

The family history presented is worrisome for Lynch II syndrome. Approximately 5% of endometrial cancers are hereditary, with the majority being Lynch II (hereditary nonpolyposis colorectal cancer syndrome). Lynch syndrome is caused by a defect in mismatch repair genes. Women who carry one of these abnormal genes have a 22% to 60% chance of developing endometrial cancer, which is similar to their risk of developing colorectal cancer. Patients with the diagnosis of endometrial cancer with a strong family history should be counseled and offered genetic testing. Families with BRCA1 or BRCA2 mutations confer an increased risk in breast and ovarian cancer. There is no convincing evidence that these patients are at an increased risk for the development of endometrial cancer. Endometrial cancer is not related to familial adenomatous polyposis syndrome.

Answer 23.2.29.   **The answer is C.**

Staging of endometrial cancer is typically surgical. Both a clinical and a surgical staging system exist. A minority of patients with major medical comorbidities would typically not undergo surgical management and require staging via the older clinical staging system. Since 1988, the surgical staging system has been used as directed by FIGO. This patient is correctly staged as IIIC.

Answer 23.2.30.   **The answer is D.**

Adjuvant therapy for patients with stage IIIC disease remains controversial. GOG-122 compared whole abdomen/pelvic radiation therapy with chemotherapy (cisplatin plus doxorubicin × eight cycles) and demonstrated a progression-free and overall survival benefit to chemotherapy. GOG-184 evaluated "volume-directed" radiation therapy that included pelvic and para-aortic lymph nodes when indicated, followed by chemotherapy. Patients were randomized to two differing chemotherapy arms (cisplatin plus doxorubicin vs. cisplatin, doxorubicin, and paclitaxel). There was no significant benefit to the addition of paclitaxel for these patients. Methods to reduce toxicity of radiation therapy including intensity-modulated radiotherapy (IMRT) are being investigated. Lower toxicity with potentially sparing the pelvic bone marrow should allow for combination of radiation and chemotherapy to maximize efficacy.

Answer 23.2.31.   **The answer is D.**

Recurrent endometrial cancer occurs most often in patients with high-risk histologic subtypes (serous, clear cell, or carcinoma) or initial advanced stage. Patients are typically followed after adjuvant therapy and evaluated for recurrence with pelvic examination and serum CA-125. One-third of recurrences in patients with early-stage disease have recurrence with disease apparently confined to the pelvis. Isolated vaginal and pelvic recurrences are important to identify because these patients have a favorable cure rate with therapy. Patients with systemic disease would rarely be cured, and treatment is palliative.

Answer 23.2.32.   **The answer is C.**

The Gynecologic Oncology Group (GOG) has conducted several randomized trials in patients with advanced or recurrent endometrial cancer. GOG-177 demonstrated the combination of cisplatin, doxorubicin, and paclitaxel to have an improved progression-free and overall survival benefit that was statistically significant. This regimen had a response rate of 57% compared with 34% in the cohort treated with cisplatin and doxorubicin alone. Ifosfamide plus paclitaxel is a regimen that has been developed and demonstrated superiority in uterine carcinosarcomas.

Answer 23.2.33.   **The answer is C.**

There are many different types of uterine sarcomas, including endometrial stromal sarcoma, leiomyosarcoma, malignant mixed mullerian tumor, and adenosarcoma. They each have differing presentations and prognosis. Typically all are treated surgically when possible. Adjuvant therapy is controversial, but there does not appear to be a survival benefit to adjuvant radiation therapy for most uterine sarcomas. Uterine leiomyosarcoma has been shown to have a reasonable response to chemotherapy. The combination of gemcitabine and docetaxel in a group of previously treated patients demonstrated a response rate of 53%.

Answer 23.2.34.   **The answer is A.**

GTN includes rare gynecologic tumors that represent less than 1% of gynecologic malignancies. These tumors are potentially life-threatening but usually should be highly curable when treated appropriately. The most common pathologic entity in GTN is complete hydatidiform mole.

Answer 23.2.35.   **The answer is D.**

Beta-hCG is an extremely sensitive and specific marker used in the management of these patients. Patients are typically followed post evacuation with weekly beta-hCG determinations. The diagnosis of persistent GTN is based on the following: a plateau in the level for at least 3 weeks, a 10% or greater increase in the level for three or more values during a 2-week time period, persistence of beta-hCG levels greater than 6 months after evacuation, or histologic evidence of choriocarcinoma.

Answer 23.2.36.   **The answer is C.**

Phantom hCG has only recently been recognized. Heterophile antibodies interfere with some immunoassays used to determine hCG levels. This has led to dramatic overtreatment and loss of fertility (hysterectomy) for some patients. If phantom hCG is suspected, urine hCG should be obtained. The heterophile antibodies are not present in the urine, and this test should be negative.

Answer 23.2.37.   **The answer is C.**

Treatment for GTN is based on risk assessment either by the WHO or the FIGO guidelines. Low-risk disease is typically treated with methotrexate or actinomycin-D. Treatment is continued until the hCG levels are normal for 3 consecutive weeks. The patient is then followed monthly for 12 months. Hysterectomy can be offered for patients who have completed childbearing.

CHAPTER 24 CANCER OF THE BREAST

KATHY D. MILLER

DIRECTIONS   Each of the numbered items below is followed by lettered answers. Select the ONE lettered answer that is BEST in each case unless instructed otherwise.

QUESTIONS

Question 24.1.   What percentage of breast cancers is caused by germ line mutations?

A. 5%
B. 10%
C. 15%
D. 2%

Question 24.2.   Which of the following about PARP1 is TRUE?

A. PARP 1 is a cellular enzyme involved in the base excision repair.
B. Tumors arising in patients with BRCA1, but not BRCA 2, mutations may be sensitive to PARP inhibitors.
C. A and B.
D. None of the above.

Question 24.3.   Characteristic features of *BRCA1*-associated breast cancers include the following except:

A. Aggressive features
B. Estrogen receptor (ER) positive
C. HER 2 negative
D. Young age at presentation

Question 24.4.   Which of the following statements about HER2 is FALSE?

A. Lapatinib is a pure HER inhibitor.
B. The addition of trastuzumab to chemotherapy in the adjuvant setting reduces the rate of recurrence by over 50%.
C. HER2 signaling is effected through homodimer formation.
D. A and C.

Corresponding chapters in *Cancer: Principles & Practice of Oncology,* Ninth Edition: 105 (Molecular Biology of Breast Cancer), 106 (Malignant Tumors of the Breast).

Question 24.5.   Which syndrome is characterized by the presence of breast cancer, soft tissue sarcoma, leukemia, and prostate cancer?

    A. Li-Fraumeni syndrome
    B. Cowden syndrome
    C. Peutz-Jeghers syndrome
    D. Ataxia-telangiectasia

Question 24.6.   Which frequently mutated gene is present in 17q21?

    A. *BRCA1*
    B. *BRCA2*
    C. *PTEN*
    D. *P53*

Question 24.7.   Which of the following factors is NOT associated with a relative risk higher than 4 for developing breast cancer?

    A. Radiation exposure before age of 40
    B. *BRCA1* mutation
    C. *CHEK2* mutation
    D. Lobular carcinoma in situ

Question 24.8.   Based on the Women's Health Initiative Study, the use of postmenopausal combined estrogen and progestin therapy:

    A. Increased the frequency of abnormal mammograms after 1 year
    B. Doubled the risk of developing breast cancer after 4 years
    C. Doubled the risk of developing breast cancer after 2 years
    D. Did not alter the likelihood of having nodal involvement at diagnosis

Question 24.9.   Which of the following is associated with the highest risk of breast cancer?

    A. Postmenopausal obesity
    B. Dense breasts on mammogram
    C. Postmenopausal estrogen plus progestin therapy
    D. Nulliparity

Question 24.10.   Current evidence does NOT support the addition of screening breast magnetic resonance imaging (MRI) for which of the following patients?

    A. A 25-year-old woman with a deleterious mutation in BRCA2
    B. A 66-year-old woman who underwent lumpectomy and radiation for a high-grade ductal cancer in situ (DCIS) 2 years ago
    C. A 32-year-old woman whose sister tested positive for a deleterious mutation in BRCA1 (she has declined testing)
    D. A 35-year-old woman who underwent mantle radiation for Hodgkin's disease at age 16 years

Question 24.11.   The Gail model includes all of the following risk factors, EXCEPT:

    A.   First-degree relatives with breast cancer
    B.   Previous breast biopsies
    C.   Age at menarche
    D.   Age at menopause

Question 24.12.   You are advising a 42-year-old premenopausal woman with a history of atypical hyperplasia on prevention strategies. Which of the following is CORRECT?

    A.   Tamoxifen reduces her risk by ∼50%.
    B.   Oophorectomy reduces her risk by ∼50% to 65%.
    C.   Bilateral mastectomy completely eliminates her risk of breast cancer.
    D.   Raloxifene would provide similar benefit as tamoxifen.

Question 24.13.   A 58-year-old woman presents to your office with a new palpable breast mass; a biopsy has been recommended based on the results of mammogram and ultrasound. In discussing the options, you explain that:

    A.   A biopsy can be deferred if a breast MRI does not show significant enhancement.
    B.   The false-negative rate of core biopsy is 5% to 10%.
    C.   Diagnosis by core biopsy decreases the number of surgical procedures required, even in women ultimately found to have cancer.
    D.   A fine-needle biopsy can distinguish DCIS from invasive cancer.

Question 24.14.   You are asked to advise a woman who underwent core-needle biopsy for evaluation of suspicious microcalcifications detected on screening mammogram. A surgical biopsy should be recommended in all of the following, EXCEPT:

    A.   Ductal hyperplasia without atypia, calcifications are seen associated with the hyperplasia
    B.   Radial scar
    C.   Lobular carcinoma in situ
    D.   Sclerosing adenosis, no calcifications are identified in the specimen

Question 24.15.   All of the following statements about DCIS are true, EXCEPT:

    A.   DCIS accounts for 15% to 30% of mammographically detected cancers.
    B.   DCIS is most common in premenopausal women.
    C.   Younger women have a higher rate of local recurrence after breast-conserving therapy.
    D.   Preoperative MRI does not improve surgical planning.

Question 24.16.   The use of radiation therapy (RT) after lumpectomy in patients with DCIS:

    A. Improves overall survival (OS)

    B. Reduces the risk of recurrent DCIS, but not invasive disease, in the treated breast

    C. Does not decrease local recurrence when tamoxifen therapy is administered

    D. None of the above

Question 24.17.   Which of the following are pathologic subtypes of breast cancer associated with a more favorable prognosis?

    A. Metaplastic

    B. Scirrhous

    C. Tubular

    D. Medullary

Question 24.18.   What stage describes a patient with a 3 cm primary breast tumor metastatic to a movable ipsilateral lymph node?

    A. T1N1M0 (IIA)

    B. T2N1M0 (IIA)

    C. T2N1M0 (IIB)

    D. T3N1M0 (IIB)

Question 24.19.   For which of the following there is insufficient evidence to recommend annual MRI screening?

    A. *BRCA* mutation

    B. Radiation to the chest between ages 10 and 30

    C. First-degree relatives of Cowden syndrome

    D. Personal history of breast cancer

Question 24.20.   Which of the following patients is at greatest risk of local recurrence after breast-conserving therapy?

    A. A 65-year-old with a 2-cm grade 1, ER + tumor, closest margin 3 mm, treated with whole breast radiation therapy (WBRT) (no boost), and an aromatase inhibitor (AI)

    B. A 25-year-old with a 2-cm grade 3, ER – tumor, closest margin <1 mm, treated with WBRT (with boost) and no systemic therapy

    C. A 35-year-old with a 2-cm grade 2, ER – tumor, closest margin 6 mm, treated with WBRT (with boost) and adjuvant chemotherapy

    D. A 65-year-old with a 4-cm grade 1, ER + tumor, closest margin 4 mm, treated with WBRT (with boost) and an AI

Question 24.21.   Which of the following is an absolute contraindication to breast-conserving surgery (BCS)?

    A. Two or more primary tumors in separate quadrants

    B. Collage vascular disease

    C. Large tumor in a smaller breast

    D. Primary tumor size of 4.8 cm

Question 24.22.   Compared with the use of adjuvant therapy, the use of neoadjuvant therapy:

A. Increases the potential for BCS
B. Does not provide an opportunity to test the chemosensitivity of the tumor
C. Increases OS
D. Decreases the risk of local recurrence

Question 24.23.   Which of the following statements regarding autologous tissue breast reconstruction is FALSE?

A. Autologous reconstruction may be performed in patients who will require postmastectomy RT without an excessively high risk of flap loss.
B. Immediate autologous reconstruction does not delay the administration of systemic chemotherapy and may be performed in patients with stage II or III disease.
C. Skin-sparing mastectomy should be avoided because there is a 2% to 4% increase in the risk of local recurrence.
D. Patients undergoing autologous tissue reconstruction may still require a complementary prosthetic implant to achieve a satisfactory cosmetic result.

Question 24.24.   Which of the following factors is associated with failure to identify the sentinel node?

A. Tumor located in the lower inner quadrant
B. Increased body mass index
C. Excisional biopsy before sentinel node biopsy (SNB)
D. Invasive lobular carcinoma

Question 24.25.   Which statement regarding SNB is TRUE?

A. SNB can be safely performed during pregnancy.
B. SNB is less accurate in patients with multicentric tumors.
C. The incidence of lymphedema is <2% at 12 months.
D. The false-negative rate in multicenter trials is ~10%.

Question 24.26.   Identify the CORRECT statement:

A. Radiation after BCS reduces the risk of local recurrence but does not improve OS.
B. Radiation after BCS improves breast cancer-specific survival but does not improve OS.
C. Radiation improves OS when administered after BCS but does not improve OS in patients who underwent mastectomy.
D. Improved local control at 5 years results in a proportional improvement in OS at 15 years.

Question 24.27.   Which of the following is both a prognostic and predictive factor?

   A. Axillary node involvement
   B. ER
   C. Patient age
   D. Lymphovascular invasion

Question 24.28.   The gains associated with adjuvant tamoxifen:

   A. Are independent of patient age
   B. Are less in patients who also receive adjuvant chemotherapy
   C. Are dependent on patient menopausal status
   D. Decline 10 years after diagnosis

Question 24.29.   The use of AIs in the adjuvant treatment of postmenopausal women:

   A. Improves OS when used as initial therapy, but not when used after 2 to 5 years of tamoxifen
   B. Increases the risk of fracture for 10 years
   C. Effectively lowers estrogen levels by 90%
   D. Provides increased benefit when administered for 10 years

Question 24.30.   You are seeing a 42-year-old premenopausal patient with newly diagnosed stage I, ER+/HER2–breast cancer. Her surgeon had requested an Onco-typeDX recurrence score assay, which returned with a score of 36. On the basis of her recurrence score, the absolute improvement in her risk of recurrence with the addition of adding cyclophosphamide (CMF) to tamoxifen is predicted to be:

   A. <5%
   B. 14%
   C. 22%
   D. 30%

Question 24.31.   You are seeing a 58-year-old woman with stage I breast cancer. She has been taking tamoxifen for 30 months and you have advised switching her hormonal therapy to exemestane on the basis of the IES trial results. In discussing the potential benefits of this strategy compared with continuing tamoxifen for the planned 5 years, you tell her that exemestane:

   A. Improved disease-free survival (DFS) by ~25%
   B. Improved OS in patients with ER+ disease
   C. Reduced contralateral breast cancers by ~40%
   D. All of the above

Question 24.32.   You are seeing a 52-year-old woman with newly diagnosed stage III breast cancer (5.5 cm tumor, 6+ LN, grade 3, ER–/PR–/HER2+ by FISH with ratio 8.7). She asks about the benefits of trastuzumab. On the basis of the updated analysis of the Intergroup adjuvant trials (N9831 and B31), you tell her that the addition of trastuzumab to adjuvant ACT chemotherapy:

A. Improves relative DFS by 35%
B. Improves relative OS by 40%
C. Reduces the probability of distant recurrence by 50%
D. Results in death from congestive heart failure in 5%

Question 24.33.   On the basis of the overview analysis, the relative benefits of adjuvant chemotherapy are:

A. Independent of ER status
B. Independent of administration of hormone therapy
C. Greater with anthracycline compared with CMF-type regimens
D. All of the above

Question 24.34.   Identify the correct statement regarding the use of taxanes in the adjuvant setting:

A. Concurrent administration with anthracyclines provides superior efficacy compared with sequential regimens.
B. Sequential anthracycline > taxane therapy is superior to anthracycline therapy alone.
C. Docetaxel administered every 3 weeks has greater efficacy than paclitaxel administered weekly.
D. Incorporation of taxanes into adjuvant therapy increases the risk of cardiotoxicity.

Question 24.35.   The addition of bevacizumab to paclitaxel as initial chemotherapy for metastatic breast cancer increases all of the following, EXCEPT:

A. DFS
B. OS
C. Response rate
D. Hypertension

Question 24.36.   The addition of lapatinib to capecitabine in patients with advanced HER2+ breast cancer increases all of the following, EXCEPT:

A. Time to progression (TTP)
B. Rash
C. Diarrhea
D. OS

Question 24.37.   A 67-year-old woman has been taking anastrozole as adjuvant therapy for stage I breast cancer for 4 years. She was recently found to have bone metastases. After RT to a painful lesion at T8, she is asymptomatic. You recommend:

A. Fulvestrant
B. Exemestane
C. Either will be equally effective
D. Neither will be effective

Question 24.38.   In a recently reported phase III trial, the addition of ixabepilone to capecitabine

A. Increased progression-free survival from 4.2 to 5.8 months
B. Increased objective response rate based on investigator, but not independent review facility, assessment
C. Increased neutropenia, but not neutropenic fevers
D. All of the above

Question 24.39.   A urologist tells you his mother has just been diagnosed with Paget's disease based on a punch biopsy of an area of crusting on her nipple. You tell him:

A. It is associated with in situ or invasive breast cancer in only 50% of cases.
B. Approximately half of Paget's disease cases are hormone-receptor positive.
C. It tends to be associated with underlying low-grade disease.
D. Underlying breast cancers are almost always located within 2 cm of the nipple.

Question 24.40.   Which of the following regarding treatment of breast cancer in the pregnant patient is FALSE?

A. Breast irradiation is contraindicated in the pregnant patient.
B. Mastectomy has no place in the treatment of pregnant patients who have tumors amenable to breast conservation.
C. Adjuvant chemotherapy should be avoided in the first trimester, because almost all chemotherapeutic agents cross the placenta and are associated with a 15% to 20% risk of fetal malformation.
D. Chemotherapy can generally be administered safely during the second and third trimesters of pregnancy; the risk of fetal malformation is 1% to 3% during this time, similar to the risk of fetal malformation in healthy women.

Question 24.41. Which of the following regarding locally advanced breast cancer is TRUE?

A. Chemotherapy given in the adjuvant setting obviates the need for postmastectomy radiation.
B. Hormonal therapy does not improve outcome.
C. There is no difference in outcomes regardless of whether chemotherapy is given in the neoadjuvant or the adjuvant setting.
D. Surgery should be done first to debulk disease and achieve local control.

Question 24.42. Which of the following does NOT accurately characterize inflammatory breast cancer (IBC)?

A. Almost all women with IBC have lymph node involvement.
B. The 10-year survival rate exceeds 30%.
C. IBC is staged as T4d, overall stage IIIC.
D. Dermal lymphatic invasion must be seen on biopsy to confirm IBC.

Question 24.43. With regard to the clinical and pathologic characteristics of male breast cancer, which of the following is FALSE?

A. Male breast cancer is found, more often than female breast cancer, to be estrogen-receptor positive, and the older a man is with breast cancer, the more likely the cancer is estrogen-receptor positive.
B. Both lobular carcinoma in situ and invasive lobular carcinoma have been reported in male patients.
C. The most common presenting symptom is a painless, firm subareolar mass, seen in more than 75% of patients.
D. In addition to a palpable mass, common physical examination findings include changes in the areola with nipple retraction, inversion or fixation, or eczematous skin changes.

Question 24.44. Concerning the staging and treatment of male breast cancer, which of the following is FALSE?

A. The same TNM staging system is used to stage male breast cancer.
B. Stage and axillary node status are the more important prognostic indicators in male breast cancer.
C. In cases of DCIS in men, simple mastectomy with axillary node dissection is the treatment of choice.
D. For localized disease, a simple mastectomy, or modified radical mastectomy, with local radiation treatment is an effective therapy; there are no data to suggest that more extensive surgical resection improves survival.

Question 24.45.   **With regard to surveillance for patients with early-stage breast cancer, all of the following are true, EXCEPT:**

A. Screening mammography and breast ultrasound are the only imaging studies recommended for routine surveillance.

B. There is no role for intense surveillance, because early detection of relapse has not been shown to improve OS or other meaningful clinical end points.

C. Survival data from surveillance strategies to detect early recurrence of disease may be affected by lead-time bias.

D. Survival data from surveillance strategies to detect early recurrence of disease may be affected by length bias.

ANSWERS

Answer 24.1.   **The answer is B.**

Approximately 10% of all breast cancers are associated with germ line mutations, while other 90% occur sporadically.

Answer 24.2.   **The answer is A.**

PARP1 is a cellular enzyme involved in the single-strand DNA repair through the base excision repair. Since both BRCA 1 and BRCA2 are important in DNA repair via the homologous combination repair pathway, patients with mutations of either BRCA1 or BRCA2 may be sensitive to PARP inhibition.

Answer 24.3.   **The answer is B.**

BRCA1-associated breast cancers usually occur in younger women, have aggressive features, and are characterized by a "triple negative" phenotype (ER, PR, and HER2 negative).

Answer 24.4.   **The answer is D.**

The addition of trastuzumab to chemotherapy in the adjuvant setting decreases recurrence rates to over 50%. Lapatinib is a dual EGFR and HER2 receptor and HER2 activation occurs through homo- and heterodimer formation.

Answer 24.5.   **The answer is A.**

Li-Fraumeni syndrome is characterized by breast cancer, soft tissue sarcoma, CNS tumors, adrenal cancer, leukemia, and prostate cancer. Adrenal cancer, prostate cancer, and leukemia are not common in Cowden, Peutz-Jegher syndromes or ataxia-telangiectasia.

Answer 24.6.   **The answer is A.**

BRCA1 is the gene at locus 17q21. *BRCA2, PTEN,* and *P53* are located on 13q12.3, 10q23.3, and 17p13.1, respectively.

Answer 24.7.   **The answer is C.**

The factors associated with an increased relative risk above 4 for the development of breast cancer include *BRCA* mutations, lobular carcinoma in situ, atypical hyperplasia, and radiation exposure before the age of 40. *CHEK2* mutations are associated with a relative risk between 2 and 4.

Answer 24.8.   **The answer is A.**

In the Women's Health Initiative study, combined estrogen and progestin increased the risk of developing breast cancer with a hazard ratio of 1.24. The increase in breast cancer was detected at 2 years, but an excess of abnormal mammograms was apparent at 1 year. Hormone replacement therapy users were more likely to have nodal involvement or distant metastases at diagnosis.

Answer 24.9.   **The answer is B.**

Hormonal risk factors typically have relative risks of less than 2. Mammographic breast density is an underappreciated risk factor with a relative risk of 2 to 4. Factors associated with a relative risk more than 4 include atypical hyperplasia, LCIS, BRCA1, or BRCA2 mutation and radiation exposure before age 40 years.

Answer 24.10.   **The answer is B.**

American Society of Clinical Oncology guidelines for MR screening were revised in 2007. Current evidence supports screening MR in patients with a known BRCA mutation, untested first-degree relatives of BRCA mutation carriers, or patients with an estimated 20% to 25% lifetime risk of breast cancer (e.g., someone who received mantle radiation at age 16 years). There is currently insufficient evidence to recommend for or against MR screening for patients with a personal history of breast cancer.

Answer 24.11.   **The answer is D.**

The Gail model estimates a woman's risk of developing breast cancer on the basis of age at menarche, age at first live birth, number of previous breast biopsies and presence of atypia, and the number of first-degree female relatives with breast cancer. It may underestimate the risk in women with a strong family history because it does not include second-degree relatives, men with breast cancer, or relatives with ovarian cancer.

Answer 24.12.   **The answer is B.**

In the P1 trial, tamoxifen reduced the risk of breast cancer by 84% in patients with atypical hyperplasia. Although raloxifene provided similar benefits with a more favorable safety profile than tamoxifen in the STAR trial, this trial only included postmenopausal women. Oophorectomy before menopause decreases the risk of breast cancer by 50% to 65% depending on age at the time of surgery. Although bilateral mastectomy decreases the risk by more than 90%, the risk is not completely eliminated.

Answer 24.13.   **The answer is C.**

If cytopathologist expertise is available, FNA can reliably diagnose cancer but cannot distinguish DCIS from invasive disease. The false-negative rate is 5% to 10% for FNA but less than 4% for core biopsy. In a prospective study of 1550 patients undergoing biopsy for mammographic abnormalities, core biopsy reduced the number of surgical procedures.

Answer 24.14.   **The answer is A.**

Ductal hyperplasia without atypia (a.k.a. usual type hyperplasia) is not an indication for surgical biopsy.

Answer 24.15.   **The answer is B.**

DCIS is most common among women ages 49 to 69 years. Several studies have reported an increased risk of local recurrence in younger women. Initial studies suggested that MRI can both over- and underestimate the extent of DCIS and does not improve surgical planning.

Answer 24.16.   **The answer is D.**

The use of RT after BCS for DCIS reduces both invasive and noninvasive recurrences but does not alter OS.

Answer 24.17.   **The answer is C.**

Subtypes with a more favorable prognosis include breast cancers with tubular, mucinous, papillary, or cribriform features.

Answer 24.18.   **The answer is C.**

The patient has T2 (tumor size between 2 and 5 cm), N1 (movable ipsilateral level 1 lymph node) M0. T2N1M0 represents stage IIB.

Answer 24.19.   **The answer is D.**

There is not enough evidence in favor or against annual screening MRI in patients with personal history of breast cancer. The recommendation for annual screening MRI in *BRCA* mutation is evidence-based whereas it is based on expert opinion for previously radiated patients between ages of 10 and 30 and first-degree relatives of Cowden syndrome.

Answer 24.20.   **The answer is B.**

This patient has multiple risk factors for local recurrence, including young age (<35 to 40 years), close (though not frankly involved) margins, high-grade histology, and lack of use of systemic therapy.

Answer 24.21.   **The answer is A.**

The absolute contraindications for breast-conserving therapy include pregnancy, more than one primary in different quadrants, previous radiation to the breast, and persistent margins after a reasonable number of surgical attempts. Collagen vascular disease, tumor size, and relationship between the sizes of the tumor and breast are all relative contraindications.

Answer 24.22.   **The answer is A.**

Although administering chemotherapy in the neoadjuvant setting does not confer a survival benefit, it may allow breast conservation in patients who would have otherwise required mastectomy. However, there is a slightly higher risk of local recurrence in patients who require neoadjuvant chemotherapy to undergo BCS compared with patients who are initial candidates for BCS.

Answer 24.23.   **The answer is C.**

Skin-sparing mastectomy does not alter the risk of local recurrence. Contrary to initial concerns, immediate reconstruction does not alter the risk of local recurrence, limit ability to detect local recurrence, or delay initiation of systemic therapy. Although fat necrosis, fibrosis, and volume loss are common with RT after autologous reconstruction, complete flap loss is rare.

Answer 24.24.   **The answer is B.**

In the ACOSOG Z10 trial, increasing age, body mass index, and surgical sites with fewer than 50 patients enrolled were associated with a decrease in sentinel node identification rate.

Answer 24.25.   **The answer is D.**

Pregnancy and lactation are contraindications to SNB. Although T3 and multicentric tumors were initially thought to be contraindications, recent data suggest that SNB is accurate in these situations. Although lymphedema is less common after SNB than with traditional axillary dissection, lymphedema was reported in approximately 5% of patients at 12 months in the ALMANAC trial.

Answer 24.26.   **The answer is D.**

On the basis of the most recent Early Breast Cancer Trialists' Collaborative Group findings, improved local control at 5 years results in a proportional improvement OS at 15 years. This was true whether improved local control was obtained by more extensive surgery or the addition of radiation.

Answer 24.27.   **The answer is B.**

A prognostic factor is defined as a measurement taken at diagnosis that is associated with outcome. A predictive factor is a measurement that predicts response or lack of response to a specific therapy. ER is both prognostic and predictive of benefit from hormonal therapies. The other factors are prognostic but not predictive.

Answer 24.28.   **The answer is A.**

Adjuvant tamoxifen results in an improvement in OS for at least 15 years. The benefits are independent of age, menopausal status, and the use of chemotherapy.

Answer 24.29.   **The answer is C.**

AIs lower estrogen levels by 90% in postmenopausal women. To date, no study has shown a survival advantage, and the optimal duration of therapy is unknown. AIs increase the risk of fracture during therapy, but that risk appears to revert to baseline levels once therapy has been discontinued.

Answer 24.30.   **The answer is C.**

The OncotypeDX assay classifies patients by expression of 16 cancer-related genes (normalized to the expression of five reference genes) into low-, intermediate-, and high-risk groups. In NSABP B-20, the addition of chemotherapy to tamoxifen did not improve distant recurrence-free survival at 10 years in patients with a low or intermediate recurrence score. However, in patients with a high recurrence score, the distant recurrence-free survival at 10 years improved from 60% to 82% with the addition of CMF.

Answer 24.31.   **The answer is D.**

DFS was improved by 24%, and time to contralateral breast cancer was reduced by 43%. Although OS was not improved in the entire study population ($p = .08$), analysis of patients with known ER+ disease did find a significant improvement in survival. (See text: Adjuvant Endocrine Therapy. See also Coombes RC, Hall E, Gibson LJ, et al. A randomized trial of exemestane after two to three years of tamoxifen therapy in postmenopausal women with primary breast cancer. N Engl J Med. 2004;350:1081–1092; Coombes R, Paridaens R, Jassem J, et al. First mature survival analysis of Intergroup Exemestane Study: A randomized trial in disease-free patients with early breast cancer randomized to continue tamoxifen or switch to exemestane following an initial 2–3 years of adjuvant tamoxifen. Proc Am Soc Clin Oncol. 2006;24:9s.)

Answer 24.32.   **The answer is C.**

Despite the crossover effects after the trial was unblinded, the most recent update of the combined analysis continued to show a similar impact on DFS ($\sim$50%), distant DFS ($\sim$50%), and OS ($\sim$30%). Among 875 patients randomized to trastuzumab and chemotherapy, there were 22 cases of congestive heart failure but no cardiac deaths. In the control arm there was only one case of CHF, and one cardiac death was reported. (See text: Adjuvant Trastuzumab. See also Romond EH, Perez EA, Bryant J, et al. Trastuzumab plus adjuvant chemotherapy for operable HER2-positive breast cancer. N Engl J Med. 2005;353:1673–1684.)

Answer 24.33.   **The answer is D.**

The relative benefits of chemotherapy are independent of age, ER status, and use of hormonal therapy, although the absolute benefits will differ according to baseline risk.

Answer 24.34.   **The answer is B.**

Approximately 12 studies have evaluated the incorporation of the taxanes, either sequentially or concurrently, into anthracycline-based adjuvant therapy. Although most studies report an improved outcome, no clearly superior regimen has emerged. In the E1199 trial, no difference was identified with docetaxel or paclitaxel administered weekly or every 3 weeks.

Answer 24.35.   **The answer is B.**

The addition of bevacizumab to paclitaxel significantly prolonged progression-free survival (11.8 vs. 5.9 months; hazard ratio [HR] = 0.60, $p < .001$) and increased objective response rate (36.9% vs. 21.2%; $p < .001$), but median OS was similar in both groups (26.7 vs. 25.2 months; HR = 0.88, $p = .16$). Grade 3/4 hypertension (15% vs. 0%; $p = .001$) and cerebrovascular ischemia (2% vs. 0%; $p = .009$) were both more frequent in patients receiving paclitaxel + bevacizumab. (See text: Antiangiogenesis Therapy for Advanced Breast Cancer. See also Miller K, Wang M, Gralow J, et al. Paclitaxel plus bevacizumab versus paclitaxel alone for metastatic breast cancer. N Engl J Med. 2007;357:2666–2676.)

Answer 24.36.   **The answer is D.**

The addition of lapatinib to capecitabine in patients with advanced HER2+ breast cancer increased TTP (HR 0.49; $p < .001$). The most common toxicities were diarrhea, hand-foot syndrome, nausea, fatigue, vomiting, and rash. Diarrhea and rash were significantly more frequent in patients receiving combined therapy. Although OS data are not yet mature, to date there is no improvement in OS. (See text: Anti-HER2 Therapy for Metastatic Breast Cancer. See also Geyer CE, Forster J, Lindquist D, et al. Lapatinib plus capecitabine for HER2-positive advanced breast cancer. N Engl J Med. 2006;355:2733.)

Answer 24.37.   **The answer is C.**

The EFECT trial compared fulvestrant and exemestane in post-menopausal women progressing on a nonsteroidal AI. Response rate, clinical benefit, and TTP were identical, suggesting either fulvestrant or exemestane would be reasonable options. However, the EFECT trial used a loading dose of fulvestrant (500 mg on day 0, 250 mg on days 14 and 28, and then monthly) to achieve steady-state potentially therapeutic levels within the first month. (See text: Endocrine Therapy for Metastatic Breast Cancer. See also Gradishar W, Chia S, Piccart-Gebhart M, et al. Fulvestrant versus exemestane following prior non-steroidal AI therapy: First results from EFECT, a randomized phase II trial in post-menopausal women with advanced breast cancer. Breast Cancer Res and Treat. 2006;100:S8–S9.)

Answer 24.38.   **The answer is A.**

Ixabepilone increased objective response rate by both the investigator (23% vs. 42%) and independent radiologic review (14% vs. 35%). Ixabepilone causes significantly more neutropenia (11% vs. 68%) than capecitabine alone. Neutropenic fevers were uncommon but were increased with ixabepilone (<1% vs. 4%, $p < .001$). (See Thomas ES, Gomez HL, Li RK, et al. Ixabepilone plus capecitabine for metastatic breast cancer progressing after anthracycline and taxane treatment. J Clin Oncol. 2007;25:5210–5217.)

Answer 24.39.   **The answer is B.**

An underlying malignancy is found in approximately 97% of patients with Paget's disease, frequently with high-grade histology. It is not uncommon for an underlying tumor to be several centimeters away from the nipple. Half of cases are hormone-receptor negative, consistent with the higher rate of underlying high-grade tumors. (See text: Paget's Disease. See also Chaudary Ma, Millis RR, Lane EB, et al. Paget's disease of the nipple: A ten year review including clinical, pathological, and immunohistochemical findings. Breast Cancer Res. 1986;8:139–146; Marshall JK, Giffith KA, Haffty BG, et al. Conservative management of Paget disease of the breast with radiotherapy; 10- and 15-year results. Cancer. 2003;97:2142–2149.)

Answer 24.40.   **The answer is B.**

Because breast irradiation is contraindicated in the pregnant patient, mastectomy may prove to be a more appropriate management approach even in patients with tumors amenable to breast conservation, particularly in women early in pregnancy.

Answer 24.41.   **The answer is C.**

Neoadjuvant chemotherapy plays a multifaceted role in the treatment of locally advanced breast cancer. It may downsize a tumor, making it more amenable to breast-conserving treatment or helping to achieve a more acceptable cosmetic result. It may downstage the patient's disease by decreasing the number of positive axillary lymph nodes, thereby improving survival. Giving neoadjuvant chemotherapy allows the oncologist to gauge the chemosensitivity of the tumor. Regardless of whether chemotherapy is given in the neoadjuvant or adjuvant setting, postsurgical radiation is still required, and the outcome is the same. Hormonal therapy improves outcome and should be given after any additional adjuvant treatment.

Answer 24.42.   **The answer is D.**

IBC is a clinical diagnosis. Dermal lymphatic invasion on full-thickness skin biopsy is often seen but is not required for diagnosis. Most women will have lymph node involvement. In the absence of distant metastases, IBC is staged as T4d, stage IIIC disease.

Answer 24.43.   **The answer is A.**

Approximately 80% of cases of male breast cancer are estrogen-receptor positive, presumably because men are effectively postmenopausal. There does not appear to be a difference in the chances a tumor will be estrogen-receptor positive depending on the age of a male patient with breast cancer.

Answer 24.44.   **The answer is C.**

As in women, DCIS is primarily a local disease with excellent prognosis, and axillary node dissection is not necessary.

Answer 24.45.   **The answer is A.**

It is not clear that early detection of distant metastatic disease improves clinically important outcomes. As such, screening mammography is the only imaging study recommended for routine surveillance in asymptomatic patients. A woman should have a mammogram of her conserved breast annually, beginning no more than 6 months after completion of radiotherapy.

RAMI Y. HADDAD • MOUHAMMED AMIR HABRA

DIRECTIONS   Each of the numbered items below is followed by lettered answers. Select the
ONE lettered answer that is BEST in each case unless instructed otherwise.

QUESTIONS

Question 25.1.   A 37-year-old woman presents with a right anterior neck mass. She denies
dysphagia or hoarseness. There is no history of radiation exposure or
family history of cancer, and no palpable nodes are detected on physical
examination. Neck ultrasound reveals a 2.5-cm right thyroid solid nodule without enlarged cervical lymph nodes. Fine-needle aspiration (FNA)
suggests the diagnosis of papillary thyroid carcinoma. You recommend
which one of the following as the initial management plan?

   A.   Total thyroidectomy
   B.   Right thyroid lobectomy
   C.   Total thyroidectomy with modified right neck dissection
   D.   Total thyroidectomy with bilateral neck dissection

Question 25.2.   A 39-year-old woman underwent right thyroid lobectomy and isthmusectomy after the incidental discovery of a 0.8-cm right thyroid nodule
with indeterminate FNA. On preoperative neck ultrasound, the left thyroid lobe appeared normal and there was no evidence of abnormal lymph
nodes. Pathologic examination revealed a 0.75-cm intrathyroidal papillary carcinoma. The most appropriate management now is:

   A.   Thyroid hormone replacement if needed without further resection.
   B.   Radioactive iodine scan followed by radioactive iodine ablation if
        there is neck uptake.
   C.   Surgical resection of remaining thyroid tissue followed by radioactive
        iodine ablation.
   D.   Radioactive iodine ablation followed by thyroid hormone suppres-
        sion.

Corresponding Chapters in *Cancer: Principles & Practice of Oncology*, Ninth Edition: 107 (Molecular Biology of
Endocrine Tumors), 108 (Thyroid Tumors), 109 (Parathyroid Tumors), 110 (Adrenal Tumors), 111 (Pancreatic Neu-
roendocrine Tumors), 112 (Neuroendocrine (Carcinoid) Tumors and the Carcinoid Syndrome), and 113 (Multiple
Endocrine Neoplasias).

Question 25.3.   A 42-year-old woman underwent FNA of a 3-cm left thyroid mass. No palpable nodes were detected on physical examination or imaging. FNA was suspicious of thyroid malignancy. What is the most appropriate next step?

A. Total thyroidectomy
B. Left lobectomy but with fresh-frozen section to plan immediate further resection
C. Left complete lobectomy and isthmusectomy, to be followed by total thyroidectomy later if malignancy is confirmed
D. Plan to repeat FNA for further tissue evaluation

Question 25.4.   A 41-year-old woman, who was treated 4 years ago for papillary thyroid carcinoma with total thyroidectomy and bilateral neck dissection followed by radioactive iodine ablation, is found on follow-up to have an elevated thyroglobulin (TG) level (16 ng/mL) with negative TG antibodies. Diagnostic whole-body iodine scan is negative, and thyroid-stimulating hormone (TSH) is suppressed. What is the most appropriate next step?

A. Chest radiograph
B. Positron emission tomography (PET) scan
C. Surveillance
D. Neck imaging

Question 25.5.   A 24-year-old woman underwent FNA of a left thyroid nodule, which showed cells suspicious of neuroendocrine origin. She has been experiencing intermittent diarrhea for the past 4 months. Family history includes kidney stones in several members. The rest of the history and physical examination results are normal. What is the most appropriate next step?

A. Obtain metanephrines and catecholamines/serum calcium/serum calcitonin/carcinoembryonic antigen (CEA)/RET proto-oncogene.
B. Obtain serum calcitonin/thyroglobulin/calcium/RET proto-oncogene, and then perform a total thyroidectomy.
C. Measure metanephrines and catecholamines/serum calcium/calcitonin/CEA.
D. Perform a total thyroidectomy now, and then obtain postoperative evaluation.

Question 25.6.   A 54-year-old man underwent total thyroidectomy for suspected papillary thyroid carcinoma on FNA. Pathologic examination confirmed a 3-cm papillary carcinoma in the right lobe, without extracapsular extension; all nodes examined were free of cancer. You recommend which one of the following?

A. Radiation therapy
B. Radioactive iodine ablation
C. Chemotherapy
D. Concurrent chemotherapy and radiotherapy
E. Observation only

Question 25.7.   A 64-year-old man was found to have an abnormal PET scan on follow-up. He was diagnosed with papillary thyroid carcinoma 10 years ago. He was treated with total thyroidectomy and radioactive iodine ablation; follow-up iodine scans have always been normal. He presents now with dysphagia. TG level is found to be 80 ng/mL with negative anti-TG antibodies and suppressed TSH. Computed tomography (CT) chest scan reveals a 3-cm mass in the upper chest causing mild esophageal compression corresponding to PET findings. You recommend which one of the following as the best initial approach?

A. Esophageal stent placement
B. External beam radiotherapy
C. Cytotoxic chemotherapy
D. Radioactive iodine ablation
E. Surgical resection to achieve local control, possibly followed by external beam radiation therapy

Question 25.8.   A 34-year-old woman who was treated with external beam radiation for Hodgkin's lymphoma when she was 14 years old was recently diagnosed with papillary thyroid carcinoma. Which genetic defect is expected to be found in this case?

A. BRAF mutation
B. APC gene mutation
C. RET proto-oncogene mutation
D. RET/PTC rearrangement

Question 25.9.   Which of the following factors is (are) considered poor prognostic features of papillary thyroid carcinoma?

A. Age; men >40 years
B. Tumor size >5 cm
C. Extracapsular invasion
D. All of the above

Question 25.10.   A 35-year-old woman is found to have bilateral lung nodules on chest CT scan. Six years ago she underwent total thyroidectomy for a 3-cm papillary thyroid carcinoma, followed by radioiodine ablation. She was lost to follow-up until she recently presented with a cough. Serum TG level is found to be 192 ng/mL. Chest CT with intravenous (IV) contrast shows small bilateral lung nodules. Biopsy obtained by thoracoscopy shows papillary histology. A whole-body radioiodine scan reveals no iodine-avid lesions. TSH is suppressed. A well-healed scar is seen on the neck, with no palpable nodes detected, and the rest of the examination shows normal results. Which is the most appropriate next step?

A. Chemotherapy
B. Repeat iodine scan in 6 to 8 weeks
C. Surgical resection of the lung nodules
D. External beam radiation

Question 25.11.   Which of the following is TRUE regarding medullary thyroid carcinoma (MTC)?

  A.   Genetic testing is not indicated in the absence of family history of MTC.
  B.   Plasma metanephrines should be obtained within a few weeks after thyroidectomy.
  C.   It is associated with radiation exposure.
  D.   It arises from the parafollicular C cells in the thyroid gland.

Question 25.12.   A 67-year-old man presents with a rapidly growing mass on the anterior part of the neck that is associated with progressive hoarseness. He also reports a 12-lb weight loss. The remainder of his history is significant for hypertension. Physical examination reveals mild respiratory distress, a 6-cm mass on the anterior part of the neck, and adequate air entry. Core needle biopsy confirms anaplastic thyroid carcinoma. CT scan shows a thyroid mass with local invasion and multiple bilateral lung nodules. Laboratory test results are normal. What is the most appropriate management now?

  A.   Surgical debulking followed by adjuvant radioiodine
  B.   Radioactive iodine alone
  C.   Concurrent chemoradiation
  D.   Doxorubicin-based chemotherapy

Question 25.13.   Which one of the following should be considered in the staging of MTC?

  A.   Complete contrast-enhanced CT scan
  B.   Serum CEA and calcitonin
  C.   Bone survey
  D.   Octreoscan
  E.   All of the above

Question 25.14.   All of the following are true regarding Hurthle cell carcinoma, EXCEPT:

  A.   It is a papillary carcinoma variant.
  B.   It is also known as Oxyphil cell carcinoma.
  C.   It has a worse prognosis than papillary or follicular carcinoma.
  D.   It is less iodine-avid than papillary or follicular carcinoma.

Question 25.15.   Which of the following is TRUE about anaplastic thyroid carcinoma?

  A.   6% of all thyroid cancers
  B.   Always stage IV
  C.   Slow growing and can be curable
  D.   Treated mainly with radioactive iodine

Question 25.16. The most commonly used chemotherapeutic agent(s) in metastatic thyroid carcinoma is (are):

A. Methotrexate
B. Cisplatin
C. 5-Fluorouracil
D. Doxorubicin (Adriamycin)

Question 25.17. Parathyroid carcinoma is suspected in a 48-year-old man. He presented with symptoms of hypercalcemia and was treated with standard approach. Parathyroid hormone (PTH) level is markedly elevated; calcium level is 16 mg/dL on presentation. PTH sestamibi scan showed an intense uptake in the left superior parathyroid gland. CT of the neck showed a 3-cm mass corresponding to the PTH scan findings. What is the most appropriate management?

A. Total or subtotal parathyroidectomy
B. Single gland resection followed by external beam irradiation to the neck
C. External beam irradiation alone
D. Radioactive iodine ablation

Question 25.18. Which of the following can be used to treat malignant hypercalcemia related to metastatic parathyroid carcinoma?

A. Cinacalcet (Sensipar)
B. Mithramycin
C. IV hydration
D. IV bisphosphonates
E. All of the above

Question 25.19. Which of the following genetic defects is most likely associated with parathyroid carcinoma?

A. Mutations of the HRPT2 gene (1q25-31)
B. Allelic loss in several chromosomes
C. RET proto-oncogene mutation
D. All of the above

Question 25.20. Which of the following is a TRUE statement regarding parathyroid carcinoma?

A. If a neck mass is palpated, parathyroid carcinoma should be suspected.
B. Reported overall 5-year survival rate is approximately 30%.
C. TNM staging corresponds to prognosis.

Question 25.21.   A 36-year-old man presents to his primary physician reporting reduced libido for the past 9 months. He also reports periodic epigastric pain associated with occasional heartburn. His medical history includes two episodes of kidney stones in the past 10 years. Family history includes kidney stone formation in his father. Physical examination results are unremarkable. Laboratory evaluation showed prolactin level of 180 ng/mL, testosterone level of 90 ng/dL, serum calcium of 10.9, and PTH level of 110 pg/mL. Magnetic resonance imaging of the brain revealed a 1.5-cm mass in the sella without evidence of damage of the surrounding structures. CT scan of the abdomen did not reveal any abnormality. What is the appropriate management of this patient?

A. Subtotal parathyroidectomy
B. Dopamine agonists (bromocriptine) with subtotal parathyroidectomy
C. Transsphenoidal pituitary resection with subtotal parathyroidectomy

Question 25.22.   All of the following are considered to be part of MEN1, EXCEPT:

A. Pituitary adenoma
B. Carcinoids
C. MTC
D. Benign adrenal tumors

Question 25.23.   The following are considered to be part of MEN2A syndrome, EXCEPT:

A. MTC
B. Pheochromocytoma
C. Parathyroid adenoma
D. Diffuse neuronal hypertrophy

Question 25.24.   What is the best approach to individuals with kindreds with MEN2A who are interested in screening and prevention?

A. Screen for RET mutation
B. Periodic imaging
C. Periodic laboratory tests
D. Clinical surveillance

Question 25.25.   What is the genetic defect that is likely to be associated with MEN1?

A. RET proto-oncogene
B. MENIN gene
C. APC gene
D. HRPT2 gene

Question 25.26.   RET proto-oncogene mutation is associated with which of the following condition(s)?

A. MEN2
B. Hirschsprung disease
C. MTC
D. A and B

Question 25.27.   A 48-year-old woman presents with amenorrhea for the past 5 months. She also reports appearance of facial hair, development of new acne lesions on the face, and recent unexplained weight gain. Medical history is unremarkable. On physical examination, blood pressure is 130/82 mm Hg, weight is 195 lbs, thick facial hair, and multiple acne-like lesions on the face are noted, and the remainder of the examination is normal. CT scan of the abdomen reveals a 6-cm mass in the left adrenal gland without other identified lesions. What is the most appropriate plan of management?

A. Percutaneous image-guided needle biopsy
B. Metabolic workup followed by surgical resection
C. Observation and reassurance that symptoms are related to menopause
D. Metabolic workup followed by mitotane

Question 25.28.   Recurrent metastatic pheochromocytoma can be treated by all of the following, EXCEPT:

A. Systemic chemotherapy combination chemotherapy cyclophosphamide, vincristine, and doxorubicin
B. High-dose meta-iodo-benzyl-guanidine therapy
C. External beam radiation
D. Mitotane

Question 25.29.   All of the following are true regarding carcinoid tumors, EXCEPT:

A. The most common site is the small bowel, followed by the rectum.
B. Diarrhea, flushing, and bronchospasm are classic features.
C. Complete surgical resection of all neoplastic tissue is the preferred therapy.
D. Diarrhea can be controlled with long-acting octreotide.
E. External beam radiation is ineffective in treating this disease.

Question 25.30.   Adrenocortical carcinoma is favored over adenoma by which of the following CT scan features?

A. Size >6 cm
B. Density of <10 Hounsfield units on nonenhanced CT
C. Washout of >50% at 15 minutes after contrast
D. Homogenous appearance

Question 25.31.   All of the following are true about pheochromocytoma, EXCEPT:

A. It arises from the adrenal medulla in 50% of the cases.
B. Most tumors of adrenal origin are not malignant.
C. Extra-adrenal tumors have increased risk of malignancy.
D. It may be associated with mutated RET proto-oncogene.

Question 25.32.   All of the following statements are true regarding mitotane, EXCEPT:

A. It treats metastatic adrenocortical carcinoma.
B. It has significant gastrointestinal and neurological side effects.
C. It can improve hormonal production.
D. Mitotane levels should be monitored.
E. Overall survival benefit has been confirmed.

Question 25.33.   All of the following statements are true regarding insulinoma, EXCEPT:

A. Whipple's triad consists of symptoms of hypoglycemia when blood glucose decreases and relief of symptoms with correction of glucose levels.
B. It is frequently malignant.
C. Surgery is indicated in most cases.
D. MEN1 should be suspected.

Question 25.34.   Excessive secretion of all the following will lead to diarrhea, EXCEPT:

A. Gastrin
B. Serum vasoactive intestinal peptide
C. 5-Hydroxy indole acetic acid
D. Insulin

Question 25.35.   All of the following are true regarding pancreatic endocrine tumors, EXCEPT:

A. Classified as APUDomas.
B. Gastrinoma is the least malignant.
C. Malignancy is established by the presence of metastasis.
D. Glucagonoma arises from alpha cells.
E. Insulinoma arises from beta cells.

Question 25.36.   All of the following are true regarding papillary thyroid carcinoma EXCEPT:

A. More common in women.
B. Follicular variant papillary thyroid carcinoma carries a worse prognosis.
C. Orphan Annie eye nuclei are characteristic feature of papillary thyroid carcinoma.
D. Median age at diagnosis is about 40 years.

Question 25.37.   All of the following are indications to biopsy a thyroid nodule less than 1 cm, EXCEPT:

A. History of thyroid carcinoma in first-degree relatives
B. History of neck irradiation
C. Nodules that are "hot" on 2-deoxy-2[^{18}F]fluoro-D-glucose positron emission tomography (^{18}FDG-PET) imaging.
D. Normal TSH level

Question 25.38.   All of the following are true regarding thyroid lymphoma, EXCEPT:

A. Usually non-Hodgkin's type
B. Accounts for 1% of all lymphomas
C. More common in men
D. Rarely associated with hyperthyroidism

ANSWERS

Answer 25.1.   **The answer is A.**

Total thyroidectomy alone and without neck dissection is the appropriate initial management in this patient with well-differentiated papillary thyroid carcinoma, especially in the absence of palpable lymph nodes or abnormal lymph nodes on ultrasound.

Answer 25.2.   **The answer is A.**

The patient has microscopic papillary thyroid carcinoma, typically defined as a solitary tumor, less than 1.0 to 1.5 cm, with the absence of lymph node involvement. There is no need for further surgical resection beyond lobectomy and intraoperative examination of the contralateral lobe in this case. Thyroid hormone replacement might be needed postoperatively.

Answer 25.3.   **The answer is C.**

The appropriate management is complete lobectomy and isthmusectomy, to be followed by total thyroidectomy later if malignancy is confirmed. This is especially true in cases of suspected follicular carcinoma because FNA does not distinguish benign from malignant follicular pathology. Intraoperative frozen section would not be of great help in this regard. The finding of vascular or capsular invasion on final pathologic examination will help to determine the diagnosis.

Answer 25.4.   **The answer is B.**

Patients with thyroid carcinoma are typically followed up with TG levels and iodine scan. TG levels are very sensitive, particularly when TSH is suppressed. In the face of negative iodine scan, and particularly when TG level is greater than 10, distant metastatic disease is suspected. PET scan is most helpful in these cases where thyroid cancer dedifferentiates and loses iodine uptake.

Answer 25.5.   **The answer is A.**

MTC is a neuroendocrine tumor. The hallmark is elevated serum calcitonin, which is produced by the parafollicular cells (thyroid C cells). CEA is another tumor marker of this disease, but less specific because it can be elevated in other malignancies. MTC can be part of MEN2A, which includes pheochromocytoma, and it must be ruled out before any surgery. Germ line mutation causes familial non-MEN MTC, MEN2A, and MEN2B. RET proto-oncogene has become a standard test in the evaluation of newly diagnosed MTC.

Answer 25.6.   **The answer is B.**

Radioactive iodine ablation is indicated in patients with high-risk features despite complete excision. Male patients aged more than 40 years are considered to be in this category. Other high-risk features include female patients aged more than 50 years, incomplete excision, capsular invasion, and tumor size more than 5 cm.

Answer 25.7.   **The answer is E.**

This is an example of dedifferentiated papillary thyroid carcinoma, where the cancer no longer shows uptake of iodine but can be detected on PET scan. Another caveat in this case is the recognition of recommended long-term follow-up, perhaps indefinitely. In thyroid carcinoma, TG level is very sensitive, particularly when TSH is suppressed, and this is also true in dedifferentiated thyroid carcinoma. Chemotherapy has been disappointing in this disease. Surgical resection, and perhaps external beam radiation, is his best option to achieve local control and relief of symptoms.

Answer 25.8.   **The answer is D.**

RET/PTC rearrangements are found in about 20% of papillary thyroid carcinoma in general, and in 60% to 80% of those occurring after irradiation. BRAF mutation can be found in patients with papillary thyroid carcinoma, but it is not associated with radiation exposure. APC gene mutation is found in patients with familial adenomatous polyposis, and some of these patients might develop differentiated thyroid carcinoma. RET proto-oncogene mutations are associated with MEN2.

Answer 25.9.   **The answer is D.**

All of the listed features indicate poor prognosis. Additional poor prognostic features include women aged more than 50 years and the presence of distant metastasis. These features can be remembered by the acronym AMES (age, metastasis, extracapsular invasion, size).

Answer 25.10.   **The answer is B.**

This case highlights the importance of the fact that IV contrast with diagnostic CT scan interferes with the thyroid cancer uptake of iodine during radioactive iodine scan. This test should be done at least 6 to 8 weeks after iodine-contrast CT scan to allow the excretion of the circulating iodine pool; 24-hour urinary iodine can be measured before repeat iodine scanning in these cases.

Answer 25.11.   **The answer is D.**

MTC arises from the parafollicular C cells in the thyroid gland and is not associated with radiation exposure. RET proto-oncogene testing is indicated even in the absence of family history. Pheochromocytoma must be ruled out before any surgical resection by measuring metanephrine levels.

Answer 25.12.   **The answer is C.**

Anaplastic thyroid carcinoma remains an incurable cancer. It grows rapidly, and 20% to 50% of cases are associated with distant metastasis.

Median survival is between 3 and 4 months. Surgery is typically reserved for local disease control, particularly in the absence of distant disease. Radioactive iodine is ineffective in the treatment of anaplastic thyroid cancer, and chemotherapy alone has modest effects on local response. This patient is best served with concurrent chemoradiation.

Answer 25.13.   **The answer is E.**

MTCs tend to metastasize early to cervical and mediastinal lymph nodes and later to the liver, bones, and lungs. CEA and calcitonin are useful tumor markers reflecting the disease burden. MTC is of neuroendocrine origin and expresses a high level of somatostatin receptors; thus, it binds to pharmacologic-radiolabeled somatostatin analogs. Octreoscan can be used in selected cases with elevated calcitonin. Only limited evidence showed that PET scan can also be helpful in the imaging of MTC.

Answer 25.14.   **The answer is A.**

Hurthle cell carcinoma, or Oxyphil cell carcinoma, is a variant of follicular cell carcinoma. It has the same malignant features, is known to have poorer outcomes, and is less apt to concentrate radioactive iodine.

Answer 25.15.   **The answer is B.**

Anaplastic thyroid carcinoma represents 1% to 3% of all thyroid cancers and is typically fast growing. It is treated mainly with chemoradiation and perhaps debulking surgery in selected cases, but is considered incurable. It is always considered stage IV because of its extremely poor prognosis, with a median survival of only 3 to 4 months.

Answer 25.16.   **The answer is D.**

Doxorubicin is the most commonly used single chemotherapeutic agent in metastatic thyroid carcinoma, with a modest partial response rate reported to be approximately 30%. Taxanes are another group of agents that has also been used in the treatment of metastatic thyroid carcinoma.

Answer 25.17.   **The answer is B.**

Parathyroid carcinoma is a rare cancer. Surgery is the standard treatment approach. Adjuvant external beam irradiation has been shown to reduce the rate of recurrence. Resection of other uninvolved parathyroid glands is not indicated because parathyroid carcinoma typically originates from one parathyroid gland. Radioactive iodine, as well as chemotherapy, is not generally effective in the treatment of parathyroid carcinoma. Bone pain, pathologic fracture, or other evidence of bone disease occurs in approximately 90% of patients, and renal stones occur in 50% to 80% of patients.

Answer 25.18.   **The answer is E.**

All of the mentioned options can be used in this case, but perhaps not all are needed at the same time. IV hydration and IV bisphosphonate represent the most widely used methods to treat malignant hypercalcemia. Mithramycin has been used in the past to treat metastatic parathyroid carcinoma. Cinacalcet (Sensipar) directly lowers PTH levels by increasing the sensitivity of calcium-sensing receptors on chief cells of the parathyroid gland to extracellular calcium. It also results in concomitant serum calcium decrease. Calcitonin can also be used to treat hypercalcemia and has an analgesic effect in cases of pathologic fracture.

Answer 25.19.   **The answer is A.**

Several genetic defects have been reported to be associated with parathyroid cancer. Mutations of the HRPT2 gene (1q25-31) have been described in this disease, most commonly in association with the hyperparathyroidism jaw tumor syndrome. However, many sporadic parathyroid carcinomas exhibit defects in this gene. This gene codes for a tumor suppressor protein called "parafibromin," whose function is not yet known. Allelic loss in several chromosomes has been noted, but other than HRPT2, no gene has definitively been associated with parathyroid carcinoma. RET proto-oncogene mutation is not associated with parathyroid carcinoma.

Answer 25.20.   **The answer is A.**

Parathyroid cancer is rare enough that no staging system has been established. A palpable mass is virtually never present with benign parathyroid adenomas or hyperplasia. The reported overall 5-year survival rate is approximately 50% to 75%.

Answer 25.21.   **The answer is B.**

This patient has MEN1 syndrome because his presentation includes pituitary adenoma and hyperparathyroidism. Prolactin-producing pituitary adenomas are treated initially with dopamine agonists; transsphenoidal resection is reserved as a second-line treatment. Subtotal parathyroidectomy (or total parathyroidectomy with autotransplantation of a parathyroid tissue in the arm) is the standard approach in treating hyperparathyroidism in MEN1 syndrome. Further evaluation is warranted to exclude pancreatic neuroendocrine tumors possibly producing gastrin, especially in the presence of gastrointestinal symptoms.

Answer 25.22.   **The answer is C.**

Hyperparathyroidism is the most common manifestation in this disorder. The other endocrine disorders include pituitary adenomas, pancreatic neuroendocrine tumors, carcinoid tumors, and occasionally adrenocortical adenomas. Other manifestations include lipomas, collagenomas, and angiofibromas.

Answer 25.23.   **The answer is D.**

Virtually 100% of patients with MEN2A have C-cell hyperplasia or MTC; 50% have pheochromocytoma, and 20% to 30% have hyperparathyroidism. Diffuse neuronal hypertrophy is part of MEN2B.

Answer 25.24.   **The answer is A.**

The gene MEN2A is the RET proto-oncogene, located at the centromeric region of chromosome 10 (10q11-2). Data are accumulating regarding genotype-phenotype correlations and mutations in various RET codons. A negative family history is not reliable because of the variable age of clinical presentation that can affect the identification of clinical cases. Thus, family members should be screened.

Answer 25.25.   **The answer is B.**

The MENIN gene was recently identified, and it is localized on the long arm of chromosome 11.

Answer 25.26.   **The answer is D.**

The RET proto-oncogene mutation is associated with MEN2 and Hirschsprung disease.

Answer 25.27.   **The answer is B.**

The development of amenorrhea, acne, hirsutism, and rapidly progressive Cushing's syndrome in a woman is a typical presentation of adrenal carcinoma. Complete metabolic workup is indicated before any intervention. Approximately 50% of adrenocortical neoplasms have features of hormonal hypersecretion. Surgical resection represents the standard treatment in localized tumors. Mitotane is given in metastatic disease and as adjuvant therapy. Hormonal hypersecretion can be medically controlled: Effective agents include ketoconazole, aminoglutethimide, and metyrapone.

Answer 25.28.   **The answer is D.**

The cyclophosphamide, vincristine, and doxorubicin regimen has been the most used chemotherapy regimen in patients with metastatic pheochromocytoma. External beam radiation can palliate metastatic bone lesions. I131 meta-iodo-benzyl-guanidine leads to a response rate of approximately 40%. Mitotane is used to treat metastatic adrenocortical carcinoma and not pheochromocytoma.

Answer 25.29.   **The answer is E.**

Carcinoid tumors are responsive to higher doses of external beam radiation, with a response rate of 40% to 50%.

Answer 25.30.   **The answer is A.**

Size more than 6 cm should raise the possibility of adrenocortical carcinoma. The other features are suggestive of benign adrenal adenoma.

Answer 25.31.   **The answer is A.**

Pheochromocytoma arises from the adrenal medulla in 90% of cases, where most are not malignant. Extra-adrenal lesions have increased risk of malignancy. The diagnosis is based on measuring catecholamines and metabolites in the serum and/or urine. Mutated RET proto-oncogene has been associated with bilateral pheochromocytomas, but it has not been associated with extra-adrenal pheochromocytoma.

Answer 25.32.   **The answer is E.**

Only limited evidence from retrospective reviews suggested improved disease-free survival with adjuvant mitotane therapy. Mitotane is associated with a wide range of side effects, especially gastrointestinal and neurologic symptoms. Mitotane levels must be followed closely to guide therapy.

Answer 25.33.   **The answer is B.**

Insulinomas are usually benign, with only 5% to 10% of cases being malignant. Documentation of metastasis is the only definitive way to diagnose malignant disease.

Answer 25.34.   **The answer is D.**

Secretory diarrhea is commonly associated with all the listed hormones except insulin.

Answer 25.35.   **The answer is B.**

The percentage of tumors of the endocrine pancreas that are malignant ranges from 10% for insulinoma, to 50% for glucagonoma, and to at least 65% for gastrinoma.

Answer 25.36.   **The answer is B.**

Papillary thyroid carcinomas are more common in women than men and the median age at diagnosis is 40 and 41 years. Orphan Annie nuclei are a characteristic histologic feature of papillary thyroid carcinomas. The prognosis for follicular variant papillary thyroid cancer is similar to papillary thyroid carcinomas.

Answer 25.37.   **The answer is D.**

Thyroid nodules less than 1 cm in size are not routinely biopsied; however, there are specific situations where a biopsy may be indicated. Patients with family history of thyroid cancer, neck irradiation, and nodules that are positive on the PET scan are all indication for biopsy. A normal TSH level is not indicative of malignancy.

Answer 25.38.   **The answer is C.**

Thyroid lymphomas are rare disease accounting for 1% of all lymphomas and the vast majority is non-Hodgkin's type. There is a female predominance with this disease and it is usually associated with hypothyroidism, not hyperthyroidism.

CHAPTER 26 SARCOMAS

DOUGLAS R. ADKINS • BRIAN A. VAN TINE • TONI B. RACHOCKI

DIRECTIONS   Each of the numbered items below is followed by lettered answers. Select the ONE lettered answer that is BEST in each case unless instructed otherwise.

QUESTIONS

Question 26.1.   Which of the following inherited syndromes represent a predisposing factor for the development of soft tissue sarcoma?

A. Retinoblastoma
B. Li-Fraumeni syndrome
C. Neurofibromatosis type I
D. All of the above

Question 26.2.   Which of the following is NOT true about radiation-induced sarcomas?

A. Cancer history usually includes breast cancer, lymphoma, and cervical cancer.
B. These sarcomas have a favorable prognosis.
C. Osteogenic sarcoma, malignant fibrous histiocytoma (MFH), angiosarcoma, and lymphangiosarcoma are the usual histologic subtypes.
D. They usually occur 10 to 30 years after radiation exposure.

Question 26.3.   Which clonal cytogenetic abnormality is associated with the correct sarcoma subtype?

A. Ewing's sarcoma and $t(11; 22)$ (q24; q12)
B. Synovial sarcoma and $t(12; 16)$ (q13; p11)
C. Myxoid liposarcoma and $t(x; 18)$ (p11; q11)
D. Alveolar rhabdomyosarcoma and $t(17; 22)$ (q22; q13)

Question 26.4.   A 20-year-old man presents with right knee pain. X-ray reveals a "sunburst" appearance in the distal femur. Biopsy reveals high-grade osteosarcoma. No distant metastases are identified. Which of the following is the most appropriate treatment?

A. Limb-sparing resection
B. Limb-sparing resection and adjuvant chemotherapy
C. Definitive radiation
D. Neoadjuvant chemotherapy, limb-sparing resection, and adjuvant chemotherapy

---

Corresponding Chapters in *Cancer: Principles & Practice of Oncology*, Ninth Edition: 114 (Molecular Biology of Sarcomas), 115 (Soft Tissue Sarcoma), and 116 (Sarcomas of Bone).

Question 26.5.   In addition to site, which of the following variables is used to estimate the risk of sarcoma-specific death for a given patient?

A. Tumor grade and histology
B. Tumor size and depth
C. Age
D. All of the above

Question 26.6.   Which of the following is NOT true regarding the staging of soft tissue sarcomas?

A. Stage II includes small (<5 cm) high-grade tumors without metastases.
B. Stage IV includes distant but not nodal metastases.
C. All low-grade tumors are classified as stage I if not metastatic.
D. Histologic grade, size, depth, and presence or absence of nodal and distant metastases are variables used to determine tumor stage.

Question 26.7.   A 52-year-old man underwent resection of a 3-cm mass from the lateral left thigh. Pathology revealed a high-grade leiomyosarcoma, and the lateral surgical margin was positive. The most appropriate next step in the treatment of this patient's cancer would be:

A. Radiation
B. Adjuvant chemotherapy
C. Re-resection
D. Observation

Question 26.8.   A 68-year-old woman presented with a purplish nodular lesion in the occipital scalp. Resection revealed an angiosarcoma measuring 3 cm. Surgical margins were negative. What is the most appropriate next step in the treatment of this patient's cancer?

A. Radiologic imaging to look for nodal metastases and referral for adjuvant radiation
B. Monitoring
C. Adjuvant chemotherapy with an anthracycline
D. Adjuvant chemotherapy with paclitaxel

Question 26.9.   A 65-year-old woman presented with abdominal pain and iron-deficiency anemia. Workup revealed a gastric mass and multiple large intra-abdominal masses and liver hypodensities. Biopsy of the gastric mass revealed a spindle cell neoplasm thought to be a leiomyosarcoma. After three cycles of doxorubicin and ifosfamide, imaging showed disease progression. The appropriate next step in the management of this patient's cancer would be:

A. Docetaxel and gemcitabine
B. Dacarbazine
C. Request the pathologist to perform a CD117 (c-Kit) stain
D. Palliative radiation

Question 26.10. A 55-year-old man presented with a 10-cm mass in the medial left thigh. Biopsy revealed a high-grade liposarcoma. Imaging revealed no evidence of distant metastases. The most appropriate treatment of this patient's cancer would be:

A. Definitive radiation
B. Definitive radiation and concurrent doxorubicin
C. Limb-sparing resection followed by adjuvant radiation
D. Preoperative chemotherapy followed by resection

Question 26.11. A 52-year-old man with metastatic unresectable gastrointestinal stromal tumor (GIST) was treated with imatinib (400 mg/d). Imaging showed initial disease response; however, the disease progressed after 28 months on therapy. The most appropriate treatment would be:

A. Erlotinib
B. Sunitinib
C. Doxorubicin
D. Imatinib 600 or 800 mg/d

Question 26.12. The following factors are independent predictors of poorer disease-specific survival in patients with nonmetastatic soft tissue sarcoma, EXCEPT:

A. Large tumor size (>10 cm)
B. High-grade histology
C. Extremity site
D. Older age (>60 years)

Question 26.13. A 48-year-old woman underwent complete resection of a 9-cm high-grade leiomyosarcoma arising in the lower extremity. Postoperative adjuvant radiation was administered. Two years later, a chest computed tomography (CT) scan revealed a new single 3-cm, round, noncalcified pulmonary nodule. What is the most appropriate next treatment?

A. Complete resection of the lung nodule
B. Radiation
C. Ifosfamide and doxorubicin
D. Docetaxel and gemcitabine

Question 26.14. Which of the following are FALSE about patients with metastatic or locally recurrent soft tissue sarcoma?

A. Median survival is 12 months, although 20% to 25% of patients are alive 2 years after diagnosis.
B. Complete resection of oligometastases to the lung can result in 5-year survivorship in 20% to 30% of patients.
C. Re-resection is the preferred treatment of a locally recurrent sarcoma.
D. Combination chemotherapy improves overall survival compared with single-agent chemotherapy.

Question 26.15.   Which of the following is TRUE about chemotherapy treatment of metastatic soft tissue sarcoma?

A. Escalating doses of doxorubicin or ifosfamide do not improve tumor response rates over standard doses of these agents.
B. Leiomyosarcoma is uniquely sensitive to ifosfamide, whereas synovial cell sarcoma is not.
C. Paclitaxel shows broad-spectrum activity.
D. Dacarbazine has modest activity.

Question 26.16.   A 30-year-old man presents with a permeative bone tumor in the distal femur. Open biopsy reveals a MFH. Radiologic imaging does not find distant metastases. What is the most appropriate treatment?

A. Limb-sparing resection with wide margins
B. Definitive radiation
C. Chemotherapy
D. Preoperative chemotherapy, limb-sparing resection, and adjuvant chemotherapy

Question 26.17.   Which of the following is NOT true regarding osteosarcoma?

A. Approximately 20% of patients with localized high-grade disease treated with resection alone remain disease free 5 years later.
B. Approximately 60% to 80% of patients with localized high-grade disease treated with resection and chemotherapy remain disease free 5 years later.
C. Parosteal (low-grade cortical) osteosarcoma is best treated with resection and chemotherapy.
D. Periosteal osteosarcoma is best treated with resection and chemotherapy.

Question 26.18.   A 45-year-old man presents with a left-sided pelvic pain. CT reveals a 5 cm mass with appearance of chondroid matrix, arising from the left side of the pelvic girdle. Bone biopsy reveals chondrosarcoma. Which of the following is NOT true regarding chondrosarcomas?

A. Most are low-grade tumors.
B. Most are treated with resection.
C. Children have a poorer prognosis than adults.
D. Adjuvant chemotherapy has no role in the management of non-metastatic disease.

Question 26.19.   A 22-year-old woman presents with a giant cell tumor (GCT) of the distal femur. Appropriate treatment would be:

A. Curettage and debridement
B. Amputation
C. Radiation
D. Preoperative chemotherapy, resection, and adjuvant chemotherapy

Question 26.20.   A 16-year-old female patient presents with a painful rapidly growing scapular mass. Core needle biopsy reveals a Ewing's sarcoma. Staging evaluation shows no evidence of metastatic disease. The most appropriate therapy is:

A. Resection
B. Preoperative chemotherapy (with vincristine, doxorubicin, and cyclophosphamide alternating with ifosfamide and etoposide, IE), resection, and adjuvant chemotherapy
C. Resection and radiation
D. Preoperative chemotherapy (with vincristine, doxorubicin, and cyclophosphamide), resection, and adjuvant chemotherapy

Question 26.21.   A 25-year-old woman presents with a painless right thigh mass, which has been slowly growing over a span of 8 years. Core needle biopsy reveals alveolar soft part sarcoma. What cytogenetic abnormality would you expect to see in this tumor?

A. $t(11,22)$ (q24;q12)
B. $t(12;16)$ (q13;p11)
C. der (17) $t(X;17)$ (p11;q25)
D. $t(X;18)$ (p11,q11)

Question 26.22.   Which of the following targeted agents is used to treat alveolar soft tissue sarcoma?

A. Imatinib
B. Sunitinib
C. Dasatinib
D. Nilotinib

Question 26.23.   Which of the following sites of soft tissue sarcomas carries the best prognosis?

A. Head and neck
B. Extremity
C. Visceral
D. Retroperitoneal

ANSWERS

Answer 26.1.   **The answer is D.**

Patients with Li-Fraumeni syndrome have an increased risk for developing soft tissue sarcomas. Neurofibromatosis type I increases the risk for the development of malignant peripheral nerve sheath tumors. Patients with retinoblastoma also have an increased risk for developing soft tissue sarcomas.

Answer 26.2.   **The answer is B.**

Radiation-induced sarcomas usually occur 10 to 30 years after exposure to radiation. The most common cancers for which radiation was administered include breast and cervical cancer, and lymphoma. Most radiation-induced sarcomas are osteogenic sarcoma or MFH, and the prognosis is poor.

Answer 26.3.   **The answer is A.**

Ewing's sarcoma is associated with five known cytogenetic abnormalities, including $t(11; 22)$ $(q24; q12)$. Synovial sarcoma is associated with $t(x; 18)$ $(p11; q11)$, whereas myxoid liposarcoma is associated with $t(12; 16)$ $(q13; p11)$. Alveolar rhabdomyosarcoma is associated with $t(2; 13)$ $(q35; q14)$.

Answer 26.4.   **The answer is D.**

The current standard of care for the treatment of osteosarcomas is neoadjuvant chemotherapy, followed by limb-sparing resection and adjuvant chemotherapy. The percentage of tumor cell necrosis on pathology from the resection gives an idea of prognosis and helps determine the adjuvant chemotherapy regimen. Surgery alone, or definitive radiation, offers lower chances of success.

Answer 26.5.   **The answer is D.**

The Memorial Sloan Kettering Cancer Center (MSKCC) nomogram for sarcoma-specific mortality incorporates the following variables: age, tumor size, depth, histology, grade of tumor, and site. Zero points are assigned for the low-risk features (age 16, size ≤5 cm, superficial depth, fibrosarcoma histology, low grade and upper extremity site). A sum of the points assigned for each variable helps predict the risk of sarcoma-specific death.

Answer 26.6.   **The answer is B.**

Stage IV disease includes the presence of nodal or distant metastases. The prognosis of patients with small (<5 cm) high-grade soft tissue sarcomas without metastases is similar to that of other patients with stage II disease. Stage I disease includes only low-grade tumors. Staging of soft tissue sarcoma requires knowledge of histologic grade, size, depth, and presence of metastatic disease.

Answer 26.7.   **The answer is C.**

Positive surgical margin predicts a higher risk of local recurrence. Re-resection in an attempt to achieve negative surgical margins would be the next most appropriate step in the management of this patient. If negative surgical margins are achieved after re-resection, adjuvant radiation would not be required. Adjuvant chemotherapy would have no clear benefit in this case.

Answer 26.8.   **The answer is A.**

Soft tissue sarcoma of the head and neck is associated with a poor prognosis. Angiosarcoma has a higher risk of nodal metastases and local recurrence after resection alone. Adjuvant radiation reduces the risk of local and regional disease recurrence. Although angiosarcomas tend to be sensitive to anthracyclines and taxanes, there would be no known benefit of adjuvant chemotherapy in this case.

Answer 26.9.   **The answer is C.**

Intra-abdominal leiomyosarcomas and GISTs have similar characteristics by light microscopy; however, GISTs stain positive for the CD117 (c-Kit) protein, whereas leiomyosarcomas usually do not. Leiomyosarcomas frequently respond to chemotherapy, whereas GISTs do not. However, GISTs are uniquely responsive to c-Kit inhibitors. In this case, a c-Kit immunostain should be requested to determine whether the sarcoma is a GIST and not a leiomyosarcoma. Because this patient has metastatic disease, systemic therapy would be favored over palliative radiation.

Answer 26.10.   **The answer is C.**

Resection of the primary tumor with intent to achieve negative surgical margins followed by adjuvant radiation would be the most appropriate treatment of a large high-grade extremity liposarcoma. Definitive radiation with or without concurrent chemotherapy would be less effective treatment. Preoperative chemotherapy may be used when the tumor is marginally resectable, but its role in this situation is controversial.

Answer 26.11.   **The answer is D.**

Studies have demonstrated that approximately one-third of patients with GIST resistant to imatinib 400 mg/d will benefit with increasing the dose of imatinib to 600 or 800 mg/d. Should that step fail, sunitinib would be the next most appropriate therapy. GIST is generally resistant to chemotherapy drugs, such as doxorubicin. Epidermal growth factor receptor inhibitors, such as erlotinib, would not be expected to benefit patients with GIST.

Answer 26.12.   **The answer is C.**

Independent predictors of prognosis of patients with nonmetastatic soft tissue sarcoma include age, histologic subtype, histologic grade, tumor site, and tumor size. Factors predictive of better disease-specific survival include younger age, selected histologic subtypes (fibrosarcoma), low histologic grade, smaller (<5 cm) tumor size, and extremity location. Nomograms are available that accurately predict the prognosis of patients with nonmetastatic soft tissue sarcoma treated with surgery with or without adjuvant radiation.

Answer 26.13.   **The answer is A.**

In this patient, the most likely cause of the new lung nodule is metastases of the leiomyosarcoma. Retrospective series have observed that 20% to 30% of such patients who undergo complete resection of the lung metastases were alive 5 years later. Factors that predict for a lower success rate with resection in such patients include more than four lung nodules, bilateral lung nodules, and a disease-free interval of less than 12 months. Chemotherapy and radiation provide only palliative intent in this case.

Answer 26.14.   **The answer is D.**

For locally recurrent sarcoma without distant metastases, re-resection is the preferred treatment. For patients with metastatic sarcoma, median survival is 1 year; however, a subset of these patients live for more than 2 years. It is important to consider complete resection of oligometastases to the lung because approximately 25% of those patients will be alive 5 years later. Nearly all randomized trials have shown no overall survival benefit with combination (vs. single agent) chemotherapy, although tumor response rates were consistently higher. A single, recent randomized trial demonstrated a modest survival benefit with the addition of docetaxel to gemcitabine in patients with metastatic sarcoma.

Answer 26.15.   **The answer is D.**

Several studies have shown higher tumor response rates (but not improved survival) with larger doses of doxorubicin and ifosfamide; however, this does result in greater toxicity. Ifosfamide is an active agent in synovial cell sarcoma but has little activity in leiomyosarcoma. Paclitaxel appears to only be effective in the treatment of angiosarcoma and Kaposi's sarcoma. Perhaps the first drug identified to be active in adult soft tissue sarcoma, dacarbazine resulted in tumor response rates of 10% to 30%.

Answer 26.16.   **The answer is D.**

In contrast with MFH of soft tissue, which is primarily treated with resection, MFH of bone is treated like high-grade osteosarcoma with preoperative chemotherapy, limb-sparing resection, and adjuvant chemotherapy. Outcomes of patients with MFH of bone and with osteosarcoma are similar when treated this way. Limb-sparing resection alone or definitive radiation would offer lower chances of success. Chemotherapy alone would provide palliation, but the chance of cure is unclear.

Answer 26.17.   **The answer is C.**

Parosteal osteosarcoma is usually a low-grade tumor that involves the bone cortex and is associated with a better prognosis than classic osteosarcoma. Resection is the preferred treatment, and there is no clear role for chemotherapy. In contrast, periosteal osteosarcoma is an aggressive, high-grade cortical sarcoma that is best treated like classic osteosarcoma with resection and chemotherapy. For classic high-grade osteosarcoma, resection alone is curative in 20%, but the addition of chemotherapy to resection improves cure rates to 60% to 80%.

Answer 26.18.   **The answer is D.**

The preferred therapy for chondrosarcoma is resection. Although chondrosarcomas as a group are known to be resistant to chemotherapy, mesenchymal and dedifferentiated chondrosarcomas have a high metastatic potential and appears to benefit from adjuvant chemotherapy. Most chondrosarcomas are low grade and usually occur in patients aged more than 40 years. Children have a worse prognosis than adults.

Answer 26.19.   **The answer is A.**

GCT of bone is a tumor with a high risk for local recurrence but a low risk for distal metastases. Appropriate treatment is resection, preferably by curettage and debridement. Amputation is reserved for massive local recurrences. Radiation is reserved for lesions of the spine that can lead to cord compression. There is no benefit of preoperative or adjuvant chemotherapy for GCT of bone.

Answer 26.20.   **The answer is B.**

A randomized trial of patients with Ewing's sarcoma treated with either vincristine, doxorubicin, and cyclophosphamide (VAC) alone or alternating with IE given as preoperative and adjuvant chemotherapy clearly showed an overall survival and progression-free survival advantage with the alternating regimen of VAC and IE versus VAC alone in patients with nonmetastatic (but not in patients with metastatic) disease. Resection alone or with radiation would be significantly less effective than when used in combination with chemotherapy.

Answer 26.21.   **The answer is C.**

Alveolar soft part sarcoma is associated with der (17) t(X;17) (p11,q25). Ewing's sarcoma is associated with five known cytogenetic abnormalities, including t(11; 22) (q24; q12). Synovial sarcoma is associated with t(X;18) (p11; q11), whereas myxoid liposarcoma is associated with t(12; 16) (q13; p11).

Answer 26.22.   **The answer is B.**

Sunitinib is an oral small molecule, multitargeted receptor tyrosine kinase inhibitor that is an active agent in the treatment of alveolar soft part sarcoma. Imatinib, dasatinib, and nilotinib are tyrosine kinase inhibitors that have activity against GIST. Sunitinib also is used to treat GIST.

Answer 26.23.   **The answer is B.**

Extremity soft tissue sarcomas have the best prognosis, followed by visceral and retroperitoneal. Head and neck soft tissue sarcomas carry the worst prognosis.

GERALD P. LINETTE

QUESTIONS

Question 27.1.   **What are the most common sites of melanoma in men?**

    A. Trunk and head and neck
    B. Head and neck and upper limb
    C. Upper limb and trunk
    D. Lower limb and upper limb
    E. Lower limb and trunk

Question 27.2.   **Recent epidemiologic data suggest that the incidence and mortality of melanoma is increasing in which of the following populations:**

    A. Young adults
    B. Women aged 50 to 64 years
    C. Infants
    D. Men aged 65 to 74 years

Question 27.3.   **Which of the following statements regarding the anatomic distribution of melanoma is FALSE?**

    A. Cutaneous melanoma can occur at any site.
    B. Acral and mucosal melanoma occur at a much higher frequency in non-Caucasians compared with Caucasian populations.
    C. Ocular melanoma is more common in Caucasians.
    D. The most common sites for cutaneous melanoma in women are the back and head and neck area.

Question 27.4.   **Risk factors for cutaneous melanoma include all of the following, EXCEPT:**

    A. Prior scalp radiation
    B. Inherited mutation of p16(CDKN2A)
    C. Higher socioeconomic status
    D. Pregnancy

Corresponding Chapters in *Cancer: Principles & Practice of Oncology,* Ninth Edition: 117 (Cancer of the Skin) and 118 (Molecular Biology of Cutaneous Melanoma), and 119 (Cutaneous Melanoma).

Question 27.5.   A healthy 42-year-old woman was recently found to have a 2.4-mm Breslow thickness nonulcerated primary cutaneous superficial spreading melanoma. The pigmented lesion was excised from her left lower extremity by her local dermatologist. The physician calls you for advice regarding further evaluation. Your recommendation is which of the following:

A. Referral to a medical oncologist for a clinical trial
B. Body positron emission tomography/computed tomography (PET-CT) scan for initial staging
C. Referral to a surgeon for wide local excision and sentinel lymph node mapping
D. Annual follow-up for skin checks

Question 27.6.   A 56-year-old man was recently diagnosed with a stage IIa primary cutaneous melanoma (T2b N0 Mx). What is the most appropriate recommendation for clinical follow-up?

A. Annual visit with a dermatologist
B. Office visits with a dermatologist every 3 months for 3 years, every 6 months for 2 years, and then annually for life
C. Office visits with a dermatologist every 3 months for 3 years, every 6 months for 2 years, and then annually for life plus body PET-CT imaging every 6 months for life
D. Office visits with a dermatologist every 3 months for life

Question 27.7.   Indications for radiation therapy in the treatment of melanoma include which of the following:

A. Symptomatic brain metastases
B. Choroidal melanoma
C. Symptomatic bone metastases
D. All of the above

Question 27.8.   The MOST common first metastatic site for ocular melanoma is:

A. Brain
B. Lung
C. Liver
D. Skin

Question 27.9.   What stage best defines a patient with a 3 mm ulcerated tumor, 4 regional lymph nodes involved and no detectable distant metastases?

A. T3bN2b (IIIA)
B. T3aN2b (IIIB)
C. T3bN3 (IIIB)
D. T3bN3 (IIIC)

Question 27.10. Which of the following statements regarding adjuvant therapy is TRUE?

A. Isolated limb perfusion has been shown to increase the overall survival for patients with surgically resected stage III melanoma in randomized clinical trials.

B. High-dose interferon has been shown to increase the relapse-free survival for patients with surgically resected stage III melanoma.

C. Radiation therapy has been shown to increase the overall survival for patients with surgically resected stage III melanoma.

D. High-dose chemotherapy with hematopoietic stem cell transplantation can increase the overall survival for patients with stage III surgically resected melanoma.

Question 27.11. Surgical resection for metastatic melanoma may be appropriate in which of these instances?

A. Symptomatic brain metastases

B. Bowel obstruction caused by small bowel metastases

C. Symptomatic adrenal metastases

D. All of the above

Question 27.12. Ipilimumab (human anti-CTLA-4 monoclonal antibody) was approved in 2011 for the treatment of unresectable or metastatic melanoma. Ipilimumab is administered intravenously over 90 minutes, every 3 weeks (for up to 4 doses). Which of the following statements is TRUE regarding ipilimumab?

A. Immune-mediated enterocolitis is the most common serious adverse event seen in patients treated with ipilimumab.

B. Premedication with ondansetron and dexamethasone is recommended prior to each dose of ipilimumab.

C. Weekly monitoring of complete blood count (CBC) is recommended during treatment with ipilimumab.

D. Ipilimumab is contraindicated in patients over 65 years of age due to poor efficacy.

Question 27.13. Which of the following statements regarding BRAF is TRUE?

A. The BRAF mutation V600E is more common in chronically sun-damaged skin.

B. BRAF is a downstream target of the phosphatidylinositol 3-kinase (PI3K) pathway.

C. The response rate to PLX4032 (the oral BRAF inhibitor, vemurafenib), in patients with metastatic melanoma, is 50%, using the RECIST criteria.

D. A and C.

Question 27.14.   A 65-year-old man with metastatic Merkel cell carcinoma is referred to you for evaluation. CT imaging reveals bilateral pulmonary metastases. What is the MOST appropriate initial therapy?

A. High-dose interleukin-2
B. Platinum-based chemotherapy
C. Imatinib
D. Referral to a surgical oncologist

Question 27.15.   Which statement regarding actinic keratosis (AK) is NOT TRUE?

A. AKs are caused by ultraviolet (UV) B.
B. AKs may progress to invasive squamous cell carcinomas.
C. Cure rates for cryosurgery in solitary lesions are 98%
D. None of the above.

Question 27.16.   Which statement regarding basal cell carcinoma is NOT TRUE?

A. It is a slow growing neoplasm.
B. Most common human cancer.
C. The most common subtype is the superficial.
D. May occur in areas not exposed to the sun.

Question 27.17.   A 45-year-old woman was recently diagnosed with metastatic melanoma. The CT examination reveals bilateral lung metastases and a 2-cm solitary liver metastasis. The brain MRI examination is normal. The tumor is negative for the BRAF V600E mutation. You recommend ipilimumab (anti-CTLA-4 antibody) as the initial treatment. Two weeks after the second dose, the patient reports 4 loose stools per day. After imodium, the frequency decreases to twice a day. The patient receives the third dose of ipilimumab on schedule. Three days later, she calls complaining of abdominal cramping, subjective fever, and eight loose stools per day. What is the most appropriate management for this patient?

A. Increase the imodium dose and have her call you back in 2 days.
B. A clinical evaluation is necessary to rule out infectious etiology and bowel perforation.
C. Observation for 7 days. If no improvement, the patient should call back with an update.
D. Check CBC and CMP. If normal, prescribe lomotil.

ANSWERS

Answer 27.1.   **The answer is A.**

The most common sites for melanoma in men are trunk and head and neck.

Answer 27.2.   **The answer is D.**

SEER statistics continue to show increasing rates for older men. The median age at diagnosis is 59 years. The age-adjusted incidence is 19.4 per 100,000 men and women per year. The most recent age-adjusted incidence rate for men (aged 65 to 74 years) is 91 (per 100,000) and has increased steadily since 1975. In comparison, the rate for women (aged 65 to 74 years) is 37 (per 100,000).

Answer 27.3.   **The answer is D.**

The most common site of primary cutaneous melanoma in women is the lower extremities. In men, the most common sites are the head and neck area and the back.

Answer 27.4.   **The answer is D.**

Prior scalp radiation (during childhood), familial p16 mutation, and higher socioeconomic status have all been shown to be risk factors for cutaneous melanoma. In contrast, pregnancy is not considered to be a risk factor for the development of primary or recurrent melanoma.

Answer 27.5.   **The answer is C.**

The management of primary cutaneous melanoma is straightforward. It is essential that primary care providers have a firm understanding of the guidelines to expedite referral to the appropriate surgical specialist. Excisional biopsy is the preferred method for diagnosis of most pigmented lesions and permits the accurate assessment of primary depth (Breslow thickness). Intraoperative lymphatic mapping with sentinel node biopsy remains the standard approach at major centers. Sentinel node mapping is performed for primary lesions 1 mm or more in depth and selected thin (<1 mm) lesions with features of regression or ulceration, high mitotic rate, and positive deep margin.

Body fluorodeoxyglucose (FDG) PET-CT imaging as an initial staging procedure is not recommended unless clinically indicated on the basis of history and physical examination. Clinical research provides strong evidence that the sensitivity of standard FDG-PET imaging is inadequate to detect micrometastasis in draining nodal basins. Finally, there is no standard adjuvant therapy currently recommended for patients with stage IIA (T3a N0 Mx) cutaneous melanoma. Oncology referral should be made after the pathologic staging is completed.

Answer 27.6.   **The answer is B.**

The current National Comprehensive Cancer Network (NCCN) guide-lines call for physical examination focused on skin and regional lymph nodes plus any new areas of clinical concern based on patient history. Routine imaging is limited to annual chest radiography in asymptomatic patients. Routine surveillance PET-CT scans every 6 months are not indicated in stage I/II melanoma. However, if clinically indicated (i.e., new symptoms), appropriate imaging is warranted for patients with a history of stage I-II-IIIA melanoma. For patients at higher risk for recurrence (stage IIIB to IIIC and surgically resected stage IV), periodic surveillance imaging is warranted.

Answer 27.7.   **The answer is D.**

Palliative radiation therapy is indicated for these three indications. In addition, patients with symptomatic cutaneous or subcutaneous metastases can often be palliated by radiation therapy.

Answer 27.8.   **The answer is C.**

Liver metastases are common in recurrent ocular melanoma. More than 90% of patients with metastatic ocular melanoma have liver metastases, often as the initial and sole site of distant disease. Brain metastasis from ocular melanoma is less frequent (>5%) compared with cutaneous melanoma and typically occurs late in the disease course. The median survival for patients with metastatic ocular melanoma is 7 months.

Answer 27.9.   **The answer is D.**

The involvement of four or more regional lymph nodes characterizes N3. In the absence of distant metastases, patients with N3 disease have stage IIIC.

Answer 27.10.   **The answer is B.**

Various clinical trials provide convincing evidence for the relapse-free survival benefit of adjuvant interferon. There are no data to suggest that limb perfusion, radiation therapy, or high-dose chemotherapy can improve survival in patients with surgically resected melanoma.

Answer 27.11.   **The answer is D.**

The three clinical situations listed are all accepted indications for surgical resection in selected patients with metastatic melanoma.

Answer 27.12.   **The answer is A.**

CTLA-4 is a cell surface molecule that regulates T cell activation. Ipili-mumab blocks the interaction of CTLA-4 (present on activated T cells) and its ligands CD80 and CD86 (present on dendritic cells/monocytes) to promote T cell activation and proliferation. Immune-mediated enterocolitis is indeed the most common serious adverse event seen in ipilimumab-treated patients and typically manifests as diarrhea and abdominal pain/cramping. Bowel perforation is uncommon but was seen in less than 1% of patients treated in the phase III trial (NEJM, 2010). In addition, immune-mediated hepatotoxicity, dermatitis, neuropathy, and endocrinopathy (including hypopituitarism) are also seen in patients. Premedication is not necessary; in fact, corticosteroids are contraindicated in patients receiving ipilimumab unless used to treat autoimmune-related toxicities. Myelosuppression is not seen in patients receiving ipilimumab so weekly CBC is unnecessary. Routine laboratories drawn prior to each dose of ipilimumab include CBC, CMP, and TSH. Interestingly, patients over 65 years had similar outcomes in terms of safety and overall survival compared to younger patients.

Answer 27.13.   **The answer is C.**

BRAF, downstream target of Kras in the mitogen-activated protein kinase MAPK pathway, is commonly mutated in melanomas. The V600E mutation appears to occur more commonly in sites of intermittent exposure to UV, whereas melanomas from chronically sun-damaged skin are usually BRAF wild type. The partial response rates according to RECIST criteria to PLX4032 in a phase I trial were 80%. The confirmed response rate to PLX4032 (the oral BRAF inhibitor, vemurafenib) in patients with metastatic melanoma is 48% by RECIST criteria in the phase III trial.

Answer 27.14.   **The answer is B.**

Although response rates are relatively high (>50%) with platinum-based chemotherapy, it is unclear if chemotherapy prolongs survival. In addition to platinum and etoposide, topotecan and doxorubicin are considered active agents in Merkel cell carcinoma. Interleukin-2 and imatinib have not been extensively studied for this disease. Surgical resection would appear to be an option for selected patients with a single distant site in instances that could be rendered disease free; however, most patients with bilateral pulmonary metastases are not generally considered for surgery.

Answer 27.15.   **The answer is D.**

AKs are common lesions in sun-exposed areas and caused by UVB. Treatment is usually indicated since there are no reliable predictors for progression into invasive squamous cell carcinomas. Cure rates from cryosurgery are 98%.

Answer 27.16.   **The answer is C.**

Basal cell carcinoma, the most common human malignancy, has a slow growth and, although more common in sun-exposed areas, may occur in any part of the body. The most common type is the nodular, which accounts for approximately 50% of the cases.

Answer 27.17.   **The answer is B.**

The patient has grade 3 immune-mediated enterocolitis until proven otherwise. A clinical evaluation is necessary prior to the start of treatment in order to rule out bowel perforation by clinical exam as well as any potential infectious cause (stool Clostridium difficile toxin, ova, and parasites). Colonoscopy should be performed if there is a clinical concern or uncertainty. Systemic corticosteroids are indicated in patients with grade 3 immune-mediated enterocolitis at a dose of 1 to 2 mg/kg/day of prednisone or equivalent. Upon improvement to grade 1 or less, the steroids should be tapered slowly over at least 1-month interval. In patients with grade 3 or higher immune-mediated toxicity, the ipilimumab should be permanently discontinued.

CHAPTER 28 NEOPLASMS OF THE CENTRAL NERVOUS SYSTEM

JANAKIRAMAN SUBRAMANIAN • GERALD LINETTE

DIRECTIONS   Each of the numbered items below is followed by lettered answers. Select the ONE lettered answer that is BEST in each case unless instructed otherwise.

QUESTIONS

Question 28.1. Linkage studies have identified genes associated with neurofibromatosis type 2 (NF2), Turcot syndrome, and Li-Fraumeni syndrome in which of the following chromosomes?

A. 10q, 22q, and 17q
B. 22q, 5q, and 17p
C. 5q, 10q, and 17p
D. 5q, 10q, and 17q

Question 28.2. Of the following, the MOST common primary brain tumor in adults in the United States is:

A. Glioblastoma
B. Meningioma
C. Astrocytoma
D. Oligodendroglioma

Question 28.3. The gene that is frequently altered and plays a key role in the development of diffuse fibrillary astrocytoma is:

A. p53
B. K-ras
C. MDM2
D. MDM4

Question 28.4. Primary (de novo) glioblastoma multiforme (GBM) is commonly associated with all of the following, EXCEPT:

A. PTEN inactivation
B. p53 mutation
C. CDKN2A deletion
D. Median age <60 years

Corresponding Chapters in *Cancer: Principles & Practice of Oncology*, Ninth Edition: 120 (Molecular Biology of Central Nervous System Tumors) and 121 (Neoplasms of the Central Nervous System).

Question 28.5.   Which gene mutation identified in GBM is frequently seen in younger patients, and is associated with better prognosis:

    A. EGFR
    B. p53
    C. IDH1
    D. Gain in chromosome 4

Question 28.6.   Loss of heterozygosity of chromosomes 1p and 19q is common in:

    A. GBM
    B. Ependymoma
    C. Oligodendroglioma
    D. Meningioma

Question 28.7.   The central nervous system (CNS) tumor that is commonly associated with NF2 mutations is:

    A. GBM
    B. Spinal ependymoma
    C. Cerebral ependymoma
    D. Oligodendroglioma

Question 28.8.   Patients with GBM have a higher likelihood of responding to therapy with epidermal growth factor receptor tyrosine kinase (EGFR-TK) inhibitors if which of the following biomarkers is present?

    A. Methyl guanine methyl transferase (MGMT) gene cytosine methylation
    B. Activated EGFRvIII
    C. Retained PTEN function
    D. B and C

Question 28.9.   The primary CNS neoplasm that is associated with Epstein-Barr virus (EBV) is:

    A. Primary CNS lymphoma
    B. Ependymoma
    C. Oligodendroglioma
    D. GBM

Question 28.10.   Which of the following tumors exhibit contrast enhancement on magnetic resonance imaging (MRI) scan?

    A. Pilocytic astrocytoma
    B. Grade 2 oligodendroglioma
    C. Grade 2 astrocytoma
    D. None of the above

Question 28.11.   All of the following are associated with poor prognosis in patients with low-grade gliomas, EXCEPT:

A. Age ≥40 years
B. Tumor diameter ≥6 cm
C. Tumor crossing midline
D. Oligodendroglioma

Question 28.12.   A 45-year-old man presents with generalized seizures, and MRI of the brain reveals a nonenhancing mass measuring 7 cm. Biopsy is done, and the tumor histology is reported as grade 2 astrocytoma. The patient undergoes surgery, and a partial (85%–90%) tumor resection is achieved. Further treatment should include:

A. Watchful waiting
B. Chemotherapy
C. Radiotherapy, 50.4 Gy in 1.8 Gy fractions
D. Radiotherapy with chemotherapy (procarbazine, CCNU, and vincristine)

Question 28.13.   In patients with GBM, who have disease recurrence following initial treatment with temozolomide and radiation, the second-line treatment of choice is:

A. Erlotinib
B. Imatinib
C. Topotecan
D. Bevacizumab

Question 28.14.   A 55-year-old man presents with headache and mental status changes. MRI scan of the brain reveals a 5-cm contrast-enhancing mass with surrounding edema. He undergoes stereotactic biopsy revealing GBM. The patient undergoes resection of the tumor, and further treatment should include:

A. Focal external beam irradiation with 45 Gy in 30 fractions plus concurrent temozolomide
B. Focal external beam irradiation with 60 Gy plus a 10 Gy boost plus concurrent temozolomide
C. Focal external beam irradiation with 60 Gy in 30 fractions plus concurrent temozolomide
D. Hyperfractionated dose of 72 Gy in 1.2 Gy fractions plus concurrent temozolomide

Question 28.15.   A 62-year-old man presents with nausea, vomiting, and severe headache. MRI scan of the brain reveals a 5-cm mass in the posterior fossa. The patient undergoes surgical resection of the mass, and pathology is reported as ependymoma. Further treatment should include:

A. Radiation therapy
B. Concurrent chemoradiation with temozolomide
C. Check MGMT methylation status
D. Chemotherapy alone with cisplatin plus etoposide

Question 28.16.   A 53-year-old woman presents with mental status changes; brain MRI identifies a left frontal tumor with dural marginal thickening. She undergoes a resection of the tumor and the involved dural attachments. The histopathology is meningioma, WHO grade I. Further treatment should include:

A. Watchful waiting
B. Adjuvant radiation therapy
C. Chemotherapy
D. Radiosurgery

Question 28.17.   In immunocompetent patients with primary CNS lymphoma, with good performance status and adequate renal function, appropriate first-line therapy comprises of:

A. High-dose methotrexate
B. R-CHOP
C. Whole brain radiation
D. None of the above

Question 28.18.   Long-term follow-up data showed improved survival for patients with GBM, receiving brain radiation with temozolomide compared to radiation alone, with the exception of patients with:

A. Age >50 years
B. Unmethylated MGMT
C. EGFR mutation positive
D. None of the above

Question 28.19.   Which of the following is LEAST commonly associated with craniopharyngioma?

A. Sexual dysfunction
B. Visual dysfunction
C. Hypothyroidism
D. Diabetes insipidus

Question 28.20.   In adult patients diagnosed with ependymoma, the indication for adjuvant radiation therapy after resection is:

A. Supratentorial location
B. High-grade tumors
C. Incomplete resection
D. Poor performance status

Question 28.21.   In patients with anaplastic oligodendrogliomas which gene mutation is an independent prognostic factors for overall survival?

A. IDH1
B. Alk
C. Myc
D. NF2

ANSWERS

Answer 28.1.   **The answer is B.**

Linkage studies have revealed the NF1 gene to reside in chromosome 17q and the NF2 gene to reside in chromosome 22q. For Turcot syndrome, the APC gene has been identified in chromosome 5q. For Li-Fraumeni syndrome, the cancer disposition has been shown to be associated with chromosomes 17p and 22q.

Answer 28.2.   **The answer is B.**

According to data from the Central Brain Tumor Registry of the United States (1998 to 2002), the proportionate distribution of incidence is 30.1% for meningioma, 20.3% for glioblastoma, 9.8% for astrocytoma, and 2.3% for ependymoma.

Answer 28.3.   **The answer is A.**

Alterations of p53 gene are found in 30% of all three grades of astrocytoma. Other reported gene alterations include the amplification of MDM2 or MDM4 gene. Chromosome 9p deletions resulting in loss of the p14 product of the CDKN2A gene have also been reported.

Answer 28.4.   **The answer is D.**

Primary (de novo) GBM is associated with age greater than 62 years, amplified EGFR, wild-type p53, PTEN inactivation, CDKN2A deletion, and decreased survival.

Answer 28.5.   **The answer is C.**

A comprehensive effort to sequence the tumor genome of GBM involved the sequencing of 20,661 genes for somatic mutations from 22 GBM samples. This study also integrated results from copy number and expression analysis of tumor tissue. In addition, to identify previously known dysregulated gene pathways such as p53, EGFR, and PTEN, this study identified mutations involving the isocitrate dehydrogenase 1 (IDH1) gene in 11% of GBM samples. Patients with mutated IDH1 gene were more likely to be younger and had better prognosis than patients with wild-type IDH1, the median survival was 3.7 years versus 1.1 years, respectively ($p < .001$).

Answer 28.6.   **The answer is C.**

Allelic loss of chromosome 1p and 19q occurs in 40% to 80% of grade 2 and 3 oligodendrogliomas. The loss of tumor suppressor genes from these chromosomes is believed to play an important role in the early stage of oligodendroglial tumorigenesis.

Answer 28.7.   **The answer is B.**

Chromosome 22q loss is common in ependymomas; in spinal ependymomas, this loss is associated with mutations of the NF2 gene. In cerebral ependymomas, loss of chromosome 22q is not associated with NF2 mutations.

Answer 28.8.   **The answer is D.**

In a randomized phase III trial, patients with GBM who were positive for MGMT gene methylation and treated with combined temozolomide and radiation had significantly improved survival when compared with patients who were either negative for MGMT gene methylation or received radiation only. In another study, patients with GBM had improved survival when treated with EGFR-TK inhibitors when the tumors expressed the common form of mutated EGFR (activated EGFRvIII) and retained PTEN function compared with patients not expressing both of these biomarkers.

Answer 28.9.   **The answer is A.**

Primary CNS neoplasms are not usually associated with viral infections in humans, except for primary CNS lymphoma, which is strongly associated with EBV. The majority of primary CNS lymphomas are large B-cell histology, and EBV DNA is detectable in most of these tumors. In addition, the incidence of primary CNS lymphoma is higher in patients with HIV infection.

Answer 28.10.   **The answer is A.**

Contrast-enhanced MRI images help differentiate between different types of CNS tumors. MRI also helps to differentiate between high- and low-grade tumors. Low-grade CNS tumors generally do not enhance, except for pilocytic astrocytoma and pleomorphic xanthoastrocytoma.

Answer 28.11.   **The answer is D.**

Multivariate analysis from two large European phase III trials have reported age greater than or equal to 40 years, tumor diameter greater than or equal to 6 cm, tumor crossing the midline, astrocytoma histology, and neurologic deficits to be associated with adverse prognosis.

Answer 28.12.   **The answer is C.**

Radiotherapy is not routinely recommended in patients undergoing resection for low-grade gliomas. In the European Organization for Research and Treatment of Cancer (EORTC) 22845 trial, patients receiving immediate postoperative radiotherapy had a progression-free survival advantage compared with those receiving radiation therapy on tumor progression (5.3 vs. 3.4 years, $p < .0001$). There was no significant difference in overall survival (7.4 years vs. 7.2 years). In another study, age greater than or equal to 40 years, tumor diameter greater than or equal to

6 cm, astrocytoma histology, and incomplete resection were identified as adverse prognostic factors, with the presence of three or more of these factors conferring poor prognosis. In such patients, immediate postoperative radiotherapy is recommended.

Answer 28.13.   **The answer is D.**

The prognosis for recurrent GBM is poor with a median survival of 3 to 9 months when using traditional chemotherapeutic agents. However, several recent publications have demonstrated a significant improvement in patients with recurrent GBM using the angiogenesis inhibitor bevacizumab.

Answer 28.14.   **The answer is C.**

For patients with GBM, standard radiation therapy is 60 Gy in 30 or 33 fractions. The Medical Research Council study reported a survival advantage in patients receiving a 60 Gy dose versus a 45 Gy dose (12 vs. 9 months, $p = .007$). In an RTOG/ECOG study, patients receiving 60 Gy followed by a 10 Gy boost did not have a survival advantage over patients receiving the standard 60 Gy dose. Hyperfractionated and accelerated regimens have likewise not shown survival advantage. In the phase I/II RTOG 8302 study, hyperfractionated doses with 64.8 Gy, 72 Gy, 76.8 Gy, and 81.6 Gy in 1.2 Gy twice daily fractions did not show a survival benefit between the different treatment arms. This study included treatment arms with accelerated hyperfractionated regimens of 48 Gy and 54.4 Gy in 1.6 Gy twice daily fractions, which also did not lead to survival benefit. Adjuvant temozolomide with radiation was shown to improve overall survival compared with radiation alone in a randomized, phase III trial for patients with GBM (14.6 vs. 12.1 months).

Answer 28.15.   **The answer is A.**

Surgical resection is the primary treatment of patients with ependymoma. There are no definitive recommendations for the addition of radiotherapy to the treatment. However, tumors in the posterior fossa cannot always be fully resected, and patients undergoing resection alone have a very high incidence of local recurrence. Therefore, adjuvant focal radiotherapy to the site of the tumor may be added in the treatment of patients with ependymoma. In one study, patients receiving focal radiotherapy of more than 45 Gy to the tumor bed had 5- and 10-year survival rates of 67% and 57%, respectively. The addition of focal radiotherapy has been shown to improve 10-year survival from 67% in patients treated with gross total resection (GTR) alone to 83% in patients treated with GTR and radiotherapy. MGMT gene methylation is associated with better survival in patients with GBM. In ependymomas, there has been no reported association between MGMT gene methylation and survival. There is no evidence to date supporting the use of chemotherapy for treating ependymoma.

Answer 28.16.   **The answer is A.**

Surgical resection is the mainstay for the treatment of meningioma, and it is classified into Simpson grades based on the extent of surgery. Grade 1 is GTR of the tumor, with removal of the dural attachments and hyperostotic bone. The relapse rate after this procedure is 9%. Grade 2 does not include removal of hyperostotic bone (relapse rate 19%). Grade 3 is GTR of the tumor alone (relapse rate 29%). Grade 4 is partial resection (relapse rate 44%). Grade 5 refers to biopsy alone without resection. Adjuvant radiotherapy is not recommended for patients with low-grade meningioma who undergo Simpson grade 1 to 2, and sometimes grade 3, resection. The patient in this case has undergone grade 2 resection for a low-grade meningioma and therefore does not require further radiotherapy. For patients with resected anaplastic and malignant meningioma, adjuvant radiotherapy is recommended. Radiosurgery can be used in patients with unresectable disease, but there is no evidence to support the use of chemotherapy in patients with meningioma. Tamoxifen, mifepristone, and hydroxyurea have not been shown to be effective in this disease.

Answer 28.17.   **The answer is A.**

High-dose methotrexate is the treatment of choice for immunocompetent patients with primary CNS lymphoma. The 5-year survival with high-dose methotrexate treatment is approximately 20%. Whereas whole brain radiation therapy is effective but is associated with serious neurotoxicity and 5-year survival is only 5%. Whole brain radiation is used upfront in patients who are not candidates for methotrexate, due to poor renal function and poor PS. In a phase III, noninferiority trial comparing high-dose methotrexate with or without whole brain radiation therapy showed no significant overall survival benefit to combining whole brain radiation with high-dose methotrexate. R-CHOP is not an appropriate choice for frontline therapy, though it is used to treat many types of non-Hodgkin's lymphoma.

Answer 28.18.   **The answer is D.**

Long-term follow-up data from the phase III EORTC-NCIC trial showed improved survival in all patients treated with combined temozolomide and radiation, followed by adjuvant radiation compared to patients treated with radiation alone.

Answer 28.19.   **The answer is D.**

Some degree of sexual dysfunction occurs in approximately 90% of all adult patients presenting with craniopharyngioma. Visual dysfunction occurs in 40% to 70% of these patients. Hypothyroidism occurs in 40% of patients, and diabetes insipidus occurs in 10% to 20% of patients. However, the incidence of diabetes insipidus after surgical resection increases substantially; in one study, it increased from 16.1% in the preoperative setting to 59.4% after surgery.

Answer 28.20.   The answer is C.

Several retrospective case series have shown that incomplete tumor resection, high tumor grade, supratentorial location, and poor performance status to be associated with poor outcomes in patients with intracranial ependymoma. However, improvement in overall survival with adjuvant radiation is limited to patients with incomplete tumor resection.

Answer 28.21.   The answer is A.

In a retrospective analysis of tumor tissue samples from patients with oligodendrogliomas who received treatment on the EORTC study 26951, both IDH1 and IDH2 mutations were found to be a prognostic marker for overall survival.

# CHAPTER 29 CANCERS OF CHILDHOOD

SHALINI SHENOY

DIRECTIONS   Each of the numbered items below is followed by lettered answers. Select the
ONE lettered answer that is BEST in each case unless instructed otherwise.

QUESTIONS

Question 29.1.   Pediatric malignancies exhibit all of the following characteristics, EXCEPT:

A. Aggressive, rapid growth
B. Short latency period
C. Associated with exposure to carcinogens
D. Familial association in 10% to 15% of cases

Question 29.2.   Genetic abnormalities predispose to malignant disorders in children because of:

A. Abnormal mechanisms of genomic DNA repair
B. Constitutional activation of molecular pathways of deregulated cellular growth and proliferation
C. Increased function of oncogenes or inactivation of tumor suppressor genes
D. All of the above

Question 29.3.   Which of these cancer predisposition syndromes do not have associated physical stigmata?

A. Beckwith-Wiedemann syndrome
B. Fanconi anemia
C. Li-Fraumeni syndrome
D. Von Hippel-Lindau disease

Question 29.4.   All cancer predisposition syndromes listed below have a dominant mode of inheritance, EXCEPT:

A. Neurofibromatosis type I
B. Xeroderma pigmentosum
C. Peutz-Jeghers syndrome
D. Multiple endocrine neoplasia (MEN) 2

Corresponding Chapters in *Cancer: Principles & Practice of Oncology*, Ninth Edition: 122 (Molecular Biology of Childhood Cancers), 123 (Solid Tumors of Childhood), and 124 (Leukemias and Lymphomas of Childhood).

Question 29.5.   Which of the following cytogenetic abnormalities is associated with Ewing sarcoma?

A. $t(11;22)$
B. $t(X;11)$
C. del13q14
D. del11p13

Question 29.6.   Retinoblastoma is a heritable tumor that is often bilateral. All of the following statements regarding retinoblastoma are true, EXCEPT:

A. Loss of heterozygosity (LOH) of the wild-type allele at the Rb1 locus results in the disease.
B. Rb1 loss abrogates control of cell-cycle regulation from the G1 to S phase.
C. Both Rb1 and EWS genes are implicated in the development of retinoblastoma.
D. In a developing retina, inactivation of Rb1 is necessary and sufficient for tumor formation.

Question 29.7.   Which of the following pediatric conditions is NOT associated with known genetic events that predispose to tumor development in children?

A. Retinoblastoma
B. Neuroblastoma
C. Ewing sarcoma
D. Hodgkin's lymphoma

Question 29.8.   Which of the following syndromes is associated with predisposition for developing renal cell carcinoma?

A. Von Hippel-Lindau
B. Beckwith-Weidemann
C. WAGR
D. Simpson-Golabi-Behmel

Question 29.9.   Patients with MEN1 syndrome are predisposed to developing all of the following endocrine tumors, EXCEPT:

A. Parathyroid adenoma
B. Pancreatic islet cell tumor
C. Pheochromocytoma
D. Pituitary adenoma

Question 29.10.   WAGR, a syndrome complex with deletions at chromosome 11q13, the locus of the WT1 gene, predisposes to Wilms' tumor and involves the following structures (choose one answer):

A. Iris, genitourinary (GU) system, IQ
B. Ovaries, gut, and central nervous system (CNS)
C. CNS, heart, and kidneys
D. None of the above

Question 29.11.   Strong correlations are present between all of the following, EXCEPT:

A. Wilms' tumor, intersex disorders, and progressive renal failure
B. Macroglossia, hyperinsulinemia, and Wilms' tumor
C. Neurofibromas, café au lait spots, and optic glioma
D. Mental retardation, spinal abnormalities, and neuroblastoma

Question 29.12.   The NF1 gene on chromosome 17 has which of the following functions:

A. Encoding a ubiquitously expressed protein neurofibromin
B. Facilitating the hydrolysis of GTP to GDP by ras oncoprotein
C. Sending inhibitory signals to cell division
D. All of the above

Question 29.13.   Each of the following is associated with poor prognosis neuroblastoma, EXCEPT:

A. N-myc amplification
B. trkA gene activation
C. LOH at 1p36 and 11q23
D. Telomerase expression and increased telomere length

Question 29.14.   The fusion transcript associated with $t(11;22)$, EWS-ETS, or EWS-FLI-1, and loss of p53 and/or p16 signaling are associated with all of the following tumors, EXCEPT:

A. Osteosarcoma
B. Ewing sarcoma
C. Askin's tumor
D. Peripheral primitive neuroectodermal tumor (pPNET)

Question 29.15.   Which of the following statements regarding the molecular basis for the development of embryonal rhabdomyosarcoma (RMS) is FALSE?

A. They are characterized by LOH at the 11p15 locus.
B. Insulin-like growth factor (IGF)-2 gene activity is increased twofold.
C. IGF-2 tumor suppressor gene activity is lost with the LOH.
D. There is loss of paternal imprinting of IGF-2.

Question 29.16.   Alveolar RMS has all of the following molecular characteristics, EXCEPT:

A. $t(2;13)$ or $t(1;13)$ translocation (PAX-3-FKHR or PAX-7-FKHR fusion)
B. Increased expression of myoblast growth factor (MGF)
C. Increased c-met expression
D. Increased hepatocyte growth factor expression

Question 29.17.   The Li-Fraumeni syndrome is characterized by the following:

A. Germ line mutations in the tumor suppressor gene p53
B. Expression of a stabilized mutant protein in affected cells
C. Mutation or deletion of the second wild-type p53 allele in tumors
D. All of the above

Question 29.18.   Therapeutic interventions targeted at known molecular abnormalities and pathways are being tested using the following intervention strategies:

A. Agents blocking growth hormone IGF-1 pathways
B. Agents targeting mutant transcription factors
C. Agents targeting tyrosine kinase enzymes that transduce growth factor signals
D. All agents listed

Question 29.19.   A 2-year-old girl is brought to the doctor after her mother feels a hard lump near the umbilicus that is not painful. On physical examination, she is noted to be a large child with hemihypertrophy. A large (6 × 6-cm) hard mass is palpable in the left flank. The remainder of his examination is normal. Laboratory evaluation of blood counts, urinalysis, serum electrolytes, and liver and renal function test results are normal. An ultrasound confirms the presence of a mass involving the superior pole of the left kidney. Which of the following anatomic areas are unlikely to be involved by this tumor?

A. Lung
B. Muscle
C. Lymph nodes
D. Renal vein

Question 29.20.   Which of the tests listed below is necessary to correctly stage this tumor?

A. Head computed tomography (CT)
B. Bone scan
C. Plain chest radiograph
D. Skeletal survey

Question 29.21.   The patient is taken to surgery. Which of the following is the ideal surgical approach for accurate diagnosis and staging?

A. Start preoperative chemotherapy followed by resection at a later date because of the size of mass.
B. Biopsy the mass and sample draining lymph nodes.
C. Resect the mass and renal vein if involved.
D. Resect the mass with renal vein if involved, explore the opposite kidney, and sample draining lymph nodes.

Question 29.22.   After surgical resection and staging, the tumor is confirmed to be consistent with stage III favorable histology Wilms' tumor. Treatment should include which of the following:

A. Surgical resection only
B. Surgery and radiation therapy to kidney
C. Radiation and chemotherapy
D. Surgery, radiation, and chemotherapy

Question 29.23.   Factors associated with a good prognosis during the evaluation of Wilms' tumor include which of the following:

A.   Tumor size <550 g
B.   Favorable histology with only focal anaplasia
C.   Isolated single pulmonary metastatic nodule
D.   Limited extension into renal vein

Question 29.24.   A 2-year-old child is brought to the emergency department with low-grade fever, pallor, lethargy, extensive bruising, and "raccoon" eyes (periorbital hematomas). On examination, it is noted that the child appears ill and has a left-sided abdominal mass that is firm and nontender. He also has involuntary rapid eye movements, noticed over 2 to 3 weeks. A biopsy of the mass confirms the presence of a neuroblastoma. All of the following procedures are helpful for further staging and workup, EXCEPT:

A.   CT scan of the chest and abdomen, bone scan, and skeletal survey
B.   Splenectomy, liver biopsy, and exploratory laparotomy
C.   Biopsy of local lymph nodes, bone marrow aspiration/biopsy
D.   Radiolabeled (123)I-metaiodobenzylguanidine (MIBG) scan and determination of urine catecholamines

Question 29.25.   Staging workup reveals stage IV neuroblastoma involving the periorbital area, multiple bones, and bone marrow. Treatment modalities include all of the following, EXCEPT:

A.   Combination chemotherapy: carboplatinum, cyclophosphamide, doxorubicin, and etoposide
B.   High-dose chemotherapy and autologous stem cell rescue
C.   Allogeneic stem cell transplant
D.   Radiotherapy and biologic response modifiers, such as 13-cis retinoic acid

Question 29.26.   Therapy planning for infants with a small adrenal mass and bone marrow involvement and non-myc amplification includes:

A.   Resection of the mass and short-course chemotherapy
B.   Resection of the mass, radiation if residual disease, and short-course chemotherapy
C.   Monitoring for spontaneous regression
D.   13-cis retinoic acid therapy only

Question 29.27. Which of the following statements about the genetics of retinoblastoma transmission is NOT true?

A. It is transmitted as a highly penetrant autosomal-dominant trait and is the most common pediatric ocular tumor.

B. The majority of retinoblastomas are hereditary, bilateral, and caused by germ line mutations of 13q14; only 10% to 15% are sporadic and unilateral.

C. All sporadic bilateral retinoblastomas also have a germ line mutation transmitted in an identical manner as familial retinoblastoma.

D. The parents and siblings of all patients with retinoblastoma should have a thorough ophthalmoscopic evaluation whether or not there is family history of the disease.

Questions 29.28.–29.31. An 11-month-old boy who has just learned to walk is noticed to consistently bump into objects in his path. There is no history of major medical illness in this healthy child. The parents report a "white-looking" eye on the right side that was not observed during a regular pediatric checkup at 6 months of age. There is no family history of ophthalmic disease or tumors. On examination, he has a white pupillary reflex on the right side. In addition, mild proptosis and a sixth nerve palsy are noticed in the right eye. The remainder of the physical examination is normal. A biopsy confirms the presence of retinoblastoma.

Question 29.28. All patients with retinoblastoma should undergo the following staging studies, EXCEPT:

A. CT of the orbit

B. Magnetic resonance imaging (MRI) of the orbit and head to include the optic nerve

C. Meticulous inspection under general anesthesia of both eyes

D. Lumbar puncture and cerebrospinal fluid (CSF) cytology

Question 29.29. Further staging studies reveal complete visual loss in the affected eye and tumor involving the right orbit and optic nerve. The left eye is normal. CSF, bone, and bone marrow studies are normal. Therapy should include:

A. Cryotherapy or hyperthermia

B. Plaque radiotherapy and chemotherapy

C. Enucleation with a sufficient length of the affected optic nerve

D. Enucleation with a sufficient length of the affected optic nerve and local radiation

Question 29.30. Enucleation instead of vision-sparing interventions is indicated for all of the following, EXCEPT:

A. Bilateral neuroblastoma with multiple lesions in both eyes

B. Unilateral retinoblastoma that completely fills the globe

C. Painful glaucoma and loss of vision in one eye

D. Bilateral retinoblastoma with no useful vision in either eye

Question 29.31.   The potential side effects of therapy for this patient include all of the following, EXCEPT:

A. Second cancers
B. Orbital hypoplasia
C. Cataract formation in the contralateral eye
D. Recurrent disease

Question 29.32.   Which of the following inherited cancer syndromes is/are associated with increased risk of developing RMS?

A. Li-Fraumeni syndrome
B. Beckwith-Wiedemann syndrome
C. Costello syndrome
D. All of the above

Question 29.33.   Survival is excellent (>70%) with current therapy in all of the following groups of patients, EXCEPT:

A. Embryonal extremity Group III tumors
B. Group III orbital tumors
C. Embryonal Group III nonorbital tumors
D. Embryonal tumors in children between 1 and 10 years of age

Question 29.34.   Staging studies for RMS should include all of the following, EXCEPT:

A. CT or MRI of the primary site
B. MIBG scan
C. Bone scan and bilateral bone marrow sampling
D. Lymph node sampling

Question 29.35.   A 6-year-old boy presents with a soft tissue mass involving the right cheek, noticed by his mother to cause facial asymmetry and proptosis, worsening over 3 to 4 weeks. He has no other systemic symptoms. Physical examination reveals a large, hard, right, lower orbital mass. An upper cervical lymph node is also palpable on the right side of his neck, measuring 2 cm in diameter. CT scan of the face and neck confirms the presence of a large tumor involving the right orbit and maxillary sinus. An incisional biopsy confirms the presence of embryonal RMS, and the lymph node is positive for tumor. Which of the following would NOT be appropriate therapy for this child?

A. Gross total resection of tumor with facial reconstruction at initial diagnosis
B. Chemotherapy: vincristine, dactinomycin, and cyclophosphamide
C. Radiation therapy to the site of tumor and lymph node metastasis
D. Second-look surgery to assess chemotherapy responsiveness to chemotherapy

Question 29.36.   **All of the following statements about treatment of RMS are true, EXCEPT:**

A. Treatment of parameningeal RMS with intracranial extension should include radiation.
B. Local radiation should be used for all patients with microscopic or gross residual RMS.
C. Hyperfractionated radiotherapy is better than conventional fractionated radiation for control of local, regional, or metastatic RMS.
D. Surgical intervention in RMS should aim for complete tumor resection with negative margins whenever possible.

Question 29.37.   **Small round blue cell tumors of childhood include all of the following, EXCEPT:**

A. Ewing sarcoma
B. Neuroblastoma
C. RMS
D. Wilms' tumor

Question 29.38.   **The most frequent site of metastasis in Ewing sarcoma is:**

A. Liver
B. Lung
C. Spleen
D. Lymph nodes

Question 29.39.   **The most important feature that distinguishes osteosarcoma from Ewing sarcoma, chondrosarcoma, and fibrosarcoma is:**

A. Metaphyseal rather than diaphyseal origin
B. The production of osteoid
C. A "sunburst" pattern on radiologic examination
D. Specificity of chromosomal translocations by karyotyping

Question 29.40.   **All of the following treatment modalities are useful in osteosarcoma, EXCEPT:**

A. Isolated surgery in low-grade tumors
B. Chemotherapy regimen that includes cisplatin, doxorubicin, and methotrexate
C. Ifosfamide combined with biologic response modifier liposomal muramyl tripeptide phosphatidylethanolamine (MTP-PE)
D. Radiation therapy

Question 29.41.   **All of the following are good prognostic factors in the outcome of Ewing sarcoma, EXCEPT:**

A. Localized tumor <8 cm in diameter and volume <100 mL
B. Primary pelvic tumors
C. Low serum lactate dehydrogenase level
D. Type 1 EWS-FLI1 fusion transcripts

Question 29.42. All of the following treatment approaches have decreased recurrence rates in Ewing sarcoma, EXCEPT:

A. The addition of ifosfamide and etoposide in nonmetastatic patients
B. The addition of irradiation to both the primary tumor and whole lung and/or bone in the case of metastatic disease
C. Preoperative chemotherapy followed by surgical resection
D. Myeloablative chemotherapy and stem cell rescue

Questions 29.43.–29.45. A 12-month-old boy who had hemihypertrophy at birth presents with abdominal distension and a right-sided abdominal mass. The mass is confirmed to be arising from the right lobe of the liver by ultrasound of the abdomen. No calcification is identified. The serum alpha-fetoprotein (AFP) level is increased markedly.

Question 29.43. The most likely histologic diagnosis of this mass is:

A. Hepatoblastoma
B. Neuroblastoma
C. Hepatocellular carcinoma (HCC)
D. Choriocarcinoma

Question 29.44. Which of the following hereditary syndromes is associated with predisposition for developing this tumor?

A. Beckwith-Wiedemann syndrome
B. Von Hippel-Lindau syndrome
C. Neurofibromatosis type 1
D. Peutz-Jeghers syndrome

Question 29.45. Staging workup for this patient should include the following, EXCEPT:

A. Liver and renal function tests
B. Chest radiograph or chest CT
C. MRI of the head
D. CT and/or MRI with magnetic resonance (MR) angiography of the abdomen

Question 29.46. The most important treatment of hepatoblastoma is:

A. Adjuvant chemotherapy
B. Concomitant radiation
C. Cryoablation or radio frequency ablation of tumor
D. Complete resection of tumor and liver transplantation, if necessary

Question 29.47.   **Which of the following statements is NOT true?**

A. Gonadal tumors are commonly germ cell tumors in adults.
B. Extragonadal germ cell tumors are more frequent in adults than in children.
C. The sacrococcygeal region is the most common site for extragonadal germ cell tumors in children.
D. Extragonadal germ cell tumors may involve the pineal gland, mediastinum, vagina, or retroperitoneum.

Question 29.48.   **Which of the following is NOT a variety of germ cell tumor?**

A. Teratoma or teratocarcinoma
B. Seminomas or dysgerminomas
C. Embryonal carcinoma
D. Cholangiocarcinoma

Question 29.49.   **Which of the following statements about germ cell tumors is NOT true?**

A. Staging should include CT or MRI scans of the mass and the lymph node region involved, the chest for metastatic disease, a bone scan, and tumor markers.
B. A transscrotal biopsy of a testicular mass should be performed to confirm the diagnosis of a germ cell tumor.
C. Cisplatinum-based chemotherapy (cisplatin, vinblastine, and bleomycin [PVB] or cisplatin, etoposide, and bleomycin [PEB]) has resulted in excellent survival, even in advanced-stage disease in children but does not need to be considered in completely resected pediatric germ cell tumors, especially if tumor markers such as AFP return to normal.
D. Radiation therapy is indicated as second-line therapy for patients who have relapsed after surgery and chemotherapy.

Question 29.50.   **Which of the following pediatric germ cell tumors would be characterized as low risk?**

A. A localized completely resected testicular tumor by high inguinal orchiectomy
B. An ovarian tumor that is completely resected and with only microscopic residual disease
C. An extragonadal germ cell tumor that has metastasized only to locally draining lymph nodes
D. An extragonadal germ cell tumor that is fully resected with only microscopic residual disease

Question 29.51.   Which of the following cytogenetic abnormalities is associated with retinoblastoma?

A. $t(11;22)$
B. $t(X;11)$
C. del13q14
D. del11p13

Question 29.52.   Which of the following hereditary leukemia/lymphoma predisposition syndromes is associated with increased risk of squamous cell carcinoma of the head and neck?

A. Shwachman–Diamond syndrome
B. Ataxia telangiectasia
C. Fanconi anemia
D. All of the above

ANSWERS

Answer 29.1. **The answer is C.**

Pediatric malignancies generally cannot be traced to long-term exposure to known carcinogens because they occur in the young, without time for prolonged exposure and transition to a malignant change.

Answer 29.2. **The answer is D.**

The mechanisms listed above are some of the known pathways of carcinogenesis in the pediatric age group and predispose to specific groups of malignant disorders.

Answer 29.3. **The answer is C.**

Many hereditary premalignant disorders, such as Li-Fraumeni, hereditary retinoblastoma, and familial adenomatous polyposis, are devoid of physical stigmata making them difficult to diagnose without a detailed family history.

Answer 29.4. **The answer is B.**

Xeroderma pigmentosum predisposes to melanoma and leukemia and is caused by multiple gene mutations.

Answer 29.5. **The answer is A.**

Ewing sarcoma is associated with $t(11;22)$ and synovial sarcoma is associated with $t(x;11)$. Cytogenetic abnormalities seen in Wilm's tumor include del11p13 and $t(3;17)$, and retinoblastoma is associated with del13q14.

Answer 29.6. **The answer is C.**

EWS is not implicated in retinoblastoma formation but is involved in the development of Ewing sarcoma. Amplification of MDMX results in retinoblastoma progression.

Answer 29.7. **The answer is D.**

Retinoblastoma is associated with deletions or mutations of Rb1. In neuroblastoma, there are deletions or mutations in the short arm of chromosome 1, and rarely chromosomes 10, 14, 17, and 19; neuroblastoma is also associated with amplification of the N-myc oncogene. Ewing sarcoma is characterized by a reciprocal $t(11;22)$ translocation, fusing a transcription factor FLI-1 with oncogene EWS.

Answer 29.8. **The answer is A.**

Von Hippel-Lindau syndrome is associated with predisposition for developing renal cell carcinoma, whereas Beckwith-Wiedemann, WAGR, and

Simpson-Golabi-Behmel syndromes are all associated with predisposition for developing Wilm's tumor.

Answer 29.9.   **The answer is C.**

MEN1 syndrome results from an autosomal-dominant mutation in the MEN1 gene. Patients with MEN1 syndrome are predisposed to developing multiple endocrine tumors. These include pancreatic islet cell tumors, pituitary adenomas, and parathyroid adenomas. Pheochromocytomas are associated with MEN2 syndrome, but not MEN1 syndrome.

Answer 29.10.   **The answer is A.**

Three hereditary syndromes genetically predispose to Wilms' tumor. WAGR manifests with aniridia, GU abnormalities, and mental retardation. Denys-Drash syndrome manifests with intersex disorders and progressive renal failure. Beckwith-Wiedemann syndrome, the most common, is a hereditary overgrowth syndrome characterized by macroglossia, visceromegaly, and hyperinsulinemia.

Answer 29.11.   **The answer is D.**

Wilms' tumor and neurofibromatosis are often associated with syndromic manifestations that are easy to recognize. No association is described between neurologic abnormalities and neuroblastoma.

Answer 29.12.   **The answer is D.**

Loss of neurofibromin activity (on both alleles) because of mutations in NF1 results in elevated levels of GTP-bound ras oncoprotein that transduces signals for cell division. This is one of the mechanisms of tumor development in neurofibromatosis type 1. The gene located on chromosome 22 has been implicated in tumor genesis due to interference of the function of the protein it encodes, called "merlin."

Answer 29.13.   **The answer is B.**

Nerve growth factor receptor trkA gene amplification shows ganglionic differentiation and has a favorable prognosis. All other markers, including trkB receptor expression, herald poor prognosis neuroblastoma.

Answer 29.14.   **The answer is A.**

EWS-ETS fusion transcripts or related variants can be found in greater than 90% of peripheral PNET group of tumors by reverse transcriptase polymerase chain reaction or fluorescence in situ hybridization.

Answer 29.15.   **The answer is C.**

Paternal gene duplication or loss of imprinting of the normally transcriptionally silent maternal allele results in overexpression of IGF-2 in embryonal RMS.

Answer 29.16.   **The answer is B.**

Except for MGF, all other statements regarding alveolar RMS are true. Additional mutations on p53 are also described. Interestingly, the mouse model with overexpression of PAX-3-FKHR develops no tumors, but mice expressing an hepatocyte growth factor transgene develop embryonal RMS.

Answer 29.17.   **The answer is D.**

Some 60% to 80% of Li-Fraumeni families have detectable germ line mutations in p53. The others may be associated with modifier genes, promoter defects, or involvement of other as yet unknown candidate genes involved in the p53 tumor suppressor pathway. hCHK2, a checkpoint kinase, is a potential candidate.

Answer 29.18.   **The answer is D.**

Identification of various altered molecular signaling pathways (e.g., growth factor, tumor suppressor, and tyrosine kinase) have shown that novel and more effective treatment approaches may lie within reach when these pathways are targeted against tumors.

Answer 29.19.   **The answer is B.**

The presentation is classic for Wilms' tumor. This often silent tumor can metastasize or invade all the structures listed and can perforate through the capsule if very large. It is, however, unlikely to invade muscle tissue. The common pathologic variety is termed "favorable histology Wilms' tumor."

Answer 29.20.   **The answer is C.**

Pulmonary metastasis is the most common site of distant dissemination. The need for a chest CT in addition to a chest radiograph is controversial because small nodules identified by CT scans are often negative on biopsy. Pulmonary nodules should be biopsied to prove tumor dissemination. Brain and bone imaging are only necessary if the diagnosis includes rare renal tumors, such as clear cell sarcoma or rhabdoid tumor.

Answer 29.21.   **The answer is D.**

The National Wilms Tumor Study Group (NWTSG) supports tumor resection. There is a 19.8% operative complication rate that includes intestinal obstruction and hemorrhage. Although the SIOP has promoted the use of preoperative chemotherapy before biopsy, there is a 7.6% to 9.9% rate of benign or other malignant disorders involving the kidney in children. The risk of rupture of the tumor during surgery is 14% and may be associated with an increased risk of local recurrence. Preoperative chemotherapy after a biopsy is recommended for solitary kidneys, bilateral renal tumors, tumor in a horseshoe kidney, or patients who are at anesthesia risks because of extensive lung involvement. Exploring the opposite kidney is also recommended by the NWTSG because there is a small chance that involvement of the opposite kidney may be missed by all other imaging studies.

Answer 29.22.   **The answer is D.**

Surgical resection of the tumor is combined with lymph node sampling and examination of the contralateral kidney (bilateral tumor is present in 5% of patients) to complete staging. Stage III disease involves the presence of residual nonhematogenous tumor confined to the abdomen. The chemotherapy combination used through serial NWTSG trials is vincristine and dactinomycin for patients with a low stage (I and II) and doxorubicin with or without cyclophosphamide for patients with a higher stage and those with unfavorable histology, such as anaplastic Wilms' tumor or clear cell sarcoma.

Answer 29.23.   **The answer is A.**

Some of these prognostic factors no longer pertain because of the development of effective therapy via the NWSTG (trials 1 to 5) and other international trials. Histology and lymph node involvement remain the most important prognostic factors. Survival for most children with favorable histology Wilms' tumor now approaches 90%. The presence of extension or metastatic spread results in intensification of therapy.

Answer 29.24.   **The answer is B.**

Neuroblastoma, a tumor of the sympathetic nervous system, disseminates frequently to the bone, bone marrow, and lymph nodes. Clinical symptoms depend on the location of the tumor and may include Horner syndrome and spinal cord compression. Hematogenous dissemination is evident in 62% of patients at diagnosis. Undifferentiated tumor (Shimada histology), low DNA ploidy, N-myc amplification, and disseminated disease are associated with poor prognosis. Other poor prognostic markers include low Trk A and high Trk B expression, chromosome 1p deletion, and chromosome 17q gains. In a unique small group of infants, small primary tumors with metastatic disease restricted to the liver, skin, and bone marrow without bone involvement (stage IV S) have favorable prognosis. Tumors in infants often have the capacity to regress spontaneously. For the new International Neuroblastoma Staging System (INSS), see *PPO* Table 50.2.2 on page 2047.

Answer 29.25.   **The answer is C.**

Intense chemotherapy alone achieves a remission rate of 22% ± 4% in disseminated neuroblastoma and can be improved to 34% ± 4% with autologous bone marrow transplant. The addition of 13-cis retinoic acid improves the 3-year relapse-free survival rate to 46% ± 6% in these patients. Those with residual disease or positive lymph nodes have better control with local radiation therapy (24 to 30 Gy) to involved areas. Low-risk patients (stage I, stage II with N-myc amplification <10 or >10 with favorable Shimada histology, stage IVS, and hyperdiploidy) often require no treatment. Allogeneic transplants have not demonstrated a definite benefit to date.

Answer 29.26.   **The answer is C.**

Neuroblastoma as described in the question is a special entity. It has a high rate of spontaneous remission and excellent survival. Intermediate-risk neuroblastomas, a rare subgroup (10% to 15%) generally in older children, are generally large and localized. Surgery and moderately intense chemotherapy results in 4-year event-free survival (EFS) rates of 54% to 100%.

Answer 29.27.   **The answer is B.**

The majority of retinoblastomas are sporadic and unilateral (70% to 75%). The median age at diagnosis is 1 to 2 years. Between 10% and 15% of patients with unilateral retinoblastoma have germ line mutations of chromosome 13q14. Between 25% and 30% of children with sporadic retinoblastoma have bilateral disease and carry germ line mutations of 13q14. The median age at diagnosis is less than 12 months.

Answer 29.28.   **The answer is D.**

The risk of dissemination of retinoblastoma is determined by the extent of ocular tumor and is increased by involvement of the choroid, optic nerve, anterior chamber, ciliary body, and orbit. Lumbar puncture, bone marrow, and bone scan should only be performed in patients with extraocular involvement or in the presence of symptoms and signs of involvement of distant sites.

Answer 29.29.   **The answer is D.**

Cryotherapy, hyperthermia, and photocoagulation can be used instead of enucleation for unilateral or bilateral localized disease that does not involve the globe or the anterior chamber to preserve vision. Enucleation, where indicated, should include a 10- to 15-mm length of optic nerve to obtain a tumor-free margin. External beam radiation including the entire orbit and optic nerve up to the optic chiasm (44 to 50 Gy) is indicated for orbital involvement. For intraocular or recurrent disease, chemotherapy agents (vincristine, etoposide, cyclophosphamide, doxorubicin, cisplatinum, and cyclosporin A as an multidrug resistance-reversing agent) are used in combination with other modalities to preserve vision or avoid enucleation, or as salvage. They are most useful in group I to IV tumors. However, chemotherapy alone rarely achieves durable control.

Answer 29.30.   **The answer is A.**

There is excellent response to vision-sparing interventions in retinoblastoma. These include photocoagulation, cryotherapy, hyperthermia, plaque radiotherapy, and so forth. Enucleation should only be undertaken if there is severe inflammation, no salvageable vision, or extraocular extension at risk for metastatic disease. For staging and classification of retinoblastoma see *PPO* Tables 50.2.6 and 50.2.7 on page 2055.

Answer 29.31.   **The answer is D.**

Radiation therapy increases the risk of second malignancies, especially bone tumors in the area of radiation, predisposes to cataracts, and interferes with normal development of the orbit.

Answer 29.32.   **The answer is D.**

Most cases of RMS are sporadic. Inherited cancer predisposition syndromes that increase the risk of developing RMS include Li-Fraumeni, Beckwith-Wiedemann, and Costello syndromes.

Answer 29.33.   **The answer is A.**

Recent analyses of prognostic factors in patients with nonmetastatic disease have identified distinct risk groups for failure-free survival. For staging and grouping classifications see *PPO* Tables 50.2.10 and 50.2.11. Stage I group I/IIa or III orbit (90% survival), stage II group I and II embryonal tumors, and stage III group I and II embryonal tumors have greater than 85% survival. Survival is poor (<50%) despite all treatment modalities in patients with embryonal extremity or alveolar tumors (see *PPO* Table 50.2.12 on page 2070), and children with metastatic disease. Younger children aged less than 10 years fare better.

Answer 29.34.   **The answer is B.**

MIBG scans are indicated for neuroblastoma and not RMS. The other scans and bone marrow samples are necessary in view of dissemination patterns of RMS that include both hematogenous spread and lymphatic spread to the draining lymph nodes. Treatment decisions are based on TNM staging (see *PPO* Table 50.2.10 on page 2069), and clinical group is based on extent of resection (see *PPO* Table 50.2.11 on page 2070). Prognosis depends on stage, age, clinical group, histology, and primary site. Orbital, vaginal, and paratesticular tumors have the best prognosis, whereas extremity and parameningeal tumors are unfavorable. Tumors that are more than 5 cm and that present in children less than 10 years of age have a worse prognosis.

Answer 29.35.   **The answer is A.**

Orbital tumors are usually of embryonal histology and have excellent response to radiation and chemotherapy. Surgical resection is only indicated for recurrent disease. The dose of radiation is 45 to 55 Gy over 5 to 6 weeks. Children with group II or III RMS of the orbit have a 5-year progression-free survival rate of 90%. Parameningeal disease (usually group III) has a 5-year progression-free survival rate of 78% without CNS involvement and 70% with CNS involvement. Extensive surgeries are not necessary to sites that produce significant surgical morbidity.

Answer 29.36.   **The answer is C.**

Radiation therapy for RMS is indicated only for gross or microscopic residual disease or regional and metastatic extension. The dose for microscopic residual disease is 41 to 50 Gy. Tested in IRS IV, hyperfractionated radiation had no added benefit over conventional fractionated radiation. Surgical resection should be attempted in the place of an incisional biopsy upfront only if the tumor is completely resectable. No radiation is necessary in the event of complete resection of the tumor without microscopic residual or regional extension.

Answer 29.37.   **The answer is D.**

All the other tumors have similar light microscopy features that group them into this category.

Answer 29.38.   **The answer is B.**

The lung, bones, and bone marrow are the most common sites of hematogenous spread of Ewing sarcoma. Lesions that originate in long bones characteristically involve the diaphysis. Parallel lamellated periosteal new bone formation frequently presents with an "onion skin" appearance. Radionuclide scans determine the presence of bone metastases. CT or MRI scans detect the presence of associated soft tissue masses and lung lesions.

Answer 29.39.   **The answer is B.**

The main feature that distinguishes osteosarcoma from other tumors that arise from primitive mesenchymal cells is the production of osteoid and thus is the sine qua non for this tumor.

Answer 29.40.   **The answer is D.**

Osteosarcomas are not very sensitive to radiation therapy. All other treatment modalities are used. Adjuvant chemotherapy has increased osteosarcoma survival rates to more than 60%. Juxtacortical osteosarcomas (parosteal and periosteal) that do not invade the medullary cavity may be treated with surgical resection alone.

Answer 29.41.   **The answer is B.**

Pelvic tumors, even when nonmetastatic, herald a poor prognosis perhaps because of poor resectability at this location. Patients with type 1 fusion transcripts of EWS-FLI1 have a 5-year EFS of 70% in contrast with 20% for all other types of fusion transcripts. Low lactate dehydrogenase levels and good response to therapy are other predictors of a better prognosis in Ewing sarcoma.

Answer 29.42.   **The answer is D.**

Although it is still being explored, previous studies have shown no benefit to adding myeloablative chemotherapy and stem cell rescue to standard chemo/radiotherapy and surgery in patients with high-risk disease.

Answer 29.43.   **The answer is A.**

Hepatoblastoma is the most common primary hepatic tumor in the young with a median age at presentation of 1 year. In contrast, the median age at which HCC presents is 12 years. Both demonstrate a male predominance. Patients with hepatoblastoma frequently have additional abnormalities, such as hemihypertrophy, congenital absence of the kidney or adrenal gland, and umbilical hernia. AFP levels are increased in 90% of patients with hepatoblastoma and in 78% of adult patients with HCC. HCC is associated with hepatitis B, biliary atresia, galactosemia, Fanconi anemia, and alpha 1-antitrypsin deficiency. Malignant tumors of the liver are rarely calcified.

Answer 29.44.   **The answer is A.**

Beckwith-Wiedemann syndrome is associated with hereditary predisposition for developing Wilm's tumor, hepatoblastoma, adrenal carcinoma and RMS.

Answer 29.45.   **The answer is C.**

Intracranial metastasis is not a common feature of malignant hepatic tumors. The grouping system used in therapeutic studies segregates patients according to resectability and lymph node or hematogenous metastases. Laboratory tests are not useful for a differential diagnosis of malignant hepatic tumors in children. Pulmonary metastases are identified on a plain chest radiograph in approximately 10% of patients with hepatic tumors. The PRETEXT staging system by the European liver study group divides the liver into four sectors and characterizes tumors by the sectors involved; it was devised to facilitate the assessment of neoadjuvant chemotherapy in rendering tumors resectable and appears to have prognostic value.

Answer 29.46.   **The answer is D.**

Resection is the primary treatment of hepatoblastoma and HCC. Long-term survival is rare in the absence of successful resection. Hepatoblastoma is generally unifocal, and approximately one half of all hepatoblastomas are resectable at initial presentation. HCC has an invasive pattern of spread across anatomic planes and is unresponsive to current forms of chemotherapy. Complete resection of HCC is frequently difficult because of multifocality and invasiveness. Only 30% of HCC tumors can be fully resected at diagnosis.

Answer 29.47.   **The answer is B.**

Only 5% to 10% of germ cell tumors are extragonadal in adults, whereas 60% are extragonadal in children. Forty percent of all childhood germ cell tumors involve the sacrococcygeal region. Germ cell tumors are relatively rare in children and account for 3% of pediatric malignancies.

Answer 29.48.   **The answer is D.**

All the others are varieties of germ cell tumors, each with characteristic histologic features. High AFP levels are common in pediatric patients with testicular, ovarian, presacral, and vaginal primary yolk sac tumors. AFP is a glycoprotein produced in the liver, gastrointestinal tract, and yolk sac of the human fetus. It has a long half-life of 7 days. Human chorionic gonadotropin (hCG) is a glycoprotein secreted by the placenta. Patients with non-yolk sac tumors, such as embryonal carcinoma, choriocarcinoma, and malignant germ cell tumors of the ovary, have elevated hCG levels. hCG has a short half-life of 24 to 36 hours.

Answer 29.49.   **The answer is B.**

Transscrotal biopsy contaminates the scrotum and the lymphatic drainage to the inguinal lymph nodes and prevents high ligation of the spermatic cord. All scrotal masses should be explored through an inguinal incision. If the tumor is malignant, high ligation of the spermatic cord should be performed at the internal ring. With adjuvant chemotherapy consisting of PVB or PEB, 5-year survival rates for germ cell tumors are more than 80%, even for advanced-stage disease. Radiation is reserved only for recurrent or refractory disease.

Answer 29.50.   **The answer is A.**

A localized testicular tumor that is resected in the right fashion by high orchiectomy qualifies for close observation only. All others use adjuvant chemotherapy.

Answer 29.51.   **The answer is C.**

Ewing sarcoma is associated with $t(11;22)$ and synovial sarcoma is associated with $t(x;11)$. Cytogenetic abnormalities seen in Wilm's tumor include del11p13 and $t(3;17)$, and retinoblastoma is associated with del13q14.

Answer 29.52.   **The answer is C.**

Fanconi anemia is associated with a high risk of developing MDS, AML, and squamous cell carcinoma of the head and neck.

CHAPTER 30 LYMPHOMAS

CAMILLE N. ABBOUD

DIRECTIONS Each of the numbered items below is followed by lettered answers. Select the ONE lettered answer that is BEST in each case unless instructed otherwise.

QUESTIONS

Question 30.1. **Which is NOT true of leukemias and lymphomas of childhood?**

A. Demonstrate better outcomes than adults with leukemia and lymphomas.

B. Cure rates range from 60% to 90%, and more than two-thirds of children are treated in clinical trials.

C. Young adults (<30 years) display similar clinical and molecular features as seen in children.

D. Young adults are not eligible for enrollment in pediatric clinical trials.

Question 30.2. **Which of the following is NOT a common translocation in Burkitt's lymphoma?**

A. $t(1;14)$

B. $t(8;14)$

C. $t(2;8)$

D. $t(8;22)$

Question 30.3. **All of the following statements about childhood leukemias are true, EXCEPT:**

A. Bloom's, ataxia telangiectasia, Shwachman-Diamond, Sotos, Noonan's syndromes, and neurofibromatosis are associated with increased incidence of leukemia.

B. ALL relapses involve testicular and central nervous system (CNS) extramedullary sites, requiring localized therapy and a second full course of systemic therapy.

C. Down syndrome (trisomy 21) is associated with ALL in the neonatal period.

D. ALL treatment protocols contain an intensive induction/consolidation phase within 6 to 12 months followed by prolonged maintenance/continuation phases lasting 2 to 3 years.

Corresponding Chapters in *Cancer: Principles & Practice of Oncology,* Ninth Edition: 125 (Molecular Biology of Lymphomas), 126 (Hodgkin's Lymphoma), 127 (Non-Hodgkin's Lymphomas), 128 (Cutaneous Lymphomas), and 129 (Primary Central Nervous System Lymphoma).

Question 30.4.   All of the following inherited syndromes are associated with a higher risk of childhood lymphomas, EXCEPT:

A. Wiskott-Aldrich
B. X-linked lymphoproliferative syndrome
C. Ataxia telangiectasia
D. Human immunodeficiency virus (HIV)-acquired immunodeficiency syndrome (AIDS)

Question 30.5.   The following are true regarding anaplastic large cell lymphomas, EXCEPT:

A. Primary systemic ALCL often have a *t*(2;5)(p23;q35).
B. Prognosis in ALK-positive cases is worse than in ALK negative.
C. ALK protein is detected in the majority of cases.
D. ALK-positive cases are most common in children.

Question 30.6.   Which B-cell malignancy is associated with the highest percentage of patients with Ann Arbor stage IV:

A. Follicular lymphoma.
B. Burkitt's lymphoma.
C. Small lymphocytic lymphoma (SLL)
D. Mantle cell lymphoma (MCL)

Question 30.7.   Regarding the epidemiology of lymphoma, all of the following are true, EXCEPT:

A. Non-Hodgkin's lymphoma (NHL) and HL are the most commonly occurring hematologic malignancies in the United States and the fifth leading cause of cancer death in the United States.
B. Nasal T-cell lymphomas are more common in China.
C. The largest increases have occurred in low-grade lymphomas.
D. Higher rates of gastric lymphoma have been reported in Northern Italy.

Question 30.8.   Which of the following is not a poor risk factor in the International Prognostic Index (IPI)?

A. Age > 60
B. Ann Arbor stage IV
C. Hemoglobin 10
D. Performance status (PS) 3

Question 30.9.   Which of the following diseases is caused by human herpesvirus-8?

A. Castleman's disease.
B. Burkitt's lymphoma
C. Monocytoid B-cell lymphoma
D. A and C

Question 30.10.   Which of the following is not a mature B-cell neoplasm?

    A. Primary effusion lymphoma
    B. Anaplastic large cell lymphoma
    C. Hairy cell leukemia
    D. Lymphomatoid granulomatosis

Question 30.11.   Genetic abnormalities in CLL/SLL can influence prognosis and include all of the following, EXCEPT:

    A. $t(11;18)(q21;q21)$ and/or $i(7q)(q10)$
    B. 11q23 deletion involving the ATM gene, which is also seen in T-cell prolymphocytic leukemia (T-PLL)
    C. 17p13 deletion involving the p53 tumor suppressor gene
    D. Trisomy 12 and/or 13q14 deletion (the latter also seen in myeloma)

Question 30.12.   All of the following are true about CLL/SLL, EXCEPT:

    A. Deletion 17p13 predicts poor survival and fludarabine resistance.
    B. CD38 expression and ZAP-70 are associated with poor prognosis.
    C. Unmutated Ig V region is associated with good prognosis.
    D. Autoimmune hemolytic anemia and immune thrombocytopenia require therapy with glucocorticoids, intravenous gammaglobulin, and/or rituximab.

Question 30.13.   Which of the following B-cell lymphomas may have CD10 positive and $t(14;18)$ translocation:

    A. Lymphoplasmacytic lymphoma
    B. Follicular lymphoma
    C. Diffuse large B-cell lymphoma (DLBCL)
    D. B and C

Question 30.14.   All of the following apply to lymphoplasmacytic lymphomas, EXCEPT:

    A. It is a neoplasm of small B lymphocytes, plasmacytoid lymphocytes, and plasma cells lacking CD5, CD10, and CD23, with strong expression of sIg and CD20, differentiating it from CLL/SLL.
    B. Translocation of $t(9;14)(p13;q32)$ and rearrangement of the PAX-5 gene.
    C. Thalidomide (an immunomodulatory agent derivative) and bortezomib (a proteosome inhibitor) are not active in these lymphomas.
    D. Monoclonal serum IgM paraproteinemia, with or without hyperviscosity, characterizes Waldenstrom's macroglobulinemia. Clinical presentation commonly involves the marrow, nodes, and spleen, but rarely involves pulmonary, small bowel, and renal sites (the latter seen with mixed cryoglobulinemia and hepatitis C virus).

Question 30.15.   Which of the following T-cell malignancies is associated with the presence of T cell receptor γδ?

A. Large granular lymphocytic leukemia
B. Hepatosplenic T-cell lymphoma
C. Angioimmunoblastic lymphoma
D. Mycosis fungoides (MF)

Question 30.16.   **Higher risk of CNS relapse may occur in all of the following large cell lymphoma presentations, EXCEPT:**

A. Paranasal sinus involvement; epidural involvement
B. Bone marrow involvement and high IPI score
C. Testicular involvement
D. Tonsillar involvement

Question 30.17.   **Regarding the staging workup of NHL and HL, all are true, EXCEPT:**

A. The fluorodeoxyglucose (FDG) positron emission tomography (PET) scan is highly reliable in finding disease activity in intermediate/high-grade lymphoma and HL.
B. The FDG-PET scan is less reliable in detecting extranodal marginal zone lymphoma.
C. The FDG-PET scan has replaced gallium scans in staging lymphoma.
D. The FDG-PET scan is not useful in the evaluation of splenic involvement.

Question 30.18.   **Regarding splenic marginal zone lymphoma (SMZL), all are true, EXCEPT:**

A. Patients can have circulating "villous" lymphocytes; most tumors are CD5 negative and express CD19, CD20, CD22, and bcl-2.
B. Hemoglobin <12 g/dL, LDH > normal, and albumin <3.5 g/dL are risk factors predicting a shorter survival of 50%.
C. Disease is confined only to the spleen.
D. Observation, splenectomy, and chemotherapy with alkylating agents and purine analogs similar to follicular lymphoma are used in these patients.

Question 30.19.   **Regarding follicular lymphoma, all are true, EXCEPT:**

A. Radiotherapy (RT) is the standard of care in early-stage disease (CS I and II).
B. Radioimmunotherapy, novel monoclonal antibodies, proteosome inhibitors, and tumor vaccines have all been associated with responses.
C. Autologous stem cell transplantation is curative for patients with advanced-stage disease.
D. Translocations involving BCL6 are seen in DLCBL transformation.

Question 30.20.   **All of the following apply to MCL, EXCEPT:**

A. *t*(11;14)(q13;q32) is seen in MCL, along with cyclin D1 overexpression.

B. Bortezomib and temsirolimus have not shown activity in MCL.

C. MCL accounts for 7% of adult NHL in the United States and Europe, and most patients present in stage IV disease (70%).

D. Hyper-CVAD + rituximab and/or clinical trials incorporating autologous or allogeneic stem cell transplantation with or without bortezomib maintenance should be considered in MCL in younger patients.

Question 30.21.   **All of the following are true about MCL, EXCEPT:**

A. Tumor cells strongly express sIgM and IgD (often of lambda light chain type) and B-cell–associated antigens, and arises from antigen-naïve B cells of the inner mantle zone.

B. Genetic abnormalities in addition to *t*(11;14) are uncommon.

C. Nuclear cyclin D1 protein is present in all cases and is the gold standard for the diagnosis.

D. More common in males.

Question 30.22.   **All of the following are true of DLBCL, EXCEPT:**

A. It is the most common lymphoma (31% in REAL series); patients often have rapidly enlarging nodal masses and B symptoms. Up to 40% of DLBCLs are extranodal, and marrow involvement is seen in 16%.

B. At least two subtypes have been defined by gene expression profiling (GEP), germinal center B cell (GCB), and activated B cell (ABC). GCB survival is better than ABC survival and has the *t*(11;14)(q32;q21) translocation, supporting the hypothesis that this DLBCL subtype is of follicular cell origin.

C. GCB and ABC DLBCL subtypes cannot be differentiated by immunochemistry.

D. Known subtypes of DLBCL include T-cell–rich B histiocyte cell variant, plasmablastic type seen in HIV-positive patients, and a rare ALK-positive variant.

Question 30.23.   **Regarding DLBCL, which of the following statements is NOT correct?**

A. Abbreviated CHOP chemotherapy plus involved field RT is excellent therapy for patients with low-risk, nonbulky, early-stage DLBCL.

B. Standard initial treatment of advanced-stage DLBCL is CHOP plus rituximab; ongoing clinical trials are focusing on the role of upfront autologous stem cell transplantation in patients with high IPI.

C. In a subset analysis of the GELA R-CHOP trial, rituximab appeared to confer greater benefit in patients with DLBCL who do not express bcl2 on immunocytochemistry.

D. Autologous stem cell transplantation is the treatment of choice for patients with relapsed DLBCL that is shown to be chemosensitive.

Question 30.24.   Which of the following regarding testicular lymphoma is false?

A. Most common testicular neoplasia in men older than 60 years
B. The most common histology is follicular lymphoma
C. Orchiectomy is recommended as the initial therapy
D. A and B

Question 30.25.   A 25-year-old college student has had a sore throat for 4 weeks associated with pain on swallowing. A 4-cm mass in the right tonsil is found showing DLBCL by biopsy. Further staging reveals no other adenopathy or hepatosplenomegaly. CT scan of the neck, chest, and abdomen reveals no further abnormality. The patient is classified as Eastern Collaborative Oncology Group (ECOG) PS 0. A bone marrow biopsy does not reveal evidence of lymphoma involvement. The CBC and LDH are normal. You recommend:

A. CHOP every 3 weeks for eight cycles
B. CHOP and rituximab every 3 weeks for eight cycles
C. CHOP for three cycles followed by RT
D. CHOP and rituximab for three cycles followed by RT

Question 30.26.   A 42-year-old woman presents with enlarged cervical lymph nodes 16 months after initial therapy with R-CHOP chemoimmunotherapy for DLBCL, stage IVB. She now has no "B" symptoms and her physical examination results are unremarkable except for multiple enlarged left cervical lymph nodes, the largest being 2.5 × 4 cm. CBC shows a hemoglobin level of 11 g/dL, WBC of 4300/μL with absolute neutrophil count of 3000/mm^3, and platelet count of 300,000/μL. LDH is normal. The patient is classified as ECOG PS 0. A biopsy of a left cervical lymph node reveals DLBCL. PET-CT scan of the chest, abdomen, and pelvis shows no detectable disease elsewhere. A bone marrow biopsy does not reveal evidence of lymphoma. What would you recommend?

A. CHOP and rituximab for three cycles followed by RT
B. Radioimmunotherapy (Bexxar or Zevalin)
C. Two cycles of rituximab-ifosfamide, cisplatin, and etoposide (R-ICE) chemotherapy followed by autologous peripheral blood stem cell transplantation with BEAM
D. Fludarabine, busulfan, and thymoglobulin reduced-intensity allogeneic stem cell transplantation

Question 30.27.   Primary mediastinal (thymic) large B-cell lymphomas (PMBCLs) are characterized by all of the following, EXCEPT:

A. Involve the thymus. Tumor cells correspond to B cells in the thymic medulla and are Ig negative but express B-cell–associated antigens CD19, CD20, CD22, CD79a, and CD45. Most cases are BCL6 positive and Ig heavy, and light-chain genes are rearranged, whereas BCL2 and BCL6 are germ line.

B. Express FIG1 and amplified REL oncogene on chromosome 9p and overexpress the MAL gene at chromosome 2p13-15.

C. GEP of PMBCL is similar to DLCBL with overexpression of the MAL and FIG1 genes.

D. OS at 5 years in patients aged less than 65 years treated with MACOP-B/VACOP-B, R-CHOP, and CHOP is 87%, 81%, and 71%, respectively (Vancouver series). Addition of RT did not improve survival in this series.

Question 30.28.   Which statement is FALSE about natural killer (NK)/T-cell neoplasms?

A. Extranodal NK/T-cell lymphoma is EBV+, is common in Asia and Peru, and can affect children and adults. Hemophagocytic syndrome may occur.

B. Extranodal sites involve the nose, palate, upper airway, gastrointestinal tract, and skin.

C. Atypical cells are CD2+, CD56+, surface CD3–, cytoplasmic CD3+, and many are CD4– CD8– and express cytoplasmic granule proteins (granzyme B and TIA-1).

D. Relapse after RT alone is rare. Patients with disseminated disease are cured by CHOP therapy.

Question 30.29.   Which statement is FALSE about T-cell neoplasms?

A. Enteropathy-type T-cell lymphoma occurs in adults with gluten-sensitive enteropathy (antigliadin antibodies). Outcomes in patients with advanced celiac disease are very poor.

B. Anaplastic large T/null cell lymphoma expresses ALK-1, CD30, and usually CD25; therapy with DLCBL active regimen without Rituxan is used; the outcome of ALK– patients is worse (31% to 37%) than that of ALK+ patients (71% to 95%). Responses have been seen with CD30-directed monoclonal antibodies.

C. Subcutaneous panniculitis T-cell lymphoma is a cytotoxic T-cell neoplasm that infiltrates subcutaneous tissues. Hemophagocytic syndrome is common with fever and serositis, myalgias, and joint pains. Disease prognosis is very good with chemotherapy.

D. Hepatosplenic T-cell lymphoma is rare, and diagnosis is often difficult. Patients present with organomegaly and sinusoidal infiltrates in the liver, spleen, or marrow. It is CD2+CD3+CD5–, CD4–CD8–CD16+CD56+/–. TCRg and TCRd genes are rearranged; isochromosome 7 is common and trisomy 8 may be seen.

Question 30.30.   **Which statement about CTCL is FALSE?**

    A. The skin is the most common extranodal site of lymphomas.

    B. The World Health Organization European Organization for Research and Treatment of Cancer (WHO-EORTC) classification identifies three groups as CTCL: cutaneous T/NK cell lymphoma (MF) and its Sézary subtype, now viewed as a distinct entity; the cutaneous B-cell lymphomas; and the precursor hematologic neoplasms.

    C. B-cell CTCL includes marginal zone (mucosa-associated lymphoid tissue) lymphoma, primary cutaneous follicular cell lymphoma, diffuse cutaneous B-cell lymphoma, intravascular large B-cell lymphoma, lymphomatoid granulomatosis, and cutaneous involvement of MCL, chronic lymphocytic leukemia (CLL), and Burkitt's lymphoma.

    D. Precursor hematologic neoplasms include the blastic NK/cell dermal neoplasms, precursor lymphoblastic leukemia/lymphomas, and myeloid leukemia.

Question 30.31.   **All is true about Sézary syndrome (SS), EXCEPT:**

    A. Sézary cells are peripheral blood atypical lymphocytes with hyperconvoluted nuclei. SS is defined as diffuse erythroderma with circulating neoplastic SS cells at >1000 cells/mm^3.

    B. IL-11 is an autocrine and paracrine growth factor for Sézary cells.

    C. Loss of antigens CD2, CD7, and CD4 is seen in MF/SS.

    D. CTCL express cutaneous T-cell antigen (CLA) that binds E selectin on activated endothelial venules and facilitates homing to the skin via CCL17/CCR4 chemokine receptor interactions.

Question 30.32.   **All are true about MF, EXCEPT:**

    A. Outcome of MF/SS is not correlated with clinical stage.

    B. Features include patches, plaques, erythroderma, and cutaneous tumors or ulcers. T-cell receptor rearrangement is used in the differential diagnosis (psoriasis, eczema, large plaque parapsoriasis, and drug eruptions).

    C. Therapy for localized disease includes topical carmustine or mechlorethamine, bexarotene, ultraviolet B, plus near ultraviolet light ± interferon alpha, and electron beam radiation.

    D. Systemic therapy may include chemotherapy (EPOCH, pentostatin, fludarabine + interferon alpha, gemcitabine, and doxorubicin), extracorporeal photochemotherapy, denileukin diftitox ± bexarotene, histone acetylase inhibition (vorinostat), and the monoclonal antibodies alemtuzumab and zanolimumab.

Question 30.33.   **Which statement is FALSE regarding primary CNS lymphoma (PCNSL)?**

    A. PCNSL was once a rare tumor accounting for 0.5% to 1.25% of intracranial neoplasms, usually associated with congenital, acquired, or iatrogenic immunodeficiency states.

    B. PCNSL has increased threefold from 1985 to 1997 in immunocompetent individuals. This increase was part of an overall increase in all extranodal NHLs.

    C. Frontal lobe presentation is the least frequent in brain PCNSL.

    D. Brain lesions are multifocal in 40% of normal patients and 100% of patients with AIDS. The frequency of AIDS PCNSL has dramatically decreased since the institution of highly active antiretroviral therapy.

Question 30.34.   **Which statement is FALSE regarding PCNSL?**

    A. The eye distinct from the orbit is a direct extension of the brain, and approximately 20% of patients with PCNSL have ocular involvement at presentation.

    B. Ocular lymphoma involves the vitreous, retina, or choroid, but optic nerve infiltration does not occur.

    C. Primary leptomeningeal lymphoma in the absence of a brain mass is rare, approximately 7% of PCNSL. Symptoms of progressive leg weakness, urinary incontinence or retention, cranial neuropathies, and confusion may be present for months before diagnosis; delayed therapy is common because of difficulty of diagnosis.

    D. MRI should be the standard imaging technique for patients with PCNSL. Prominent contrast enhancement is characteristic in 90% of patients.

Question 30.35.   **Management and therapy of PCNSL include all, EXCEPT:**

    A. Corticosteroids should be avoided before diagnostic biopsy, and resection should be avoided.

    B. Polymerase chain reaction for EBV on cerebrospinal fluid in AIDS-associated PCNSL.

    C. RT must be whole brain (3600 to 4500 cGy) and may be deferred in patients >60 years of age. Primary treatment of ocular disease is 3500 to 4500 cGy RT to both eyes.

    D. Chemotherapy should be considered at diagnosis for every patient, must penetrate the blood–brain barrier (high-dose methotrexate and leucovorin rescue), must be lipophilic (procarbazine), and should be administered after RT.

Question 30.36.   **ALL are true of HL, EXCEPT:**

    A. The malignant cells known as Hodgkin cells or Reed-Sternberg (HRS) cells represent 0.15% to 1% of the entire cell population in classic Hodgkin's lymphoma (cHL).

    B. In lymphocyte-predominant Hodgkin's lymphoma (LPHL), HRS cells express B-cell antigens like CD19 and CD20.

    C. In cHL, these HRS cells express the activation marker CD30, and in many cases are CD15 positive and lack major B- and T-cell lineage antigens.

    D. HRS cells express IL-13 but lack IL-5.

Question 30.37.   **All of the following statements are true, EXCEPT:**

    A. The activator protein (AP)-1 and the nuclear factor-kappa B (NF-kB) transcription factors are constitutively active in cHL.

    B. NF-kB is the central mediator of survival and proliferation of HRS cells in cHL.

    C. Mutations of the NF-kB inhibitory gene IkBa are not important transforming events in cHL in the absence of EBV or other viruses.

    D. Activation of the signal transducer and activator of transcription family (STAT3, STAT6, and STAT5a) have been found in cHL. STAT3 activation was constitutive and did not depend on IL-6, whereas STAT6 depended on IL-13 signaling.

Question 30.38.   **All statements are true about the immunology of HL, EXCEPT:**

    A. Eosinophils stimulated by IL-5 and attracted by eotaxin inhibit the Th2 response.

    B. T cells within the HL lymphoma are CD4+, TCRab+, express the CD38, CD69, and CD71 activation markers, but lack CD26 and the IL-2 receptor CD25.

    C. Secretion of IL-10 and TGF-βb by HRS cells and the inability of T cells to secrete IL-2 suppress an effective immune response.

    D. HRS cells are not able to mount an effective immune response.

Question 30.39.   **NLPHL differs in several ways from the subtypes of cHL, nodular sclerosing, mixed cellularity, and lymphocyte depleted. All of the following statements about NLPHL are true, EXCEPT:**

    A. Approximately 80% of patients with NLPHL have stage I or II disease at the time of diagnosis.

    B. In contrast with cHL, the atypical cells in NLPHL are CD45+, express B-cell antigens (CD19, CD20, CD22, CD79a, and PAX5), the transcription factors Oct2 and BOB.1, and the germinal center-associated proteins Bcl6 and EMA, but lack CD15 and CD30.

    C. NLPHL does not transform to DLCBL.

    D. NLPHL accounts for 5% of the cases of HL. More than 90% of patients have a clinical remission and are alive at 10 years.

Question 30.40.   The term "lymphocyte rich classic Hodgkin's lymphoma" (LRCHL) has been proposed in the Revised European–American Lymphoma (REAL) classification for cases of HL with RS cells that appear classic by morphology and immunophenotype and have a background infiltrate consisting predominantly of lymphocytes, with rare or no eosinophils. True statements about LRCHL include all of the following, EXCEPT:

A. LRCHL can closely resemble NLPHL morphologically, and immunophenotyping may be required to differentiate the two entities. Cases of LRCHL have the same immunophenotype of cHL with expression of CD15 and CD30 by the HRS cells. CD20 is coexpressed in 3% to 5% of cases.

B. Follicular meshworks of follicular dendritic cells are seen with antibodies to CD21 or CD35, and RS cells are found within the mantle and interfollicular regions.

C. Patients with LRCHL usually lack bulky disease or B symptoms and tend to present with early-stage disease. The clinical features at presentation seem to be intermediate between those of NLPHL and cHL.

D. OS of LRCHL is slightly better than that of NLPHL in the German Hodgkin Study Group (GHSG) studies.

Question 30.41.   All are true about the association of cHL with other lymphomas, EXCEPT:

A. cHL can be associated with high-grade DLCBL, Burkitt's, or Burkitt's-like lymphoma.

B. Cases of cHL associated with follicular lymphoma or DLCBL may precede, follow, or occur simultaneously with the lymphoma.

C. B-cell CLL does not transform into HL.

D. Mediastinal gray zone lymphoma has features of both cHL and DLCBL at diagnosis.

Question 30.42.   Staging procedures for HL have become simpler and less invasive with the advent of new staging modalities and the use of combined modality treatment. Which of the following statements is TRUE?

A. Patients with large mediastinal adenopathy, mediastinal mass >50% of the thoracic diameter at T5-6, or a ratio >50% of the transverse diameter of the mediastinal mass over the diameter of the diaphragmatic thorax have increased risk of relapse (nodal or extranodal sites) after RT alone.

B. For a patient with early-stage HL treated initially with chemotherapy, if a PET scan is subsequently negative, there is good evidence that the patient does not need adjuvant-involved field RT after chemotherapy.

C. Staging laparotomy has been replaced by FDG-PET scanning but should be used in rare circumstances in early-stage HL, in which the use of limited RT alone depends on pathologic staging.

D. Evidence of contiguous spread of HL is most convincing in patients with LP disease.

Question 30.43.   A 25-year-old man with stage IIA nodular sclerosing HL was treated with total nodal RT 3 years ago. The patient now presents with a new enlarged lymph node in the groin. A biopsy of the node confirms a diagnosis of recurrent HL, nodular sclerosing type. The patient has no "B" symptoms. A restaging workup includes a CT scan of the chest, abdomen, and pelvis, and PET scanning. Recurrent disease is found in nodes above and below the diaphragm. A bone marrow biopsy is negative for HL. The patient is classified with clinical stage IIIA. Which of the following statements is TRUE?

A.   Because the patient has recurrent disease after initial curative therapy, he should be treated with high-dose chemotherapy and allogeneic or autologous stem cell transplant.

B.   Patients with early-stage HL who relapse after RT fare worse than patients who relapse after initial conventional chemotherapy, suggesting that RT affects drug resistance and can compromise chemotherapy outcome.

C.   Treatment with Adriamycin, bleomycin, vinblastine, dacarbazine (ABVD) chemotherapy results in superior disease-free survival compared with nitrogen mustard, Oncovin, procarbazine, prednisone (MOPP) regimen in patients with recurrent HL after RT.

D.   Advanced relapsing patients with "B" symptoms after prior RT have a low 10-year survival when treated with conventional salvage chemotherapy (<10%) and should be considered for autologous stem cell transplant as initial therapy rather than conventional chemotherapy.

Question 30.44.   The following statements about standard treatment strategy in HL are true, EXCEPT:

A.   Early stages, favorable patients: radiation alone (extended field).

B.   Early stages, unfavorable patients: moderate amount of chemotherapy (typically four cycles) plus radiation.

C.   Patients who receive pelvic irradiation for subdiaphragmatic HL have a high risk of loss of fertility. The risk of loss of fertility in women is minimal, particularly in women aged less than 25 years at the time of treatment.

D.   Advanced stages: extensive chemotherapy (typically eight cycles) with or without consolidation RT (usually local).

Question 30.45. All of the following statements about HL during pregnancy are true, EXCEPT:

A. CT scanning is to be avoided because it exposes the fetus to ionizing radiation. MRI may be used for staging because it is nonteratogenic.

B. Chemotherapy drugs that act as antimetabolites, such as methotrexate, have a high risk of causing teratogenesis. The long-term survival of women with HL who were pregnant at the time of initial presentation is worse than that of nonpregnant women with similar stages of disease.

C. In the second or third trimester of pregnancy, if there is rapid progression of supradiaphragmatic lymphadenopathy, RT alone can be used. If involved field or mantle radiation is used with abdominal shielding, the risk of adverse sequelae for the fetus is low.

D. If HL is diagnosed in the first trimester of pregnancy, therapeutic options in early pregnancy are limited and include supradiaphragmatic irradiation or pregnancy termination. If the woman wants to continue the pregnancy, treatment should be deferred until at least the second trimester, if possible.

Question 30.46. Patients with HL develop treatment-related complications after curative therapy for HL. All of the following statements such as secondary malignancies are true, EXCEPT:

A. Secondary AML appears to be higher in patients treated with ABVD regimen, compared with patients treated with MOPP.

B. Treatment-related AML has a latency period of 3 to 5 years, and most cases occur within 10 years of the initial treatment.

C. Most cases of NHL occurring after HL have intermediate or high-grade histology.

D. Solid tumors tend to occur in the second decade after therapy and include lung cancer in smokers and breast cancer in women.

Question 30.47. All of the following statements about long-term complications in patients with HL are true, EXCEPT:

A. Myocardial damage from radiation and anthracycline exposure can be serious.

B. Lung fibrosis is not seen after exposure to RT plus bleomycin or BCNU-based high-dose therapy (i.e., BEAM or BEC)/autologous SCT.

C. Hypothyroidism after mantle RT can be detected by finding an elevated thyroid-stimulating hormone level.

D. The risk of postsplenectomy sepsis can be minimized by immunization with pneumococcal vaccine; vaccines have also been developed against Neisseria and Haemophilus, which are also associated with postsplenectomy sepsis.

Question 30.48.   The GHSG recently conducted a series of clinical trials to look at the role of dose intensification in advanced HL. The BEACOPP regimen (bleomycin, etoposide, doxorubicin, cyclophosphamide, vincristine, procarbazine, and prednisone) was used as a standard combination for dose escalation. The GHSG designed a three-arm study comparing COPP/ABVD, standard BEACOPP, and escalated BEACOPP in patients with advanced HL. Approximately two-thirds of the patients also received consolidation RT. In 1996, at an interim analysis, the COPP/ABVD arm was closed to accrual because it was inferior to the BEACOPP arm. All of the following statements about the GHSG trial are true, EXCEPT:

A.   At a median of 5 years, the freedom from treatment failure rate was 69% for COPP/ABVD, 76% for standard BEACOPP, and 87% for the escalated BEACOPP.

B.   There were nine cases of AML/MDS in the escalated BEACOPP arm, whereas there were two cases in the standard BEACOPP arm; also, the total rate of second neoplasms was highest in the escalated BEACOPP arm.

C.   Escalated BEACOPP was associated with greater hematologic toxicity, requiring more red cell and platelet transfusions, but there were no differences in hematologic toxicity between the standard BEACOPP arm and the COPP/ABVD arm.

D.   Rates of early progression were significantly lower with the escalated BEACOPP compared with standard BEACOPP and COPP/ABVD.

Question 30.49.   Several trials have looked at the use of less-toxic chemotherapy combined with RT. These combinations would allow a reduction in the amount and toxicity of chemotherapy and the use of smaller radiation volumes. All of the following statements are true, EXCEPT:

A.   A less-toxic regimen, vinblastine, bleomycin, and methotrexate (VBM) was developed at Stanford. A trial treating patients with PS IA to IIIA compared subtotal nodal/total nodal irradiation with involved field irradiation followed by VBM. There was no significant difference in OS.

B.   The British National Lymphoma Investigation (BNLI) trial found that the combination of VBM with involved field irradiation produced unacceptable pulmonary and hematologic toxicity.

C.   In a later Stanford trial, patients with CS IA-IIIA HL received subtotal nodal and splenic irradiation or two cycles of VBM, followed by regional mantle irradiation and then four more cycles of VBM with dose-reduced bleomycin. There was no difference in PFS or OS.

D.   The GHSG HD7 (1994 to 1998) trial randomized 643 CS IA-IIB patients to either subtotal nodal and splenic irradiation alone or to two courses of ABVD and the same RT. No difference was seen in the freedom from treatment failure between the two groups.

Question 30.50.   All of the following statements about new treatment modalities in HL are true, EXCEPT:

A. Vinorelbine, idarubicin, and gemcitabine have been found to have activity in HL.

B. Native monoclonal antibodies have been tested in HL: CD20-based antibodies are not active in LPHL.

C. Anti-CD30 antibodies and bispecific anti-CD30 antibodies (CD16/CD30; CD30/CD64) are currently under development.

D. In EBV-positive HL, mostly LMP2a-specific autologous cytotoxic CD8 T cells have been generated in vitro and shown to be active in vivo.

Question 30.51.   All of the following statements about novel therapies are true, EXCEPT:

A. SGN-35 (brentuximab vedotin) is active in both Hodgkin's disease and anaplastic large cell lymphoma.

B. SGN-35 is an antibody-drug conjugate combining an anti-CD30 antibody with a synthetic antimitotic agent monomethyl auristin that enhances its antilymphoma activity as compared to SGN-30 that consists of the anti-CD30 antibody alone.

C. CD30 is expressed only in ALK-positive anaplastic large cell lymphoma and Hodgkin's disease.

D. Lenalinomide (a thalidomide-derivative immune modulator), panabinostat (a histone deacetylase class I and II inhibitor), and everolimus (an mTOR inhibitor) have shown activity in Hodgkin's disease and are currently under development for relapsed disease and for maintenance after autologous stem cell transplantation.

ANSWERS

Answer 30.1.   **The answer is D.**

Patients aged less than 30 years are eligible for treatment in pediatric clinical trials. Many findings and methods first shown to be useful in pediatric oncology (including the clinical trial mechanism itself) have been successfully applied to adult oncology.

Answer 30.2.   **The answer is A.**

The classic translocations in Burkitt's lymphoma are $t(2;8)$, $t(8;14)$, and $t(8;22)$. The translocation $t(1;14)$ may be seen in MALT lymphoma.

Answer 30.3.   **The answer is C.**

Patients with trisomy 21, Down syndrome, have a higher risk for ALL up to age 13 years, but not in the neonatal period. Extra copies of chromosome 21 are a common finding but carry no prognostic meaning. In neonates, a transient myeloproliferative disease is seen that resolves spontaneously. AML M7 develops in patients with Down syndrome aged less than 2 years and is associated with GATA-1 mutations.

Answer 30.4.   **The answer is D.**

HIV infection is an acquired infection and is associated with increased secondary lymphomas possibly related to EBV infection and a low CD4 count. Common variable immunodeficiency is also a risk factor, but its cause is not known and may be a function of environmental exposure and genetic predisposition.

Answer 30.5.   **The answer is B.**

ALK, is detected in more than half of the patients, is more common in children and is associated with better prognosis.

Answer 30.6.   **The answer is C.**

According to the Non-Hodgkin's Lymphoma Classification Project, small lymphocytic lymphoma/chronic lymphocytic leukemia is the lymphoma subtype most commonly associated with stage IV at diagnosis (83%), followed by MCL (71%) and peripheral T-cell lymphoma (65%).

Answer 30.7.   **The answer is C.**

The largest NHL increase is in patients with aggressive histologies. In primary CNS lymphoma, diffuse large B-cell NHL occurs increasingly in patients with AIDS. Adult T-cell leukemia/lymphoma (ATL) is common in Southern Japan and the Caribbean, whereas certain small intestinal lymphomas are commonly seen in the Middle East.

Answer 30.8.   **The answer is C.**

The poor prognostic factors in the IPI include age greater than 60, PS greater than or equal to 2, increased LDH, Ann Arbor stage III or IV, and greater than or equal to 2 extranodal sites. Hemoglobin less than 12 is a poor risk factor in the Follicular Index.

Answer 30.9.   **The answer is A.**

HHV-8 is the putative etiology of Castleman's disease. Endemic Burkitt's lymphoma and monocytoid B-cell lymphoma have been associated with EBV and hepatitis C viruses, respectively.

Answer 30.10.   **The answer is B.**

Primary effusion lymphoma, hairy cell leukemia and lymphomatoid granulomatosis are mature B-cell neoplasms, whereas anaplastic large cell lymphoma is a mature T-cell neoplasm.

Answer 30.11.   **The answer is A.**

The $t(11;18)(q21;q21)$ translocation seen in MALT lymphomas produces the antiapoptotic API2-MLT fusion protein, which is activated as a consequence of the fusion. Isochromosome 7q deletion is characteristic of hepatosplenic T-cell lymphoma and not CLL.

Answer 30.12.   **The answer is C.**

Unmutated Ig V region is associated with aggressive disease and correlates with ZAP-70 expression (a tyrosine kinase protein normally expressed in T and NK cells) and CD38 antigen expression. (Rassenti LZ, Jain S, Keating MJ et al. Relative value of ZAP-70, CD38, and immunoglobulin mutation status in predicting aggressive disease in chronic lymphocytic leukemia. Blood 2008;112:1923–1930.)

Answer 30.13.   **The answer is D.**

Although CD10 and $t(14;18)$ are characteristic features of follicular lymphoma, they may also be present in DLBCL. Lymphoplasmacytic lymphoma is CD 10 negative and is associated with the $t(9;14)$ translocation.

Answer 30.14.   **The answer is C.**

IMIDs such as thalidomide and lenalinomide, as well as bortezomib, have demonstrated activity in lymphoplasmacytic lymphomas. Like most CD20 positive B-cell lymphomas, the combined use of chemotherapy and immunotherapy with rituxan has improved the disease-free interval and led to greater complete remissions.

Answer 30.15.   **The answer is B.**

The most common TCR subtype observed in lymphomas is the αβ. TCR γδ is seen in hepatosplenic T-cell lymphoma and some cases of enteropathy-type T-cell lymphoma.

Answer 30.16.   **The answer is D.**

Patients with paranasal sinus, testicular involvement, epidural lymphoma, and bone marrow involvement with large cells are especially prone to meningeal spread and should have a diagnostic lumbar puncture unless their therapy includes agents that penetrate the cerebrospinal fluid, such as high-dose methotrexate and leucovorin rescue. In addition, a lumbar puncture is favored for highly aggressive large cell lymphoma in immuno-compromised patients with HIV infections.

Answer 30.17.   **The answer is D.**

The majority of studies evaluating FDG-PET in intermediate/high-grade NHL and HL have shown high standardized uptake value in areas of active disease. FDG-PET is highly reliable in detecting splenic involvement and has rendered laparotomy obsolete in the staging workup of these patients. Many studies have shown the lack of reliability in detecting marginal zone lymphoma, particularly the extranodal marginal type. The available data strongly demonstrate increased sensitivity of FDG-PET compared with the gallium scan in the staging of NHL and has supplanted that test in the workup of patients with lymphoma.

Answer 30.18.   **The answer is C.**

SMZL accounts for up to 25% of low-grade B-cell neoplasms in splenectomy samples and 1% to 2% of chronic lymphoid leukemia. The lack of CD103 and CD25 differentiates it from hairy cell leukemia. SMZL is not only found in the spleen but also involves the bone marrow, peripheral blood, and unusual sites, such as the CNS (leukemic meningitis).

Answer 30.19.   **The answer is C.**

Follicular lymphoma arises from the GCBs (centrocytes and centroblasts). Tumors are CD10+, CD20+, CD5–. Most cases are bcl-2+, and some neoplastic cells have nuclear bcl-6. Rituxan immunotherapy has improved all chemotherapy modalities in this disease, and radioimmunotherapy with I131 Tositumomab (Bexxar) or Ytrium90 ibritumomab tiuxetan (Zevalin) has produced objective responses and is currently under evaluation when combined with chemotherapy (CHOP) and/or autologous stem cell transplantation. Myelodysplastic syndrome has been reported after radioimmunotherapy and high-dose therapy and autologous stem cell transplantation. The latter is not curative in follicular lymphoma, but the addition of rituxan purging has improved disease-free survival and delayed onset of relapses. Rituxan maintenance therapy has been used in various stages of the disease, but its ultimate benefit may reside in patients who are receiving chemotherapy for relapsing disease. Reduced-intensity allogeneic stem cell transplantation has been successfully applied to patients with advanced relapsed follicular lymphoma.

Answer 30.20.   **The answer is B.**

Bortezomib and the mTOR inhibitor temsirolimus have demonstrated activity in MCL and are under evaluation in clinical trials. Bortezomib maintenance after autologous stem cell transplantation is being evaluated in clinical trials.

Answer 30.21.   **The answer is B.**

More than 90% of the patients with MCL have cytogenetic abnormalities in addition to the classic $t(11;14)(q13;q32)$.

Answer 30.22.   **The answer is C.**

A panel of three immunohistochemical stains (CD10, BCL6, and MUM1) has been validated for distinction of the CGB and ABC subtypes of DLCBL. Localized stage I and II extranodal disease is seen in 30% of cases. Host response, B-cell receptor/proliferation, and oxidative-phosphorylation have been found by GEP to be associated with favorable outcome.

Answer 30.23.   **The answer is C.**

The benefit of rituximab was greater in patients with lymphoma that overexpressed bcl-2 on immunochemistry.

Answer 30.24.   **The answer is B.**

Primary testicular lymphomas is the most common testicular neoplasm in men older than 60, and orchiectomy is the initial therapy of choice. The most common histologies are diffuse large cell and immunoblastic lymphoma. Although described in the literature, primary testicular follicular lymphoma is rare.

Answer 30.25.   **The answer is D.**

The Southwest Oncology Group Trial in a recent pilot study has shown that R-CHOP × 3 plus RT led to outstanding results. The mabThera International Trial (Min T) used six cycles of CHOP-like chemotherapy in young patients with favorable risk factors (75%) with early-stage disease. In that study, the rituximab-containing arm had outstanding results without added RT. Ongoing clinical trials are comparing radioimmunotherapy with and without radiation and increasingly relying on FDG-PET imaging to define optimal amount of therapy.

Answer 30.26.   **The answer is C.**

Abbreviated chemotherapy followed by RT has been shown to be superior to a full course of chemotherapy in patients with untreated limited-stage DLBCL, but this has not been shown to be beneficial in patients relapsing after chemotherapy. The role of R-CHOP (a regimen that was previously used) in the treatment of relapsed aggressive lymphoma is less optimal and may expose the patient to increased cardiac toxicity. On the basis of the Parma trial, this patient would benefit from cytoreductive chemotherapy followed by autologous stem cell transplantation if her lymphoma is still chemosensitive. The addition of granulocyte-macrophage colony-stimulating factor/granulocyte colony-stimulating factor to augment antibody-mediated cellular cytotoxicity may be used to purge residual circulating DLCBL cells before peripheral blood stem cell collection. Radioimmunotherapy is active in large-cell lymphoma, but its role as a single agent in this disease has not been studied prospectively. Reduced-intensity allogeneic stem cell transplantation may be used in patients with less optimal responses or in whom autologous stem cell collection is not possible.

Answer 30.27.   **The answer is C.**

The GEP in PMBCL shows a distinct signature from nodal DLCBL, whereas MAL and FIG1 genes were observed; similarities to HL were apparent with loss of B-cell receptor signaling genes and activation of the JAK-2 and NF-kb pathways. Ongoing studies are evaluating bortezomib in combination with R-CHOP therapy in PMBCL.

Answer 30.28.   **The answer is D.**

Patients with localized NK/T-cell lymphoma in the nasal pharynx can be cured with a combination of chemotherapy and local RT. With RT alone, treatment failure is frequent. Genetic abnormality includes del(6) (q21;q25); T-receptor genes are germ line. Patients with disseminated NK/T-cell lymphoma have an extremely poor outlook and should be enrolled in clinical trials. Early application of high-dose chemotherapy and autologous stem cell transplantation may be curative in some patients after relapse from standard therapy.

Answer 30.29.   **The answer is C.**

Subcutaneous panniculitis T-cell lymphoma is associated with atypical lymphoid cells and often with necrosis and karyorrhexis. Responses to RT and chemotherapy are transient, and the long-term outlook is very poor. Early consideration of aggressive approaches, such as autologous or allogeneic stem cell transplantation, is recommended.

Answer 30.30.   **The answer is A.**

CTCLs are a heterogeneous group of both T and B lymphocytes that localize to the skin, which is the second most common site of extranodal lymphoma estimated at 1:100,000.

Answer 30.31.   **The answer is B.**

Sézary cells are clonal CD4+CD45RO+ T cells; some CTCL variants are CD8+. Antigen loss is characteristic of the disease (loss of CD7, CD5, or CD2 and dim CD3) and display a Th2 phenotype secreting IL-4, 5, 6, 10, and 13. The pruritus characteristic of this disease is related to IL-5 and other chemokines. IL-7, not IL-11, is an autocrine and paracrine growth factor for these cells. Clinical features of SS include extensive skin involvement with erythroderma that may progress to lichenification, palmoplantar hyperkeratosis, and diffuse exfoliation.

Answer 30.32.   **The answer is A.**

Overall outcome in MF is correlated with clinical stage (skin involvement and visceral stage). Staging for MF is based on estimating the degree of skin involvement and the amount of infiltration of lymph nodes and viscera. T1 and T2 are disease patches or plaques on less than 10% of the skin surface, whereas T4 is erythroderma flat and patch-like with diffusely infiltrated skin and thickening and fissuring of the palms and soles of the feet. LN4 nodes are effaced by tumor cells and characterize patients with poor prognosis.

Answer 30.33.   **The answer is C.**

The most common presentation of primary CNS lymphoma is the frontal lobe and is associated with changes in personality and level of alertness. Headaches and symptoms of increased intracranial pressure are seen frequently. Many lesions are periventricular, allowing tumor cells to gain access to the cerebrospinal fluid.

Answer 30.34.   **The answer is B.**

Optic nerve involvement can occur.

Answer 30.35.   **The answer is D.**

The risk of multifocal leukoencephalopathy is higher in older patients and when chemotherapy and RT are overlapping. Radiation boost to affected areas should be avoided. Most often chemotherapy is administered before RT in PCNSL to avoid cognitive damage and decrease neurotoxicity. The blood–brain barrier after completion of cranial RT may remain open weeks to months, thereby increasing the risks of leukoencephalopathy when drugs accumulate in brain tissue.

Answer 30.36.   **The answer is D.**

HRS cells express many cytokines and chemokines, thereby explaining the inflammatory infiltrates seen in affected lymph nodes. IL-5 is expressed in 95% of HRS cells and 63% of elaborate eotaxin, thereby providing proliferation and chemotactic signals to recruit eosinophils to the site(s) of HL. Genes like IL (IL-13, 6, 12, and 10), interferon-γ, tumor necrosis factor (TNF)-α, and IL-1 are expressed by HRS cells and mediate the B symptoms and immune dysregulation seen in patients with HL at presentation.

Answer 30.37.   **The answer is C.**

Mutations of IκBα were found in 15 of 26 primary cHL cases, 11 of which were EBV-negative.

Answer 30.38.   **The answer is A.**

HRS cells effectively escape the host immune system by modulating the immune response in the direction of an impaired Th2 response. Surrounding eosinophils inhibit an effective Th1 response in favor of a primarily humoral Th2 response, which helps the growth of malignant cells in cHL.

Answer 30.39.   **The answer is C.**

Transformation of NLPHL to DLCBL occurs in 2% to 6% of cases. The complete response rate after initial therapy is more than 90%. The immunophenotype is an important part of the definition of NLPHL. Unlike typical B-cell lymphomas, however, they are usually immunoglobulin-negative by routine techniques.

Answer 30.40.   **The answer is D.**

In the GHSG, the OS of LRCHL was significantly worse than that of NLPHL.

Answer 30.41.   **The answer is C.**

Rare cases of B-cell CLL may contain RS cells, and others may evolve into HL (HL variant of Richter syndrome). These cases may or may not be clonally related to the CLL. Lymphomas are presumed to arise in the setting of immune deficiency (estimated risk 1% to 5%), and cases of MF, lymphomatoid papulosis, and HL have been reported. Recent GEP data suggest that mediastinal large B-cell lymphoma is closely related to cHL.

Answer 30.42.   **The answer is D.**

Patients with nodular sclerosis (NS) and mixed cellularity (MC) most convincingly display contiguous HL spread. The left and right sides of the neck were each involved in greater than 60% of patients with NS and MC histologies. These sites were at least four times more common as other nodal sites above and below the diaphragm. Most patients with NS or MC HL have a central pattern of nodal involvement (cervical, mediastinal, para-aortic). In MC histology, the spleen is more frequently involved, along with adenopathy below the diaphragm and B symptoms.

Answer 30.43.   **The answer is C.**

Patients who relapse after RT alone for conventional HL have satisfactory results with conventional combination chemotherapy. Prior RT does not cause drug resistance or a clinically significant compromise of chemotherapy dose intensity. Patients who relapse with stage IV disease or "B" symptoms have a 10-year disease-free survival as high as 34% and should be treated initially with conventional chemotherapy. It does appear that ABVD gives a better disease-free survival when compared with MOPP in patients with recurrence after radiation (81% with ABVD vs. 54% with MOPP).

Answer 30.44.   **The answer is C.**

Women also have a high risk of loss of fertility with pelvic irradiation. There is a lower risk of loss of fertility in women aged less than 25 years who are treated with chemotherapy, not RT.

Answer 30.45.   **The answer is B.**

HL is the fourth most common cancer diagnosed during pregnancy and has been reported in 1 of every 1000 to 6000 deliveries. Several studies have shown that pregnancy does not worsen the clinical course of HL, and that the long-term survival of pregnant women with HL is not different from that of nonpregnant women. The ABVD regimen may be used when chemotherapy is indicated beyond the first trimester. Because drugs accumulate in the milk, mothers are advised not to breastfeed during treatment.

Answer 30.46.   **The answer is A.**

More cases of secondary AML are seen after MOPP chemotherapy because of exposure to alkylating agents. DLBCL is more often seen after HL treatment.

Answer 30.47.   **The answer is B.**

RT, bleomycin, and high-dose BCNU exposure are all associated with a higher risk of late complications, including severe pulmonary fibrosis.

Answer 30.48.   **The answer is B.**

The total rate of secondary neoplasms was highest in the COPP/ABVD arm.

Answer 30.49.   **The answer is D.**

In the GHSG HD7 trial, the patients who received two cycles of ABVD had a statistically significant improvement in freedom from treatment failure (91% vs. 75% for irradiation alone, $p < .0001$). This study raised several questions. Is the benefit in freedom from treatment failure worth the risk of long-term toxicity from the exposure to doxorubicin and bleomycin? Will it be more difficult to salvage the patients who relapse after the irradiation if they have already received two cycles of ABVD? Only longer follow-up will answer these questions.

Answer 30.50.   **The answer is B.**

The CD20 antigen is expressed on all malignant cells in nodular LPHL. Two phase II trials with rituximab showed promising results with high overall response rates (86% to 100%).

Answer 30.51.   **The answer is C.**

CD30 is expressed both in ALK-positive and ALK-negative anaplastic large cell lymphomas, embryonal and nonembryonal carcinoma, leiomyosarcomas, rhabdomyosarcoma, aggressive fibromatosis, and malignant fibrous histiocytoma (Durkop H et al. Journal of Pathology 2000;190:613–618), peripheral T cell lymphomas (PTCL-NOS) (Weisenburger DD et al. Blood 2011;117:3402–3408), and on mast cells in systemic mastocytosis (Valent P et al. Leukemia lymphoma 2011;52:740–744).

CHAPTER 31 ACUTE LEUKEMIAS

JOHN WELCH • AMANDA F. CASHEN

DIRECTIONS   Each of the numbered items below is followed by lettered answers. Select the ONE lettered answer that is BEST in each case unless instructed otherwise.

QUESTIONS

Question 31.1.   The favorable cytogenetic rearrangement in acute myeloid leukemia (AML) resulting from the t(8;21) juxtaposes which genes?

A.   AML1-ETO
B.   RUNX1-RUNX1T1
C.   A core-binding factor and a zinc finger protein
D.   All of the above

Question 31.2.   You are caring for a 25-year-old woman with AML-M2 and normal cytogenetics. She receives 7 + 3 induction therapy, and her day-14 bone marrow biopsy is ablated. She returns to clinic and her day-45 bone marrow shows normal hematopoeisis, however, she relapses after 18 months. Which of the following likely contributed to her relapse?

A.   DNMT3A mutation
B.   CEBPA mutation
C.   NPM mutation without FLT3-ITD
D.   Her age

Question 31.3.   Your well-read 30-year-old patient with AML asks you how you will follow her disease once she is in remission. She asks which is the most sensitive test for minimal residual disease? In which order are these assays most sensitive (least to most sensitive)?

A.   Cytopathology   <fluorescence   in   situ   hybridization   (FISH) <polymerase chain reaction (PCR)
B.   FISH <cytogenetics <PCR
C.   PCR <cytopathology <FISH
D.   Cytogenetics <PCR <flow cytometry

Corresponding Chapters in *Cancer: Principles & Practice of Oncology*, Ninth Edition: 130 (Molecular Biology of Acute Leukemias) and 131 (Management of Acute Leukemias).

Question 31.4.   Mutations in which pair of transcripts would be expected to cooperatively contribute significantly to leukemia?

A. FLT3 and ABL
B. A core-binding factor and the retinoic acid receptor alpha
C. FLT3 and the retinoic acid receptor alpha
D. Tel-PDGFβR and FLT3

Question 31.5.   A 52-year-old man presents with AML. On day 2 of induction therapy, he develops diffuse alveolar hemorrhage. An expected physical finding on examination would be:

A. Diffuse ecchymosis
B. Diffuse intravascular coagulopathy
C. Swollen gums
D. Cardiac rub

Questions 31.6.   You have been following a 75-year-old woman in clinic with mild renal
–31.7.   insufficiency and progressive anemia. She presents to clinic with a 3-day history of progressive fatigue and new headaches. Her white blood cell (WBC) count is 53,000 with 50% blasts.

Question 31.6.   Given her history, you might expect to find what on her cytogenetics?

A. $t(15;17)$
B. -7
C. inv(16)
D. $t(8;21)$

Question 31.7.   Which of these improves her prognosis?

A. Probable leukostasis
B. Her age
C. Prior myelodysplastic syndrome (MDS)
D. Good performance status

Question 31.8.   You are caring for a 70-year-old man with newly diagnosed AML. According to his cytogenetics, you give him an unfavorable prognosis based on which result:

A. -7
B. $t(15;17)$
C. inv(16)
D. $t(8;21)$

Question 31.9.   All of the following are considered to be poor prognosis factors in adult ALL, EXCEPT:

A. Age >55 years
B. Leukocytosis
C. Diploid chromosomes on karyotyping
D. $t(4;11)$

Question 31.10.   A 70-year-old man presents with newly diagnosed AML-M4 with eosinophilia. Choice of treatment will be based on all, EXCEPT:

A. His age
B. His performance status
C. His cytogenetics
D. Excellent response to $7 + 3$ induction therapy in the elderly

Question 31.11.   You have been following a 54-year-old woman with acute promyelocytic leukemia (APL) in clinic. After 2 years she returns to clinic with fatigue, an elevated WBC, and increased promyelocytes. Peripheral blood PCR confirms recurrence of her t(15;17) translocation. Before starting arsenic salvage therapy you obtain which test?

A. Liver function test
B. Erythrocyte sedimentation rate
C. D-dimer
D. Electrocardiogram

Question 31.12.   You have been caring for a 65-year-old woman with a distant history of breast cancer treated with adjuvant cyclophosphamide and Adriamycin. During the last year, she developed progressive anemia and thrombocytopenia. She also recently developed leukopenia. Her bone marrow biopsy shows decreased cellularity with dysplastic features and 25% blasts. Which of the following cytogenetic changes might you expect to find?

A. $t(15;17)$
B. $t(9;21)$
C. Complex cytogenetics
D. Trisomy 21

Question 31.13.   All of the following statements are true regarding elderly patients (age >60 years) with AML, EXCEPT?

A. In general, older patients with AML have poor outcomes when compared to younger patients.
B. Treatment with low-dose cytarabine leads to better outcomes than best supportive care.
C. Single-agent tipifarnib treatment did not improve survival compared to best supportive care alone.
D. Treatment with decitabine leads to better survival outcomes compared to low-dose cytarabine.

Questions 31.14.
–31.18.
You are consulted to see a 20-year-old Hispanic woman who presented with progressive fatigue during the last week and then significant epistaxis. Her WBC is 12,000/μL with 40% promyelocytes and a platelet count of 15,000/μL. Her international normalized ratio (INR) is 2.7 with a prothrombin time of 45 and partial thromboplastin time of 65. Her fibrinogen is 82. On review of her peripheral smear, you observe many promyelocytes with large granules and multiple Auer rods.

Question 31.14.
After review of her peripheral smear, you suspect that she has APL. Your initial therapy would include all of the following, EXCEPT:

A. Fresh-frozen plasma
B. Cryoprecipitate
C. All-trans retinoic acid (ATRA)
D. Arsenic trioxide

Question 31.15.
Three days after starting daunorubicin and ATRA, her coagulopathy has improved. She has shortness of breath in the morning and rapidly becomes hypoxic over the course of the day. Which of the following would prove most helpful in treating her hypoxia?

A. High-flow facemask oxygen
B. Lasix
C. Methylprednisolone
D. Albuterol

Question 31.16.
Fifteen days into treatment she develops a severe headache. Her neurologic examination results are normal, as are her funduscopic examination results. Review of her morning laboratory tests reveal a WBC of 0.6/μL, hematocrit of 9.8, platelet count of 25,000/μL, INR of 1.4, and fibrinogen of 190. You obtain a noncontrast head computed tomography scan but are more worried that this is a result of:

A. Relapse
B. ATRA
C. Daunorubicin
D. Transfusion reaction

Question 31.17.
Six months later you are reviewing her chart. Her CBC has normalized, and she has tolerated consolidation therapy. Her most recent PCR showed no sign of residual disease. You are most concerned about relapse because of:

A. Her microgranular variant presentation
B. Her presenting coagulopathy
C. Her presenting WBC
D. Her ethnicity

Question 31.18.   Three years later she presents to clinic with an elevated leukocyte count. PCR of peripheral blood confirms the presence of her initial $t(15;17)$ translocation. Treatment options at this point include all of the following, EXCEPT:

A. Arsenic trioxide
B. Gemtuzumab ozogamicin
C. Autologous transplant after achieving CR
D. Clofarabine

Question 31.19.   A 30-year-old, otherwise healthy woman is diagnosed with AML. Cytogenetics reveal inv(16). She undergoes induction therapy. Day-14 bone marrow biopsy shows an ablated marrow. Her day-45 marrow shows restored cellularity without evidence of disease. Repeat cytogenetics do not reveal the inv(16) rearrangement. Appropriate consolidation therapy would be:

A. Allogeneic transplant if a matched sibling donor is available
B. High-dose cytarabine (HIDAC) 3 g/m^2 every 12 hours on days 1, 3, and 5 for four 28-day cycles
C. Intermediate-dose cytarabine (IDAC) 300 mg/m^2 every 12 hours on days 1, 3, and 5 for four 28-day cycles
D. Arsenic 0.15 mg/kg on days 1 to 5 for four 28-day cycles

Question 31.20.   Which of the following regimens require graft-versus-tumor effects to remove residual AML blasts?

A. Busulfan-cyclophosphamide
B. Cyclophosphamide-TBI
C. Busulfan-fludarabine
D. Busulfan-VP16

Question 31.21.   High-dose busulfan used in myeloablative preparative regimens for stem cell transplantation may result in all of the following side effects, EXCEPT:

A. Seizures
B. Mucositis
C. Pancytopenia
D. MDS

Question 31.22.   Central nervous system (CNS) prophylaxis should be considered in which of the following patients?

A. A 25-year-old Latina woman with APL who presents with a WBC of 2500/μL, an INR of 2.5, and fibrinogen of 100
B. A 78-year-old man with AML evolved from MDS
C. A 30-year-old woman with AML who develops headaches while receiving ondansetron for nausea on day 9 of induction therapy
D. A 20-year-old man with Down syndrome and ALL who presents with leukocytosis (WBC 120,000/μL)

Question 31.23.   Dexamethasone has replaced prednisone in ALL induction therapy because of improved penetration in which tissue?

A. Testes
B. Spleen
C. Bone marrow
D. Brain

Question 31.24.   Maintenance therapy for ALL with daily 6-mercaptopurine, weekly methotrexate, and monthly vincristine and prednisone should be continued for how long?

A. 6 months
B. 12 months
C. 24 to 36 months
D. Until relapse

Question 31.25.   Which of the following targeted agents have been shown to be beneficial in adult ALL?

A. Imatinib
B. Alemtuzumab
C. Gemtuzumab ozogamicin
D. Sunitinib

Question 31.26.   For which of the following patients would you consider myeloablative stem cell transplantation in CR1?

A. A 30-year-old woman with inv(16) AML-M4 with eosinophilia
B. A 50-year-old man with complex cytogenetics AML-M1
C. A 65-year-old man with complex cytogenetics AML-M1
D. A 50-year-old woman with *t*(15;17) AML-M3

Question 31.27.   All of the following statements are true regarding the nucleophosmin 1 (NPM1) mutation in AML EXCEPT:

A. NPM1 gene encodes a protein that functions as chaperone between the nucleus and cytoplasm.
B. NPM1 mutations are found only in patients with AML with normal karyotype.
C. NPM1 mutations in the absence of FLT3-ITD have good prognosis.
D. Aberrant cytoplasmic localization of NPM1 is associated with mutation in the gene.

ANSWERS

Answer 31.1.   **The answer is D.**
The favorable t(8;21) translocation results in the juxtaposition of the initially named AML1 gene with the ETO gene (the AML gene and the eight-twenty-one gene). These two have recently been renamed RUNX1 and RUNX1T1, respectively. RUNX1 is a member of the core-binding factor family of transcription factors, which regulate differentiation of normal blasts. This fusion protein creates a dominant negative protein, which results in a differentiation block. Inv(16) and the t(16;16) rearrangements likewise result in dominant negative effects on core-binding factors and are associated with a favorable prognosis.

Answer 31.2.   **The answer is A.**
The DNMT3A gene encodes the DNA (cytosine-5)-methyltransferase 3A enzyme that catalyzes the addition of a methyl group to the cytosine residue of CpG dinucleotides. In patients with AML with normal cytogenetics, the presence of DNMT3A mutations is independently associated with poor outcomes. CEBP/α is a transcription factor involved in myeloid differentiation thought to be activated by ATRA treatment in APL. Mutations in the CEBPA gene have been noted in other FAB-AML classifications and have been associated with a superior outcome compared with the wild-type transcript. NPM mutations, in the absence of the FLT3-ITD, have also been associated with improved prognosis. Age is a strong prognostic factor. However, it is patients who are older than 65 years who have a worse prognosis. Her young age would be a marker of a good prognosis.

Answer 31.3.   **The answer is A.**
Cytopathology requires greater than 5% blasts on a bone marrow biopsy to diagnose AML relapse. This results in a sensitivity of 1 in 20. A cytogenetic review of 30 metaphases results in a 1 in 30 sensitivity. FISH has a sensitivity of approximately 1 in 500. PCR techniques allow sensitivity of approximately 1 in 10^4. However, both FISH and PCR require screening for defined cytogenetic changes. Because initial cytogenetic changes typically recur during AML relapse, this is generally not a significant barrier, unless patients present with uncommon cytogenetic changes for which FISH and PCR probes are not commercially available.

Answer 31.4.   **The answer is C.**
Current models of leukemia suggest that two separate classes of mutations are required for leukemogenesis: an activating mutation and a differentiation mutation. Activating mutations result in dysregulation of proliferative signaling pathways and thus lead to hyperproliferation. Important targets of activating mutations in leukemia include FLT3-ITD, RAS, BCR-ABL, TEL-PDGFβR, and PTPN11. Many of these contain tyrosine kinase domains. Leukemogenic mutations often result in constitutive kinase activity and thus constitutive activity in signal transduction

pathways leading to growth and proliferation. Important targets of differentiation mutations include core-binding factors (RUNX1 or AML1, CBFβ), retinoic acid receptor alpha, HOXA9, and MOZ. Mutations in these transcripts (frequently resulting from balanced chromosomal rearrangements) result in blocks in differentiation. Current paradigms suggest that leukemia requires both a differentiation block and a dysregulated proliferation. Thus, the common combination of FLT3-ITD and the *t*(15;17) PML-RARα translocation may be involved in APL leukemogenesis, whereas the other combinations are each within the same functional group.

Answer 31.5.   **The answer is C.**
Diffuse alveolar hemorrhage is a rare complication of induction therapy in AML, which carries significant mortality risk. However, it is most commonly reported in patients with AML and myelomonocytic or monocytic features (M4 or M5). These myelomonoblasts and monoblasts display a predilection for tissue invasion, such as in the gums, as well as into the lungs. This is thought to result from their high expression of adhesion molecules: intercellular adhesion molecule and vascular cell adhesion molecule. During initial treatment, activation and death of circulating blasts may lead to pulmonary inflammation and alveolar hemorrhage. Because of the rarity of such events, treatment options remain poorly studied. In small series, high-dose steroids have shown benefit.

Answer 31.6.   **The answer is B.**
AML, which has evolved from MDS, is especially recalcitrant to therapy. It may be associated with –5 or –7 cytogenetic abnormalities but is most commonly associated with complex cytogenetics. This patient is presenting with many poor-risk features (age >60 years, symptoms suggestive of leukostasis, and underlying organ insufficiency), which will make response to therapy difficult.

Answer 31.7.   **The answer is D.**
There are many prognostic factors for AML. Of particular note are age, cytogenetics, and performance status. Age greater than 65 years has been associated with worse outcomes independently of cytogenetics. AML evolving from prior MDS also confers a worse prognosis. Leukostasis at presentation presents significant early morbidity and mortality, especially in an older patient. An elevated peripheral blast count, which may be associated with leukostasis, is also associated with a poor long-term prognosis.

Answer 31.8.   **The answer is A.**
AML prognosis is currently separated into three broad categories based on cytogenetic results: favorable (inv[16]; *t*[8;21] and *t*[15;17]); intermediate (normal, +8); and unfavorable (–5, –7, complex with ≥5 chromosomes involved). Some studies have also included 11*q*, +8, del(20*q*), *t*(6;9), and 17*p* abnormalities in the unfavorable risk group.

Answer 31.9.   **The answer is C.**
Age greater than 50 years, poor performance status, African American ethnicity, and leukocytosis (>30,000/μL B-lineage or >100,000/μL T-lineage) are associated with high-risk ALL. Immunophenotypes including early and mature-T ALL and pro-B ALL are also considered high risk. Cytogenetics including the Philadelphia chromosome *t*(9;22) and *t*(4;11) are both high-risk prognostic factors. Normal diploid chromosomes on karyotyping is not associated with poor prognosis.

Answer 31.10.   **The answer is D.**
Treatment of AML in the elderly (>65 years) is difficult because of the heterogeneous nature of response and the generally high rate of treatment-related mortality. Older patients at MD Anderson with a performance status >2, bilirubin greater than 1.9 mg/dL, or serum creatinine greater than 1.9 mg/dL had a treatment-related mortality of 62% and only a 27% complete remission rate. Thus, decision to undergo standard induction therapy must be based on a careful assessment of the patient's ability to tolerate the therapy and his/her prognosis. The patient's age, performance status, and low-risk cytogenetics might influence a physician to recommend standard therapy.

Answer 31.11.   **The answer is D.**
Arsenic trioxide has demonstrated considerable activity in salvage therapy for APL. Arsenic trioxide has been associated with prolonged QTc syndrome. Because of this, Electrocardiograms should be performed before and during therapy. Electrolytes should also be monitored and corrected. Additional medications that may prolong the QTc should be eliminated if possible.

Answer 31.12.   **The answer is C.**
Prior alkylator therapy increases the risk of MDS and treatment-related AML. Her recent history of progressive anemia and thrombocytopenia, with dysplastic features seen in her marrow, are all suggestive of an underlying MDS. Her blast count greater than 20% meets criterion for AML under current World Health Organization standards. AML evolved from MDS could carry a loss of chromosome 5 or 7 associated with the prior MDS, but most often is associated with complex cytogenetics. It also carries an unfavorable prognosis in multiple studies. *t*(15;17) is associated with APL but is not associated with prior breast cancer or alkylator therapy. *t*(9;21) is associated with the Philadelphia chromosome and seen in chronic myelocytic leukemia or acute lymphocytic leukemia, but is rarely associated with AML or MDS. Trisomy 21 is associated with AML-M7 with increased megakaryocytes. Recent data suggest this may be associated with the concomitant overexpression of an miRNA carried on chromosome 21.

Answer 31.13.   **The answer is D.**
Older patients with AML have worse outcomes when compared to younger patients irrespective of their performance status or comorbidities. Treatment with low-dose cytarabine has been shown to improve survival

when compared to best supportive care alone. More recently, hypomethylating agents have been used in the treatment of AML in the elderly. However, they have not been shown to be superior to treatment with low-dose cytarabine. Treatment with tipifarnib, a farnesyl transferase inhibitor, did not improve outcomes for elderly patients with AML when compared to best supportive care alone. Treatment with decitabine is associated with better response rate, but not improved survival, compared to low-dose cytarabine.

Answer 31.14.   **The answer is D.**
Patients with APL are at considerable risk of early morbidity and mortality because of disseminated intravascular coagulation and bleeding complications. Aggressive management of coagulopathy is mandatory, with the goal of maintaining the fibrinogen greater than 150, INR less than 1.5, and platelet count greater than 30,000. Patients with WBC greater than 10,000/μL are at a higher risk of differentiation syndrome once ATRA is started. Typically, ATRA is held while daunorubicin is started until the WBC is less than 10,000/μL. Arsenic trioxide has demonstrated significant efficacy in the setting of relapsed APL. Ongoing studies are evaluating its efficacy during induction therapy in conjunction with ATRA. However, it is not currently standard of care during induction therapy.

Answer 31.15.   **The answer is C.**
Differentiation syndrome can be a life-threatening complication of APL and ATRA treatment. As the granule-laden promyelocytes differentiate, the granular products stimulate pulmonary edema and fluid retention. Fevers and weight gain are common symptoms of differentiation syndrome. Treatment includes steroids and management of coagulopathy. Differentiation syndrome may affect as many as 10% to 25% of patients with APL.

Answer 31.16.   **The answer is B.**
Headache is a common side effect from ATRA. Treatment options include dose reduction and symptom management with analgesics. Unfortunately, patients occasionally require drug discontinuation because of this side effect.

Answer 31.17.   **The answer is C.**
The greatest risk of relapse in APL is associated with an elevated WBC greater than 10,000/μL on presentation. Patients with presenting WBC less than 10,000/μL achieve CR approximately 90% of the time.

Answer 31.18.   **The answer is D.**
Clofarabine is being studied in relapsed AML, but it has not been evaluated in APL. Arsenic trioxide has demonstrated significant efficacy in relapsed APL and in consolidation protocols. APL promyelocytes commonly express high levels of CD33, and gemtuzumab ozogamicin (anti-CD33) has demonstrated efficacy in relapsed APL. APL is one of the few cases in AML in which autologous transplantation has demonstrated significant benefit, and it is often used in a salvage consolidation protocol.

Answer 31.19.   **The answer is B.**
Although most patients with AML will relapse without consolidation therapy, the appropriate consolidation therapy remains unclear for the majority of these patients. Young patients with good-risk cytogenetics are one of the few cohorts with AML in whom specific consolidation recommendations are supported by clinical data. A study sponsored by the Cancer and Leukemia Group B (CALGB) found that young patients with inv(16) had a 78% CR rate at 5 years after four cycles of HIDAC therapy, whereas 57% remained in CR in the IDAC arm and only 16% remained in CR with conventional 100 mg/m^2 dosing. Patients with normal cytogenetics fared less well as a group with equivalent outcomes (47% vs. 37% CR at 5 years) in the HIDAC and IDAC arms and worse outcomes with conventional dosing (20%). Patients with unfavorable cytogenetics should be considered for allogeneic transplant in first CR. Arsenic has shown benefit in a consolidation protocol for APL, but it has not been evaluated in general AML consolidation protocols.

Answer 31.20.   **The answer is C.**
Nonmyeloablative conditioning regimens require a graft-versus-leukemia effect to improve the clearance of residual AML blasts not eliminated by the conditioning regimen.

Answer 31.21.   **The answer is D.**
High-dose busulfan decreases the seizure threshold of patients, and therefore seizure prophylaxis is commonly used. Mucositis commonly follows busulfan therapy, especially during prolonged neutropenia. Pancytopenia naturally follows a myeloablative regimen. Risk for MDS may increase after alkylator and topoisomerase II inhibitor therapy. However, MDS is not a risk of myeloablative preparatory regimens.

Answer 31.22.   **The answer is D.**
CNS prophylaxis may consist of intrathecal chemotherapy (methotrexate, cytarabine, corticosteroids), high-dose chemotherapy (methotrexate, cytarabine, L-asparaginase), or CNS irradiation. Patients with ALL with increased risk for CNS disease include those with an elevated WBC count, an elevated lactate dehydrogenase, a traumatic lumbar puncture, and T-lineage ALL. Although APL may relapse in the CNS, relapse is uncommon in patients with a presenting WBC less than 10,000/μL. CNS evaluation and prophylaxis are not routinely recommended in patients with APL. There is no role for CNS prophylaxis in elderly patients with AML without neurologic deficits. Although CNS disease must be considered in a patient with AML and headaches, a new headache caused by CNS leukemia on day 9 of induction therapy would be unusual and treatment could be delayed until proper evaluation is completed.

Answer 31.23.   **The answer is D.**
Dexamethasone has improved penetration in the CNS. Given the high risk of CNS disease in patients with ALL, dexamethasone is preferred over prednisone.

Answer 31.24.   **The answer is C.**
Attempts have been made to shorten maintenance therapy to 12 to 18 months, with inferior results. Current recommendations are for 2 to 3 years.

Answer 31.25.   **The answer is A.**
Philadelphia chromosome positive ALL carries a high-risk prognosis, but this has improved with the ABL tyrosine kinase inhibitor imatinib. Second-generation inhibitors such as dasatinib and nilotinib may also prove of value in the future. Alemtuzumab is an anti-CD52 monoclonal antibody that has demonstrated significant efficacy in the treatment of CLL. It has not been evaluated in ALL, which typically does not express CD52. Gemtuzumab ozogamicin is an anti-CD33 monoclonal antibody cross-linked to a cytotoxin, calicheamicin. It has been shown to improve outcomes in relapsed AML. Sunitinib is a nonspecific tyrosine kinase inhibitor. It has significant activity against FLT3 and may prove of value in the treatment of AML with FLT3-ITD.

Answer 31.26.   **The answer is B.**
Stem cell transplantation for AML remains a developing field. Current studies and meta-analysis have not found benefit in CR1 for patients with favorable cytogenetics (e.g., inv[16] and *t*[15;17]). Benefit is uncertain in patients with normal cytogenetics. Future trials may be able to assess the benefit of transplant in CR1 in higher-risk subpopulations of normal cytogenetics (e.g. FLT3-ITD or DNMT3A mutations). Patients aged less than 55 years who have unfavorable cytogenetics (e.g., –5, –7, complex cytogenetics) appear to benefit from myeloablative transplantation in CR1. However, older patients tolerate this approach less well, with increased treatment-related morbidity and mortality. Decision making in older patients must be individualized, and nonmyeloablative transplant approaches are being explored.

Answer 31.27.   **The answer is B.**
NPM1 gene encodes a protein that functions as a molecular chaperone between the nucleus and cytoplasm. Mutations involving this gene are found in 50% to 60% of all AML patients with normal karyotype. Aberrant cytoplasmic localization of NPM1 is associated with point mutations in the gene. In the absence of FLT3-ITD, the NPM1 mutation is associated with favorable prognosis.

CHAPTER 32 CHRONIC LEUKEMIAS

JAMES C. MOSLEY III • KEITH STOCKERL-GOLDSTEIN

DIRECTIONS   Each of the numbered items below is followed by lettered answers. Select the ONE lettered answer that is BEST in each case unless instructed otherwise.

QUESTIONS

Question 32.1.   A 54-year-old white man with chronic-phase chronic myeloid leukemia (CML) has quickly obtained a complete hematologic response while receiving imatinib 400 mg daily. He has been receiving therapy for 5 months, but you have noticed that his neutrophil count has gradually decreased to 0.9×10^9/L and now has a platelet count of 42×10^9/L. What is the MOST appropriate therapeutic intervention?

A. Decrease dose of imatinib to 200 mg by mouth every day
B. Interrupt therapy until recovery of blood counts
C. Discontinue therapy with imatinib and initiate therapy with dasatinib
D. Discontinue therapy with imatinib and initiate therapy with interferon

Question 32.2.   Which of the following statements is correct, regarding response to imatinib therapy in patients with CML?

A. Patients with low-risk Sokal scores have a 91% rate of complete cytogenetic response.
B. In patients who achieve a complete cytogenetic response, Sokal risk score is not predictive of disease progression.
C. Of patients who have a complete cytogenetic response after 12 months, 97% remain in chronic phase at 5 years.
D. All of the above.

Question 32.3.   Which of the following mechanisms is responsible for relapse in patients with CML?

A. Point mutations in the BCR-ABL kinase
B. BCR-ABL gene amplification
C. Clonal evolution
D. All of the above

Corresponding Chapters in *Cancer: Principles & Practice of Oncology,* Ninth Edition: 132 (Molecular Biology of Chronic Leukemias), 133 (Chronic Myelogenous Leukemia), and 134 (Chronic Lymphocytic Leukemias).

Question 32.4.   Which of the following is TRUE concerning patients treated with imatinib before allogeneic stem cell transplantation (ASCT) compared with
patients directly proceeding to ASCT in CML?

A. Treatment with imatinib during the chronic phase before transplantation is associated with a worse overall survival after ASCT.
B. Treatment with imatinib before transplantation results in more organ
toxicity in the posttransplant setting.
C. Patients treated with imatinib before transplant have no difference in
overall survival or progression-free survival.
D. Patients with imatinib-resistance mutations display inferior overall
survival compared with cohorts with advanced stages of disease.

Question 32.5.   A 34-year-old man was diagnosed with chronic-phase CML 3 years ago.
He was initially treated with imatinib and rapidly obtained a partial cytogenetic response. Unfortunately, the patient was noted to have developed
a relapse of disease. The patient has a human leukocyte antigen-matched
sibling, and the decision was made to undergo a myeloablative stem cell
transplant. Six months after transplantation, the patient is noted to have
developed evidence of BCR-ABL fusion by qualitative reverse transcriptase polymerase chain reaction assessment. Which of the following is the
MOST appropriate initial course of action?

A. Continued observation because reemergence of the leukemic clone is
common up to 1 year after transplantation
B. Donor lymphocyte infusion
C. Retransplantation from an unrelated donor
D. Initiation of imatinib 400 mg daily

Question 32.6.   Which of the following orally administered tyrosine kinase inhibitors is
indicated for the treatment of patients with newly diagnosed Ph+ chronic-
phase CML?

A. Imatinib 400 mg daily
B. Dasatinib 100 mg daily
C. Nilotinib 300 mg twice daily
D. All of the above

Question 32.7.   Which of the following is TRUE regarding chronic lymphocytic leukemia
(CLL)?

A. ZAP-70 overexpression is correlated with mutated VH genes.
B. Deletion 13q is the most common genetic aberration by fluorescence
in situ hybridization (FISH) in CLL.
C. 11q deletion is thought to be associated with Bcl-2 overexpression.
D. Patients with 17p deletions usually present with early-stage disease
that follows an indolent course.

Question 32.8. A 71-year-old white woman presents with a white blood cell of 39 × 10^9/L, with 78% mature lymphocytes. Flow cytometry is remarkable for the cells being CD5+, CD19+, CD23+, CD10–. The patient has palpable lymphadenopathy in the cervical region, axillary region, and bilateral groins, with no splenomegaly. Her hemoglobin is 13.9 g/dL, and her platelet count is 315 × 109/L. Which of the following is the MOST appropriate therapy at this time?

A. Observation with monitoring of complete blood count and physical examination every 3 to 6 months
B. Initiation of single-agent chlorambucil
C. Initiation of single-agent fludarabine
D. Initiation of combination fludarabine, cyclophosphamide, and rituximab

Question 32.9. A 54-year-old man with Rai stage 0 CLL has been followed by you for 2 years. He presents for a routine visit. His physical examination reveals no new lymphadenopathy or splenomegaly. Which of the following findings would be an indication for initiation of systemic therapy?

A. Recent hospitalization for pneumococcal pneumonia and diagnosis of hypogammaglobulinemia
B. An increase in his absolute lymphocyte count from 15 × 10^9/L to 33 × 10^9/L over the last 2 years
C. An increase in his absolute lymphocyte count from 24 × 10^9/L to 38 × 10^9/L in the previous 2 months
D. Fever of 38°C for the last 1 week without evidence of infection

Question 32.10. Which of the following is NOT true?

A. In trials comparing fludarabine versus fludarabine with rituximab, grade 3/4 neutropenia was more common with the combination therapy.
B. In patients with previously untreated CLL, complete remission (CR) rates approaching 70% have been seen with combination fludarabine, cyclophosphamide, and rituximab.
C. Combination therapy with fludarabine plus cyclophosphamide has demonstrated superior overall survival compared with fludarabine alone.
D. Patients with 17q and 11q deletions have demonstrated inferior progression-free survival rates when treated with combination regimens including fludarabine and cyclophosphamide.

Question 32.11.   A 71-year-old woman presents with a mature lymphocytosis, diffuse lymphadenopathy, splenomegaly, thrombocytopenia, and an autoimmune hemolytic anemia. Workup is consistent with CLL. Treatment is initiated with four cycles of fludarabine and cyclophosphamide with a partial response (PR). The patient elects to undergo a treatment break for the next 6 months. She is then noted to have return of her lymphocytosis, lymphadenopathy, and thrombocytopenia. Fludarabine and cyclophosphamide are reinitiated, but she demonstrates continued disease progression. What is the MOST appropriate next line of therapy?

A. Chlorambucil
B. Single-agent rituximab
C. Combination fludarabine, cyclophosphamide, with addition of rituximab
D. Alemtuzumab

Question 32.12.   Which of the following cytogenetic abnormalities is associated with poor prognosis in patients with CML?

A. Iso-17q
B. Trisomy 8
C. Trisomy 19
D. Duplication of Philadelphia chromosome

Question 32.13.   The Philadelphia chromosome and BCR-ABL fusion gene are observed in all of the following hematologic malignancies, EXCEPT:

A. Acute myeloid leukemia (AML)
B. Acute lymphocytic leukemia (ALL)
C. Chronic myeloid leukemia (CML)
D. Chronic lymphocytic leukemia (CLL)

Question 32.14.   Which of the following treatments are curative in patients with CML?

A. Imatinib
B. Dasatinib
C. Nilotinib
D. None of the above

Question 32.15.   Which of the following statements is CORRECT regarding BCR-ABL in CML?

A. The breakpoint in ABL is highly variable, and is almost always upstream of exon 2.
B. The BCR-ABL fusion protein resides in the cytoplasm.
C. BCR breakpoints occur either between exon 13 and 14 or between exon 14 and 15.
D. All of the above.

ANSWERS

Answer 32.1.   **The answer is B.**
Nonhematologic toxicities are the most frequently observed toxicities during treatment with imatinib and include nausea, diarrhea, muscle cramping, edema, rashes, and fatigue. Grade 3 or 4 myelosuppression occurs in a minority of treated patients and is the result of the predominant Philadelphia chromosome positive stem cell clone that is driving the majority of the hematopoiesis. The appropriate therapy is to interrupt the dose if the absolute neutrophil count decreases to less than 1.0×10^9/L or platelets decrease to less than 50×10^9/L. Dose reductions are not appropriate because the normal hematopoiesis is minimally affected by imatinib and may allow for emergence of resistant clones.

Answer 32.2.   **The answer is D.**
Cytogenetic responses on imatinib therapy have a significant impact of disease progression. Of patients who achieve a complete cytogenetic response to imatinib therapy at 12 months, 97% will not progress to the accelerated phase or blast crisis. For patients with a partial cytogenetic response, the estimate is 93%. Sokal risk score at diagnosis predicts rate of complete cytogenetic response: patients with a low-risk Sokal score have a 93% rate of complete cytogenetic response, compared with an 81% rate in patients with a high-risk Sokal score. For patients who obtain a complete cytogenetic response, pretreatment Sokal scores are not predictive of disease progression at 5 years.

Answer 32.3.   **The answer is D.**
Point mutations in the BCR-ABL kinase are the most common cause of relapse in patients with CML. These mutations render the BCR-ABL kinase less sensitive to imatinib. Other mechanisms mediating disease relapse include BCR-ABL gene amplification, drug efflux, and finally clonal evolution.

Answer 32.4.   **The answer is C.**
Although allogeneic stem cell transplantation is the only potentially curative therapy in CML, most patients with chronic-phase disease are treated with imatinib therapy initially. Concerns have been raised that exposure to such kinase inhibitors could result in poorer outcomes if patients were to later proceed with stem cell transplantation as was demonstrated with prolonged exposure to interferon. Large observational studies have suggested that there is no detrimental effect to prior imatinib exposure in patients proceeding with stem cell transplantation. These patients do tend to undergo transplant with more advanced stages of disease and higher EBMT scores, but there has been no evidence for inferior overall survival, disease-free survival, transplant-related mortality, acute graft-versus-host disease (GVHD), engraftment kinetics, or organ toxicity compared with patients who were not exposed to imatinib before transplant. Furthermore, in small case studies, it appears that patients harboring

imatinib-resistant mutations have outcomes that are similar to what would be expected in clinically advanced disease.

Answer 32.5.   **The answer is D.**

Allogeneic hematopoietic stem cell transplantation is the only potentially curative therapy in CML. Induction of molecular remission after transplantation is more durable than that obtained with imatinib alone. After allogeneic hematopoietic stem cell transplantation, evidence of the leukemic clone can be detected in many patients, but will disappear over time, with very few patients continuing to have molecular evidence of CML at 2 years when undergoing transplantation in the chronic phase. The relapse rate after transplantation in the chronic phase is less than 10% in most series with greater than 50% of relapses occurring within the first year and less than 5% occurring after the fifth year.

Early intervention at first documentation of relapse confers the greatest chance of controlling the disease. Initial institution of imatinib 400 mg daily can restore complete molecular remission in 83% of patients with molecular relapse and 56% of patients with cytogenetic relapse. Up to 25% of patients who attain a complete molecular remission can be withdrawn from the imatinib therapy within 6 to 24 months, whereas others may require long-term therapy with imatinib or donor leukocyte infusions (DLIs). Because of the exquisite sensitivity of CML to graft-versus-leukemia effects, patients who relapse into chronic phase by cytogenetics or hematologic criteria, 60% to 80% can be treated with DLI alone with 5-year disease-free survival rates of 50%. Patients who relapse again after initial DLI can often be retreated with DLI as well. However, DLI carries significant risks with treatment-related mortality of 8% to 20% and adverse effects of acute and chronic GVHD, infectious complications, and others.

Answer 32.6.   **The answer is D.**

Imatinib was the first tyrosine kinase inhibitor approved for treating patients diagnosed with chronic-phase CML. Two newer tyrosine kinase inhibitors, nilotinib and dasatinib, are more potent inhibitors of BCR-ABL kinase than imatinib, and were initially developed for use in patients with resistance or intolerance to imatinib. They both have recently been approved by the FDA for treating patients with newly diagnosed Ph+ chronic-phase CML, based on randomized trials comparing these agents with imatinib in the first-line setting, which demonstrated superiority of the newer agents in the rates of major molecular response.

Answer 32.7.   **The answer is B.**

Much insight has been gained into the molecular abnormalities associated with CLL. Various chromosomal abnormalities can be reliably detected by FISH, with greater than 80% of cases demonstrating abnormalities. The most commonly encountered abnormality is a deletion of chromosome 13q, found in approximately 55% of cases. Further investigation of this common abnormality has led to the observation that this is often associated with deletion or downregulation of two microRNA genes (miR15 and miR16), which may downregulate the antiapoptotic protein, bcl-2.

Other less common chromosomal abnormalities occur, such as 11q deletion, trisomy 12, and 17p deletion. Of these, 11q and 17p deletions tend to present at more advanced stages and follow more aggressive courses. Early investigations have noted that approximately 50% of patients have unmutated VH genes, which has been associated with a poorer prognosis in retrospective analyses compared with cohorts with mutated VH genes. Further investigation noted that patients with unmutated VH genes had high expression of the T-cell receptor signal transduction protein, ZAP-70.

Answer 32.8. **The answer is A.**

This patient has Rai stage I CLL as evidenced by her lymphadenopathy, lack of splenomegaly, and lack of anemia or thrombocytopenia, placing her at intermediate risk. Her flow cytometry studies are typical of CLL. Despite the diagnosis of CLL, immediate treatment in this situation is not warranted. It is believed that CLL is not curable with current treatment approaches, so treatment is directed at symptomatic disease or patients who are likely to have poor prognosis. Most patients with CLL will have a prolonged course, and many studies have demonstrated that treatment with combinations of therapies can prolong progression-free survival and increase response rates compared with single-agent therapies, but no survival advantage has been noted in early intervention trials. Continued observation of patients with early-stage disease with attention to prognostic factors, such as lymphocyte doubling time, ZAP-70 expression, and karyotype, is indicated.

Answer 32.9. **The answer is C.**

Because CLL can be a heterogeneous disease, the National Cancer Institute-sponsored Working Group has established guidelines addressing indications to initiate treatment of patients. These include constitutional symptoms attributable to CLL, including weight loss of greater than 10% of baseline weight within the preceding 6 months, extreme fatigue, Eastern Cooperative Oncology Group performance status of 2 or greater, temperature greater than 38°C or 100.5°F for at least 2 weeks, or night sweats without evidence of infection; evidence of progressive bone marrow failure characterized by the development or progression of anemia or thrombocytopenia, or both; autoimmune hemolytic anemia or autoimmune thrombocytopenia, or both, which are poorly responsive to corticosteroid therapy; massive or progressive splenomegaly; massive or progressive lymphadenopathy; progressive lymphocytosis, defined as an increase in the absolute lymphocyte count by greater than 50% over a 2-month period, or a lymphocyte doubling time predicted to be less than 6 months. Diagnosis of hypogammaglobulinemia is not an indication for initiation of therapy.

Answer 32.10. **The answer is C.**

Studies of chemotherapy regimens in CLL have repeatedly demonstrated the activity and tolerability of the purine analog fludarabine as the most effective single-agent chemotherapy. Not surprisingly, this agent has been used as the backbone of other combination regimens in clinical trials. With various clinical trials including fludarabine in combination with other agents, CR and overall response rates have been superior with the combination arm. However, because of the usually long duration of disease that most patients experience, no trials have consistently demonstrated superior overall survival rates with one chemotherapy regimen over another. In the CALGB 9712 trial of sequential fludarabine and rituximab versus concurrent therapy, there was a significant increase in the CR rate, but there was also an increase in the incidence of grade 3 and 4 neutropenia. The combination of fludarabine, cyclophosphamide, and rituximab has been evaluated in both treatment-naïve and previously treated patients. In treatment-naïve patients, a CR rate of 70% was observed with a projected failure-free survival at 4 years of 69%; this is the highest response rate reported for any regimen for previously untreated patients in CLL. Unfortunately, patients carrying deletions in 17p or 11q have repeatedly demonstrated inferior outcomes with respect to progression-free survival in these studies.

Answer 32.11.   **The answer is D.**
Alemtuzumab is a humanized monoclonal antibody targeting CD52, which is highly expressed on CLL cells in addition to normal B and T lymphocytes. In a pivotal study of patients who were previously treated with fludarabine, second-line therapy with alemtuzumab was able to induce a CR in 2% of patients and a PR in 31% of patients. Some 59% of patients achieved stable disease as well. This led to the FDA approval of single-agent alemtuzumab for patients with fludarabine-refractory CLL. Alemtuzumab is effective at treatment of marrow and peripheral blood disease; however, it is less effective at treating patients with bulky lymphadenopathy. Of note, this agent is associated with an increased risk of cytomegalovirus infections and is also effective in patients with 17p deletion, which has generally been resistant to therapy with other agents.

Another monoclonal antibody, rituximab, directed against CD20 on malignant and normal B cells, has very limited activity as a single agent in CLL. This is likely because CLL cells demonstrate relatively low levels of expression of CD20 compared with normal lymphocytes, as well as the demonstration of increased levels of soluble CD20 in patients with CLL, which may interfere with rituximab's ability to induce antibody-dependent cellular cytotoxicity on target cells. Because this patient has progressed on combination therapy with fludarabine and cyclophosphamide, continuation with this regimen with addition of rituximab is unlikely to be of much clinical benefit.

Answer 32.12.   **The answer is A.**
The most common clonal cytogenetic abnormalities in patients with CML, in addition to t(9;22), which are found at diagnosis include duplication of the Philadelphia chromosome, trisomy 8, iso-17q, and trisomy 19. Although iso-17q has been associated with a poorer prognosis, the prognostic significance of the other chromosomal abnormalities is less clear.

Answer 32.13. **The answer is D.**
The Philadelphia chromosome and BCR-ABL fusion gene are not pathognomonic for CML. They are also observed in 25% to 50% of adult patients with ALL and in rare cases in AML.

Answer 32.14. **The answer is D.**
Tyrosine kinase inhibitors, such as imatinib, nilotinib and dasatinib, can lead to good long-term disease control in patients with CML; however, they are not curative. The only curative treatment of CML is hematologic stem cell transplantation.

Answer 32.15. **The answer is D.**
The breakpoint in ABL is highly variable, and is almost always upstream of exon 2, which results in translocation of all but exon 1. BCR breakpoints occur in two sites, between exon 13 and 14, or between exon 14 and 15; both of which carry a similar prognosis. The BCR-ABL fusion protein resides in the cytoplasm.

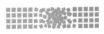

CHAPTER 33 MYELODYSPLASTIC SYNDROMES

SAIAMA N. WAQAR

DIRECTIONS   Each of the numbered items below is followed by lettered answers. Select the ONE lettered answer that is BEST in each case unless instructed otherwise.

QUESTIONS

Question 33.1.   Which of the following cytogenetic abnormalities in a patient with myelodysplastic syndromes (MDS) are indicative of a favorable prognosis?

A. del(5q)
B. del (20q)
C. −Y
D. All of the above

Question 33.2.   Which of the following is NOT a prognostic variable in the International Prognostic Scoring System (IPSS) for MDS?

A. Karyotype
B. Age
C. Percentage of blasts in the bone marrow
D. Number of cytopenias

Question 33.3.   A 55-year-old postmenopausal woman presents with anemia. Her hemoglobin is 10 g/dL, mean corpuscular volume is 105 fL, white blood cell count is 7,000/μL, and platelet count is 450,000/μL. Her ferritin is 400μg/L and erythropoietin level is 600U/L. Her serum creatinine, liver enzymes, iron studies, B12, and folate levels are normal. Bone marrow biopsy shows dyserythropoiesis and hypolobulated megakaryocytes, with 2% blasts. Cytogenetics reveal del (5q). Which of the following is the most appropriate therapy?

A. Azacitidine
B. Decitabine
C. Lenalidomide
D. Vorinostat

Corresponding Chapter in *Cancer: Principles & Practice of Oncology*, Ninth Edition: 135 (Myelodysplastic Syndromes).

Question 33.4.   Which of the following is correct regarding the IPSS for MDS?

A. IPSS does not distinguish patients with moderate or severe cytopenias.
B. IPSS includes patients with 21% to 30% blasts in the bone marrow.
C. Normal cytogenetics are assigned an intermediate risk score.
D. All of the above.

Question 33.5.   Which of the following genes is frequently mutated in patients with therapy-related MDS?

A. AML/RUNX1
B. JAK2
C. c-kit
D. All of the above

Question 33.6.   Which of the following statements is correct regarding therapy-related MDS resulting from prior treatment with alkylating agents?

A. MDS occurs within the first 2 years after treatment with alkylating agents.
B. Therapy-related MDS carries a good prognosis.
C. 90% of patients have aberrations of chromosomes 5 and/or 7.
D. All of the above.

Question 33.7.   Which of the following has been implicated in the development of MDS?

A. Defective growth of stromal progenitors
B. Decreased mitochondrial cytochrome c mediated activation of caspase-9
C. Decreased expression of Fas and Fas ligand
D. Decreased TNF-α-mediated signaling

Question 33.8.   Which of the following is correct regarding the role of allogeneic hematopoietic stem cell transplantation (HSCT) in MDS?

A. High-dose chemotherapy and allogeneic HSCT are the only known curative therapy for patients with MDS.
B. Allogeneic HSCT is indicated at the time of presentation, in patients with high-risk MDS, who have a matched sibling donor.
C. In pediatric MDS, diepoxybutane test must be performed prior to transplant.
D. All of the above.

ANSWERS

Answer 33.1.   **The answer is D.**
Cytogenetic abnormalities that confer a good prognosis in patients with MDS include del(5q), del(20q), and –Y. Abnormalities in chromosome 7 and complex abnormalities are associated with poor prognosis. Intermediate-risk cytogenetics include all the other cytogenetic abnormalities, which cannot be classified as good or poor.

Answer 33.2.   **The answer is B.**
The three prognostic variables used in the IPSS for MDS are percentage of marrow blasts, karyotype, and number of cytopenias. The overall IPSS score is based on the sum of the scores for these three variables.

Answer 33.3.   **The answer is C.**
This woman has 5q- syndrome. The typical presentation is refractory macrocytic anemia in a woman, with normal or elevated platelet count and normal white blood cell count. Bone marrow biopsy reveals dyserythropoiesis and hypolobulated megakaryocytes and cytogenetics show del(5q). Patients with 5q- syndrome have a good prognosis and respond to lenalidomide.

Answer 33.4.   **The answer is D.**
A limitation of the IPSS is that it does not distinguish patients with severe or moderate degrees of cytopenias, which may influence outcome. Furthermore, it includes patients with 21% to 30% blasts, which would be defined as AML per the WHO system. Normal cytogenetics are considered to be intermediate risk on karyotype scoring.

Answer 33.5.   **The answer is A.**
Somatic mutations in AML1/RUNX1 are common in therapy-related MDS. JAK2 mutations are seen in less than 5% of patients with MDS, but are common in myeloproliferative diseases such as polycythemia vera and essential thrombocytosis. c-kit mutations are seen in 13% of high-risk MDS, and are thought to play a role in transformation to AML.

Answer 33.6.   **The answer is C.**
Alkylating agents are associated with therapy-related MDS. This usually occurs 3 to 7 years after treatment and carries a poor prognosis. Most patients (90%) have monosomy 5/del (5q) and/or monosomy 7/del (7q).

Answer 33.7.   **The answer is A.**
Inhibitory cytokines and increased apoptosis contribute to the development of MDS. Bone marrow cells from patients with MDS have increased expression of Fas and Fas ligand. TNF-α is thought to play a role, and anti-TNF-α therapy results in increased numbers of hematopoietic colonies. Spontaneous release of mitochondrial cytochrome c in patients with MDS may result in activation of caspase-9, triggering the apoptotic pathway.

Finally, defects in the bone marrow microenvironment, such as defective or reduced growth of stromal progenitors, are thought to play a role.

Answer 33.8.   **The answer is D.**
High-dose chemotherapy and allogeneic HSCT are the only known curative therapy in MDS. It is indicated at presentation in patients with high-risk MDS, who have a matched sibling donor. In lower risk disease, it may be considered at the time of progression. It is the treatment of choice for pediatric MDS; however, Fanconi anemia should be excluded prior to transplant, with diepoxybutane testing.

CHAPTER 34 PLASMA CELL NEOPLASMS

RAVI VIJ • GIRIDHARAN RAMSINGH

DIRECTIONS Each of the numbered items below is followed by lettered answers. Select the ONE lettered answer that is BEST in each case unless instructed otherwise.

QUESTIONS

Question 34.1. An 80-year-old woman presents to the emergency department with progressive low back pain for 3 weeks. On examination, she has tenderness at multiple levels on her spine but no neurological deficits. She has an Eastern Cooperative Oncology Group (ECOG) performance status of 2. Laboratory testing shows a hemoglobin (Hb) of 7.8 g/dL, creatinine of 2.1 mg/dL, calcium of 8.8 mg/dL, and albumin of 4.1 g/dL. She has a skeletal survey showing multiple osteolytic lesions, including multiple vertebral compression fractures. She has a serum protein electrophoresis (SPEP) showing a monoclonal protein of 6.2 g/dL. Serum immunofixation shows a monoclonal immunoglobulin (Ig)G kappa light chain protein. Her beta-2 microglobulin level is 5.3 mg/L. She has a bone marrow biopsy that shows a hypercellular marrow with 60% plasma cells, and cytogenetic analysis reveals a normal female karyotype. Of the following treatment options, which would be considered the MOST appropriate?

A. Melphalan and prednisone (MP)
B. Melphalan, prednisone, and thalidomide (MPT)
C. Thalidomide and dexamethasone (TD)
D. Melphalan 100 mg/m^2 followed by autologous stem cell transplantation

Corresponding Chapter in *Cancer: Principles & Practice of Oncology*, Ninth Edition: 136 (Plasma Cell Neoplasms).

Question 34.2.   A 59-year-old man is evaluated for anemia with an Hb of 9.2 g/dL. He has no other medical comorbidities and is asymptomatic. His clinical examination reveals no abnormality. He is found to have a high total protein of 12 g/dL and albumin of 3.2 g/dL. His serum creatinine is 1.0 mg/dL and serum calcium is 9.3 mg/dL. He has an SPEP that shows a monoclonal protein level of 8.6 g/dL, and serum immunofixation shows an IgG lambda monoclonal protein. His skeletal survey is normal. His serum beta-2 microglobulin is 4.3 mg/L. He has a bone marrow examination that shows 40% plasma cells, and cytogenetic analysis reveals a normal male karyotype. He is being considered for autologous stem cell transplantation. Which of the following induction regimens would give the best chance of complete remission after autologous stem cell transplantation?

A. Vincristine, Adriamycin, and dexamethasone (VAD)
B. TD
C. Bortezomib and dexamethasone (VD)
D. Bortezomib, thalidomide, and dexamethasone (VTD)

Question 34.3.   A 52-year-old woman is evaluated for progressive fatigue. Clinical examination is remarkable only for pallor. Further investigation reveals an Hb of 8.2 g/dL with mean corpuscular volume of 88 fL. Her iron studies, vitamin B_{12} levels, and folate levels are normal. Her serum creatinine is 0.8 mg/dL. Her SPEP reveals a monoclonal protein level of 3.8 g/dL, and serum immunofixation shows a monoclonal IgG kappa light chain protein. Further investigation reveals a calcium of 8.8 mg/dL, albumin of 4.2 g/dL, and beta-2 microglobulin of 2.1 mg/L. Skeletal survey shows multiple lytic lesions. She has a bone marrow examination that shows 80% cellular marrow with 50% plasma cells. Cytogenetic analysis shows normal female karyotype, and a fluorescence in situ hybridization (FISH) panel is positive for 13q deletion in 50% of plasma cells. Which of the following treatment options would be considered MOST appropriate for the patient?

A. Bortezomib/dexamethasone induction followed by high-dose melphalan and autologous stem cell transplantation (HDCT)
B. Bortezomib and dexamethasone with no option for HDCT
C. MP
D. MPT

Question 34.4.   A 58-year-old woman is incidentally found to have a monoclonal protein on SPEP with a monoclonal protein concentration of 1.7 g/dL, and on immunofixation she is found to have monoclonal IgG kappa free light chains. She is asymptomatic, and clinical examination results are normal. Her laboratory investigations show an Hb of 13.1 g/dL, creatinine of 0.7 mg/dL, serum albumin of 4.7 g/dL, calcium of 9.3 mg/dL, and beta-2 microglobulin of 1.7 mg/L. The skeletal survey was negative for any lytic lesions. Bone marrow examination shows 13% plasma cells, and cytogenetics shows normal female karyotype. What is the chance of this patient developing multiple myeloma at 5 years?

A. 5%
B. 10%
C. 30%
D. 50%

Question 34.5.   A 78-year-old male presents with history of severe back pain. X-rays of the spine show multiple lytic lesions. Laboratory investigations reveal an Hb of 13.2 g/dL, creatinine of 1.1 mg/dL, calcium of 8.6 mg/dL, and albumin of 4.2 g/dL. Serum electrophoresis shows a 3.8 g/dL M-protein, IgG Kappa on immunofixation. His bone marrow reveals 40% plasma cells. He is started on I.V bortezomib 1.3 mg/m^2 (days 1, 4, 8 and 11 of 28 days cycle) and dexamethasone. After completing the first cycle, he presents with a burning sensation and tingling in the hands and feet. On examination, he has decreased sensation in upper and lower extremities. His current SPEP shows a monoclonal protein level of 3.4 g/dL. All of the following would be appropriate regarding continuing with bortezomib therapy except:

A. Decrease the dose of bortezomib
B. Change bortezomib to once weekly administration
C. Change bortezomib to subcutaneous route
D. Make no change

Question 34.6.   A 58-year-old woman was diagnosed with IgG kappa multiple myeloma 8 months ago when she presented with bone pain, multiple lytic lesions, and an M-protein level of 5.8 g/dL. She was treated with lenalidomide along with dexamethasone for four cycles following which her M-protein decreased to 1.2 g/dL. She then underwent an autologous stem cell transplant following which her M protein levels decreased further to 0.2 g/dL. Of the following maintenance options, all have been shown to improve survival EXCEPT:

A. Thalidomide
B. Lenalidomide
C. Pomalidomide
D. Bortezomib

Question 34.7.   A 48-year-old male presents with anemia, hypercalcemia, and multiple lytic lesions. His bone marrow examination shows 60% plasma cells with high-risk chromosomal changes including loss of 13q on metaphase cytogenetics and FISH showing t(4,14). He is started on bortezomib and dexamethasone therapy. He enquires about the possibility of having stem cell transplantation. Which of the following is true in this population?

A. Allogenic transplantation should be considered standard of care for patients with high-risk chromosomal features.

B. Tandem autologous transplantation followed by reduced intensity allogeneic transplantation results in lower response rates in patients with high-risk cytogenetics.

C. Autologous transplantation results in lower response rates in patients with high-risk cytogenetics than patients with normal cytogenetics.

D. These patients may benefit from maintenance therapy after autologous transplantation.

Question 34.8.   A 60-year-old female presents with Hb of 9 g/dL and a creatinine of 1.5 mg/dL. SPEP shows a monoclonal spike of 3.7 g/dL with an IgG kappa monoclonal protein on immunofixation. Bone marrow examination shows 27% plasma cells. A skeletal survey shows no lytic lesions. All the following investigations have been shown to provide additional information that could be potentially clinically useful except:

A. MRI spine/pelvis

B. Whole body PET scan

C. Gene expression profiling

D. Serum free light chain (SFLC) assay

Question 34.9.   A 58-year-old male with anemia is diagnosed with light chain disease. His SFLC assay shows a kappa light chain level of 100 mg/dL and lambda light chain level of 2.0 mg/dL with a kappa/lambda ratio of 50. The patient starts treatment with lenalidomide and dexamethasone. The SFLC assay can be used to monitor response to treatment using:

A. Decrease in the level of involved light chain

B. Decrease in the level of the difference between involved and uninvolved light chain

C. Decrease in kappa/lambda ratio

D. The SFLC assay cannot be used to assess response

Question 34.10.   A 60-year-old female presents with pain in the left arm. X-rays show a large lytic lesion in the shaft of the left humerus. Biopsy of the lesion reveals a kappa restricted plasma cell population. The patient has normal blood counts and renal function. A skeletal survey fails to reveal any additional lesions. SPEP shows an IgG kappa monoclonal spike measuring 0.4 g/dL. UPEP fails to reveal any monoclonal protein. Bone marrow biopsy shows 3% nonclonal plasma cells. All of the following statements are true, EXCEPT:

A. Age has no impact on overall survival (OS).
B. An MRI of the spine and pelvis is indicated.
C. African Americans have a poorer survival compared with Caucasian population.
D. Patients with solitary bone plasmacytomas have a worse outcome compared to patients with solitary extramedullary plasmacytomas.

Question 34.11.   A 47-year-old male presents with fatigue. The patient is found to be anemic with an Hb of 6.7 g/dL. He has a WBC of 2000 with 21% circulating plasma cells and a platelet count of 79,000. He has a serum creatinine of 1.8 mg/dL with a normal serum calcium. SPEP and UPEP fail to reveal a monoclonal protein. Skeletal survey shows no lytic lesions. Bone marrow biopsy shows a lambda restricted clonal plasma cell population constituting 40% of marrow cellularity. Which of the following statements is correct?

A. For a diagnosis of plasma cell leukemia, the absolute WBC has to be >10,000.
B. As is the case with multiple myeloma, OS of patients with plasma cell leukemia has improved significantly.
C. The incidence of plasma cell leukemia is equal in males and females.
D. Autologous stem cell transplantation is of no utility in this situation.

ANSWERS

Answer 34.1.   **The answer is B.**

The choice of initial therapy for elderly patients with multiple myeloma has been a subject of several clinical trials. There have been three randomized controlled trials (IFM 99-06: Facon T, Mary JY, Hulin C, et al. Lancet. 2007;370[9594]:1209–1218; IFM 01-01: Hulin C, Virion J, Leleu X, et al. Am J Clin Oncol. 2007;25[18S]:8001; GIMEMA: Palumbo A, Bringhen S, Caravita T, et al. Lancet. 2006;367[9513]:825–831.) comparing MPT and MP regimens. All three studies showed superiority of MPT over MP on the basis of response including complete remission (13% to 16% vs. 2% to 2.4%) and progression-free survival (24 to 27.5 months vs. 17.8 to 19 months). In the IFM studies, the improved response rate of MPT over MP translated into improved OS (45 to 50 months vs. 27 to 33 months). The VISTA trial (San Miguel, et al. Blood [ASH Annual Meeting Abstracts] 2007;110[11]:2712) recently showed the melphalan, prednisone, and bortezomib (MPV) combination to be superior to MP (CR rate: 35% vs. 5%, 2-year OS: 83% vs. 70%). There is no study comparing MPV with MPT. The combination of TD has been compared with MP (Ludwig H, et al. Hematologica. 2007;92[10]:1411–1414). Although TD showed a better response rate (CR/near CR: 30% vs. 14%), it resulted in inferior survival (OS: 44.6 vs. 57.9 months) secondary to its toxicity. HDCT with melphalan 200 mg/m^2 has emerged as standard of care for transplant-eligible patients. However, patients aged more than 75 years are usually not considered for transplantation because of the toxicity of the treatment in this group. In the IFM 99-06 study, patients who received MPT showed a superior survival compared with reduced-dose melphalan 100 mg/m^2 followed by autologous stem cell transplantation (OS: 51.6 vs. 38.3 months). Thus, the MPT regimen would be the most appropriate for this patient.

Answer 34.2.   **The answer is D.**

The choice of the optimal induction therapy before autologous stem cell transplantation for patients with multiple myeloma has been the subject of several randomized clinical trials. VAD chemotherapy had been the most popular induction chemotherapy regimen in the United States until the 1990s. Several randomized trials have recently compared various regimens for induction therapy before transplantation. Marco et al. (Blood [ASH Annual Abstracts] 2007;110[11]) compared TD with VAD as induction regimen before HDCT and reported a good partial response (VGPR) with TD compared with VAD before transplant (35% vs. 12%). However, there was no difference in VGPR at 6 months post-HDCT (44% vs. 41%). Horousseau et al. (Blood [AHS Annual Abstracts] 2007;110[11]) reported a higher CR+ near CR postautologous transplantation with VD as induction therapy compared with VAD as induction therapy (41% vs. 29%). In a phase 3 study, Carvo et al. (ASH 2007) reported that VTD induction therapy resulted in higher CR+ near CR postautologous transplantation when compared with TD (57% vs. 28%). Phase 2 trials have reported that lenalidomide and dexamethasone are an appropriate induction regimen pretransplant (Lacy et al. Blood [ASH Annual Abstracts] 2006;108[11]). However, there are increasing data on the adverse impact of lenalidomide on stem cell mobilization, and it is recommended that stem cells be collected within the first 4 months of starting a lenalidomide-based regimen. Unfortunately, we do not have any long-term follow-up from these trials showing survival data. However, previous studies such as MRC VII and IFM 90-06 on high-dose chemotherapy reported that patients achieving CR after high-dose chemotherapy had longer progression-free survival and OS compared with those with less than CR. Therefore, the VTD regimen with the highest reported CR rate may be the most appropriate induction regimen.

Answer 34.3.   **The answer is A.**

The optimal initial therapy for a young patient with multiple myeloma is currently a subject of controversy. HDCT has been compared with conventional chemotherapy in several randomized controlled trials. The IFM 90-06 and MRCVII established HDCT as standard of care for these patients. The introduction of novel drugs such as thalidomide, lenalidomide, and bortezomib has improved the CR rate in patients with myeloma and led several experts to question the continued role of upfront HDCT for all patients with multiple myeloma. However, regimens containing these novel drugs have not been directly compared with HDCT in randomized trials, and most investigators think that these novel agents should be incorporated with HDCT in the treatment paradigm. Some investigators have suggested delaying the HDCT option for the time of progression. This may be an appropriate strategy because a randomized trial (Fermand JP. Blood. 1998;92[9]:3131–3136) showed that HDCT at first progression resulted in OS comparable to patients who underwent HDCT as initial therapy. However, there are no data on delaying HDCT beyond first progression. Other investigators have proposed a risk-stratified approach to HDCT for patients with multiple myeloma. Deletion 13 by conventional cytogenetics was seen in approximately 15% of patients with multiple myeloma and has been shown to be an adverse prognostic factor. Trials with HDCT have reported a median time to progression of 8 to 9 months in this population. However, deletion of chromosome 13 by FISH is detected in 40% to 50% of patients. Individuals with deletion 13 detected by FISH in the absence of deletion 13 by conventional cytogenetics do not seem to have the same adverse impact. Therefore, we think that this patient with deletion 13 detected by FISH alone should be offered HDCT as part of her regimen. Bortezomib has been shown in several studies to negate the adverse impact of deletion 13 detected by conventional cytogenetics. However, because there are no randomized controlled trials comparing bortezomib-based combination regimen alone with HDCT, we think that HDCT cannot be excluded from the treatment paradigm. Melphalan-based regimen should be avoided in a patient eligible for HDCT.

Answer 34.4.   **The answer is D.**

The diagnostic criterion for plasma cell dyscrasias was recently revised. Multiple myeloma is defined as a plasma cell dyscrasia associated with end-organ dysfunction (acronym CRAB: hyperCalcemia, Renal failure, Anemia, or Bone lesions). Patients should also have greater than or equal to 10% clonal plasma cells and a monoclonal protein in serum and/or urine. In the absence of organ involvement, the plasma cell dyscrasia is classified as monoclonal gammopathy of undetermined significance (MGUS) if the monoclonal protein levels are less than 3 g/dL and the bone marrow contains less than 10% clonal plasma cells, and as smoldering myeloma if the bone marrow has greater than or equal to 10% clonal plasma cells and/or monoclonal protein of greater than or equal to 3 g/dL. On the basis of the above criteria, this patient has a smoldering myeloma. Recently, the natural history of these indolent plasma cell dyscrasias has been better defined. MGUS transforms to a clinically significant plasma cell dyscrasia at a constant rate of approximately 1% per year (Kyle et al. N Engl J Med. 2002;346[8]:564–569). The serum level of the monoclonal protein and the type of monoclonal protein (IgA and IgM >IgG) were risk factors for progression in the same study. In a subsequent study, Rajkumar et al. (Blood. 2005;106[3]:812–817) proposed a risk stratification model that included three risk factors (abnormal SFLC ratio, non-IgG-type monoclonal protein, and monoclonal protein concentration >1.5 g/dL) to further help predict progression of MGUS to a clinically significant plasma cell dyscrasia. Kyle et al. (N Engl J Med. 2007;356[25]:2582–2590) reported that the overall risk of progression of smoldering myeloma is approximately 10% per year in the first 5 years, 3% per year in the next 5 years, and decreases to 1% per year thereafter. On the basis of this study, this patient has a 5-year risk of progression of approximately 50%. Kyle et al. further classified smoldering myeloma into three risk groups with different rates of progression: group (1) bone marrow plasma cell greater than or equal to 10%, monoclonal M protein greater than or equal to 3 g/dL: 15-year progression rate 87%; group (2) bone marrow plasma cells greater than or equal to 10%, monoclonal M protein less than or equal to 3 g/dL: 15-year progression rate 70%; and group (3) bone marrow plasma cells greater than or equal to 10%, monoclonal M protein greater than or equal to 3 g/dL: 15-year progression rate 39%.

Answer 34.5.   **The answer is D.**

Decreasing the dose of bortezomib to 1 mg/m^2 is effective in decreasing neuropathy as shown in the CREST trial and is recommended as per the FDA guidelines. Decreasing the frequency of administration of bortezomib has also been shown to decrease the rates of neuropathy (Mateos et al. Lancet Oncol. 2010 Oct;11(10):934–941 and Palumbo et al. J Clin Oncol. 2010 Dec 1;28(34):5101). However, both these studies showed that efficacy was not compromised by reducing bortezomib to once weekly in the context of bortezomib use in three or four drug combination regimens. Recently in a phase 3 randomized controlled trial (Moreau et al. Lancet Oncol. 2011;12(5):431–440) I.V bortezomib was compared to subcutaneous bortezomib and was found to be equally efficacious but with significantly decreased toxicity including a much lower incidence of peripheral neuropathy. Since the patient is already symptomatic with painful neuropathy, not altering the current regimen is likely to make the neuropathy worse and would not be appropriate.

Answer 34.6.   **The answer is C.**

Thalidomide has been shown to improve survival postautologous transplant (Attal et al. Blood. 2006 Nov 15;108(10):3289–3294 and Spencer et al. J Clin Oncol. 2009 Apr 10;27(11):1788–1793). Two randomized clinical trials IFM 2005-02 (Attal et al. Blood. Nov 2010;116:310) and CALGB 100104 (McCarthy et al. Blood. Nov 2010;116:37.) have studied lenalidomide maintenance after autologous stem cell transplantation. Both trials have shown a progression-free survival advantage for lenalidomide versus observation following autologous stem cell transplantation with the CALGB trial also showing superior survival for patients receiving lenalidomide maintenance. In the HOVON-65/GMMG-HD4 randomized phase III trial comparing bortezomib, doxorubicin, dexamethasone (PAD) versus VAD followed by high-dose melphalan and maintenance with bortezomib or thalidomide in patients with newly diagnosed multiple myeloma patients who received bortezomib maintenance achieved a superior survival that indirectly provides evidence supporting bortezomib maintenance following autologous transplantation (Sonnoveld et al. Blood. Nov 2010;116:40). Pomalidomide, a third-generation immunomodulatory drug, is being studied in patients with relapsed/refractory myeloma. There is currently no evidence to support pomalidomide maintenance after autologous stem cell transplantation.

Answer 34.7.   **The answer is D.**

At this time, there is no data to suggest that allogeneic transplantation improves outcomes in patients with multiple myeloma with high-risk chromosomal features. Three randomized trials have shown no benefit to tandem autologous allogeneic transplantation: the PATHEMA trial (Rosinol et al. Blood. 2008 Nov 1;112(9):3591–3593), the French IFM99-03 trial (Garbon et al. Blood. 2006;107(9):3474–3480), and the BMT CTN 0102 trial (Krishnan et al. Blood. Nov 2010;116:41). These studies that compared tandem autologous transplantation with autologous transplantation followed by reduced intensity allogeneic stem cell transplantation showed no difference in survival between the two groups. Only Bruno et al. (NEJM, 15;356(11):1110-20.2007) demonstrated superior survival with allogeneic stem cell transplantation compared to autologous stem cell transplantation in newly diagnosed patients with multiple myeloma less than 65 years old. High-risk patients have similar response rates following autologous and allogeneic stem cell transplantation but shorter progression-free survival compared to patients with standard-risk cytogenetics. There is emerging evidence supporting the use of maintenance therapy following autologous transplantation. Maintenance therapy trials with bortezomib and lenalidomide suggest that this benefit is apparent even for patients with high-risk cytogenetic features

(Sonnoveld et al. Blood. 2010 Nov;116:40 and Attal et al. Blood. 2010 Nov;116:310).

Answer 34.8.   **The answer is D.**

The International Myeloma Working Group (IMWG) consensus guidelines on diagnostic workup in plasma cell neoplasms was recently published (Dimopoulos et al. Blood. 2011;117:4701–4705). These recommend MRI of spine and pelvis as mandatory workup of patients with solitary plasmacytoma. An MRI should also be considered in patients with smoldering myeloma because it can detect occult lesions and if positive can predict for more rapid progression to symptomatic myeloma. An MRI of the spine is indicated in case of back pain to exclude any soft tissue mass arising from a bone lesion or for the investigation of patients with a suspicion of cord compression. An MRI of the spine may also be valuable in defining the etiology of new, painful collapsed vertebra. An MRI is also strongly indicated in patients with nonsecretory myeloma for the initial assessment and follow-up of response to treatment. PET-CT has been shown to provide prognostic information at diagnosis in myeloma (Bartel et al. Blood. 2009;114(10):2068–2076). A PET-CT is helpful for detection of extraosseous soft tissue masses and evaluation of rib and appendicular bone lesions. PET-CT is especially useful in patients with elevated LDH, Bence Jones protein escape, and otherwise rapidly recurrent disease or with suspected extramedullary plasmacytoma. Unlike MRI, PET-CT obviates the need for a skeletal survey (Durie BG, et al. J Nucl Med. 2002;43(11):1457–1463). In a large study studying gene expression profiling, it was shown that 70 genes linked to shorter durations of complete remission, even-free survival, and OS (Shaughnessy et al. Blood. 2007 Mar 15;109(6):2276–2284). This 70-gene chip is now approved for clinical use by Medicare. The SFLC assay is unlikely to provide any additional useful information in a patient with a quantifiable M spike on SPEP at this time.

Answer 34.9.   **The answer is B.**

In patients with light chain myeloma, the IMWG recommends monitoring the difference between the involved and uninvolved light chains to monitor response (Dimopoulos et al. Blood. 2011;117:4701–4705). A decrease of greater than or equal to 50% in the difference between involved and uninvolved FLC levels is considered a partial response. In amyloidosis, it is recommended to follow the absolute level of light chains for assessment of response. The kappa/lambda light chain ratio is of prognostic importance in patients with MGUS and multiple myeloma (Kyle RA, et al. N Engl J Med. 2007 Jun 21;356(25):2582–2590 and Rajkumar SV, et al. Blood. 2005 Aug 1;106(3):812–817).

Answer 34.10.   **The answer is A.**

This patient has a solitary bone plasmacytoma. A large retrospective study using the SEER database reported on prognostic factors and survival of patients with plasmacytoma (Ramsingh et al. Br J Haematol. 2009

May;145(4):540–542). It was identified that older age, African American race, and extramedullary plasmacytomas were all associated with worse survival. As per the recent IMWG consensus guidelines (Dimopoulos et al. Blood. 2011;117:4701–4705) MRI of spine is part of the mandatory workup of patients with solitary plasmacytoma.

Answer 34.11.   **The answer is C.**

The diagnostic criterion for plasma cell leukemia is a plasma cell count of more than 2000 if the WBC is less than 10,000 or 20% plasma cells if the WBC is less than 10,000. A large retrospective study using the SEER database (Ramsingh et al. Cancer. 2009 Dec 15;115(24):5734–5739) reported no improvement in survival of patients with plasma cell leukemia between 1973 and 2004. The same study also reported that the sex ratio was equal in plasma cell leukemia. Autologous stem cell transplantation can be useful therapy even in patients with plasma cell leukemia. A large retrospective study of patients from European Group for Blood and Marrow Transplantation (Haematologica. 2010 May;95(5): 804–809) showed a median OS of 25.7 months that is significantly higher than historical controls treated with conventional therapy.

CHAPTER 35 CANCER OF UNKNOWN PRIMARY SITE

MUHAMMAD ATIF WAQAR

DIRECTIONS   Each of the numbered items below is followed by lettered answers. Select the ONE lettered answer that is BEST in each case unless instructed otherwise.

QUESTIONS

Question 35.1.   In patients with cancer of unknown primary, what is the most common histology seen on initial light microscopic exam?

    A.   Adenocarcinoma
    B.   Poorly differentiated carcinoma
    C.   Squamous cell carcinoma
    D.   Neuroendocrine carcinoma

Question 35.2.   Which of the following statements is CORRECT regarding aggressive neuroendocrine carcinomas of unknown primary site?

    A.   Patients with thyroid transcription factor-1 (TTF-1) positive tumors should undergo bronchoscopy.
    B.   They rarely secrete bioactive substances.
    C.   Colonoscopy should be considered in patients whose tumors stain positive for CDX2.
    D.   All of the above.

Question 35.3.   Which of the following immunohistochemical (IHC) stains is the most specific in guiding the diagnostic workup for carcinoma of unknown primary?

    A.   Common leukocyte antigen
    B.   TTF-1
    C.   Chromogranin
    D.   Cytokeratin 7 (CK-7)

Corresponding Chapter in *Cancer: Principles & Practice of Oncology*, Ninth Edition: 137 (Cancer of Unknown Primary Site).

Question 35.4.   Which of the following subgroups of patients diagnosed with carcinoma of unknown primary is NOT associated with a favorable outcome?

A. Men with tumor in the mediastinum or retroperitoneal lymph nodes
B. Men with bilateral lung nodules and tumor in the supraclavicular lymph nodes
C. Women with poorly differentiated neuroendocrine carcinoma
D. Women with peritoneal carcinomatosis

Question 35.5.   A 19-year-old man presents with headaches, nausea, visual disturbances, and diplopia of 3-week duration. MRI of the brain reveals a mass in the pineal gland mass extending to the thalamus. Biopsy reveals poorly differentiated carcinoma. Cytogenetic analysis reveals isochromosome 12p. CT scan of the chest, abdomen, and pelvis and testicular ultrasound is normal. Serum AFP is 74 ng/dL and β-hCG is 94 mIU/mL. What is the most likely diagnosis?

A. Pilocytic astrocytoma
B. Extragonadal germ cell tumor
C. Pineoblastoma
D. Meningioma

Question 35.6.   A 40-year-old postmenopausal woman, who is a nonsmoker, presents for evaluation of an incidentally discovered 3 cm liver lesion on abdominal ultrasound. Biopsy of the lesion reveals adenocarcinoma. IHC studies demonstrate the tumor to be CK7 and CA 19-9 negative, CK20 positive, CDX2 positive, TTF-1 negative, ER and Her-2/neu negative. CT of the chest, abdomen pelvis with contrast, and PET scan fail to reveal the primary site of origin. What diagnostic test would you order next?

A. Pancreatic protocol CT scan
B. Colonoscopy
C. Breast MRI
D. Bronchoscopy

Question 35.7.   A 38-year-old premenopausal woman, who is a never smoker, presents with a left axillary lump. She reports that her mother was treated for breast cancer 5 years back. CT scan of the chest, abdomen, and pelvis reveals a 2.5 cm left axillary lymph node, but is otherwise within normal limits. Mammogram and breast ultrasound are normal. Biopsy reveals adenocarcinoma, with immunostains demonstrating the tumor to be negative for CK20, TTF-1, ER, Her-2, but positive for CK7, mammaglobin, and GCDFP-15. Which of the following tests would be helpful in determining the site of origin?

A. Bronchoscopy
B. Multiple random biopsies of both breasts
C. MRI of the breasts
D. All of the above

Question 35.8.   A 40-year-old woman is BRCA1 mutation positive and has undergone bilateral prophylactic mastectomies with reconstruction, and prophylactic oophorectomy 3 years back. She presents with a 6-month history of fatigue progressive abdominal girth distension. Physical examination demonstrates ascites. CT scan of the abdomen and pelvis reveals diffuse peritoneal carcinomatosis. CT-guided biopsy of a peritoneal nodule reveals papillary serous adenocarcinoma. Which of the following would you expect to see in this patient?

A. Psammoma bodies on histology
B. Elevated serum CA 125
C. Family history of breast and ovarian cancer
D. All of the above

Question 35.9.   A 45-year-old man, with a 20 pack-year history of smoking, presents with a right neck mass. CT of the neck with contrast reveals a 2 cm enlarged right upper cervical lymph node. Biopsy of the mass reveals squamous cell carcinoma. Which of the following tests would be helpful in identifying the primary site?

A. Examination of upper esophagus by direct endoscopy
B. Examination of the pharynx and laryngoscopy
C. PET scan
D. All of the above

Question 35.10.   A 45-year-old man presents with abdominal pain. CT of the abdomen shows multiple abdominal masses, the largest of which is 4 cm. CT of the chest is normal. Biopsy reveals poorly differentiated carcinoma. Immunoperoxidase stains show the tumor to be desmin $(+)$, vimentin $(+)$, and factor VIII antigen $(+)$. What would be the most appropriate next step?

A. Request CD117 staining
B. Surgical consultation
C. Systemic chemotherapy
D. Radiation oncology consultation

Question 35.11.   A 30-year-old woman presents for a pre-employment physical exam. She is a never-smoker, and has no significant past medical history, other than a spontaneous abortion 2 months ago. Physical exam, including breast exam, is within normal limits. Chest X-ray demonstrates multiple pulmonary nodules. CT-guided biopsy demonstrates metastatic poorly differentiated carcinoma. What is the next best step in her evaluation?

A. Request immunoperoxidase staining for CK 7, TTF-1, and CK 20
B. Request immunoperoxidase staining for ER and PR
C. Serum β-hCG
D. EGFR mutational analysis on tumor

Question 35.12.   Immunoperoxidase staining patterns may be helpful in the differential diagnosis of poorly differentiated neoplasms. Which of the following tumor types is INCORRECTLY matched with the characteristic findings on immunoperoxidase staining?

A. TTF-1 (+), Surf-A, and Surf-B (+); small cell carcinoma
B. CK 7 (+), CK20 (–), gross cystic fluid protein 15 (+), ER (+); breast carcinoma
C. CK7 (–), CK20 (+); colorectal carcinoma
D. CK7 (+), CA19-9 (+); pancreas carcinoma

Question 35.13.   The identification of characteristic cytogenetic abnormalities can help identify the site of origin of a tumor in some cases. Which of the following tumor types is INCORRECTLY matched with the characteristic cytogenetic abnormality?

A. Deletion of 1p; neuroblastoma
B. Deletion of 11p; alveolar rhabdomyosarcoma
C. Isochromosome of 12p; germ cell tumors
D. Deletion of 3p; small cell carcinoma

Question 35.14.   A 35-year-old man presents with a 3-month history of an enlarging lump in the right inguinal region. He has a 3 cm right inguinal lymph node palpable on exam. Genital exam, digital rectal exam, and anoscopy are normal. Core biopsy of the mass reveals poorly differentiated squamous carcinoma. CT of the abdomen and pelvis and chest X-ray are negative for any other sites of involvement. Which of the following is the most appropriate treatment for him?

A. Palliative chemotherapy
B. Definitive radiation therapy
C. Referral to hospice
D. Surgical consultation, radiation oncology consultation, chemotherapy

ANSWERS

Answer 35.1.   **The answer is A.**

In patients with cancer of unknown primary, the most common histology seen on initial light microscopic exam is adenocarcinoma (60%). Approximately 29% of these tumors are poorly differentiated carcinoma or poorly differentiated adenocarcinoma, 5% are squamous carcinoma, 5% are poorly differentiated malignant neoplasm, and 1% are neuroendocrine carcinoma. Further identification usually requires specialized tests including IHC staining, electron microscopy, and genetic analysis.

Answer 35.2.   **The answer is D.**

Aggressive neuroendocrine carcinomas of unknown primary site are usually found in multiple metastatic sites and rarely secrete bioactive peptides. Histologic features and IHC staining can help guide further workup. Bronchoscopy should be performed in patients with small-cell neuroendocrine carcinoma histology, or in patients with TTF-1 positive tumors. Colonoscopy should be performed in patients with tumors staining positive for CDX2, to determine the primary site.

Answer 35.3.   **The answer is A.**

Common leukocyte antigen is specific for differentiating lymphoma from carcinoma. TTF-1 is positive in 75% of cases of lung adenocarcinoma, as well as small cell carcinoma. Cytokeratin 7 and 20 staining are increasingly being used and can help guide further diagnostic workup, but are not very specific. Chromogranin staining is suggestive of neuroendocrine differentiation.

Answer 35.4.   **The answer is B.**

In a large clinical trial of 220 patients, some subsets were identified as having a more favorable prognosis. These subsets include (i) tumors in the retroperitoneum, mediastinum, or peripheral lymph nodes; (ii) two or more features associated with germ cell syndrome; (iii) women with peritoneal carcinomatosis; (iv) poorly differentiated neuroendocrine tumors; (v) poorly differentiated neoplasm not otherwise specified; and (vi) anaplastic lymphoma. Many of these patients were proven to have thymomas, germ cell tumors, primary peritoneal carcinomatosis, lymphomas, and neuroendocrine carcinomas. These tumors are very responsive to chemotherapy with a complete response rate in different clinical trials ranging from 10% to 26%.

Answer 35.5.   **The answer is B.**

Extragonadal germ cell tumors usually occur in midline locations including the mediastinum, retroperitoneum, or pineal region. This patient presented with a pineal mass, normal testicular exam, and an elevated serum hCG and AFP level, which are suggestive of an extragonadal germ cell tumors. The biopsy revealed poorly differentiated carcinoma, though cytogenetic testing revealed isochromosome 12p. Abnormalities of chromosome 12 such as i(12p) and del (12p) or multiple copies of 12p are useful in the diagnosis of germ cell tumors in this setting.

Answer 35.6.   **The answer is B.**

The patient presents with adenocarcinoma of unknown primary with liver metastasis. Her tumor stains positive for CK20 and CDX2, and negative for CK 7; this pattern is suggestive of colorectal primary and colonoscopy should be performed. Lung cancers are typically CK 7 positive and CK20 negative and TTF-1 staining is seen in approximately 75% of lung adenocarcinomas. ER positivity is suggestive of breast cancer, but up to 15% of patients are negative for ER, PR, and HER2-neu. Breast cancers are typically CK 7 positive, unlike this patient. Pancreatic cancers are typically CK 7 positive and CA 19-9 positive.

Answer 35.7.   **The answer is C.**

Isolated axillary adenopathy in a woman is suggestive of occult breast cancer, and the IHC features also suggest breast cancer. Since the mammogram and ultrasound are negative, the next step would be MRI of the breasts. Even when MRI and PET are negative for a primary lesion, modified radical mastectomy has been recommended in such patients and an occult primary has been identified in 44% to 80% of patients after mastectomy.

Answer 35.8.   **The answer is D.**

The incidence of both ovarian carcinoma and primary peritoneal carcinomatosis is increased in women with BRCA1 mutations. These patients often have a family history of breast and ovarian cancer. Prophylactic oophorectomy can prevent ovarian cancer, but these patients can still present with primary peritoneal carcinomatosis. Clinical features include elevated CA-125, but no identifiable primary on imaging or even laparotomy. They share the same histologic features as ovarian cancer, such as papillary serous features and psammoma bodies. They are treated using the same guidelines as advanced ovarian cancer with surgical cytoreduction followed by chemotherapy.

Answer 35.9.   **The answer is D.**

This patient has metastatic squamous cell carcinoma of unknown primary, with upper cervical lymph node involvement. When upper or middle cervical lymph nodes are involved, a primary tumor in the head and neck should be suspected. Clinical evaluation should include examination of the oropharynx, hypopharynx, nasopharynx, and larynx, as well as upper esophagus, by direct endoscopy. Any suspicious areas should be biopsied. PET scans are useful in this setting, and can help identify primary tumor sites.

Answer 35.10.   **The answer is A.**

The immunoperoxidase staining pattern is suggestive of sarcoma. In patients with abdominal masses with carcinoma or sarcoma histology, CD117 (C-KIT) staining should be performed on the biopsy specimen, to rule out gastrointestinal stroma tumors. In these patients, imatinib therapy may be considered.

Answer 35.11.   **The answer is C.**

In young women with poorly differentiated carcinoma and lung nodules, the possibility of metastatic gestational choriocarcinoma should be considered. The history of recent pregnancy, miscarriage, or missed periods should help guide the diagnosis. Imaging of the abdomen may show an enlarged uterus, and dilation and curettage may be indicated. Single-agent methotrexate therapy can be curative in this setting.

Answer 35.12.   **The answer is A.**

The immunoperoxidase staining pattern TTF-1 (+), Surf-A and Surf-B (+), is characteristic of adenocarcinoma of the lung. The typical pattern for small cell lung cancer is TTF-1 (+), chromogranin (+), and NSE (+). The other associations are correct.

Answer 35.13.   **The answer is B.**

The characteristic cytogenetic abnormality seen in alveolar rhabdomyosarcoma is t(2;13), while deletion of 11p is seen in Wilm tumor. The other associations are correct.

Answer 35.14.   **The answer is D.**

Most patients with a tumor in the inguinal lymph nodes have a detectable primary site in the genital or anorectal areas. In patients in whom a primary site is not identified, surgical resection, with or without radiation therapy to the inguinal area, may result in long-term survival. These patients should also be considered for neoadjuvant or adjuvant chemotherapy.

CHAPTER 36 BENIGN AND MALIGNANT MESOTHELIOMA

DANIEL MORGENSZTERN

DIRECTIONS   Each of the numbered items below is followed by lettered answers. Select the ONE lettered answer that is BEST in each case unless instructed otherwise.

QUESTIONS

Question 36.1.   What is the most common histologic subtype of malignant mesotheliomas?

    A. Epithelial
    B. Sarcomatoid
    C. Poorly differentiated
    D. Biphasic

Question 36.2.   Which of the following immunohistochemistry markers is present in malignant mesotheliomas?

    A. CEA
    B. TTF-1
    C. Moc-31
    D. Calretinin

Question 36.3.   Which of the following is NOT considered a poor prognostic factor in malignant mesothelioma?

    A. Sarcomatoid histology
    B. Biphasic histology
    C. Female gender
    D. Thrombocytosis

Question 36.4.   Which of the following findings does NOT define a technically unresectable tumor?

    A. Involvement of the endothoracic fascia
    B. Direct extension into the spine
    C. Extension into the internal surface of the pericardium without pleural effusion
    D. Direct transdiaphragmatic extension to the peritoneum

Corresponding Chapter in *Cancer: Principles & Practice of Oncology*, Ninth Edition: 138 (Benign and Malignant Mesothelioma).

Question 36.5.   A 57-year-old man with a malignant mesothelioma extending from the visceral pleura into the underlying pulmonary parenchyma and with metastatic disease restricted to a single hilar lymph node is best described at what stage?

A. T2N1M0 (stage II)
B. T2N1M0 (stage III)
C. T3N1M0 (stage III)
D. T2N2M0 (stage III)

Question 36.6.   Which of the following statements regarding solitary fibrous tumors of the pleura (FTPs) is NOT true?

A. Approximately 10% of the tumors are malignant.
B. Benign FTPs may recur and transform to the malignant variant.
C. Pleural effusion is commonly seen in the benign variant.
D. Up to 50% of cases may present with clubbing or osteoarthropathy.

Question 36.7.   Which of the following statements regarding peritoneal mesothelioma is FALSE?

A. Pleural plaques are observed in approximately 50% of patients.
B. Associated with airborne asbestos fiber exposure.
C. Median age of presentation is 60 years.
D. Account for approximately 10% to 15% of mesothelioma cases.

ANSWERS

Answer 36.1.   **The answer is A.**

Epithelial is the most common subtype of malignant mesotheliomas, comprising approximately 50% to 60% of cases. Biphasic and sarcomatoid mesotheliomas are less frequent and the uncommon tumors that cannot be categorized morphologically are called poorly differentiated.

Answer 36.2.   **The answer is D.**

Mesothelioma cells are diffusely positive for pankeratin, keratin 5/6, calretinin, and *WT1*. CEA, a nonspecific marker, Moc-31, which is commonly seen in adenocarcinomas, and TTF-1, which is seen in primary tumors of the lung and thyroid, are negative in mesotheliomas.

Answer 36.3.   **The answer is C.**

The established poor prognostic factors in malignant mesothelioma are poor performance status, male gender, anemia, thrombocytosis, leukocytosis, elevated LDH, and nonepithelial histology including sarcomatoid and biphasic subtypes.

Answer 36.4.   **The answer is A.**

Locally advanced and technically unresectable tumor (T4) is defined by a tumor involving all the ipsilateral pleural surfaces and extension of the tumor to the peritoneum, contralateral pleura, mediastinal organs, spine, chest wall, or internal surface of the pericardium with or without effusion. Involvement of the endothoracic fascia describes a locally advanced but potentially resectable disease.

Answer 36.5.   **The answer is B.**

Extension of the tumor to the underlying lung parenchyma and involvement of an ipsilateral bronchopulmonary or hilar lymph node make the tumor T2 and N1, respectively. T2N1M0 represents a stage III disease.

Answer 36.6.   **The answer is C.**

Solitary FTPs are usually benign, with the malignant variant present in approximately 10% of cases. The benign variant, however, may relapse with malignant features. Benign FTPs are associated with clubbing and osteoarthropathy in 20% to 50% of cases but rarely with effusions.

Answer 36.7.   **The answer is D.**

The incidence of peritoneal mesothelioma is increasing and it currently accounts for 25% to 33% of all mesotheliomas. This disease has a median age at presentation of 60 years and is more common in men with a ratio of 3 to 1. There is a clear relationship between peritoneal mesothelioma and heavy exposure to airborne asbestos fibers, and approximately 50% of patients have pleural plaques.

CHAPTER 37 PERITONEAL CARCINOMATOSIS

ANDREA WANG-GILLAM • DAVID D. TRAN

DIRECTIONS   Each of the numbered items below is followed by lettered answers. Select the ONE lettered answer that is BEST in each case unless instructed otherwise.

QUESTIONS

Question 37.1.   Peritoneal carcinomatosis may arise from tumors of which of the following structures?

A. The peritoneal lining
B. Intra-abdominal viscera
C. Extra-abdominal organs
D. All of the above

Question 37.2.   Which is the most common type of cancer presenting with isolated peritoneal carcinomatosis?

A. Ovarian
B. Appendiceal
C. Colon
D. Stomach
E. A and B

Question 37.3.   Unlike high-grade, poorly differentiated tumors, low-grade, well-differentiated tumors disseminate via which of the following mechanisms?

A. Cell shedding
B. Hematological spread
C. Pressure-burst phenomenon
D. Lymphatic spread

Question 37.4.   The mere presence of free-floating tumor cells within the peritoneal cavity does not universally correlate with peritoneal carcinomatosis. True or False?

A. True
B. False

Corresponding Chapter in *Cancer: Principles & Practice of Oncology*, Ninth Edition: 139 (Peritoneal Surface Malignancy).

Question 37.5.   Which imaging modality is the best tool to detect peritoneal recurrence?

A. Computed tomography (CT)
B. Magnetic resonance imaging (MRI)
C. Abdominal ultrasonogram
D. Positron emission tomography (PET)

Question 37.6.   What is the most important adverse prognostic factor associated with pseudomyxoma peritonei?

A. Presence of malignancy
B. Amount of mucin
C. Abdominal distention
D. Abdominal pain

Question 37.7.   The features of disseminated peritoneal adenomucinosis (DPAM) include:

A. Peritoneal tumor
B. Scant cellularity
C. Abundant extracellular mucin
D. Low-grade endothelial cells
E. All of the above

Question 37.8.   A 63-year-old patient presented with bowel obstruction and underwent exploratory laparotomy that revealed a ruptured appendix with abundant mucin. Scant, atypical cells without obvious malignant histology were reported by the pathologist. What treatment plan results in the best clinical outcome in this patient?

A. Maximal tumor debulking immediately followed by hyperthermic intraperitoneal mitomycin C with or without 5FU and augmented with adjuvant systemic therapy with 5FU and mitomycin C
B. Maximal tumor debulking followed by adjuvant systemic 5FU and mitomycin C
C. Systemic 5FU and mitomycin C alone without surgical resection
D. Close observation

Question 37.9.   Which of the following factors predicts the worst outcome in patients with mucinous adenocarcinoma of appendix?

A. Histologic grade
B. Age
C. Performance status
D. The use of intraperitoneal therapy

Question 37.10.   A 45-year-old woman presented with 3 months' duration of abdominal discomfort and chronic reflux. She underwent an esophagogastroduodenoscopy that showed a stomach mass at the antrum. Endoscopic ultrasound/fine-needle aspiration confirmed an adenocarcinoma with clinical staging of a T3N0 lesion. CT scans did not show any metastatic lesions. The patient is scheduled for curative surgical resection and now wants to discuss the potential use of intraperitoneal chemotherapy.

A. Postoperative intraperitoneal chemotherapy provides survival benefit when compared with surgery alone and should be offered as part of the standard of care.

B. The role of adjuvant intraperitoneal chemotherapy after complete resection of primary tumors remains to be determined.

C. 5FU and mitomycin C will be used as part of intraperitoneal treatment.

D. Cisplatin and mitomycin C are the agents of choice for intraperitoneal therapy.

Question 37.11.   A 50-year-old man was found to have a near obstructing adenocarcinoma involving the splenic flexure of his colon. His staging CT scans showed five small nodules associated with the greater omentum. No distant metastases were identified. He underwent surgical resection of the primary mass and debulking of his intraperitoneal carcinomatosis. However, complete cytoreduction was not possible because of the intraoperative discovery of multiple tumor masses firmly adhering to intra-abdominal vital organs. He now wants to know his overall prognosis and treatment plan.

A. His prognosis is the same as if he had complete cytoreduction.

B. Hyperthermic intraperitoneal chemoperfusion does not significantly improve prognosis in incomplete cytoreduction.

C. His prognosis is much poorer when compared with those with complete cytoreduction, and the need for systemic chemotherapy is inevitable.

D. Both B and C.

Question 37.12.   What is not a risk factor for malignant peritoneal mesothelioma?

A. Asbestos exposure

B. Abdominal radiation

C. Simian virus 40 exposure

D. Cigarette smoking

Question 37.13.   Which of the histologic subtypes of malignant peritoneal mesothelioma has the best prognosis?

A. Epithelial

B. Sarcomatoid

C. Mixed

Questions
37.14.–37.15.

A 55-year-old man presents with increasing abdominal girth and abdominal pain. CT scan of his chest and abdomen shows diffuse sub centimeter peritoneal nodules. Biopsy of the peritoneum is positive for carcinoma. The tumor was positive for immunohistochemical staining with calretinin, cytokeratin 5/6, and WT-1. It was negative for CEA, Ber-Ep4, LeuM1, and Bg8.

Question 37.14.   What is the most likely diagnosis in this patient?

A. Malignant peritoneal mesothelioma
B. Primary peritoneal carcinoma
C. Gastric adenocarcinoma
D. Appendiceal adenocarcinoma

Question 37.15.   The patient is in excellent health and has no significant medical comorbidities. What would be his treatment of choice?

A. Surgical cytoreduction
B. Surgical cytoreduction and intraperitoneal chemotherapy
C. Systemic cisplatin and pemetrexed
D. Single-agent pemetrexed

Question 37.16.   A 66-year-old man presented with nausea, vomiting, and abdominal pain. He was diagnosed with appendicitis and subsequently underwent appendectomy. During the surgery, he was noted to have tumor implants on his peritoneum. Biopsy of these tumors was reported as well-differentiated papillary mesothelioma. What would be the appropriate treatment option for this patient?

A. Surgical resection
B. Chemotherapy with cisplatin and pemetrexed
C. Radiation therapy
D. Intraperitoneal chemotherapy

Question 37.17.   A 40-year-old woman presented with abdominal distention and early satiety. On examination, the patient was found to have massive ascites. CT scan showed massive ascites and multiple peritoneal implants. In addition, a single 2-cm deposit was noted on the surface of the right ovary; her bilateral ovaries otherwise appear normal. The patient underwent paracentesis, which revealed malignant serous type cells. A PET scan did not reveal other metastatic sites except what appears on the CT. What is the diagnosis in this patient?

A. Primary peritoneal carcinoma
B. Peritoneal mesothelioma
C. Metastatic ovarian cancer
D. Adenocarcinoma of unknown primary

Question 37.18.   A 45-year-old woman presented with lower abdominal pain, and imaging study revealed a moderate amount of ascites with large peritoneal implants and one suspicious 3 × 5-cm heterogeneous mass in the right ovary. The patient also has high CA-125. FNA of the ovarian mass showed a malignant serous type cells. No other lesions were seen. What would be the next step of diagnosis or treatment?

A. Exploratory laparotomy with optimal surgical debulking
B. Systemic chemotherapy with platinum and paclitaxel
C. Surgical debulking and intraperitoneal chemotherapy
D. Surgical debulking and intraperitoneal chemotherapy followed by systemic chemotherapy

Question 37.19.   A 50-year-old man with a history of gastric cancer with diffuse peritoneal involvements progressed after two lines of chemotherapy, now with persistent nausea, vomiting, and constipation. An abdominal CT scan showed multiple air fluid levels but no clear obstruction transition points. The patient also has poor performance status. What would you consider to relieve his obstruction?

A. Diverting colostomy
B. Gastrostomy tube placement
C. Surgical exploration to locate the site of obstruction
D. Gastrointestinal (GI) evaluation for possible stent placement

Question 37.20.   A 65-year-old man with progressive and refractory pancreatic cancer who presented with a large amount of ascites resulted in shortness of breath at rest. The patient underwent a large-volume paracentesis but returned 1 week later with reaccumulated fluid. What would be the next step to manage his ascites?

A. Repeat paracentesis
B. Initiation of antidiuretics, such as spironolactone
C. Placement of a peritoneovenous shunt
D. Placement of a Denver catheter

Question 37.21.   A 23-year-old woman presents with worsening abdominal pain and distention. CT scan of the chest and abdomen reveals multiple rounded masses in the peritoneum and liver. Biopsy of the tumor nodule reveals small round cells that were positive for both epithelial and mesenchymal markers. Cytogenetic testing revealed t(11;12) (p13;q12). What is the diagnosis in this patient?

A. Ewings sarcoma
B. Desmoplastic small round cell tumor
C. Gastrointestinal stromal tumor
D. Clear cell sarcoma

ANSWERS

Answer 37.1.   **The answer is D.**

Peritoneal carcinomatosis can arise from tumors of all these structures with or without concurrent systemic metastases.

Answer 37.2.   **The answer is E.**

Intraperitoneal viscera, including the ovary and appendix, are the most common source of tumors presenting with isolated peritoneal carcinomatosis.

Answer 37.3.   **The answer is C.**

Low-grade, well-differentiated tumors disseminate via a pressure-burst phenomenon, common to slow-growing tumors such as mucinous tumors of the appendix and ovary, where the slow tumor growth permits the sheer volume of tumor cells to rupture through viscera and contaminate the peritoneum with tumor cells. In contrast, high-grade, poorly differentiated tumors spread through primary organ invasion with subsequent cell shedding and distant organ attachment, often with concurrent lymphatic or hematologic metastases.

Answer 37.4.   **The answer is A.**

Identification of free-floating tumor cells within the peritoneal cavity (e.g., after cytological examination of ascitic fluid) does not always mean peritoneal carcinomatosis. Attachment, implantation, and proliferation are all necessary steps in the establishment and growth of intraperitoneal disease.

Answer 37.5.   **The answer is B.**

MRI has been shown to be superior to helical CT in the assessment of bowel and mesenteric thickening. Sensitivity and specificity for MRI were demonstrated to be 84% and 100%, respectively, for the detection of peritoneal recurrence in ovarian carcinoma. PET has gained growing acceptance for assessing intraperitoneal carcinomatosis; however, its major drawback is the lack of efficacy in the evaluation of lesions less than 1 cm in diameter.

Answer 37.6.   **The answer is A.**

The presence of tumor cells in peritoneal washings obtained at the time of surgical resection correlates with increased local recurrence and decreased survival, even in the absence of nodal or systemic metastases. In DPAM, the absence of malignant cells is associated with significantly improved disease-free and overall survival.

Answer 37.7.   **The answer is E.**

DPAM includes peritoneal tumors with scant cellularity in the presence of abundant extracellular mucin. Endothelial cells present are histologically bland with low-grade adenomatous features, minimal cytologic atypia, and low mitotic activity.

Answer 37.8.   **The answer is A.**

In the series of 65 patients from Ronnet et al. (Cancer. 2001;92) and a review of 62 patients with pseudomyxoma peritonei by van Ruth et al. (Eur J Surg Oncol. 2003;29), median survival was significantly improved in patients with DPAM who were treated with maximal tumor debulking followed by intraperitoneal mitomycin C alone or in combination with 5FU. Three additional cycles of systemic 5FU/mitomycin C chemotherapy were given to all patients in the Ronnet series but was reserved only for patients with pathological evidence of malignancy in the van Ruth series. Both approaches appear to confer similar survival outcomes.

Answer 37.9.   **The answer is A.**

In mucinous adenocarcinoma of the appendix, histologic grade is the single most important prognostic indicator, with high-grade histologic atypia associated with the poorest outcome. In a series of 94 consecutive patients with adenocarcinoma of the appendix, the presence of high-grade "colonic type" tumors was reported in 45% of patients and was associated with higher grade tumors and higher stage, and ultimately poorer prognosis when compared with benign mucinous tumors (Nitecki et al. Ann Surg. 1994;219).

Answer 37.10.   **The answer is B.**

Data regarding adjuvant intraperitoneal chemotherapy for high-risk tumors have been mixed. Yu et al. (Ann Surg. 1998;64) randomized 248 patients with stage II and III gastric cancer to surgical resection alone versus resection plus postoperative intraperitoneal mitomycin C and 5FU, with an increase in survival seen only in the subset of patients with stage III cancer. Other series of similar patients using intraperitoneal cisplatin or mitomycin C did not show statistically significant improvements in local control or survival, except in patients with serosal invasion by tumors (Sautner et al. J Clin Oncol. 1994;12; Ikeguchi et al. Eur J Surg. 1995;161).

Answer 37.11.   **The answer is D.**

When complete resection of the primary tumor along with all peritoneal disease is not possible, surgical intervention merely delays the inevitable need for intravenous chemotherapy. Complete surgical cytoreduction was achieved in only 43% of the cases in one series. Compared with patients with complete surgical debulking, those without total resection of the primary and intraperitoneal disease fare much worse regardless of the use of hyperthermic intraperitoneal chemoperfusion.

Answer 37.12.   **The answer is D.**

All of these factors have been associated with increased risks for malignant peritoneal mesothelioma. Reported associations between asbestos and malignant mesothelioma range from 50% to 83%, but the link appears to be less than that seen with pleural mesothelioma.

Answer 37.13.   **The answer is A.**

The epithelial type of malignant peritoneal mesothelioma is the most common and carries the best prognosis, although significant variability in the extent of disease at presentation is common.

Answer 37.14.   **The answer is A.**

Distinguishing between adenocarcinoma and malignant mesothelioma by routine histologic examination may be difficult. Immunohistochemistry is helpful in such situations. However, there is no single specific marker to diagnose malignant mesothelioma. A panel of markers is used to differentiate between adenocarcinoma and malignant mesothelioma. Malignant mesothelioma is usually positive for WT-1, calretinin, and cytokeratin 5/6, whereas a positive CEA is seen in adenocarcinoma. Primary peritoneal carcinoma is rarely seen in men.

Answer 37.15.   **The answer is B.**

There is no clear consensus in the treatment of peritoneal malignant mesothelioma. However, in patients who are otherwise healthy with good performance status, nonbulky peritoneal disease, and no extraperitoneal spread, an aggressive surgical approach with cytoreduction followed by intraperitoneal chemotherapy is feasible. Even though there have been no randomized studies to evaluate the effectiveness of this approach, small prospective studies have shown dramatic benefit in carefully selected patients.

Answer 37.16.   **The answer is A.**

Well-differentiated papillary mesothelioma is an intermediate-grade benign tumor. The treatment of choice is surgical resection. Treatment with chemotherapy and radiation therapy does not improve outcomes.

Answer 37.17.   **The answer is A.**

Primary peritoneal carcinoma is a rare group of tumors of unclear origin arising in the peritoneal cavity. Primary peritoneal carcinoma can be distinguished from ovarian cancer by the following criteria: Both ovaries must be normal in size; the amount of extraovarian tumor must be greater than the involvement on the surface of the ovary; the ovarian component must be less than 5 × 5 mm within the ovary and otherwise confined to the surface of the ovary; and the cytologic characteristics must be of the serous type. Treatment of primary peritoneal carcinoma follows programs established for ovarian carcinoma, including operative debulking and adjuvant chemotherapy.

Answer 37.18.   **The answer is D.**

The differential diagnosis for this patient's cancer is primary peritoneal carcinoma versus ovarian carcinoma versus carcinoma of unknown origin. The elevated CA-125 and the large heterogeneous mass in the right ovary favor ovarian carcinoma, although the serous histology is more consistent with primary peritoneal carcinoma. However, treatment programs for primary peritoneal carcinoma usually follow those established for ovarian carcinoma. These regimens traditionally involve surgical debulking supported by intraperitoneal chemotherapy and followed by systemic chemotherapy with a combination of a platinum and a taxane.

Answer 37.19.   **The answer is B.**

Diffuse carcinomatosis often results in functional, not anatomic, obstruction that may only be effectively palliated through placement of a gastrostomy tube.

Answer 37.20.   **The answer is B.**

Conservative management of recurrent malignant ascites through diuretic therapy is effective in up to 47% of patients and should be initiated first. Spironolactone therapy starting at 150 mg per day may be necessary for prolonged periods to establish and maintain control of the ascites. Direct drainage of ascitic fluid through repeated paracentesis or a surgically placed peritoneovenous shunt provides immediate relief but carries increased risk of infection and protein loss. Peritoneal shunts (Denver catheter) remove ascitic fluid and return it to the systemic circulation. Successful, prolonged control of ascites is possible in up to 70% of patients; however, disseminated intravascular coagulation, pulmonary emboli, pulmonary edema, and rarely tumor emboli are the complications associated with these catheters.

Answer 37.21.   **The answer is B.**

Desmoplastic small round cell tumor commonly involves the peritoneum and can present with metastasis to the liver. The tumor is usually positive for both epithelial and mesenchymal markers. The presence of t(11;12) is specific to this tumor.

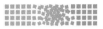

CHAPTER 38
IMMUNOSUPPRESSION-RELATED MALIGNANCIES

LEE RATNER

DIRECTIONS   Each of the numbered items below is followed by lettered answers. Select the ONE lettered answer that is BEST in each case unless instructed otherwise.

QUESTIONS

Question 38.1.   In human immunodeficiency virus (HIV)-infected patients, which of the following malignancies is considered to be an acquired immunodeficiency syndrome (AIDS)-defining cancer?

A. Colon cancer
B. Cervical cancer
C. Anal cancer
D. Penile cancer

Question 38.2.   Chemotherapy is usually well tolerated with concomitant highly active antiretroviral therapy (HAART) with which of the following exceptions:

A. Zidovudine, nucleotide reverse transcriptase inhibitor therapy
B. Protease inhibitors
C. Raltegravir, the new integrase inhibitor
D. Fuzeon, the HIV entry inhibitor

Question 38.3.   What is the response rate to HAART therapy, in a treatment-naïve patient with favorable-risk Kaposi sarcoma (KS)?

A. 20%
B. 40%
C. 60%
D. 80%

Corresponding Chapters in *Cancer: Principles & Practice of Oncology*, Ninth Edition: 141 (AIDS-Related Malignancies) and 142 (Transplantation-Related Malignancies).

Question 38.4.   **Which of the following is true about the combination of rituximab with chemotherapy for AIDS-associated lymphomas?**

    A. Adding rituximab to cyclophosphamide, doxorubicin, vincristine, and prednisone (CHOP) chemotherapy in patients with CD4 $<50/mm^3$ may result in higher rate of neutropenic infections.

    B. Rituximab is of no added benefit to CHOP or infusional etoposide, vincristine, and doxorubicin, bolus cyclophosphamide, and daily prednisone (EPOCH) chemotherapy for AIDS-associated diffuse large B cell lymphoma (DLBCL).

    C. Rituximab with chemotherapy is usually beneficial in plasmablastic lymphoma.

    D. Rituximab with chemotherapy is usually beneficial in primary effusion lymphoma.

Question 38.5.   **Which is NOT true concerning primary central nervous system (CNS) lymphoma in AIDS?**

    A. Positive cerebrospinal fluid (CSF) Epstein-Barr virus (EBV) polymerase chain reaction (PCR) test, a consistent radiological picture, and brain biopsy are necessary to diagnose primary CNS AIDS lymphoma.

    B. In patients with CD4 count $<50/mm^3$ and poor performance status, cranial radiotherapy alone may be appropriate.

    C. In patients with CD4 count $>50/mm^3$ and good performance status, the use of high-dose methotrexate with leucovorin rescue may be appropriate.

    D. Addition of HAART may increase the duration of response.

Question 38.6.   **A 38-year-old man with HIV infection presents with 3-month history of weight loss and night sweats. He is not on antiretroviral therapy and his last CD4 count 3 months ago was $300/mm^3$. On exam, he has multiple enlarged cervical lymph nodes. His hemoglobin is 10 g/dL, white blood cell count is 3.6 K/cumm, and platelet count is 190 K/cumm. Serum LDH is 300. Infectious workup is negative. CT of the neck and chest demonstrates diffuse cervical and mediastinal lymphadenopathy. You suspect lymphoma and arrange for an excisional biopsy of a neck lymph node. Which of the following lymphomas is a non-AIDS defining cancer?**

    A. Hodgkin disease

    B. DLBCL

    C. Burkitt lymphoma

    D. Primary CNS lymphoma

Question 38.7.   **Which of the following statements is correct regarding KS?**

    A. Tumor, node, metastasis (TNM) system is useful for staging KS.

    B. Extent of tumor and AIDS-related systemic illnesses is useful in stratifying patients with KS into prognostic risk groups.

    C. Response Evaluation Criteria in Solid Tumors (RECIST) is useful in assessing KS response to therapy.

    D. All of the above are correct.

Question 38.8.   How does the presentation of HIV-associated Hodgkin lymphoma (HL) differ from that of HL in immunocompetent patients?

A. Patients with HIV-associated HL present at an older age.

B. B symptoms are rare in patients with HIV-associated HL.

C. Extranodal sites are less frequently involved in patients with HIV-associated HL.

D. Mediastinal involvement is less frequent in patients with HIV-associated HL.

Question 38.9.   Which of the following is NOT correct regarding anogenital cancers in patients infected with HIV?

A. In HIV-infected women with preinvasive cervical neoplasia, standard therapy results in a twofold higher frequency of recurrence, compared to their immunocompetent counterparts.

B. In patients with a CD4 count of less than 200/mm^3, who are treated with chemotherapy and radiation for invasive anal cancer, intractable diarrhea is more common.

C. In patients with HIV, anal cancer and cervical cancer appear to be unrelated to infection with human papilloma virus (HPV).

D. In women diagnosed with HIV infection, an initial PAP smear is recommended.

Question 38.10.   Which of the following viruses are implicated in the development of cancers in patients with HIV infection?

A. EBV

B. Hepatitis C virus

C. Human herpes virus-8 (HHV-8)

D. All of the above

ANSWERS

Answer 38.1. **The answer is B.**

Anal cancer in a patient with HIV is considered to be an AIDS-defining cancer, whereas penile cancer, colon cancer, and anal cancer fall in the non-AIDS-defining cancer category.

Answer 38.2. **The answer is A.**

Zidovudine is generally poorly tolerated with chemotherapy because of myelosuppression. Protease inhibitors are generally well tolerated with chemotherapy, although they may affect metabolism of many drugs through effects on cytochrome P450-associated enzymes. Preliminary results with the most recently approved HIV drugs suggest that the integrase inhibitor raltegravir, coreceptor inhibitor maraviroc, and fusion inhibitor fuzeon are also well tolerated with chemotherapy.

Answer 38.3. **The answer is D.**

In patients with favorable-risk KS (confined to skin or lymph nodes, CD4 count >200, no B symptoms or opportunistic infections, and good performance status) who are treatment-naïve, response rates of up to 80% have been reported with HAART therapy. However, it is extremely rare for patients with extensive poor-risk KS (tumor associated edema or ulceration, extensive oral or gastrointestinal involvement, CD4 <200, opportunistic infections, B symptoms, HIV-related illness, poor PS) to respond to HAART alone. In addition, worsening of KS may occur with initiation of HAART, due to an immune reconstitution inflammatory response.

Answer 38.4. **The answer is A.**

Although the role of rituximab with chemotherapy in non-HIV-infected patients has been documented, its role in AIDS lymphoma is more controversial. Although several studies have suggested that there is a benefit to the addition of rituximab to CHOP or EPOCH chemotherapy, in patients with CD4 less than 50 to 100/mm^3 there are reports of excess neutropenic fevers and infections. Rituximab is usually not beneficial for treatment of plasmablastic lymphomas and primary effusion lymphomas, because CD20 is usually not expressed on the malignant cells.

Answer 38.5. **The answer is A.**

CSF EBV PCR is a rather sensitive (~80%) and highly specific test (>95%) for diagnosis of primary CNS lymphoma, and together with a consistent radiological picture, brain biopsy may not be required to establish the diagnosis. In patients with low CD4 counts or poor performance status, cranial radiotherapy is the treatment of choice for primary CNS lymphoma, because opportunistic infections cause much greater morbidity and mortality than recurrent lymphoma. In contrast, for patients with higher CD4 counts and good performance status, high-dose systemic methotrexate therapy with leucovorin rescue may be associated with improved responses, as reported in non-HIV-associated primary CNS lymphoma.

Answer 38.6.   **The answer is A.**

Hodgkin disease is a non-AIDS-defining cancer, whereas Burkitt lymphoma, DLBCL, and primary CNS lymphoma are considered to be AIDS-defining cancers.

Answer 38.7.   **The answer is B.**

TNM staging is not useful in KS. The most widely used staging system is the TIS system, which attempts to stratify risk of poor prognosis in patients with KS. It is based on the extent of tumor involvement (T), immune status of the patient (I), and the presence of AIDS-related system illness. In the era of HAART, assessing the immune system (CD4 count) does not provide prognostic information in patients with HIV sensitive to HAART, though is useful in patients with multidrug resistant HIV. RECIST criteria are not useful in assessing KS response to therapy. The AIDS Clinical Trials Group Oncology Committee criteria for assessing response include a 50% decrease in the total number of lesions, a 50% decrease in the area of measured cutaneous lesions, or a flattening of 50% of nodular lesions.

Answer 38.8.   **The answer is D.**

Patients with HIV-associated HL present at a younger age, B symptoms are more frequent, and they usually have higher-stage disease at presentation. Mediastinal involvement is less frequent in patients with HIV-associated HL, whereas extranodal involvement is more frequent.

Answer 38.9.   **The answer is C.**

Cervical cancer and anal cancer in patients infected with HIV appear to be related to HPV infection. In women who are newly diagnosed with HIV, cervical cancer screening is recommended. If preinvasive cervical neoplasia is found, standard therapy (cryotherapy, laser therapy, cone biopsy, and loop excision) should be used. However, the recurrence rate in patients with HIV infection is twice that of HIV-seronegative women. In HIV-infected patients with anal cancer (CD4 $<200/mm^3$), who are treated with chemotherapy and radiation, treatment-related toxicities (diarrhea, cytopenias) are also significantly higher than those in HIV-negative patients with anal cancer.

Answer 38.10.   **The answer is D.**

EBV is involved in the pathogenesis of HL and the EBV genome has been detected in tumor nuclei. Hepatitis C and HIV coinfection is common and leads to increased risk of cirrhosis and hepatocellular carcinoma. HHV-8 is implicated in the development of KS.

CHAPTER 39 ONCOLOGIC EMERGENCIES

GIRIDHARAN RAMSINGH • DANIEL MORGENSZTERN

DIRECTIONS   Each of the numbered items below is followed by lettered answers. Select the
ONE lettered answer that is BEST in each case unless instructed otherwise.

QUESTIONS

*Questions
39.1.–39.3.*

A 48-year-old white man presents with a history of progressive facial swelling and shortness of breath for 1 month. He has a 40-pack-year smoking history. On examination, the patient has cervical and thoracic venous distention. Laboratory test results revealed normal blood counts, basic metabolic profile, and liver functions. Computed tomography (CT) scan revealed a 6 × 5-cm lung mass with liver metastases.

Question 39.1.   What is the most likely cause of his condition?

A. Small cell lung cancer
B. Non-Hodgkin's lymphoma
C. Non-small cell lung cancer
D. Superior vena cava (SVC) thrombosis

Question 39.2.   Biopsy was performed and showed small cell lung cancer. Which is the best initial modality of treatment for this patient?

A. Surgery
B. Radiation therapy
C. Chemotherapy
D. SVC stent

Question 39.3.   What is the most likely location for the primary tumor?

A. Peripheral left lung
B. Peripheral right lung
C. Central left lung
D. Central right lung

Corresponding Chapter in *Cancer: Principles & Practice of Oncology,* Ninth Edition: 143 (Superior Vena Cava Syndrome), 144 (Increased Intracranial Pressure), 145 (Spinal Cord Compression), and 146 (Metabolic Emergencies).

Question 39.4. Which among the following is the earliest fundoscopic sign for increased intracranial pressure?

 A. Absence of venous pulsations within the center of the optic disk
 B. Blurring of the disk margins
 C. Disk hemorrhage
 D. Foster-Kennedy syndrome

Question 39.5. A 57-year-old man presents with severe back pain and bilateral leg weakness for 3 days. Magnetic resonance imaging (MRI) of the spine reveals metastatic lesion at T10 vertebral body with significant cord compression. What are the most likely primary tumors?

 A. Lung cancer and breast cancer
 B. Lung cancer and lymphoma
 C. Breast cancer and lymphoma
 D. Colon cancer and prostate cancer

Question 39.6. Which of the following signs indicate damage to pontine structures?

 A. Midsize pupils unresponsive to light
 B. Coma
 C. Absence of oculocephalic reflex
 D. Ataxic breathing

Question 39.7. Which of the following statements regarding rasburicase is FALSE?

 A. Mechanism of action is inhibition of urate oxidase
 B. Should be avoided in patients with glucose 6-phosphate deficiency (G6PD)
 C. Antibodies against rasburicase or its epitopes may occur in up to 20% of cases
 D. None of the above; all answers are correct

Question 39.8. A 28-year-old man presents with newly diagnosed acute myeloid leukemia. He has a white cell count of 140,000/mm^3, glucose of 96 mg/dL, sodium of 138 mEq/L, potassium of 4 mEq/L, creatinine of 1.1 mg/dL, blood urea nitrogen (BUN) of 15 mg/dL, uric acid of 4.8 mg/dL, albumin of 5.2 g/dL, and calcium of 10.2 mg/dL. He is started on induction chemotherapy, aggressive intravenous fluids and allopurinol. Twelve hours later, the patient developed cardiac arrest not responsive to cardiopulmonary resuscitation and died. What is the most likely cause of his death?

 A. Leukostasis
 B. Electrolyte imbalance
 C. Pulmonary embolism
 D. Chemotherapy-induced cardiac arrhythmia

Question 39.9.   Which of the following is NOT a component of the Kocher–Cushing reflex observed in patients with increased intracranial pressure?

    A. Changes in breathing pattern
    B. Headaches
    C. Hypertension
    D. Bradycardia

Question 39.10.   A 63-year-old man with metastatic squamous cell carcinoma of the lung presents with worsening confusion, constipation, and nausea for 3 days. Laboratory tests revealed hemoglobin of 13.5 g/dL, WBC of 12,500/mm^3, platelets of 155,000/mm^3, sodium of 149 mEq/L, potassium of 4.8 mEq/L, bicarbonate of 28 mEq/L, BUN of 44 mg/dL, creatinine of 1.8 mg/dL, albumin of 2.8 g/dL, and calcium of 13.6 mg/dL. What is the most appropriate initial therapy?

    A. Intravenous fluids and bisphosphonate
    B. Intravenous fluids, bisphosphonate, and calcitonin
    C. Intravenous fluids, bisphosphonate, and gallium nitrate
    D. Intravenous fluids, bisphosphonate, and plicamycin

ANSWERS

Answer 39.1.   **The answer is A.**

Malignant disease is the most common cause of SVC syndrome. Among the malignancies, the most common is small cell lung cancer, followed by squamous cell lung cancer and lymphoma in most series. Diffuse large B-cell lymphoma and lymphoblastic lymphoma are the most common among lymphomas that cause SVC syndrome. Although Hodgkin's disease frequently involves mediastinum, it rarely causes SVC syndrome. Breast cancer is the most common metastatic cancer that causes SVC syndrome. Nonmalignant condition causing SVC syndrome is increasingly becoming more common because of the use of vascular devices, which can result in SVC thrombosis.

Answer 39.2.   **The answer is C.**

Studies have shown that both radiation therapy and chemotherapy are equally effective in relieving symptoms in small cell lung cancer and lymphoma. Surgery is not a good option for this patient with extensive-stage small cell lung cancer, and an SVC stent may be used in case of lack of response or relapsed obstruction after initial therapy. Although radiation could be used for immediate symptomatic relief, combination chemotherapy is also very effective and preferable as initial therapy, avoiding the large radiation field and also addressing the metastatic lesions.

Answer 39.3.   **The answer is D.**

The SVC extends from the junction of the right and left innominate veins to the right atrium and is completely encircled by lymph node chains draining from the right thoracic cavity and lower part of the left thorax. Approximately 80% of the tumors causing SVC syndrome are located in the right lung. In the absence of mediastinal lymph node enlargement, the most likely cause of the SVC is direct extension from the centrally located right-sided tumor.

Answer 39.4.   **The answer is A.**

Absence of venous pulsations within the center of the optic disk is usually one of the earliest signs of increased intracranial pressure, with blurring of the optic disk and hemorrhage occurring at later stages. The Foster-Kennedy syndrome, characterized by ipsilateral optic atrophy and contralateral papilledema, is rarely seen late event.

Answer 39.5.   **The answer is B.**

Although most patients with malignant spinal cord compression (MSCC) have a history of malignancy, approximately 20% develop this complication at the initial presentation. Breast cancer is a common cause of MSCC during the course of the disease, but this manifestation rarely occurs at presentation. Colon cancer is an uncommon cause of MSCC, and prostate cancer usually affects the lumbosacral spine. The most common causes of MSCC at presentation are lung cancer, non-Hodgkin's lymphoma, and multiple myeloma.

Answer 39.6. **The answer is C.**

Midsize and nonresponding pupils indicate midbrain dysfunction, whereas coma is seen with damage to the mesencephalic reticular activating system. Ataxic breathing may be observed with cerebellar tonsil herniation and indicates a damage to the medullary respiratory center. Absence of the oculocephalic reflex (doll's head maneuver) and horizontal eye movements in response to caloric stimulation of the vestibular system are signs of pontine damage.

Answer 39.7. **The answer is A.**

Urate oxidase catalyzes the conversion of uric acid to allantoin. This enzyme is present in most mammals but not in humans. Rasburicase is a recombinant urate oxidase produced in *Saccharomyces cerevisiae*. This medicine should be avoided in patients with G6PD because it may cause hemolysis as a result of the increase in the byproduct hydrogen peroxidase, and approximately 10% to 20% of patients taking rasburicase may develop antibodies, increasing the risk of allergic reaction with subsequent treatments.

Answer 39.8. **The answer is B.**

Despite vigorous hydration, the most likely cause of death soon after initiating chemotherapy is tumor lysis syndrome (TLS). Among the metabolic complications of tumor lysis syndrome, hyperkalemia caused by the release of intracellular potassium from tumoral cells represents the most important cause of early mortality. Leukostasis, pulmonary embolism, and cardiac arrhythmia are possible causes that are far less likely in this patient.

Answer 39.9. **The answer is B.**

The Kocher–Cushing reflex is characterized by changes in breathing pattern, hypertension, and bradycardia. Despite being common in patients with increased intracranial pressure, headaches are not a component of this triad.

Answer 39.10. **The answer is B.**

This patient has severe hypercalcemia and requires prompt reduction in the calcium levels. Intravenous hydration is the most important initial step, with or without the addition of furosemide, which may enhance the renal calcium excretion. Bisphosphonates are also very effective and well tolerated. However, because the patient is symptomatic and the effect of bisphosphonates may take a few days, he will require an additional short-acting agent. Gallium nitrate is usually given by continuous infusion for 5 days, with a gradual reduction in the calcium during the infusion time.

Although plicamycin lowers the calcium levels typically within 12 hours, side effects including thrombocytopenia and nephrotoxicity limit its use in patients with severe and refractory hypercalcemia. Calcitonin is safe and relatively nontoxic, and may result in a rapid decrease in calcium levels within 2 to 6 hours. In this patient, the calcitonin may provide a fast improvement in the hypercalcemia, whereas bisphosphonate can cause a more sustainable effect.

CHAPTER 40 TREATMENT OF METASTATIC CANCER

KUMAR RAJAGOPALAN

DIRECTIONS   Each of the numbered items below is followed by lettered answers. Select the ONE lettered answer that is BEST in each case unless instructed otherwise.

QUESTIONS

Question 40.1.   Which of the following prognostic factors predicts for improved overall survival after lung metastatectomy in osteosarcoma?

A. Age
B. Histology
C. Number of tumor nodules
D. Complete resection

Question 40.2.   All of the following are true regarding liver metastases in patients with colorectal cancer, EXCEPT:

A. Synchronous liver metastases are seen in 15% to 20% of colorectal cancer.
B. Liver metastases are more common in patients over 75 years old than in younger patients.
C. Synchronous liver metastases are less common in women than men.
D. Long-term survival may be feasible after metastatectomy in certain patients with liver metastases from colorectal cancers.

Question 40.3.   All of the following are prognostic factors for survival in patients with liver metastases from colorectal cancer, EXCEPT:

A. Grade of primary tumor
B. Presence of extrahepatic tumor
C. Mesenteric lymph node involvement
D. Age and sex of the patient

Corresponding Chapters in *Cancer: Principles & Practice of Oncology,* Ninth Edition: 147 (Metastatic Cancer to the Brain), 148 (Metastatic Cancer to the Lung), 149 (Metastatic Cancer to the Liver), 150 (Metastatic Cancer to the Bone), 151 (Malignant Effusions of the Pleura and the Pericardium), 152 (Malignant Ascites), and 153 (Paraneoplastic Syndromes).

Question 40.4.   Which of the following is an appropriate indication for operative management of femoral metastases?

A. Size ≥2 cm
B. Subtrochanteric location of metastases
C. Metastasis involving 40% of the diameter of the cortex
D. All of the above

Question 40.5.   Which of the following cancers rarely metastasizes to the brain?

A. Colorectal cancer
B. Melanomas
C. Thyroid cancer
D. Prostate cancer

Question 40.6.   Which of the following malignancies has the best long-term survival outcomes after resection of lung metastases?

A. Sarcomas
B. Melanomas
C. Breast cancer
D. Germ cell tumors

Question 40.7.   All of the following statements related to whole brain radiation therapy (WBRT) are true, EXCEPT:

A. The hippocampus is the least sensitive area of the brain to the effects of radiation.
B. Myringotomy may be required in some patients to relieve radiation-induced fluid buildup behind the tympanic membrane.
C. Treatment with whole brain radiation results in complete resolution of brain metastases in a third of patients with small cell lung carcinoma.
D. Long-term side effects include dementia and cognitive problems.

Question 40.8.   All of the following factors are associated with improved median survival in patients with brain metastases, EXCEPT:

A. Karnofsky Performance Status of 70% or greater
B. Controlled primary tumor
C. Age less than 65 years old
D. Presence of extra-cranial metastasis

Question 40.9.   Overall median survival for patients with malignant pericardial effusion is:

A. Less than 1 year
B. Less than 9 months
C. Less than 6 months
D. Less than 3 months

Question 40.10.   **All of the following are TRUE about intraperitoneal chemotherapy, EXCEPT:**

    A. Achieves high peritoneal concentration of chemotherapy, while minimizing systemic absorption and systemic toxicity.

    B. Choice of drugs is determined by the chemosensitivity of the target cancer and peritoneal pharmacokinetics.

    C. Hyperthermia can enhance the cytotoxicity of intraperitoneal chemotherapy.

    D. Post-surgical residual tumor nodules' size does not determine effective tumor absorption of chemotherapy.

Question 40.11.   **Which of the following factors have prognostic significance in patients with colorectal cancer, who undergo ablative therapy of hepatic metastases?**

    A. Low pretreatment CEA levels

    B. Diameter of largest lesion <3 cm

    C. No extrahepatic disease

    D. All of the above

Question 40.12.   **All of the following statements about radionuclide treatment of bone metastases are true, EXCEPT:**

    A. Strontium-89 and Samarium-153 are commonly used radionuclides in the treatment of diffuse bone metastases.

    B. For Strontium-89 the average time to clinical response is about 7 to 14 days with a median duration of action of 18 weeks.

    C. Thrombocytopenia nadir is 1 to 2 weeks after treatment and completely recovers by 4 weeks.

    D. Retreatment is possible for both Strontium-89 and Samarium-153 after an interval of 10 to 12 weeks and 6 to 10 weeks, respectively.

Question 40.13.   **All of the following statements are correct about radiosensitizers in brain metastases treatment, EXCEPT:**

    A. Motexafin gadolinium (MGd) is a redox mediator that selectively targets tumor cells and decreases local oxygen consumption.

    B. In patients with brain metastases MGd use with WBRT did not increase median survival or median time to neurologic progression.

    C. In patients with non-small cell lung cancer and brain metastases, use of MGd with WBRT was found to improve median time to neurologic progression.

    D. Use of RSR13, an allosteric modifier of hemoglobin that facilitates O_2 release, along with WBRT in patients with breast cancer and brain metastases was not associated with improved median survival compared with WBRT alone.

Question 40.14.   All of the following risk factors are associated with shorter overall and disease-free survival after neoadjuvant chemotherapy followed by resection for patients with colorectal liver metastases, EXCEPT:

A. Preoperative tumor size >10 cm
B. Preoperative CA 19-9 >100 IU/L
C. Colon primary
D. More than three metastatic liver lesions at the time of operation

Question 40.15.   The following statements are true of bisphosphonates use in metastatic bone disease, EXCEPT:

A. Consensus recommendations indicate that all patients with myeloma and radiologically confirmed bone metastasis from breast cancer should receive bisphosphonates from the time of diagnosis and continue indefinitely.
B. Development of a skeletal-related event or progressive bone metastasis while on pamidronate is an indication of ineffectiveness of bisphosphonates and benefit will not be obtained by switching to zoledronic acid.
C. Bone resorption markers such as N-telopeptide of type I collagen (NTx) may be useful to identify patients at high risk of skeletal complications.

Question 40.16.   All of the following statements regarding peritoneovenous shunt are true, EXCEPT:

A. Has a unidirectional valve allowing flow from abdomen to chest and preventing reflux.
B. Contraindicated with loculated effusions.
C. No increased risk of spreading malignant cells into the systemic circulation.
D. Studies demonstrate control of ascites in 72% of patients with mean shunt patency of 9.6 weeks.
E. No contraindications to shunt in cases of hemorrhagic ascites.

ANSWERS

Answer 40.1.   **The answer is D.**

In patients with metastases to the lungs, complete resection of the tumor nodules in the lung, when feasible, was associated with improved overall survival when compared to patients with unresectable metastasis or partial resection of lung metastasis.

Answer 40.2.   **The answer is B.**

Synchronous liver metastases are slightly less frequent in females than males. Similarly they are less frequent in patients older than 75 years old compared to younger age patients.

Answer 40.3.   **The answer is D.**

Age and sex of the patient did not have an impact on survival outcome whereas performance status, tumor grade, lymph node involvement, and extrahepatic disease are independent prognostic factors for survival. Also percentage of liver replaced by tumor (less than 25% vs. greater than 25%) was prognostic for survival.

Answer 40.4.   **The answer is D.**

Subtrochanteric segment extends from lesser trochanter to the junction of the proximal and middle-thirds of the diaphysis, and is subject to very high axial loads of weightbearing and tremendous bending forces. All these features make it appropriate for operative management.

Answer 40.5.   **The answer is D.**

Prostate cancer along with oropharyngeal and non-melanoma skin cancers are rarely associated with tumor metastases to the brain. Lung, breast, colorectal cancers along with melanomas, kidney, and thyroid cancers have higher rates of metastases to brain.

Answer 40.6.   **The answer is D.**

The international registry of lung metastases notes up to 60% survival at 10 years for patients with germ cell tumors who underwent resection of their lung metastases, whereas the survival with the other listed cancers is not so good.

Answer 40.7.   **The answer is A.**

The hippocampus is the most sensitive area of the brain to whole brain radiation. With newer techniques it is possible to minimize the dose to the hippocampus while delivering the full dose to the brain. Treatment with WBRT is associated with a complete response rate of 37% in patients with small cell lung cancer and brain metastases.

Answer 40.8.   **The answer is D.**

Presence of extra-cranial metastases is associated with a decreased median survival in these patients, while the other factors listed are associated with improved median survival times.

Answer 40.9.   **The answer is C.**

Approximately half of all pericardial effusions that require intervention are due to malignant effusions. Like pleural effusions due to malignancy, malignant pericardial effusion is indicative of advanced, incurable malignancy. Symptoms include dyspnea, cough, chest pain, and fever. Treatment options include simple pericardiocentesis, pericardial window, pericardiectomy, and percutaneous tube pericardiostomy with or without installation of sclerosing agents like bleomycin. Radiation therapy is useful to control malignant pericardial effusions due to lymphoma/leukemia and breast cancers.

Answer 40.10.   **The answer is D.**

Tumor deposits less than 10 mm result in better drug absorption. In fact, this has served as the rationale for aggressive surgical cytoreduction. Using hyperthermic intraperitoneal therapy, Ben-Ari et al. reported complete resolution of malignant ascites in 38 of 41 patients with varying histologies.

Answer 40.11.   **The answer is D.**

All of the above factors have independent prognostic significance in patients with colorectal cancer undergoing ablative therapy for liver metastases. Additional factors include successful cryotherapy of all hepatic lesions and metachronous (vs. synchronous) liver metastases.

Answer 40.12.   **The answer is C.**

Myelosuppression, especially thrombocytopenia is the main toxicity with radionuclide treatment of bone metastases. As opposed to standard chemotherapy, radionuclide-induced thrombocytopenia is delayed with a nadir 4 to 6 weeks after treatment which may take 6 to 10 weeks for complete recovery.

Answer 40.13.   **The answer is D.**

The use of RSR13 in breast cancer primaries with brain metastases was associated with improved median survival of 8.7 months compared with 4.6 months in the control arm of WBRT alone. (Suh et al. Neuro-Oncology. 2003;5(4):345) Other responses are correct.

Answer 40.14.   **The answer is C.**

Rectal primary is associated with a shorter overall and disease-free survival in patients with liver metastases undergoing neoadjuvant therapy followed by resection. Other poor prognostic factors include disease progression on therapy, positive resection margins, less than complete tumor necrosis and history of ≤2 hepatectomies.

Answer 40.15.   **The answer is B.**

In a phase II trial involving 31 patients with breast cancer who had experienced progressive bone metastases or skeletal-related events (SRE) while on pamidronate benefit was seen by switching to the more potent zoledronic acid. Treatment with zoledronic acid was associated with significant reductions in both severity of pain (p <0.001) and urinary markers of bone turnover (P = 0.008).

Answer 40.16.   **The answer is E.**

Contraindications to peritoneovenous shunts include chylous and hemorrhagic ascites which are associated with high rates of shunt clotting and occlusion. Also underlying cardiac, pulmonary, and renal insufficiency could be exacerbated from the increased volumes draining via the peritoneovenous shunts.

CHAPTER 41 PARANEOPLASTIC SYNDROMES

C. DANIEL KINGSLEY • MICHAEL C. PERRY

DIRECTIONS   Each of the numbered items below is followed by lettered answers. Select the ONE lettered answer that is BEST in each case unless instructed otherwise.

QUESTIONS

Question 41.1.   Chronic lymphocytic leukemia (CLL) has been associated with all of the following, EXCEPT:

- A. Pure red cell aplasia
- B. Warm antibody hemolytic anemia
- C. Microangiopathic hemolytic anemia
- D. Paraneoplastic pemphigus

Question 41.2.   Which of the statements about small cell lung cancer (SCLC) is FALSE?

- A. SCLC is the second leading cause of ectopic adrenocorticotropic hormone (ACTH) production after bronchial carcinoid.
- B. SCLC is the leading cause of syndrome of inappropriate antidiuretic hormone production (SIADH).
- C. Subacute sensory neuronopathy and encephalomyeloneuritis is most frequently associated with SCLC, compared with other forms of cancer.
- D. Patients with cancer with Lambert-Eaton syndrome (LES) most frequently have SCLC as an underlying cause.

Question 41.3.   Ectopic ACTH production causes all the following, EXCEPT:

- A. Muscle wasting
- B. Moon facies
- C. Hypokalemia
- D. Hyperpigmentation

Question 41.4.   Many patients with SCLC produce ectopic ACTH, but what percentage develop clinical Cushing's syndrome?

- A. 3% to 7%
- B. 12% to 15%
- C. 20% to 25%
- D. 33% to 36%

Corresponding Chapter in *Cancer: Principles & Practice of Oncology*, Ninth Edition: 153 (Paraneoplastic Syndromes).

Question 41.5.   A 55-year-old man with a 50 pack-year history of smoking presents with a 6-month history of a cough, 20 pound weight loss, progressive proximal muscle weakness, and darkening of his skin. Laboratory studies are remarkable for a low potassium level of 2.9 mEq/dL. Chest X-ray reveals a right upper lobe mass. What is the most likely finding on biopsy of this mass?

A. Adenocarcinoma
B. Mesothelioma
C. Small cell carcinoma
D. Squamous cell carcinoma

Question 41.6.   In addition to potassium supplementation, which of the following is the most appropriate treatment for his weakness and hypokalemia?

A. Aminoglutethimide
B. Mitotane
C. Ketoconazole
D. Metyrapone

Question 41.7.   Laboratory findings of SIADH include all of the following, EXCEPT:

A. Normal volume status
B. Plasma osmolality greater than urine osmolality
C. Elevated renal excretion of sodium
D. Hyponatremia

Question 41.8.   Which of the following tumors is associated with necrolytic migratory erythema?

A. Gastric cancer
B. Glucagonoma
C. Insulinoma
D. Gastrointestinal (GI) stromal tumor

Question 41.9.   Which of the following tumors is most frequently associated with erythrocytosis?

A. Adrenal cortical tumors
B. Virilizing ovarian tumors
C. Hepatoma
D. Renal cell carcinoma

Question 41.10.   Which laboratory findings would describe the most common anemia seen in patients with cancer?

A. Low serum iron, low ferritin, elevated total iron-binding capacity (TIBC), elevated erythropoietin
B. Low serum iron, normal ferritin, elevated TIBC, low erythropoietin
C. Low serum iron, elevated ferritin, low TIBC, low erythropoietin
D. Normal serum iron, elevated ferritin, low TIBC, elevated erythropoietin

Question 41.11.   Which of the associations between red cells and disease is FALSE?

A. Pure red cell aplasia and thymoma
B. Microangiopathic hemolytic anemia and adenocarcinoma of the GI tract
C. Autoimmune hemolytic anemia and CLL
D. Cold agglutinin disease and ovarian cancer

Question 41.12.   Independent risk factors for disseminated intravascular coagulation (DIC) include all the following, EXCEPT:

A. Female gender
B. Older age
C. Advanced stage
D. Breast cancer

Question 41.13.   Which of the following renal associations is INCORRECT?

A. Minimal change disease and Hodgkin's lymphoma
B. Immunoglobulin (Ig)A nephropathy and head and neck cancer
C. Focal and segmental glomerulosclerosis and gastric cancer
D. Membranous nephropathy and lung cancer

Question 41.14.   A 54-year-old former smoker develops lung cancer and is noted to have a corrected serum calcium of 11.9. Which histological subtype is most expected?

A. Squamous cell
B. Adenocarcinoma
C. Small cell
D. Mesothelioma

Question 41.15.   Which of the following associations is INCORRECT?

A. Sudden appearance of seborrheic keratoses and gastric cancer
B. Pachydermoperiostosis and SCLC
C. Acquired ichthyosis and Hodgkin's lymphoma
D. Necrolytic migratory erythema and glucagonoma

Question 41.16.   Which of the following associations is INCORRECT?

A. Vitiligo and melanoma
B. Acrokeratosis paraneoplastica and squamous cell carcinoma of the esophagus
C. Pyoderma gangrenosum and pancreatic cancer
D. Sweet's syndrome and acute myelogenous leukemia

Question 41.17.   A relapsing high-grade fever with fever spikes that are abrupt in onset and resolution should point toward the diagnosis of:

A. Diffuse large B-cell lymphoma
B. Hodgkin's lymphoma
C. Follicular lymphoma
D. Renal cell carcinoma

Question 41.18.   Acquired von Willebrand's disease is seen in all the following, EXCEPT:

A. Plasma cell dyscrasias
B. Lymphoma
C. Gastric cancer
D. Hepatocellular carcinoma

Question 41.19.   Cancer-related thrombosis results from which of the following mechanisms?

A. Direct generation of thrombin
B. Increased platelet aggregation
C. Decreased levels of protein C, protein S, and antithrombin
D. All of the above

Question 41.20.   A 39-year-old woman presents with ptosis, diplopia, and proximal muscle weakness, which improve with rest. Tensilon challenge test is positive, with improvement in weakness following edrophonium administration. Which of the following diagnostic tests is indicated?

A. Computed tomography (CT) scan of the chest
B. Nerve conduction studies
C. Serum calcium level
D. Muscle biopsy

Question 41.21.   Which of the following about limbic encephalitis (LE) is INCORRECT?

A. Testicular cancers associated with LE have the anti-Hu antibody.
B. It may be mistaken for herpes simplex encephalitis.
C. Most cases are associated with SCLC.
D. It is one of the more treatable forms of central nervous system (CNS) paraneoplastic disorders.

Question 41.22.   The anti-Yo antibody CNS paraneoplastic disorder has all these in common, EXCEPT:

A. It is commonly associated with ovarian and breast cancer.
B. The antibody is active against the Purkinje cells.
C. It causes opsoclonus-myoclonus.
D. The disorder is subacute in onset and usually progressive.

Question 41.23.   Which of the following about LES is INCORRECT?

A. Sixty percent of patients with LES have an underlying cancer.
B. The malignancy most associated with LES is SCLC.
C. It is a pure motor syndrome.
D. Proximal weakness is the common presenting symptom.

Question 41.24.   Melanoma-associated retinopathy includes all the following, EXCEPT:

A. It most commonly appears at the metastatic stage.
B. It is more common in men.
C. Only cones are affected, sparing rods.
D. Progressive blindness is unusual.

Question 41.25.   A 59-year-old man, with 50 pack-year history of smoking, is found to have a left upper lobe mass, detected incidentally on chest X-ray. He is afebrile, and has a chronic productive cough and hemoptysis for the past 2 months. He is noted to have a white blood cell count of 20×10^9/L, with 90% neutrophils. All other cell lines are within normal limits. Leukocyte alkaline phosphatase (LAP) level is elevated. What is the most likely cause of his leukocytosis?

A. Bone marrow metastasis from lung cancer
B. Acute bronchitis
C. Hematopoietic cytokine release from his tumor
D. Chronic myelogenous leukemia (CML)

ANSWERS

Answer 41.1.   **The answer is C.**

CLL has been described in association with both warm antibody hemolytic anemia and autoimmune hemolytic anemia, but not with microangiopathic hemolytic anemia with its red cell fragmentation.

Answer 41.2.   **The answer is A.**

SCLC is the leading cause of ectopic ACTH production.

Answer 41.3.   **The answer is B.**

Classic hypercortisolism causes moon facies, but ectopic production usually does not.

Answer 41.4.   **The answer is A.**

Some 3% to 7% of patients with SCLC and ectopic ACTH production will develop Cushing syndrome.

Answer 41.5.   **The answer is C.**

Myopathy with weakness, muscle wasting, weight loss, hyperpigmentation, and hypokalemia are characteristic of ectopic ACTH production from SCLC. SCLC is the leading cause of ectopic ACTH production.

Answer 41.6.   **The answer is C.**

Ketoconazole is considered the therapy of choice because of its rapid onset of action and favorable toxicity profile. Mitotane is rarely used due to slow onset of activity and severe toxicities associated with its use (allergic reaction, dizziness, blurred vision, fainting). Aminoglutethimide has limited efficacy when used alone, and is used in combination with metyrapone to treat ectopic ACTH production from cancer.

Answer 41.7.   **The answer is B.**

Patients have a urine osmolality greater than plasma osmolality.

Answer 41.8.   **The answer is B.**

Necrolytic migratory erythema is characterized by erythema, papules, and pustules on the face, lower abdomen, perineum, and buttocks. These lesions progress to form blisters and result in epidermal necrosis. Necrolytic migratory erythema is associated solely with glucagonoma, and clears after resection of the tumor.

Answer 41.9.   **The answer is D.**

Although all of the answers listed are associated with erythrocytosis, renal cell carcinoma is the leading cause, followed by hepatoma. Both of these tumors are associated with elevated erythropoietin levels. In the case of adrenal cortical tumors and virilizing ovarian tumors, the production of androgenic hormones and prostaglandins leads to erythrocytosis.

Answer 41.10.   **The answer is C.**

Anemia of chronic disease is the most common anemia seen in patients with cancer and is reflected by a low serum iron, normal or increased ferritin, low TIBC, and low serum erythropoietin.

Answer 41.11.   **The answer is D.**

Cold agglutinin disease is most common in Waldenström's macroglobulinemia.

Answer 41.12.   **The answer is A.**

Male gender is an independent risk factor for DIC.

Answer 41.13.   **The answer is C.**

Focal and segmental glomerulosclerosis is associated with CLL, T-cell receptor lymphomas, and acute myelogenous leukemias, whereas stomach cancer is associated with membranous nephropathy.

Answer 41.14.   **The answer is A.**

Squamous cell cancers of the lung and head and neck are more commonly associated with hypercalcemia than the other subtypes.

Answer 41.15.   **The answer is B.**

Pachydermoperiostosis is most often associated with bronchogenic carcinoma.

Answer 41.16.   **The answer is C.**

Pyoderma gangrenosum is associated with hematological malignancies, as well as gastric carcinoma and other GI abnormalities.

Answer 41.17.   **The answer is B.**

This describes a Pel-Ebstein fever, which although uncommon, should lead one to look for Hodgkin's lymphoma.

Answer 41.18.   **The answer is D.**

Acquired von Willebrand's disease is seen in plasma cell dyscrasias, gastric and adrenal carcinomas, leukemias, and lymphomas.

Answer 41.19.   **The answer is D.**

Cancer-related thrombosis occurs due to a complex imbalance between coagulation and fibrinolysis. Decreased levels of protein C, protein S, and antithrombin contribute to the prothrombotic state. Increased platelet activation and platelet aggregation, activation of the coagulation cascade, and direct generation of thrombin all play a role in cancer-related thrombosis.

Answer 41.20.   **The answer is A.**

This woman's presentation is characteristic of myasthenia gravis, in which autoantibodies develop against the acetylcholine nicotinic postsynaptic receptor. Myasthenia gravis is associated with thymoma in 15% of cases, and a CT of the chest is indicated, to look for thymoma. In patients with thymoma, myasthenia gravis may remit after thymectomy.

Answer 41.21.   **The answer is A.**

SCLC is associated with the anti-Hu antibody, and testicular cancer is associated with the anti-Ma2 antibody.

Answer 41.22.   **The answer is C.**

Anti-Yo antibody causes progressive cerebellar degeneration, whereas opsoclonus-myoclonus is caused by not one antibody, but several, including anti-Hu, anti-Ri, and antineurofilament.

Answer 41.23.   **The answer is C.**

LES is not a pure motor disorder because paresthesias are frequently reported, and dry mouth and erectile dysfunction are also reported.

Answer 41.24.   **The answer is C.**

Only rods are affected, and acquired night blindness may occur.

Answer 41.25.   **The answer is C.**

This is likely to be a paraneoplastic leukocytosis associated with lung cancer. In this setting, leukocytosis occurs due to hematopoietic cytokine release from his tumor. Marrow infiltration is unlikely, as other cell lines are normal. LAP is decreased in CML, which would also make this an unlikely diagnosis. Infection is unlikely in the absence of any signs or symptoms.

CHAPTER 42 STEM CELL TRANSPLANTATION

MARK A. SCHROEDER • PETER WESTERVELT

DIRECTIONS Each of the numbered items below is followed by lettered answers. Select the ONE lettered answer that is BEST in each case unless instructed otherwise.

QUESTIONS

Question 42.1. The curative potential of allogeneic hematopoietic stem cell transplantation (HSCT) may be derived from which of the following:

A. High-dose chemotherapy
B. Graft-versus-leukemia (GVL) effect
C. Graft-versus-host effect
D. A and B

Question 42.2. The allogeneic transplant conditioning regimen serves to achieve which of the following:

A. Provide immunosuppression to prevent rejection
B. Provide immunosuppression to prevent graft-versus-host disease (GVHD)
C. Eradicate malignant cells
D. A and C

Question 42.3. Which of the following regimens is considered myeloablative?

A. Cyclophosphamide 60 mg/kg/d intravenously (IV) × 2 days plus 1200 cGy total body irradiation (TBI)
B. Cyclophosphamide 60 mg/kg/d IV × 2 days plus busulfan 3.2 mg/kg/d IV × 4 days
C. Fludarabine 30 mg/kg/d IV × 5 plus busulfan 3.2 mg/kg/d IV × 2 plus antithymocyte globulin (ATG) 2.5 mg/kg/d IV × 4
D. A and B

Corresponding Chapters in *Cancer: Principles & Practice of Oncology*, Ninth Edition: 154 (Autologous Stem Cell Transplantation) and 155 (Allogeneic Stem Cell Transplantation).

Question 42.4.   Which conditioning regimen leads to improved disease-free survival in chronic myeloid leukemia (CML)?

A. Cyclophosphamide 60 mg/kg/d IV × 2 days plus busulfan 3.2 mg/kg/d IV × 4 days
B. 1200 cGy TBI and cyclophosphamide 60 mg/kg/d IV × 2 days
C. Chemotherapy and radiation-based conditioning are equivalent
D. Fludarabine 30 mg/kg/d IV × 5 plus busulfan 3.2 mg/kg/d IV × 2 plus ATG 2.5 mg/kg/d IV × 4

Question 42.5.   Which of the following drugs used in the conditioning regimens for stem cell transplant (SCT) is the most common cause of acute cardiac toxicity?

A. Cytarabine
B. Mitoxantrone
C. Cyclophosphamide
D. Busulfan

Question 42.6.   TBI-based conditioning is associated with an increased risk of all the following, EXCEPT:

A. Cataracts
B. Growth retardation
C. Veno-occlusive disease (VOD)
D. Secondary malignancies

Question 42.7.   The GVL effect after transplant is MOST pronounced in which of the following malignancies?

A. Acute myelogenous leukemia (AML)
B. ALL
C. Chronic-phase CML
D. Accelerated-phase CML

Question 42.8.   Which of the following increases the risk of relapse after transplant?

A. Human leukocyte antigen (HLA)-mismatched transplant
B. CD34 cell dose >2 × 106 but <5 × 106/kg recipient body weight
C. Acute and chronic GVHD
D. T-cell–depleted graft

Question 42.9.   Each of the following measures is effective at reducing the indicated regimen-related toxicities, EXCEPT:

A. Hydration, mesna (sodium 2-sulfanylethanesulfonate), and forced diuresis during cyclophosphamide for prevention of hemorrhagic cystitis
B. Phenytoin before and during busulfan infusion for prevention of seizures
C. Dexamethasone and ondansetron before conditioning for nausea prophylaxis
D. Granulocyte colony-stimulating factor (G-CSF) growth factor support to decrease infection-related mortality

Question 42.10.   VOD of the liver is associated with which of the following factors:

A. Presence of acute GVHD
B. Oral busulfan conditioning
C. Advanced age
D. All of the above

Question 42.11.   All of the following are part of the clinical syndrome of VOD, EXCEPT:

A. Jaundice
B. Tender hepatomegaly
C. Weight gain and ascites
D. Diarrhea

Question 42.12.   A 50-year-old man presents to the hospital with shortness of breath and fevers 2 months after an unrelated donor HSCT for AML (M5). He is found to be hypoxic on presentation. Chest radiography shows diffuse pulmonary infiltrates. He is placed on broad-spectrum antibiotics and has been compliant with antifungal and anti-*Pneumocystis jirovecii* pneumonia prophylaxis since his transplant. Sputum culture is negative. Peripheral blood cytomegalovirus (CMV) polymerase chain reaction (PCR) shows an unquantifiable number of viral DNA copies. A bronchoscopy is performed with lavage showing bloody secretions with negative aerobic, anaerobic, fungal, and viral cultures. Bronchoalveolar lavage is tested for galactomannan, which is negative, and the tumor necrosis factor-α level is found to be elevated. His condition fails to improve with antibiotics. What is the most likely diagnosis?

A. CMV pneumonitis
B. Idiopathic pneumonitis
C. Pneumocystis pneumonia
D. Relapsed leukemia

Question 42.13.   All of the following are risk factors for developing acute GVHD post-transplant, EXCEPT:

A. T-cell replete graft
B. Mismatch at HLA-DP
C. Older age of recipient
D. Unrelated donor

Question 42.14.   Each of the following is appropriate as infection prophylaxis in a patient with chronic GVHD on corticosteroids, EXCEPT:

A. Dapsone
B. Fluconazole
C. Penicillin VK
D. Ganciclovir

Question 42.15.   The risk for graft failure is increased by all of the following, EXCEPT:

A. T-cell depletion of the product
B. Less than 1 × 106 CD34+ cells/kg recipient body weight
C. Matched sibling SCT
D. Umbilical cord blood transplant

Question 42.16.   In which setting is the risk of CMV reactivation the highest after allogeneic HCT?

A. CMV-positive donor to a CMV-negative recipient
B. CMV-negative donor to a CMV-positive recipient
C. CMV-negative donor to a CMV-negative recipient
D. CMV-positive donor to a CMV-positive recipient

Question 42.17.   Peripheral blood mobilized stem cell allografts, compared with bone marrow, are associated with which of the following:

A. Shorter period of neutropenia
B. Shorter period to platelet recovery
C. Equivalent T-cell numbers
D. Equivalent incidence of acute GVHD
E. A, B, and D

Question 42.18.   For which of the following patients with an HLA-matched donor is allogeneic stem cell transplantation MOST appropriate?

A. A 35-year-old man with AML with inversion 16 in CR1 after 7+3
B. A 40-year-old woman with AML and complex cytogenetics in first clinical remission (CR)
C. A 48-year-old woman with diffuse large B-cell lymphoma with chemosensitive relapse after initial remission of 18 months
D. A 55-year-old man with Rai stage III chronic lymphocytic leukemia (CLL) in first remission

Question 42.19.   All of the following are potential complications of donor lymphocyte infusion (DLI), EXCEPT:

A. Bone marrow aplasia
B. GVHD flare
C. VOD
D. A and B

Question 42.20.   Common manifestations of CMV reactivation after allogeneic SCT include each of the following, EXCEPT:

A. Pneumonitis
B. Colitis
C. Retinitis
D. Bone marrow suppression

Question 42.21. Limitations of autologous SCT, compared with allogeneic SCT, include all of the following, EXCEPT:

A. Lack of potential graft-versus-tumor effect
B. Higher treatment-related mortality
C. Potential graft contamination with tumor cells
D. Higher relapse risk

Question 42.22. Factors that influence the choice of conditioning regimen include:

A. Underlying malignancy and prior treatment
B. Patient age and comorbidity
C. Donor:recipient HLA compatibility
D. All of the above

Question 42.23. Potential benefits of reduced-intensity conditioning regimens for allogeneic SCT include all of the following, EXCEPT:

A. Decreased period of neutropenia
B. Improved tumor cytoreduction
C. Decreased regimen-related toxicity
D. Appropriate for older patients or with significant comorbidity

Question 42.24. Evidence supporting the existence of the graft-versus-tumor effect includes the following, EXCEPT:

A. Decreased relapse risk among patients with acute and chronic GVHD
B. Increased relapse risk among recipients of identical twin donor grafts
C. Decreased relapse risk among recipients of T-depleted grafts
D. Spontaneous remission after posttransplant relapse on tapering of immunosuppression

Question 42.25. Late complications after allogeneic SCT include:

A. Skeletal complications, including osteoporosis and avascular necrosis
B. Secondary malignancies
C. Endocrine failure
D. All of the above

Question 42.26. Risk factors for acute GVHD includes the following, EXCEPT:

A. Increased age
B. Graft T-cell depletion
C. Donor:recipient HLA disparity
D. Inadequate GVHD prophylaxis

Question 42.27. What is the most common cause of late hemorrhagic cystitis in patients undergoing allogeneic SCT?

A. Cyclophosphamide
B. BK virus
C. Adenovirus
D. B and C

Question 42.28.   Autologous stem cell transplantation is indicated in which of the following solid tumors?

    A. Testicular cancer
    B. Neuroblastoma
    C. Breast cancer
    D. A and B

Question 42.29.   Graft manipulation ex vivo to purge contaminating tumor cells is a strategy that has been successful in reducing the rate of relapse after autologous stem cell transplantation.

    A. True
    B. False

Question 42.30.   Autologous HCT is considered potentially curative in which of the following clinical scenarios?

    A. Intermediate-grade non-Hodgkin's lymphoma in chemotherapy-sensitive first relapse
    B. Multiple myeloma after complete response to initial therapy
    C. Small lymphocytic lymphoma in second CR
    D. Chemotherapy-sensitive metastatic breast carcinoma

Question 42.31.   Which of the following is present in idiopathic pneumonia syndrome?

    A. Associated with prior radiation therapy
    B. Usually occurs more than 3 months after transplant
    C. Rarely associated with CMV infection
    D. A and C

Question 42.32.   Which of the following is NOT a complication associated with autologous HSCT?

    A. Late incidence of myelodysplastic syndrome
    B. Varicella zoster reactivation
    C. *Pneumocystis carinii* pneumonia
    D. Pericarditis

ANSWERS

Answer 42.1.   **The answer is D.**

High-dose chemotherapy (and/or radiation) conditioning regimens have significant antitumor activity and are typically used in younger patients with aggressive hematologic malignancies. Historically, it was believed that the curative potential of allogeneic HCT was derived entirely from the conditioning regimen, and that the donor graft served only as hematopoietic "rescue." It is now known that the graft can mediate a powerful immunologic "GVL effect" that can contribute significantly to the curative potential of the transplant. GVHD represents the deleterious reverse of GVL, an immunologic attack on normal tissue.

Answer 42.2.   **The answer is D.**

The primary objectives of allogeneic transplant conditioning are to provide sufficient immunosuppression of the host immune system to permit donor engraftment, and particularly with fully myeloablative regimens, to achieve significant cytoreduction of tumor cells by incorporating agents with known activity against the underlying malignancy. The conditioning regimen, administered before infusion of donor cells, does not exert a significant impact on the risk of GVHD.

Answer 42.3.   **The answer is D.**

High-dose cyclophosphamide in combination with 1200 to 1350 cGy TBI or busulfan 13.8 mg/m^2 IV constitute the two most commonly used myeloablative conditioning regimens for allogeneic transplantation. Fludarabine and ATG, although significantly lymphosuppressive, have minimal myelosuppressive effects.

Answer 42.4.   **The answer is C.**

Two randomized clinical trials have failed to demonstrate differences in disease-free survival among patients with CML conditioned with either cyclophosphamide and busulfan or cyclophosphamide and TBI. Although the use of reduced-intensity conditioning regimens (answer D) has shown promise in older patients with CML, there are insufficient data comparing such approaches with traditional myeloablative regimens to recommend their routine use in younger patients who are candidates for myeloablative conditioning.

Answer 42.5.   **The answer is C.**

Although acute cardiac toxicity, characterized by cardiomyopathy, arrhythmia, or pericarditis, may be seen with cytarabine and mitoxantrone, this toxicity is most commonly caused by cyclophosphamide. Busulfan is not commonly associated with cardiac toxicity but may cause VOD and pneumonitis.

Answer 42.6.   **The answer is C.**

TBI-containing regimens are associated with an increased risk of several regimen-related toxicities, including cataracts, growth retardation, and secondary malignancies. The incidence of VOD, however, is higher among patients receiving busulfan conditioning, particularly among those with high busulfan area under the concentration-time curve. The use of intravenous busulfan has been shown to lower the incidence of VOD because of its more predictable pharmacokinetics than the traditional oral formulation.

Answer 42.7.   **The answer is C.**

It was primarily on the basis of retrospective studies of outcomes among patients with chronic-phase CML that the GVL effect was first recognized, and a majority of patients treated with DLI for posttransplant relapse of CML achieve a durable molecular remission. In contrast with CML, only a minority of patients with relapsed acute leukemias or more advanced CML are rendered long-term disease-free survivors after DLI.

Answer 42.8.   **The answer is D.**

Posttransplant disease relapse risk is inversely related to the incidence of acute and chronic GVHD. HLA-mismatched transplants, with a correspondingly higher risk of GVHD, also confer a lower risk of relapse. T-cell depletion, although an effective strategy for lowering the risk of GVHD, confers an increased risk of disease relapse.

Answer 42.9.   **The answer is D.**

G-CSF administration after stem cell infusion has been shown in randomized studies to shorten the time to sustained myeloid engraftment but has not been shown to affect treatment-related mortality. Hemorrhagic cystitis, resulting from urinary secretion of acrolein, a metabolite of cyclophosphamide, can be prevented by its inactivation with concurrent mesna administration or by dilution through hyperhydration with intravenous fluids. High-dose busulfan is known to lower the threshold for developing seizures, which can be effectively prevented by the prophylactic use of phenytoin. Concurrent ondansetron and dexamethasone is an effective and widely used regimen for nausea prophylaxis during highly emetogenic conditioning.

Answer 42.10.   **The answer is D.**

The incidence of VOD, thought to result from chemotherapy or radiation-induced injury to the small venules in the liver, is associated with advanced age, prior exposure to gemtuzumab, oral busulfan conditioning, and pre-existing liver disease.

Answer 42.11.   **The answer is D.**

The typical presentation of VOD includes isolated hyperbilirubinemia in the context of tender liver enlargement, ascites, and weight gain during the first 2 to 3 weeks posttransplant. Diarrhea is not typically associated with VOD but may be present concurrently because of other causes in the immediate posttransplant period. The diagnosis of VOD can often be reliably made solely on the basis of clinical grounds, although in complicated clinical scenarios, a liver biopsy may be helpful, demonstrating sinusoidal congestion, fibrin deposition, fibrosis, and surrounding hepatocyte damage.

Answer 42.12.   **The answer is B.**

This scenario, with pulmonary infiltrates, hypoxia, and culture-negative hemorrhagic lavage, is most consistent with idiopathic pneumonitis with diffuse alveolar hemorrhage, a complication of allogeneic HCT generally observed in the first several weeks posttransplant. High-dose corticosteroids, and more recently recombinant Factor VII, have been used with some success, although mortality remains high.

Answer 42.13.   **The answer is B.**

Although HLA-A, B, C, and DR mismatches have been associated with an increased risk of GVHD, the impact of mismatches at HLA-DP (and -DQ) is minimal. Compared with T cell-depleted grafts, T cell-replete grafts confer a higher risk of GVHD. Older recipient age is also associated with an increased risk of acute GVHD.

Answer 42.14.   **The answer is D.**

Knowledge of the types of opportunistic infections that patients with allogeneic HCT are at risk for at various time points allows for a rational, targeted strategy for prophylaxis. Patients with chronic GVHD requiring ongoing immunosuppression remain at increased risk for various opportunistic infections, including pneumocystis, fungal, and viral infections, as well as CMV. The routine use of ganciclovir as prophylaxis is not indicated, however, because of its significant myelosuppression, and instead a more rational approach to preventing CMV disease involves periodic monitoring of peripheral blood with CMV PCR and reserving ganciclovir for preemptive use in the event of detectable CMV viremia.

Answer 42.15.   **The answer is C.**

Graft failure remains a relatively uncommon complication (2% to 3%) of matched sibling allogeneic HSC, although the risk is increased in the setting of an HLA-mismatched or unrelated donor, marginal CD34+ cell dose, or T depletion. Cell doses are often limiting in cord blood products, particularly for adult recipients, which are associated with a higher risk of graft failure.

Answer 42.16.   **The answer is B.**

The risk of developing CMV infection with a CMV-negative donor and recipient is negligible. Among CMV-positive recipients, a CMV-positive donor confers a lower risk of reactivation because of the transfer of preexisting CMV immunity to the recipient, compared with a CMV-naïve donor.

Answer 42.17.   **The answer is E.**

Mobilization and harvest of hematopoietic stem cells from peripheral blood with G-CSF leads to significantly higher numbers of CD34+ cells and results in a shorter time to engraftment of both neutrophils and platelets, compared with bone marrow. Despite significantly higher numbers of T cells, there was no evidence of a significant increase in the incidence of acute GVHD in a randomized trial of peripheral blood mononuclear cell (PBMC) versus bone marrow, although a trend toward increased chronic GVHD in PBMC recipients was observed.

Answer 42.18.   **The answer is B.**

Because of its substantial treatment-related morbidity and mortality, allogeneic stem cell transplantation is generally reserved for patients with hematologic malignancies with a low likelihood of cure with lower risk alternatives, including conventional chemotherapy and/or autologous HCT. Patients with AML with inversion 16 and translocation (8;22) in remission have a favorable prognosis for cure with high-dose cytarabine consolidation and are generally only considered for allogeneic HCT in the event of relapse. In contrast, patients with AML with high-risk cytogenetics, including deletions of chromosomes 5 and 7, and complex karyotypes, are rarely cured with conventional chemotherapy or autologous HCT, and should be referred for consideration of allogeneic HCT when in remission. Relapsed patients with intermediate-grade non-Hodgkin's lymphoma who respond to salvage chemotherapy may be cured with autologous stem cell transplantation with a relatively low risk of treatment-related morbidity and mortality. Because of the generally indolent nature of CLL, initial remissions may persist for years. Although potentially curative for CLL, the early mortality risk associated with allogeneic HCT is generally not justified in this scenario, although it may be appropriate in selected patients with more advanced, multiply relapsed disease.

Answer 42.19.   **The answer is D.**

DLIs by design result in the infusion of large numbers of effector T cells with the goal of augmenting an alloimmune response directed against residual host-derived tumor cells. An unintended negative consequence, however, is the simultaneous infusion of alloreactive T-cell clones directed at normal tissue that may result in a significant flare in GVHD. In the case of relapsed CML, a substantial percentage of host hematopoiesis may be derived from the residual leukemic clone at relapse, in which case the development of the desired GVL effect may be associated with transient marrow aplasia. VOD is typically observed during the first 2 to 3 weeks posttransplant and is thought to result from endothelial damage caused by the conditioning regimen.

Answer 42.20.   **The answer is C.**

Some 40% to 60% of CMV-seropositive allogeneic HCT recipients undergo CMV reactivation posttransplant. Asymptomatic CMV viremia is often detected by regular PCR monitoring of peripheral blood, although it may be heralded by an unexplained decline in white blood cell or platelet counts. Pneumonitis is the most common manifestation of CMV-mediated disease after allogeneic HCT and is associated with a significant mortality rate. CMV colitis may mimic gastrointestinal GVHD and usually requires colonoscopic biopsy to distinguish. CMV retinitis, a common manifestation of CMV reactivation among patients with AIDS, is relatively uncommon among allogeneic HCT recipients.

Answer 42.21.   **The answer is B.**

Autologous HCT is associated with a higher risk of relapse than allogeneic HCT, likely resulting from a combination of the potential for tumor cell contamination of the autologous graft and the absence of an immune-mediated graft-versus-tumor effect associated with the latter. The major advantage of autologous HCT is its relatively low treatment-related morbidity and mortality (3% to 5% in most cases).

Answer 42.22.   **The answer is D.**

The choice of conditioning regimen is driven by multiple factors, including, for both autologous and allogeneic HCT recipients, the underlying malignancy and its predicted responsiveness to various therapeutic agents. Similarly, the age and comorbidities of the recipient may dictate the use of a regimen with a lower predicted toxicity profile. For recipients of allogeneic HCT, donor : recipient HLA mismatching may influence the use of a more immunosuppressive conditioning regimen to lower the risk of graft rejection.

Answer 42.23.   **The answer is B.**

Reduced-intensity conditioning regimens for allogeneic HCT were developed to exploit the curative potential of the GVL effect with reduced toxicity among older, sicker patients who might not otherwise be candidates for traditional myeloablative conditioning. Because reduced-intensity regimens are generally less myelosuppressive, a period of mixed myeloid chimerism often persists during the peritransplant period that may attenuate the period of absolute neutropenia. A potential limitation of these regimens is that their reduced cytotoxicity limits the tumor cell kill, rendering them less effective in the setting of refractory disease with significant tumor burdens.

Answer 42.24.   **The answer is C.**

Retrospective studies of allogeneic transplant recipients have demonstrated that the highest incidence of relapse is among patients who experienced either acute or chronic GVHD were the recipients of T-depleted grafts, or received grafts from identical twin donors. In some patients, discontinuation of immunosuppression may be sufficient to induce regression of the leukemic clone. Each of these observations provides indirect evidence of the existence of the GVL effect. Definitive evidence, however, is derived from the ability of DLIs to reinduce complete remissions in the absence of any additional cytotoxic therapy.

Answer 42.25.   **The answer is D.**

Allogeneic HCT recipients remain at risk for various long-term complications, including skeletal complications (especially with chronic steroids), infertility, secondary malignancies, and endocrine failure, for which ongoing follow-up and monitoring are indicated.

Answer 42.26.   **The answer is B.**

Several factors are associated with an increased risk of acute GVHD, including recipient age, HLA disparity, and inadequate prophylaxis. T-cell depletion of the graft decreases the incidence of GVHD.

Answer 42.27.   **The answer is D.**

Unlike the early hemorrhagic cystitis that is usually caused by high-dose cyclophosphamide, the late counterpart is usually of viral etiology, including BK virus and adenovirus.

Answer 42.28.   **The answer is D.**

Autologous stem cell transplantation has a role in the treatment of patients with various solid tumors including neuroblastoma, Ewing sarcoma, and testicular cancer. Since randomized clinical trials did not show survival improvement for autologous stem cell transplantation in breast cancer, this approach should be used only in the context of clinical trials.

Answer 42.29.   **The answer is B.**

Attempts to purge tumor cells from autologous hematopoietic stem cell grafts, using either negative or positive selection strategies, have not been proven to reduce the risk of relapse or prolong overall survival.

Answer 42.30.   **The answer is A.**

Autologous HCT is curative in approximately 40% to 50% of relapsed diffuse large cell non-Hodgkin's lymphoma cases but has not been shown to be curative in the case of low-grade lymphoproliferative disorders, multiple myeloma, or breast carcinoma.

Answer 42.31.   **The answer is A.**

Idiopathic pulmonary syndrome is an inflammatory lung disease that may occur within 3 months from transplant, is commonly associated with CMV virus infection and prior radiation therapy, and may be fatal in up to 50% of patients.

Answer 42.32.   The answer is C.

Myelodysplastic syndrome occurs in 10% to 20% of long-term survivors of autologous stem cell transplantation, although it may be impossible to dismiss the potential contribution of pretransplant chemotherapy regimens to its development. *Varicella zoster* outbreaks are commonly observed up to 6 to 12 months posttransplant and form the basis for the widespread practice of posttransplant antiviral prophylaxis. Pericarditis and myocarditis are observed in association with high-dose cyclophosphamide, usually in the immediate peritransplant period. Pneumocystis pneumonia is a frequent complication of allogeneic stem cell transplantation, because of prolonged systemic immunosuppression, but is rarely observed in the autologous transplant setting except in patients treated with chronic corticosteroids before transplant.

CHAPTER 43 INFECTIONS IN THE CANCER PATIENT

ALEX E. DENES

QUESTIONS

Question 43.1.   A patient with Hodgkin's disease who undergoes splenectomy should be immunized against which of the following organisms?

A. *Streptococcus pneumoniae*
B. *Hemophilus influenzae*
C. *Neisseria meningitidis*
D. All of the above

Question 43.2.   Randomized controlled trials of antibacterial prophylaxis in patients with neutropenia have shown which of the following?

A. No difference in fever, infection, or mortality rates
B. Decreased episodes of fever but no difference in infection or mortality rates
C. Decreased episodes of fever and infections but no difference in mortality rates
D. Decreased episodes of fever and infections, and lower mortality rates

Question 43.3.   A 32-year-old man who has received allogeneic bone marrow transplantation for acute myelogenous leukemia (AML) is now receiving immune-suppressing medications for the prevention of graft-versus-host disease. The MOST effective prophylaxis for *Pneumocystis jiroveci* (formerly carinii) is which of the following?

A. Atovaquone
B. Dapsone
C. Inhaled pentamidine
D. Trimethoprim/sulfamethoxazole (TMP/SMX)

Corresponding Chapters in *Cancer: Principles & Practice of Oncology,* Ninth Edition: 156 (Infections in the Cancer Patient) and 157 (Leukopenia and Thrombocytopenia).

Question 43.4.   A cytomegalovirus (CMV)-seronegative patient is about to receive an allogeneic hematopoietic stem cell transplant (HSCT) from a CMV-seropositive donor. Which of the following strategies are acceptable for the prevention of CMV disease?

A. Prophylaxis with an antiviral agent such as ganciclovir.
B. Treatment when CMV antigen is detected by highly sensitive polymerase chain reaction (PCR).
C. Both A and B. Both are acceptable strategies.
D. Neither A nor B. The transplantation should not be performed.

Question 43.5.   A 54-year-old male patient with stage IV diffuse large B-cell lymphoma calls with fevers and chills 9 days after receiving his third cycle of R-CHOP chemotherapy. Which of the following is the Infectious Diseases Society of America (IDSA) definition of fever in a patient with severe neutropenia?

A. Single oral temperature greater than 38.0°C
B. Single oral temperature greater than 38.3°C or greater than 38.0°C for more than 1 hour
C. Oral temperature greater than 38.3°C for more than 1 hour
D. Oral temperature greater than 37.0°C for any duration

Question 43.6.   A 56-year-old patient with breast cancer receives chemotherapy and 1 week later experiences a fever of 39.1°C (102°F). She has a complete blood count drawn that reveals a total white blood count of 1000/μL and an absolute neutrophil count of 200/μL. She has an indwelling central venous catheter that appears normal and has no localizing symptoms. Appropriate antibiotic therapy could consist of which of the following options?

A. Cefepime or ceftazidime
B. Choice A plus vancomycin
C. Choice A plus an aminoglycoside
D. Choice A plus ciprofloxacin

Question 43.7.   This patient is started on appropriate empiric antibiotics and remains clinically stable but with persistent fever after 4 days. The addition of what agent would be indicated at this time?

A. Caspofungin
B. Liposomal amphotericin B
C. Voriconazole
D. Any of the above

Question 43.8.   A 70-year-old man with metastatic non-small cell lung cancer presents with fever and neutropenia 1 week after chemotherapy. He is admitted and started on appropriate empiric antibiotics, and his fevers resolve after his first dose. For how long should his antibiotic therapy be continued?

A. Discontinue immediately
B. Until 24 to 48 hours after the last fever
C. For a total of 7 days
D. Until resolution of neutropenia

Question 43.9.   A 68-year-old man with metastatic colon cancer receiving FOLFOX chemotherapy has a fever to 102.5°F. Examination reveals tenderness and warmth at the infusion port site of his surgically implanted catheter. Blood cultures are positive for *Staphylococcus aureus,* and sensitivities are pending. What is the MOST appropriate management strategy?

A. Vancomycin
B. Vancomycin and imipenem
C. Vancomycin and removal of catheter
D. Await drug sensitivity testing for the isolated organism

Question 43.10.   A 52-year-old man with AML who has received an allogeneic HSCT presents with sinus congestion, fever, and headaches. Sinus computed tomography (CT) reveals a maxillary sinus mass with bone erosion. Zygomycosis (or mucormycosis) is isolated on fungal culture. What is the MOST appropriate management?

A. Amphotericin B, with surgical debridement as salvage therapy, if necessary
B. Amphotericin B and early surgical debridement
C. Voriconazole and early surgical debridement
D. Voriconazole, with surgical debridement as salvage therapy, if necessary

Question 43.11.   A 61-year-old woman with non-Hodgkin's lymphoma presents with fever, cough, and prolonged neutropenia. A chest CT reveals bilateral lung nodules with the "halo sign." A serum galactomannan assay is positive. What is the MOST likely causative agent?

A. Aspergillus species
B. *Pneumocysistis jiroveci*
C. *S. aureus*
D. Zygomycetes

Question 43.12.   A 56-year-old man with stage III non-small cell lung cancer is being treated with concurrent chemotherapy and radiation therapy. He has odynophagia and retrosternal chest pain that have gradually worsened over the past few weeks. He has an absolute neutrophil count of 800/μL. Which of the following causes is the LEAST likely cause of his symptoms?

A. Candida
B. Herpes simplex virus (HSV)
C. CMV
D. Radiation esophagitis

Question 43.13.   A 34-year-old woman diagnosed with AML receives induction chemotherapy. Ten days later, she experiences severe right-sided abdominal pain with nausea, vomiting, and diarrhea. On examination, she has a fever to 101°F and her abdomen is tender without rebound or guarding. Absolute neutrophil count is 0/μL. Lactic acid is not elevated, and stool *Clostridium difficile* toxin assay is negative on three separate samples. What is the MOST likely diagnosis?

   A. CMV colitis
   B. Typhlitis
   C. Bowel ischemia
   D. Bowel perforation

Question 43.14.   A 64-year-old man with pancreatic cancer is diagnosed with *C. difficile* colitis. He is treated with a course of oral metronidazole 500 mg three times per day, but he continues to have diarrhea and stool *C. difficile* toxin remains positive. What is the MOST appropriate treatment at this time?

   A. Intravenous metronidazole
   B. Oral vancomycin
   C. Intravenous vancomycin
   D. Probiotic agents

Question 43.15.   A 47-year-old woman with metastatic colorectal cancer is treated with systemic chemotherapy. She develops pain on defecation along with low-grade fevers. Laboratory tests are obtained, and her white blood cell count is 1000/μL (20% neutrophils). Visual inspection reveals a perianal fissure with erythema and induration. What should you do next?

   A. Digital rectal examination to rule out rectal abscess
   B. Recommend stool softeners, sitz baths, and analgesics
   C. Administer broad-spectrum antibiotics without anaerobic coverage
   D. Administer broad-spectrum antibiotics with anaerobic coverage

Question 43.16.   A 48-year-old man received allogeneic bone marrow transplant 2 months ago for his relapsed AML. He now presents with mental status changes, fever, and rash. A lumbar puncture reveals cerebrospinal fluid pleocytosis (mostly neutrophils) and slightly elevated protein. Gram stain is negative and cultures are pending. What would be an appropriate initial antibiotic therapy?

   A. Acyclovir, ceftriaxone, and vancomycin
   B. Acyclovir, ceftriaxone, ampicillin, and vancomycin
   C. Acyclovir, ampicillin, cefepime, and vancomycin
   D. TMP/SMX, vancomycin, and cefepime

Question 43.17.   A 62-year-old man with squamous cell carcinoma of the oral cavity in remission presents with headaches, diplopia, and low-grade fevers. Brain magnetic resonance imaging (MRI) reveals a ring-enhancing lesion within the brain parenchyma. You suspect a brain abscess and call the neurosurgeon for needle aspiration. Pending cultures, which of the following empiric regimens should be recommended?

A. Ceftriaxone
B. Vancomycin and metronidazole
C. Ceftriaxone and metronidazole
D. Voriconazole

Question 43.18.   A 45-year-old woman with hepatocellular carcinoma undergoes chemoembolization. What is the rate of infection associated with this procedure?

A. 1%
B. 10%
C. 20%
D. 30%

Question 43.19.   Vancomycin-resistant enterococcus (VRE) faecium is isolated from blood culture in a patient with cancer and normal hepatic and renal function. Which of the following choices is acceptable first-line antibiotic therapy?

A. Linezolid
B. Daptomycin
C. Quinupristin-dalfopristin
D. Any of the above

Question 43.20.   A 44-year-old man with refractory AML has multiple painful sores in his mouth, and oral swab culture is positive for HSV. He has lost 15 lbs with decreased food intake because of his painful lesions. He also has lightheadedness on standing but denies other symptoms. What is the preferred treatment?

A. Oral acyclovir 400 mg three times daily
B. Intravenous acyclovir 5 mg/kg every 8 hours
C. Intravenous acyclovir 10 mg/kg every 8 hours
D. Oral valacyclovir 1 g twice daily

Question 43.21.   Posttransplant lymphoproliferative disorder (PTLD) is induced by which pathogen?

A. Epstein-Barr virus (EBV)
B. Human herpes virus-6
C. CMV
D. Varicella-zoster virus

Question 43.22. Patients receiving alemtuzumab may experience all of the following EXCEPT:

A. Increased risk for *P. jiroveci* infection
B. Low risk of neutropenia
C. Herpes virus prophylaxis is recommended
D. Treatment results in prolonged lymphopenia

Question 43.23. A 56-year-old man was recently diagnosed with AML and received 7 + 3 induction. Ten days after treatment patient developed neutropenic fever requiring treatment with broad-spectrum antibiotics. However, his fever persisted after count recovery. Blood and urine cultures were negative and the alkaline phosphatase was elevated. CT scan of the abdomen revealed multiple discrete "bulls eye" lesions on the liver and spleen. What is the likely cause for the patient's fever?

A. Candida
B. *Escherichia coli*
C. Streptococcus
D. Pneumocystis

Question 43.24. Which of the following oral antibiotics has activity against pseudomonas species?

A. Amoxicillin/clavulanate
B. Cefdinir
C. Clindamycin
D. Levofloxacin

Question 43.25. A 23-year-old man was recently diagnosed with AML and underwent 7 + 3 induction. However, he did not recover his counts event after 4 weeks after induction. A workup revealed parvovirus B19 infection. What is the treatment of choice?

A. Intravenous immunoglobulin
B. Ribavirin
C. Foscarnet
D. Ganciclovir

ANSWERS

Answer 43.1.   **The answer is D.**

Patients without a functional spleen are at risk for overwhelming sepsis by encapsulated bacteria. The most common causative pathogens include *S. pneumoniae, H. influenzae,* and *N. meningitidis.* Asplenic patients should receive the pneumococcal polysaccharide vaccine. The conjugated meningococcal vaccine is preferred over the polysaccharide version because it provides longer lasting immunity. Immunization is ideally performed at least 2 weeks before scheduled splenectomy, but may still be administered after surgery if unable to administer prior to surgery.

Answer 43.2.   **The answer is C.**

Antibiotic prophylaxis in neutropenic patients has led to decreased episodes of fever and decreased infections, but has demonstrated no difference in mortality in randomized controlled trials. This has primarily been evaluated with oral fluoroquinolones such as levofloxacin. The benefit is more pronounced in patients with prolonged neutropenia, and prophylaxis is not routinely recommended in patients expected to have neutropenia lasting 7 days or less.

Answer 43.3.   **The answer is D.**

The most effective prophylaxis is TMP/SMX. Numerous dosing schedules, including one double-strength tablet daily, one single-strength tablet daily, and one double-strength tablet 3 days per week, appear to be effective. Second-line agents, including dapsone, inhaled pentamidine, and atovaquone, may be administered in patients unable to receive TMP/SMX because of marrow intolerance or hypersensitivity reaction, but appear to be less effective.

Answer 43.4.   **The answer is C.**

CMV disease may be prevented in the setting of preexisting infection through one of two equally acceptable approaches: prophylaxis with antiviral agents or preemptive therapy. In the latter strategy, active surveillance with highly sensitive methods of detection such as CMV DNA by PCR may be used to trigger preemptive antiviral therapy in asymptomatic patients with CMV reactivation. Both strategies are considered appropriate in guidelines published by the Centers for Disease Control and Prevention (CDC), although the preemptive approach is more widely adopted.

Answer 43.5.   **The answer is B.**

According to IDSA guidelines, fever is defined as a single oral temperature of greater than 38.3°C or a temperature of greater than 38.0°C for 1 hour or more. Severe neutropenia is defined as a neutrophil count of less than 500 cells/μL or a count of less than 1000 cells/μL with a predicted decrease to less than 500 cells/μL.

Answer 43.6.   **The answer is A.**

Neutropenic patients with fever require prompt empiric administration of a broad-spectrum B-lactam antibiotic with activity against *P. aeruginosa*, such as ceftazidime, cefepime, imipenem, or meropenem. The addition of an aminoglycoside or ciprofloxacin is warranted for patients with hemodynamic compromise. The empiric addition of vancomycin has not been shown to improve outcomes and is not indicated for initial empiric therapy in hemodynamically stable patients in the absence of clinically apparent catheter-related infections. Vancomycin should also be considered in patients with severe mucositis, previous use of fluoroquinolone antibiotic prophylaxis, and history of methicillin-resistant *S. aureus* infection.

Answer 43.7.   **The answer is D.**

In patients with persistent neutropenic fever, the addition of antifungal agents after 4 to 7 days is standard practice. Randomized prospective studies have shown decreased invasive fungal infections with this strategy. Liposomal amphotericin B, itraconazole, voriconazole, caspofungin, and micafungin are all acceptable alternatives, with no agent demonstrating higher overall efficacy than the others. Some authorities feel that fluconazole or anidulafungin are acceptable alternatives.

Answer 43.8.   **The answer is D.**

Antibiotic treatment of neutropenic fever that resolves after initiation of empiric therapy should be continued until resolution of neutropenia. For patients with prolonged neutropenia, 2 weeks of antibiotics may be sufficient. In clinically stable patients, it may be acceptable to switch initial intravenous antibiotics to an oral regimen, such as ciprofloxacin with amoxicillin/clavulanate. Some authors have also suggested that select patients can be treated on an outpatient basis with close monitoring.

Answer 43.9.   **The answer is C.**

Intravascular catheter-associated infections are common given the widespread use of central venous catheters in patients with cancer. These consist of exit-site infections, tunnel or pocket infections, and catheter-related bacteremia. Tunnel (or port) catheter infections typically require catheter removal. Although catheter salvage may be attempted with certain pathogens, IDSA guidelines suggest routine removal of catheters for infections with *S. aureus*, fungi, and mycobacteria. Attempts at catheter salvage may be considered with *S. epidermidis,* with removal of catheter should bacteremia not be resolved with antibiotics.

Answer 43.10.   **The answer is B.**

Zygomycosis (or mucormycosis) is seen most commonly in patients with prolonged neutropenia or corticosteroid use, including those with hematologic malignancies and allogeneic HSCT recipients. Sinus or pulmonary involvement is typical. Therapy should consist of lipid formulation amphotericin B along with early and aggressive surgical debridement in those with sinus or localized skin disease. Voriconazole and echinocandins are not active. Posaconazole has shown promising results as salvage therapy.

Answer 43.11. **The answer is A.**

Neutropenic patients with persistent fever are at risk for fungal pneumonia. CT imaging of the chest may disclose characteristic signs, such as the nodules, masses, or the "halo sign." This latter finding is highly suggestive of invasive aspergillosis but may also be seen with *P. aeruginosa* or other molds. The serum galactomannan assay is specific (although not highly sensitive) for aspergillus species, because invasive zygomycosis does not cause positive results. Prompt treatment with voriconazole or amphotericin B is indicated.

Answer 43.12. **The answer is C.**

The causative agents in esophagitis include candida, HSV, CMV, bacteria, and aspergillus. Erosive esophagitis caused by radiation therapy or chemotherapy-induced mucositis may also produce a similar clinical picture. CMV infections occur mainly in patients with prolonged immunosuppression, such as patients who have undergone hematopoietic stem cell transplantation.

Answer 43.13. **The answer is B.**

Typhlitis, or neutropenic enterocolitis, occurs in patients receiving chemotherapy toxic to the bowel mucosa, most commonly during treatment of acute leukemia. CT findings include bowel wall thickening, mucosa edema, pericecal fluid, and a right lower quadrant inflammatory mass. Treatment should consist of broad-spectrum antibiotics including coverage against gram-negative and anaerobic organisms. CMV infection is uncommon in patients with cancer without prior allogeneic stem cell transplantation.

Answer 43.14. **The answer is B.**

C. difficile colitis is common in patients with cancer because of their frequent exposure to broad spectrum antibiotics and recurrent hospitalizations that facilitate transmission. Treatment options for *C. difficile* colitis include oral metronidazole (or intravenous administration in those unable to receive oral medications) and oral vancomycin. The latter option may be considered in patients with severe diarrhea, significant comorbidities, or persistent infections. Intravenous vancomycin is not effective because it is not transported through the bowel wall. Fidaxomicin was recently approved for the treatment of *C. difficile* colitis. The recommended dose is 200 mg po bid for 10 days. Studies regarding the efficacy and safety of probiotics have been inconclusive to date.

Answer 43.15. **The answer is D.**

Anorectal infections are most commonly caused by organisms commonly found in the gastrointestinal tract, such as Enterobacter species, Enterococcus, *P. aeruginosa,* or anaerobes, and are often polymicrobial. Digital rectal examination should be avoided in patients with neutropenia. Broad-spectrum antibiotics are required in anorectal infections, and anaerobic coverage is also indicated in the presence of fistula formation, induration, or cellulitis. Local comfort measures may also be used, but antibiotic treatment should be initiated without delay. Pelvic CT to rule out perirectal abscess requiring surgical management should also be considered.

Answer 43.16.   **The answer is C.**

Patients with cancer who are suspected to have meningitis an appropriate initial antibiotic regimen should cover (*S. pneumoniae, N. meningitidis, H. influenzae*) along with Listeria and penicillin-resistant *S. pneumoniae*. The vancomycin, ceftriaxone, and ampicillin regimen would be an appropriate empiric antibiotic regimen. If the patient is allergic to penicillin, then TMP/SMX could be substituted for ceftriaxone. Patients who had undergone stem cell transplant within the last 2 months should be treated for possible pseudomonas infection, therefore substituting ceftriaxone with cefepime or meropenem would be appropriate. In this patient, the presence of mental status changes raises the possibility of encephalitis and intravenous acyclovir for the treatment of HSV encephalitis should be included.

Answer 43.17.   **The answer is C.**

Brain abscesses may present with symptoms including headache, neurologic deficits, or seizures, and appear as ring-enhancing lesions on MRI. In immunocompetent patients, bacterial brain abscess is frequently caused by dental flora. Third-generation cephalosporins, such as ceftriaxone and metronidazole, are recommended for empiric therapy, particularly in a patient with a suspected oral source. Voriconazole may be added to broad-spectrum antibacterial coverage in immunocompromised patients, who are more likely to have a fungal cause.

Answer 43.18.   **The answer is A.**

Liver-directed therapies, such as chemoembolization and radiofrequency ablation, are effective palliative measures in selected patients with hepatic tumors. Resultant tumor necrosis may serve as a nidus for infection, with an incidence of approximately 1% after these procedures. Prior biliary enteric anastomosis is the primary risk factor for liver abscess after chemoembolization, with an incidence of approximately 5% in these patients.

Answer 43.19.   **The answer is D.**

Enterococcus species are common pathogens in bacteremia. Colonization with VRE is frequently detected in patients with cancer with repeated hospitalizations. VRE bacteremia typically occurs in severely debilitated patients and is associated with high mortality. First-line agents include linezolid and daptomycin. Quinupristin-dalfopristin is effective in *Enterococcus faecium* infections, but not *Enterococcus faecalis*, and has moderate efficacy comparable to linezolid. Unfortunately, refractory bacteremia is not rare in this disease.

Answer 43.20.   **The answer is B.**

Oropharyngeal HSV is commonly seen in patients with prolonged chemotherapy-induced neutropenia and may lead to significant morbidity in these patients. Oral acyclovir (400 mg given five times daily) or valacyclovir for 7 to 10 days may be considered in some patients, but intravenous acyclovir (5 mg/kg every 8 hours) is preferred for patients with significant mucosal disease causing impaired oral intake. Disseminated HSV should be treated with intravenous acyclovir (10 mg/kg every 8 hours).

Answer 43.21.   **The answer is A.**

Solid-organ and HSCT recipients are at risk for PTLD, which is an abnormal proliferation of EBV-infected B cells. There are varied clinical manifestations, including a mononucleosis-like syndrome, generalized adenopathy, and extranodal organ involvement. Treatment strategies include reduction in immune suppression, rituximab, and adoptive transfer of EBV-specific cytotoxic T lymphocytes. For those with a more aggressive clinical course, combination chemotherapy may also be warranted.

Answer 43.22.   **The answer is B.**

Alemtuzumab is a humanized monoclonal antibody against CD52 and is approved for the treatment of CLL. Treatment with alemtuzumab results in prolonged lymphopenia and patients are at increased risk for *P. jiroveci* infection. There is also increased risk for CMV reactivation but CMV disease is rare. Herpes virus prophylaxis is recommended in patients receiving alemtuzumab.

Answer 43.23.   **The answer is A.**

Persistent fever despite count recovery should trigger a careful search for occult infections such as line infections, abscesses, and fungal infections. Elevated alkaline phosphatase and the characteristic findings on the liver by imaging are consistent with hepatosplenic candidiasis.

Answer 43.24.   **The answer is D.**

Fluoroquinolones are the only class of oral antibiotics with activity against pseudomonas species. As a result fluoroquinolones are the preferred agents for antibacterial prophylaxis to prevent febrile neutropenia as well as for outpatient management of febrile neutropenia.

Answer 43.25.   **The answer is A.**

Patients with acute and chronic leukemias, myelodysplastic syndrome, undergoing highly myelosuppressive chemotherapy and prolonged treatment with steroids are at increased risk for parvovirus B19 infection. Parvovirus B19 infection can result in prolonged cytopenias in immunocompromised patients. Intravenous immunoglobulin is the treatment of choice for parvovirus B19 infection.

MARIA Q. BAGGSTROM

QUESTIONS

Question 44.1.   A 40-year-old woman with breast cancer is receiving adjuvant chemotherapy with dose dense AC (doxorubicin and cyclophosphamide) with pegfilgrastim support. After 3 cycles of chemotherapy, she presents to the
emergency room with left upper quadrant abdominal pain, and is found
to be hypotensive and anemic with a hemoglobin of 9 g/dL. The most
likely reason for her anemia is:

A. Chemotherapy
B. Splenic rupture
C. Disease progression
D. Iron deficiency

Question 44.2.   Primary prophylactic G-CSF administration is recommended in which
cases?

A. Chemotherapy regimens in which the expected incidence of febrile
neutropenia is 20% or greater.
B. A decrease in dose intensity would compromise long-term outcomes,
such as survival or cure.
C. The patient is at increased risk for serious complications or death
from febrile neutropenia.
D. All of the above are true.

Corresponding Chapters in *Cancer: Principles & Practice of Oncology*, Ninth Edition: 158 (Cancer-Associated
Thrombosis), 159 (Nausea and Vomiting), 160 (Diarrhea and Constipation), 161 (Oral Complications), 162 (Pul-
monary Toxicity), 163 (Cardiac Toxicity), 164 (Hair Loss), 165 (Gonadal Dysfunction), 166 (Fatigue), 167 (Second
Primary Cancers), 168 (Neurocognitive Effects), and 169 (Cancer Survivorship).

Question 44.3.   A 50-year-old man with metastatic non-small cell lung cancer is receiving carboplatin, paclitaxel, and bevacizumab therapy. He is also receiving darbepoetin to support chemotherapy-induced anemia. He presents with right arm swelling and is found to have extensive clot extending from his central venous catheter, into his right brachiocephalic, internal jugular, and axillary veins. Which of the following factors likely contributed to deep venous thrombosis in this gentleman?

A. Presence of a central venous catheter
B. Bevacizumab
C. Darbepoetin
D. All of the above

Question 44.4.   Regarding the use of prophylactic anticoagulation for central venous catheters, which of the following statements is TRUE?

A. Fixed-dose warfarin is more effective than low-molecular-weight heparin.
B. Symptomatic catheter-related thrombosis rates of 15% were reported without the use of prophylaxis.
C. The American College of Chest Physicians (ACCP) 2008 guidelines recommend against the use of routine prophylaxis using low-molecular-weight heparin and fixed-dose warfarin.
D. The use of fixed-dose warfarin (1 mg daily) is not associated with increased bleeding risk.

Question 44.5.   Chemotherapy-induced nausea and vomiting (CINV) include which of the following types?

A. Acute CINV
B. Delayed CINV
C. Anticipatory CINV
D. All of the above

Question 44.6.   Patient-related factors important in increased risk of CINV include all of the following, EXCEPT:

A. Female gender
B. Younger age
C. History of chronic alcohol consumption
D. History of motion sickness

Question 44.7.   Recommended antiemetic therapy for the prevention of acute emesis with high emetic risk chemotherapy include all of the following, EXCEPT:

A. $5-HT_3$ receptor antagonist
B. Phenothiazine
C. Aprepitant
D. Dexamethasone

Question 44.8.   Delayed CINV appears to be mostly related to which mechanism?

A. Substance P
B. Dopamine
C. 5HT
D. All of the above

Question 44.9.   Agents commonly causing chemotherapy-induced diarrhea include all of the following, EXCEPT:

A. Fluoropyrimidines
B. Platinum agents
C. Irinotecan
D. Taxanes

Question 44.10.   A 50-year-old man with locally advanced pancreatic cancer presents with intractable abdominal pain. His last bowel movement was 1 day prior. His medications include pancrelipase and liquid morphine. His G-tube is found to be functioning normally. Imaging reveals a mass arising from the head of the pancreas, invading the superior mesenteric artery. A celiac plexus block is performed. The following day, he complains of diarrhea and his blood pressure is noted to be 89/60. His diarrhea is likely due to:

A. Pancreatic insufficiency
B. Enteral feedings
C. Celiac plexus block
D. All of the above

Question 44.11.   The somatostatin analog octreotide has all of the following actions, EXCEPT:

A. Suppresses inflammatory bowel disease
B. Suppresses release of insulin and vasoactive intestinal peptide
C. Reduces motility
D. Alters increased gastrointestinal absorption of water and electrolytes

Question 44.12.   Agents commonly causing constipation in patients with cancer include all of the following, EXCEPT:

A. Opioid analgesics
B. Antidepressants
C. Phenothiazine antiemetics
D. Diuretics

Question 44.13.   Patient-related risk factors for stomatitis include which of the following?

A. Age more than 65 years or less than 20 years
B. Inadequate nutritional status
C. Exposure to oral stressors, including alcohol and smoking
D. All of the above

Question 44.14.   Common prophylactic measures for the prevention of chemotherapy- and radiation-induced stomatitis include all of the following, EXCEPT:

A. Chlorhexidine gluconate
B. Viscous lidocaine
C. Sodium bicarbonate rinses
D. Ice

Question 44.15.   A 55-year-old man is receiving radiation therapy for head and neck cancer. Which of the following agents is NOT useful for preventing xerostomia in this gentleman?

A. Amifostine
B. Pilocarpine
C. Salt and baking soda mouth rinse
D. Drinking plenty of water

Question 44.16.   Regarding radiation pneumonitis, which is FALSE?

A. It develops in 5% to 15% of patients receiving external beam radiation for lung cancer.
B. It can be divided into early, intermediate, and late stages.
C. The use of corticosteroids can prevent the onset of radiation pneumonitis.
D. Dyspnea is the main presenting symptom.

Question 44.17.   Some factors that are associated with increased risk of chemotherapy-induced pulmonary toxicity include which of the following?

A. Total dose of chemotherapy
B. Simultaneous or prior radiation to the lungs
C. Renal function
D. All of the above

Question 44.18.   Cardiac irradiation can induce which symptoms of heart disease?

A. Pericarditis and pericardial effusion
B. Ischemic heart disease
C. Electrical conduction abnormalities
D. All of the above

Question 44.19.   Regarding early detection of cardiac dysfunction, which is NOT used?

A. Electrocardiograms
B. Measurement of left ventricular ejection fraction by echocardiography
C. Serum cardiac troponin T levels
D. Serum brain natriuretic peptide levels

Question 44.20.   Which of the following chemotherapy drugs are likely to cause complete alopecia?

    A. Docetaxel
    B. Cyclophosphamide
    C. Irinotecan
    D. All of the above

Question 44.21.   All of the following antitumor agents cause prolonged azoospermia in men, EXCEPT:

    A. Radiation to the testis
    B. Carboplatin
    C. Cyclophosphamide
    D. Melphalan

Question 44.22.   Regarding interventions for cancer-related fatigue, which of the following did NOT show improvement in fatigue?

    A. Massage therapy
    B. L-carnitine supplementation
    C. Stress-reduction intervention
    D. Omega-3 fatty acid supplementation

Question 44.23.   Chemotherapy-associated constipation may result from treatment with which of the following agents?

    A. Vinorelbine
    B. Thalidomide
    C. Vincristine
    D. All of the above

Question 44.24.   Which of the following chemotherapy agents can cause palmar-plantar erythrodysesthesia?

    A. Pegylated liposomal doxorubicin
    B. Cytarabine
    C. Sorafenib
    D. All of the above

ANSWERS

Answer 44.1.   **The answer is B.**

This lady likely has splenic rupture, a rare adverse event associated with the use of filgrastim and pegfilgrastim. Allergic-type reactions and adult respiratory distress syndrome have also been reported as rare, serious adverse events associated with the administration of these agents.

Answer 44.2.   **The answer is D.**

Primary prophylactic use of G-CSF is recommended in all of the above scenarios as per the American Society of Clinical Oncology 2006 Guidelines.

Answer 44.3.   **The answer is D.**

Patient with cancer has an increased risk of deep venous thrombosis. Factors that increase the risk of thrombosis in these patients include presence of metastatic disease, primary site of cancer (pancreatic cancer, lung cancer), presence of indwelling central venous catheter, and certain treatments such as bevacizumab and erythropoietin-stimulating agents.

Answer 44.4.   **The answer is C.**

Multiple trials have shown that the prophylactic use of either warfarin or low-molecular-weight heparin is effective in reducing symptomatic catheter-related thrombosis. These rates are approximately 4% with some possible increased bleeding complications in those on anticoagulation. Current ACCP guidelines recommend against the use of routine anticoagulation prophylaxis.

Answer 44.5.   **The answer is D.**

Acute, delayed, and anticipatory nausea and vomiting make up the three clinical syndromes of CINV. Acute CINV occurs within the first 24 hours of chemotherapy administration, whereas delayed CINV occurs more than 24 hours after chemotherapy administration. Anticipatory CINV occurs as a conditioned response to stimuli that remind patients of previous episodes of nausea and vomiting.

Answer 44.6.   **The answer is C.**

Patient-related factors that increase the risk of CINV include female gender, younger age, CINV with previous chemotherapy treatment, history of pregnancy-associated nausea and vomiting, and history of motion sickness. A history of chronic alcohol consumption is associated with a decrease in risk of CINV. Treatment-related factors that increase the risk of CINV include the agent, dose, rate, and route of administration.

Answer 44.7.   **The answer is B.**

With high emetic-risk chemotherapy, recommended antiemetic therapy includes medications from the following classes: 5-HT$_3$ receptor antagonist (dolasetron, granisetron, ondansetron, tropisetron, palonosetron), corticosteroids (dexamethasone), and NK1 receptor antagonist (aprepitant). Phenothiazines, such as prochlorperazine, have a lower therapeutic index.

Answer 44.8.   **The answer is A.**

The pathophysiology of delayed CINV may be more dependent on Substance P as seen by the efficacy of NK1 antagonists in the delayed emesis setting. Because 5-HT3 receptor antagonists and dopamine D2 antagonists have less efficacy in this setting, 5-HT and dopamine appear to have a less important role in delayed CINV.

Answer 44.9.   **The answer is B.**

Agents such as 5-fluorouracil, capecitabine, and irinotecan are chemotherapy agents that commonly cause diarrhea. Docetaxel is also associated with a mild diarrhea but can also cause severe enteritis and colitis.

Answer 44.10.   **The answer is C.**

The celiac plexus transmits the sensation of pain arising from the pancreas and also carries sympathetic nerves. Interruption of the plexus with alcohol injection may result in sympathetic blockade leading to diarrhea and hypotension from unopposed parasympathetic activity. This is usually transient and lasts for 48 hours. Though pancreatic insufficiency and enteral feeding may cause diarrhea, this is usually a chronic diarrhea and are less likely in this setting.

Answer 44.11.   **The answer is A.**

Octreotide has multiple methods of activity in the reduction of diarrhea. It can suppress the release of insulin, glucagon, vasoactive intestinal peptide, and gastric acid; reduce gastrointestinal motility and decrease pancreatic exocrine function; and alter the increased absorption of water, electrolytes, and nutrients from the gastrointestinal tract.

Answer 44.12.   **The answer is C.**

Drugs that commonly cause constipation in patients with cancer include opioid analgesics, serotonin 5HT3 receptor antagonists, vinca alkaloids, thalidomide, antidepressants, aluminum- or calcium-containing antacids, iron supplements, and diuretics.

Answer 44.13.   **The answer is D.**

Study results of chemotherapy-related stomatitis are conflicting, but some patient-related factors include age more than 65 years or less than 20 years, female gender, inadequate nutritional status, herpes simplex infection, and decreased chemotherapy metabolism. Oral factors such as periodontal disease, microbial flora, chronic low-grade mouth infection, salivary gland secretory dysfunction, ill-fitting dental prostheses, and exposure to oral stressors including alcohol and tobacco can also contribute to risk of stomatitis.

Answer 44.14.   **The answer is B.**

Chlorhexidine gluconate, saline rinses, sodium bicarbonate rinses, acyclovir, amphotericin B, and ice are common prophylactic measures used in the prevention of stomatitis. Viscous lidocaine and Carafate suspension, dicyclomine hydrochloride, opioids, and mixtures (including ingredients such as diphenhydramine, Maalox, viscous lidocaine, and nystatin) are commonly used in the treatment of stomatitis-related pain.

Answer 44.15.   **The answer is B.**

Patients undergoing radiation therapy for head and neck cancer should be advised to drink plenty of fluids and rinse their mouth with saltwater or baking soda solution to prevent xerostomia. Amifostine is beneficial in prevention of xerostomia; however, the role of pilocarpine for prophylaxis of xerostomia is less clear. Because of toxicity related to glaucoma and cardiac issues, pilocarpine is used with caution in patients with xerostomia.

Answer 44.16.   **The answer is C.**

Patients with radiation pneumonitis typically present with dyspnea, self-limited or progressive. They can also present with cough, fever, chest pain, tachypnea, and cyanosis. Corticosteroids are not used as a prophylactic measure or in the treatment of radiation fibrosis; however, prednisone is commonly used in the treatment of radiation pneumonitis, but data are mixed.

Answer 44.17.   **The answer is D.**

Many factors are associated with increased risk of chemotherapy-induced pulmonary toxicity. Bleomycin, for example, is associated with increased risk of pulmonary toxicity in terms of total dose, advanced age, oxygen therapy, simultaneous or prior radiation therapy to the lungs, combination with other drugs, and renal dysfunction.

Answer 44.18.   **The answer is D.**

Radiation-induced heart disease covers a wide clinical spectrum, including pericardial disease, acute pericarditis, pericardial effusion, constrictive pericarditis, myocardial dysfunction, valvular heart disease, electrical conduction abnormalities, and congestive heart disease.

Answer 44.19.   **The answer is A.**

Early detection of cardiac dysfunction is important in the prevention of overt cardiomyopathy during the administration of chemotherapy.

Echocardiograms or radionuclide imaging can directly measure left ventricular ejection fraction. Other measures of cardiac dysfunction include measuring serial diastolic pressures, serum cardiac troponin T levels, and brain natriuretic peptide levels. Electrocardiograms have little value in early detection of cardiac dysfunction because changes tend to occur late.

Answer 44.20.   **The answer is D.**

Systemic chemotherapy can cause hair loss through either thinning of the hair shaft or inhibition of matrix proliferation. The chemotherapy drugs most commonly associated with total alopecia include cyclophosphamide, doxorubicin, irinotecan, docetaxel, topotecan, and bleomycin.

Answer 44.21.   **The answer is B.**

Prolonged azoospermia is often seen with radiation to the testis, chlorambucil, cyclophosphamide, procarbazine, melphalan, and cisplatin. Carboplatin does not often cause prolonged azoospermia. Other agents (doxorubicin, cytosine arabinoside, vinblastine, vincristine) can be additive in causing prolonged azoospermia when combined with other agents that affect sperm production but cause only temporary reductions in sperm when used alone.

Answer 44.22.   **The answer is D.**

Several interventions have been shown to improve cancer-related fatigue. These include supplementation with mistletoe extract, L-carnitine, and high-dose vitamin C, as well as massage therapy, stress-reduction intervention, polarity therapy, and relaxation breathing. Data are mixed for progressive muscle relaxation, psychoeducation, virtual reality distraction, and yoga. The use of music therapy, omega-3 fatty acid supplementation, and reiki did not show an improvement in fatigue symptoms.

Answer 44.23.   **The answer is D.**

Constipation may occur with up to a third of patients treated with vinca alkaloids (vincristine, vinblastine, vinorelbine). Constipation usually occurs after the first dose and is most prominent between 3 and 10 days after chemotherapy, and typically resolves in a few days. Thalidomide also frequently causes constipation.

Answer 44.24.   **The answer is D.**

Hand-foot syndrome is an adverse effect seen with several chemotherapy agents including cytarabine, 5-fluorouracil, capecitabine, pegylated liposomal doxorubicin, and multitargeted tyrosine kinase inhibitors such as sorafenib and sunitinib.

CHAPTER 45 SUPPORTIVE CARE AND QUALITY OF LIFE

ANNA ROSHAL

DIRECTIONS   Each of the numbered items below is followed by lettered answers. Select the
ONE lettered answer that is BEST in each case unless instructed otherwise.

QUESTIONS

Question 45.1.   Christine is a 45-year-old woman with newly diagnosed triple negative
metastatic breast cancer. She and her husband have two school-aged children. She is beginning chemotherapy and asks you, "How much should
we share with the kids?" Your advice is:

   A.   I am sorry, this is out of my area of expertise, but I will be glad to
refer you to a social worker.

   B.   Talk as little as possible about the cancer to preserve the sense of
normalcy in the children's lives.

   C.   Sit the children down and explain her disease process, including eventual death from cancer.

   D.   Try to let the children initiate the discussion, and then answer all
of their questions in an age-appropriate manner, including fears and
concerns about their mother dying.

Question 45.2.   Christine is treated with Abraxane and bevacizumab and achieves a very
good partial response. However, she has numbness, tingling, and aching in
her hands. You diagnose her as having treatment-related grade 2 peripheral neuropathy. In addition to giving her a chemotherapy holiday, you
will also recommend:

   A.   Oxycodone 5 mg every 6 hours as needed

   B.   Gabapentin 300 mg three times per day

   C.   Dexamethasone 4 mg every 6 hours

   D.   Refer her to neurologist for electromyography (EMG)

Question 45.3.   What are the two most common causes in insomnia in dying patients?

   A.   Pain and depression

   B.   Pain and dyspnea

   C.   Anxiety and nausea

   D.   Anxiety and depression

Corresponding Chapters in *Cancer: Principles & Practice of Oncology,* Ninth Edition: 170 (Management of Cancer
Pain), 171 (Nutritional Support), 172 (Sexual Problems), 173 (Psychological Issues in Cancer), 174 (Communicating
News to the Cancer Patient), 175 (Specialized Care of the Terminally Ill), and 176 (Community Resources).

Question 45.4.   Christine completed whole brain radiation, which she tolerated poorly with worsening fatigue. Unfortunately, 2 months later, she is more short of breath. Her CT scan shows worsening pulmonary and liver metastases. Her Eastern Cooperative Oncology Group (ECOG) performance status (PS) is 3. You are convinced that there is no further standard therapy that would be of benefit to her. She is not eligible for any clinical trials available at your institution. After discussing her latest scan results, you say:

A. I am sorry, but there is nothing more I can offer you.
B. There are no other treatments against the cancer, but I will continue taking care of you and make sure your comfort remains a priority.
C. Unfortunately, you have only 2 months to live, but we will make sure you have as much quality time as possible.
D. I can offer you other chemotherapy, but it is unlikely that it will provide any benefit.

Question 45.5.   Which of the following neuroablative procedures is useful for refractory pain from tumor infiltration of cranial nerves?

A. Rhizotomy
B. Cordotomy
C. Thalamotomy
D. Mesencephalic tractomy

Question 45.6.   Which of the following is TRUE about palliative care services?

A. Patients need to abandon other forms of therapy, such as chemotherapy, to receive palliative care.
B. Palliative care has no role in management of patients with curable cancers.
C. Total costs of care are higher for patients who died in the palliative care unit, compared with those who died outside the unit.
D. Palliative care teams can assist oncology patients and their doctors with symptom management, as well as other forms of pain, at any point along the disease trajectory, beginning from diagnosis.

Question 45.7.   The MOST common symptom experienced by patients in the last days to week before death is:

A. Fatigue and/or pain
B. Restlessness/delirium
C. Dyspnea
D. Nausea and vomiting

Question 45.8.   Which of the following provides oral equivalent doses to methadone 20 mg oral?

A. Hydromorphone 15 mg
B. Oxycodone 30 mg
C. Propoxyphene 200 mg
D. Codeine 300 mg

Question 45.9.   Which statement(s) is/are TRUE regarding nausea and vomiting that occurs during treatment with opioid analgesics:

A. It is produced through chemoreceptor trigger zone.
B. Tolerance rarely develops to these side effects.
C. Switching to alternative opioid often results in improvement.
D. A and C.

Question 45.10.   Which of the following can be a cause of depression in terminally ill patients?

A. Hypercalcemia
B. Uncontrolled pain
C. Steroid treatment
D. All of the above

Question 45.11.   Which of the following factors have been shown to be associated with high rates of primary caregiver burnout?

A. Lower socioeconomic status
B. Race
C. Caring for a patient for more than 6 months
D. All of the above

Question 45.12.   Professional barriers to cancer pain management include:

A. Inadequate knowledge of pain mechanisms
B. Fear of producing iatrogenic complications
C. Time and reimbursement pressures
D. All of the above

Question 45.13.   Lisa, a 45-year-old woman with locally advanced right-sided breast cancer undergoes neoadjuvant chemotherapy, followed by modified radical mastectomy and axillary dissection. She achieves partial response and undergoes adjuvant irradiation to total dose of 55 GY. Five years later, she has no evidence of disease recurrence. However, on routine visit, she reports right shoulder ache, arm/hand numbness, and weakness. There is mild arm edema. Her symptoms have been slowly progressive during the last year. The best test to determine the cause of her symptoms is:

A. Brachial plexus magnetic resonance imaging (MRI)
B. Cervical spine MRI
C. Bone scan
D. EMG

Question 45.14.   Lisa is very relieved that her symptoms are not related to progressive disease. However, she is distressed by her pain and decreased ability to function. On her recent office visit she is tearful. Treatment approaches to this patient's problem may include:

A. Physical therapy
B. Support group
C. Antidepressants and anticonvulsants
D. All of the above

Question 45.15. John is an 80-year-old man with ECOG PS 2 and metastatic hormone refractory prostate cancer to the bones. He is treated with Taxotere, bisphosphonates, and ibuprofen. His pain is initially controlled well on 60 mg twice per day of long-acting morphine with short-acting morphine 15 mg every 6 to 8 hours as needed. If his pain is increased, all of these approaches may be reasonable, EXCEPT:

   A. Increase morphine by 50% to 100%
   B. Add corticosteroids
   C. Treatment with strontium-89 or samarium-153
   D. Change to methadone 60 mg by mouth twice per day

Question 45.16. In this patient, anticipated adverse effects of morphine include all of the following, EXCEPT:

   A. Sedation
   B. Respiratory depression
   C. Nausea and vomiting
   D. Constipation

Question 45.17. You eventually increase John's morphine to 120 mg twice per day with 30 mg as needed, which he takes every 3 hours, and add corticosteroids. Unfortunately, the patient's pain is still poorly controlled, and he develops increasing sedation and drowsiness. Further evaluation shows normal electrolytes and no evidence of further disease progression. You refer him to a palliative care specialist who recommends switching to methadone at a dose ratio of 6:1. Properties of methadone that make it somewhat difficult to use include:

   A. Cost
   B. QT prolongation
   C. Requires up to 1 week to achieve steady state
   D. B and C

Question 45.18. John achieves good pain control on methadone 40 mg/d and enjoys a good quality of life with his family. Which of the following best explains his response to methadone?

   A. He reached a maximum tolerated dose of morphine.
   B. He developed tolerance to morphine.
   C. NMDA receptor plays a critical role in opioid tolerance and may explain the dramatic reduction in dosage when his medication is switched from morphine to methadone.
   D. Both B and C.

Question 45.19. Which of the following medications are effective as adjuvants in treating neuropathic pain?

   A. Tricyclic antidepressants
   B. Anticonvulsants
   C. Local anesthetics
   D. All of the above

Question 45.20.   Which of the following is TRUE about using anesthetic and neurosurgical approaches to treat cancer pain?

    A. Celiac ganglion block is effective in 50% of patients treated.
    B. Peripheral nerve blocks are most useful in patients with somatic pain.
    C. Cordotomy is almost always complicated by motor paresis.
    D. Epidural local anesthetics delivered by continuous low-dose infusion are useful long term for cancer pain.

Question 45.21.   John eventually develops liver metastases and enters hospice care. His elderly wife is unable to manage him at home, and he is transferred to inpatient hospice after a few weeks. Eventually he becomes bed-bound and mostly unresponsive. In the last 24 hours, his respirations are becoming irregular, and he appears agitated, moaning, and restless. No recent changes to his medications have been made. Appropriate management of his condition includes:

    A. Lorazepam 1 mg every 2 hours
    B. Opioid drip to control dyspnea
    C. Haldol 1 mg intravenously administered every 2 hours
    D. All of the above

Question 45.22.   Which of the following metabolic abnormalities in humans with cachexia is TRUE?

    A. Increased total body water
    B. Increased serum lipid levels
    C. Insulin resistance
    D. All of the above

Question 45.23.   What threshold is used to define critical weight loss in patients with cancer?

    A. 10% of baseline body weight in 6 months
    B. 10% of lean body mass in 6 months
    C. 10% of baseline body weight in 3 months
    D. 10 lbs in 1 month

Question 45.24.   Which of the following metabolic abnormalities is/are present in cancer cachexia?

    A. Increased gluconeogenesis
    B. Decreased lipoprotein lipase activity
    C. Decreased body glucose consumption
    D. A and B

Question 45.25.   Which of the following statements regarding dysgeusia is FALSE:

    A. Taxanes have one of the strongest associations with dysgeusia.
    B. Dysgeusia may be caused by depression.
    C. Foods are better tolerated when they are thoroughly chewed prior to ingestion.
    D. Zinc may work best for sweet dysgeusia.

Question 45.26.   Which of the following patients is a good candidate for inpatient total parenteral nutrition (TPN)?

A. Patients with rapidly progressing cancer and no response to chemotherapy.

B. Patients who are terminally ill.

C. Mildly malnourished patients undergoing chemotherapy.

D. Severely malnourished patients who are responding to chemotherapy.

Question 45.27.   Which of the following statements regarding the pharmacological therapy of cachexia is NOT TRUE?

A. Megestrol acetate improves appetite and body weight in cancer patients.

B. Erythropoietin has a potential stimulatory effect on cancer cells.

C. Recombinant growth factor receptor has anabolic effects and no risk of promoting tumor growth.

D. C

Question 45.28.   All of the following outcomes have been consistently documented in clinical trials of psychosocial interventions aimed at patients with metastatic breast cancer, EXCEPT:

A. Improved survival

B. Reduced depression

C. Reduced pain

D. Reduced overall distress scores

Question 45.29.   Which of the following is an indication for the use of corticosteroids?

A. Refractory neuropathic pain

B. Bone pain

C. Capsular expansion

D. All of the above

Question 45.30.   Your patient with newly diagnosed early-stage breast cancer asks your opinion about complementary and alternative medicine (CAM). She has not selected any specific modality yet. She makes it clear that she wants to combine CAM with her adjuvant therapy. You advise her:

A. Not to use any modalities, because there are no data, and they are likely to be harmful.

B. She can use herbal preparations as long as she has no adverse effects.

C. She needs to select a licensed professional to administer her CAM.

D. To inform you if she decides to use CAM, so you can help her avoid unfavorable adverse effects and interactions with chemotherapy, and devise an integrated treatment plan, if possible.

ANSWERS

Answer 45.1.   **The answer is D.**

In addition to other professionals, such as social workers and school counselors, the oncology team plays an important role in helping patients explain to their children about their illness and prognosis. In 2002, Rauch et al. (Rauch PK, Muriel AC, Cassem NH. Parents with cancer: Who's looking after the children? J Clin Oncol. 2002;20(21):4399–4402) published recommendations that addressed this difficult issue. For school-aged children, the guidelines include sharing information honestly, avoiding euphemisms, encouraging the children to ask questions, and letting them initiate the discussions.

Answer 45.2.   **The answer is B.**

This patient has neuropathic pain, in this case related to her treatment. Although corticosteroids have a role in treating refractory neuropathic pain, they are generally not used first line. Likewise, opioid drugs can be useful, especially methadone, in more refractory settings and for severe pain. However, neuropathic pain has a variable responsiveness to opioids and may be less responsive than other types of pain. Most common drug classes used as first line for mild-to-moderate neuropathic pain include antidepressants and anticonvulsants. Controlled trials of gabapentin show 30% to 50% response rates in neuropathic pain. The major adverse effect is sedation.

Answer 45.3.   **The answer is A.**

The two most common causes of insomnia in terminally ill patients are pain and depression.

Answer 45.4.   **The answer is B.**

Dealing with situations when the oncologist believes treatment will do more harm than good is very challenging for both the physician and the patient. The key is in the words used and their implications, not just their literal meanings. The goal is to convey a caring attitude and hope that her quality of life will remain as good as possible, without making the patient feel abandoned or unsure in regard to goals of therapy.

Answer 45.5.   **The answer is A.**

The procedure useful in refractory somatic or neuropathic pain from tumor infiltration of the cranial nerves is rhizotomy. Cordotomy, thalamotomy, and mesencephalic tractomy are useful for unilateral pain below the waist, unilateral neuropathic pain in the chest or lower extremity, and pain in the nasopharynx or trigeminal region, respectively.

Answer 45.6.   **The answer is D.**

There are still many misconceptions regarding palliative care programs. Unlike entering hospice care, patients do not need to change or abandon their current treatment program to benefit from additional services provided by palliative care specialists. Several studies in the United States, Canada, and England demonstrated that hospital-based palliative care programs are generally cost-saving for the hospitals. For example, studies done in palliative care units demonstrated significantly decreased daily charges and decreased total costs for patients who died in the unit, compared with age and diagnosis-matched patients who died outside the unit.

Answer 45.7.   **The answer is B.**

Delirium is present in up to 80% of dying patients. Delirious patients may appear agitated or hypoactive, or may alternate between these states. Frequent symptoms of delirium include insomnia, restlessness or agitation (which can mimic uncontrolled pain), irritability, anxiety, and hallucinations.

Answer 45.8.   **The answer is B.**

Oral dose of 20-mg methadone is equivalent to 200 mg of codeine, 7.5 mg of hydromorphone, 100 mg of propoxyphene, and 30 mg of oxycodone.

Answer 45.9.   **The answer is D.**

Although the exact mechanism is unclear, it is accepted that opioid analgesics produce nausea and vomiting by action limited to the medullary chemoreceptor trigger zone. Fortunately, tolerance frequently develops to these side effects. Rotating opioids and adding antiemetics, such as Compazine, are both effective in reducing or obviating this effect.

Answer 45.10.   **The answer is D.**

Although there are many existential reasons that depression is common in the terminally ill, physical factors can also produce symptoms of depression or mimic it. Corticosteroids can trigger psychosis, as well as depressive symptoms. Hypercalcemia can result in an altered, depressed mood. Uncontrolled pain, especially if prolonged, induces a sense of helplessness and depression.

Answer 45.11.   **The answer is D.**

Race, low socioeconomic status, and prolonged time in caring for the patient have all been demonstrated to independently predict high rates of primary caregiver burnout.

Answer 45.12.   **The answer is D.**

Several studies have addressed the issue of professional barriers to effective cancer pain management. Surveys of oncologists demonstrated that both inadequate knowledge and regulatory pressures contribute to inadequate analgesia in patients with cancer.

Answer 45.13.   **The answer is A.**

The patient has chronic postradiation brachial plexopathy. It is important to recognize and effectively manage treatment-related chronic pain syndromes, because these patients frequently need integrated approach to treatment. Brachial plexus MRI is able to distinguish between tumor infiltration and radiation fibrosis. Radiation fibrosis injury typically produces low signal intensity on T2-weighted images, generally not enhancing with gadolinium.

Answer 45.14.   **The answer is D.**

Although it is consoling to the patient to realize that her symptoms are not related to recurrent cancer, the persistence of pain is a constant remainder of the previous cancer diagnosis. Psychological factors play a significant role in how these patients adapt to and function with chronic pain. A multidisciplinary approach combining a wide range of therapies is usually needed. It is also very important to select appropriate analgesics for neuropathic pain. Antidepressants and anticonvulsants will likely be most effective. Antidepressant drugs should be first-line agents, given her tearfulness and anxiety.

Answer 45.15.   **The answer is D.**

Approaches A to C are both reasonable options when dealing with a patient with uncontrolled bone pain from prostate cancer. Opioid rotation can also be attempted if tolerance to morphine is suspected. Methadone can be considered, although conversion can be more challenging than for other opioids because of prolonged plasma half-life but relatively short duration of anesthesia. When converting from another opioid to methadone, marked reduction in equianalgesic dose often results. A reasonable starting methadone daily dose for this patient would be approximately 30 mg of methadone divided into three doses (6:1 ratio for oral morphine, based on 180 mg of oral morphine per day).

Answer 45.16.   **The answer is B.**

All listed adverse effects can occur with opioids, but respiratory depression is unlikely in this setting. This adverse effect most commonly occurs after a short course of intravenous administration of an opioid. Tolerance to this effect develops rapidly with repeat drug doses, which allows prolonged use without significant risk of respiratory depression.

Answer 45.17.   **The answer is D.**

Cost is one of the biggest advantages of methadone, which is relatively inexpensive, compared with other opioids. Because of prolonged half-life, it requires careful titration and may take up to 1 week to achieve steady state. QT prolongation syndrome can occur with methadone and is a cause for concern in those with cancer, who might be taking other agents, known to prolong QT interval.

Answer 45.18.   **The answer is D.**

Development of tolerance to opioids is not well understood but is generally suspected when patients on a previously stable dosage begin to require more frequent doses. Often, there is simultaneous disease progression, complicating the issue of tolerance. However, incomplete cross-resistance among opioids often allows for "opioid rotation" and achievement of effective analgesia. Methadone is known to bind to NMDA receptors in the brain, in addition to opioid receptors. This may be one of the mechanisms that explain dramatic dose reductions when a patient's medication is switched from morphine or hydromorphone to methadone.

Answer 45.19.   **The answer is D.**

In addition to commonly used classes, such as antidepressants and anticonvulsants, the use of local anesthetics has demonstrated some efficacy in the management of chronic neuropathic pain. Mexiletine is the oral local anesthetic for which there is pilot data to support analgesic efficacy. The starting dose is low, at 150 mg/d, with gradual titration. Epidural local anesthetics (lidocaine and bupivacaine) have been widely used to manage refractory neuropathic pain, either alone or with opioid.

Answer 45.20.   **The answer is B.**

Continuous epidural low-dose infusion of local anesthetic via a pump is associated with development of tolerance within days to weeks, limiting long-term use. It is most useful in patients who experience acute pain crisis or in patients in whom the use of spinal opioids is considered but who have developed tolerance from large doses of systemic opiates. Temporary use of this technique allows for reducing systemic opioids doses, therefore partially reversing tolerance. Celiac ganglion block is reported to be effective in 70% to 85% of appropriately selected patients. Cordotomy is associated with a 10% to 20% risk of ipsilateral motor weakness, which results from inadvertent extension of the lesion anteriorly to involve corticospinal tract.

Answer 45.21.   **The answer is D.**

This patient is nearing the end of life. The goal is to control any symptoms that he is experiencing. Possible causes of his dyspnea include anxiety, tumor infiltration, and other cardiac and pulmonary conditions. Patients with continuous dyspnea benefit from opioids; if the patient is no longer able to take pills, opioid drips can be very effective. For patients with perceived anxiety, anxiolytics should be added. Haldol can also be useful to control symptoms of agitated delirium.

Answer 45.22.   **The answer is D.**

Among the many metabolic abnormalities seen in patients with cachexia, the total body water and serum free lipids are increased and there is insulin resistance.

Answer 45.23.   **The answer is A.**

Loss of excess of 10% of baseline body weight over 6 months is defined as critical weight loss.

Answer 45.24.   **The answer is D.**

Cancer cachexia is a complex process, mediated by the induction of inflammatory response to the tumor. The hallmark of cancer cachexia is increased catabolism and limited anabolism. This includes an increase in hepatic gluconeogenesis to compensate for increased body glucose consumption. Lipoprotein lipase activity is decreased, and fat breakdown is increased. Muscle proteolysis and hepatic protein synthesis are both increased as well.

Answer 45.25.   **The answer is C.**

Taxanes and depression are associated with dysgeusia and zinc may work best for sweet dysgeusia. The best tolerated food is the one that can be swallowed with little chewing and little production of saliva.

Answer 45.26.   **The answer is D.**

TPN is not indicated in patients with rapidly progressive tumor growth that is unresponsive to therapy, terminally ill patients, and patients with mild malnourishment. Brief, inpatient TPN is indicated in severely malnourished patients who are responding to chemotherapy and in whom gastrointestinal or other toxicities preclude adequate enteral intake for 7 to 10 days or longer.

Answer 45.27.   **The answer is C.**

Megestrol acetate improves body weight in cancer patients mainly due to water retention. Both erythropoietin and recombinant growth factor may promote tumor growth.

Answer 45.28.   **The answer is A.**

Even though a few small studies, including a well-known study by Spiegel in 1989, reported improved survival, more recent studies, including a large multicenter trial, did not confirm these results. However, every well-conducted study of psychotherapy in patients with cancer improved quality of life or reduced stress. A study by Goodwin in patients with metastatic breast cancer showed decreased pain scores, reduced depression, and overall reduced distress.

Answer 45.29.   **The answer is D.**

There are several indications for corticosteroids in the management of pain including neuropathic pain, bone pain, headaches due to increased cranial pressure, and pain associated with capsular expansion or duct obstruction.

Answer 45.30.   **The answer is D.**

Use of CAM among patients with cancer is frequent and growing. There is also expanding body of knowledge regarding different forms of CAM and several completed and ongoing large-scale clinical trials of various modalities. These include herbal preparations, energy-based approaches, manipulative and body-based approaches, and mind–body medicine. It is extremely important to ask patients about their use of CAM therapies and monitor side effects that may occur, as well as incorporate knowledge into the treatment plan. Several websites have been developed to aid clinicians in identifying purported mechanisms and possible adverse effects and drug interactions of various forms of CAM, especially herbal-derived preparations.

CHAPTER 46 REHABILITATION OF THE CANCER PATIENT

JANAKIRAMAN SUBRAMANIAN

DIRECTIONS Each of the numbered items below is followed by lettered answers. Select the ONE lettered answer that is BEST in each case unless instructed otherwise.

QUESTIONS

Question 46.1. Which chemotherapy is commonly associated with peripheral neuropathy resulting in sensory ataxia and pain, usually without weakness?

A. Platinum analogs
B. Vinca alkaloids
C. Taxanes
D. Methotrexate

Question 46.2. In which of the following settings exercise is NOT recommended in a patient with cancer?

A. Platelets 30,000 to 50,000/m^3
B. Bony metastases with 25% to 50% cortex involvement
C. Hematocrit <25%
D. Sodium of 127 mmol/L

Question 46.3. Therapy that is specifically directed toward helping the patient's ability to perform activities of daily living is:

A. Occupational therapy
B. Physical therapy
C. Recreational therapy
D. Speech therapy

Question 46.4. The treatments of radiation therapy-induced hyposalivation include all of the following, EXCEPT:

A. Bromhexine
B. Pilocarpine
C. Moist and soft foods
D. Anticholinergic agents

Corresponding Chapter in *Cancer: Principles & Practice of Oncology*, Ninth Edition: 177 (Rehabilitation of the Cancer Patient).

Question 46.5.   A 56-year-old Caucasian woman has recently been diagnosed with extensive-stage small cell carcinoma of the lung. She is currently undergoing chemotherapy and is having severe pain caused by metastases to her ribs. Which of the following is contraindicated?

A. Oxycodone
B. Deep heat application over the ribs
C. Rib belt
D. Topical lidocaine

Question 46.6.   The following therapies are approved for the management of lymphedema, EXCEPT:

A. Manual lymphatic drainage
B. Compression bandaging
C. Resistance exercises
D. Benzopyrones

Question 46.7.   Treatment modalities for patients with cancer who are at risk for fracture of the spine include all of the following, EXCEPT:

A. Surgery
B. Thoracolumbar corset
C. Bed rest
D. Walker

Question 46.8.   In cancer patients with foot drop and severe pain with ankle movement, the preferred ankle orthotic device is:

A. Solid ankle-foot orthosis
B. Posterior leaf spring orthosis
C. Hinged ankle-foot orthosis
D. None of the above

Question 46.9.   The employment rights of patients with cancer are mainly protected by the:

A. Americans with Disabilities Act of 1990
B. Family and Medical Leave Act of 1993
C. Federal Rehabilitation Act of 1973
D. Employee Retirement Income Security Act of 1974

Question 46.10.   All of the following are true regarding cancer-related spinal cord injury (SCI), EXCEPT:

A. 15% of all cancer patients have symptomatic SCI due to spinal metastasis.
B. Epidural-based tumor metastasis is the most common cause of SCI.
C. The most common site of spine metastasis is the vertebral body.
D. Patients with SCI above T6 are at risk for autonomic dysreflexia.

Question 46.11.   The MOST common indication for rehabilitation care in patients with cancer undergoing treatment of their malignancy is:

A. Deconditioning
B. Impaired mobility
C. Impaired activities of daily living
D. Reduced range of motion (ROM)

Question 46.12.   All of the following are associated with improved rehabilitation gains in patients with brain tumors, EXCEPT:

A. Meningioma
B. Presenting at initial diagnosis
C. Left-sided brain tumor
D. Receiving radiation therapy

Question 46.13.   The MOST common functional limitation reported by cancer survivors returning to work is:

A. Performing physical tasks
B. Analyzing data
C. Prolonged mental concentration
D. Lifting heavy loads

Question 46.14.   A 75-year-old man was recently diagnosed with cranial meningioma and underwent primary resection of the tumor. He requires active rehabilitation after his surgery. All of the following statements regarding his rehabilitation are correct, EXCEPT:

A. Impaired cognition and weakness are the most common indication for acute rehabilitation after surgery.
B. This patient's rehabilitation is likely to be shorter than patients with stroke undergoing rehabilitation.
C. He requires short-term antiseizure prophylaxis during rehabilitation.
D. Postoperative deep vein thrombosis (DVT) prophylaxis would be indicated.

Question 46.15.   All of the following interventions may be appropriate for the management of neuritic pain, EXCEPT:

A. Desensitization measures such as tapping or vibration.
B. Application of topical lidocaine.
C. Local injection of corticosteroids.
D. Treatment with gabapentin.

Question 46.16.   A 65-year-old man was recently diagnosed with prostate cancer and underwent prostatectomy. He is recovered from his surgery but suffers from sexual dysfunction including difficulty with having erections. All of the following are appropriate treatment measures, EXCEPT:

A. Body image counseling
B. Pelvic floor exercises
C. Vacuum-assisted devices
D. Penile prosthesis

Question 46.17.   All of the following are appropriate measures for rehabilitating a cancer patient with paraplegia, EXCEPT:

A. Weight shift techniques
B. Complex decongestive therapy (CDT)
C. Education regarding skin care
D. Customized wheel chair prescription

ANSWERS

Answer 46.1.   **The answer is A.**

Taxanes and vinca alkaloids cause a predominately length-dependent motor and sensory axonal polyneuropathy in a distal symmetric distribution. Resulting in paresthesias, pain, sensory ataxia, and potentially weakness, this condition usually improves when the treatment is stopped. The platinum analogs damage the cell body of the sensory nerves in the dorsal root ganglion, and at higher doses can damage the anterior horn cell within the spinal cord. As a result, it is more likely for patients treated with platinum analogs to have sensory neuropathy without motor weakness. The clinical manifestations include severe sensory ataxia and pain, usually without weakness. Peripheral neuropathy is not a commonly reported toxicity of methotrexate.

Answer 46.2.   **The answer is D.**

For platelets 30,000 to 50,000/m^3, the recommended activities are range of motion (ROM) exercises, aerobic activity, light weights, and ambulation. If hematocrit is less than 25%, ROM exercise and isometric exercises are recommended. However, aerobic exercises should be avoided. For bone metastasis involving 25% to 50% of the cortex, mild aerobic and weight-bearing exercises are recommended. In patients with sodium less than 130 mmol/L and potassium less than 3 mmol/L, no exercises are recommended until evaluated by a physician.

Answer 46.3.   **The answer is A.**

Occupational therapy is directed toward helping patients perform their activities of daily living. It involves assessing their activity level, living environment, and interventions, such as exercises for strengthening, improvement in dexterity, proper posture, energy conservation, and instruction in the use of adaptive equipment. Physical therapy involves the development of strength, promotion of mobility, and pain-control techniques. Recreational therapists provide treatment services and recreation activities for individuals with disabilities or illnesses. Speech therapists address people's speech production, vocal production, swallowing difficulties, and language needs.

Answer 46.4.   **The answer is D.**

Anticholinergic drugs are a well-known cause of hyposalivation, and as a result, they should not be used in patients with radiation-induced hyposalivation. Pilocarpine is a sialogogue that promotes saliva secretion by muscarinic stimulation of the salivary glands. Bromhexine promotes increased salivary secretion and reduces the viscosity.

Answer 46.5.   **The answer is B.**

Cancer pain control includes both pharmacologic and nonpharmacologic treatment modalities. Both opioid medications and topical anesthetics are recommended for cancer pain control. Rib belts help with pain control in patients with rib metastasis but should not be used continuously because they can affect respiratory effort. Deep-heat modalities are recommended for cancer pain control but should not be applied directly over the malignant tumor because they can cause significant tissue damage.

Answer 46.6.   **The answer is D.**

The mainstay for the management of lymphedema is CDT. This consists of manual lymphatic drainage by gentle massaging and compression bandaging. Resistance exercises can be performed safely by patients with lymphedema wearing compression garments. Benzopyrones are not approved in the United States in the management of lymphedema.

Answer 46.7.   **The answer is C.**

Both surgical and nonsurgical treatments are recommended for impending fracture of spine caused by metastasis. In patients who are not surgical candidates or refuse surgery, alternatives include thoracolumbar corset and gait aids such as walkers. However, bed rest is not recommended because this can result in further functional loss and increased risk for DVT.

Answer 46.8.   **The answer is A.**

In most patients with foot drop, a ready-made or custom-made posterior leaf spring orthosis is sufficient. In patients with severe pain caused by ankle movements, an immobilizing solid ankle-foot orthosis may be more helpful.

Answer 46.9.   **The answer is A.**

The Americans with Disabilities Act of 1990 protects the employment rights of patients with cancer. Additional protections are provided in the Family and Medical Leave Act of 1993, Federal Rehabilitation Act of 1973, and Employee Retirement Income Security Act of 1974.

Answer 46.10.   **The answer is A.**

Studies have shown that the incidence of SCI in patients with cancer ranges between 0.2% and 7.9%. Autopsy studies indicate that SCI from metastasis is present in 5% of all patients diagnosed with cancer. Epidural-based tumors are the most common cause of SCI. Patients with SCI above T6 level are at risk for autonomic dysreflexia that is characterized by a more than 20 mmHg rise in baseline blood pressure.

Answer 46.11.   **The answer is A.**

The indications for rehabilitation in patients with cancer are as follows: 76% with deconditioning, 58% with mobility impairment, 43% with reduced ROM, and 22% with impaired activities of daily living.

Answer 46.12.   **The answer is D.**

Left-sided brain lesion and meningioma are associated with favorable rehabilitation outcomes. Patients with recurrence or relapse of tumor have poor outcomes when compared with patients at initial presentation. In the case of radiation therapy, there is no clear evidence regarding whether this has an adverse or favorable impact on rehabilitation.

Answer 46.13.   **The answer is D.**

According to a study with 253 cancer survivors, the most common functional limitation reported was difficulty lifting heavy objects (26%), followed by performing physical tasks (18%), prolonged mental concentration (12%), and analyzing data (11%).

Answer 46.14.   **The answer is C.**

The role for antiseizure prophylaxis is not well established in patients with brain tumors with no history of seizure activity. On the other hand, patients with brain tumors are at high risk for DVT in the postoperative setting. The most common neurologic problems faced by patients with brain tumors in the postoperative setting are impaired cognition and weakness. Studies have shown that patients with meningioma require shorter periods of rehabilitation in the postoperative setting than patients with stroke.

Answer 46.15.   **The answer is C.**

Local injection of corticosteroids is effective for the treatment of inflamed joints or bursa and not for neuritic pain. All of the other treatments are appropriate for the management of neuritic pain.

Answer 46.16.   **The answer is B.**

Pelvic floor exercises are usually prescribed for urinary incontinence. Sexual dysfunction could result from poor body image due to altered anatomy after surgery and counseling can help address this issue. Vacuum-assisted devices and penile prosthesis may be helpful in this setting.

Answer 46.17.   **The answer is B.**

CDT is useful in the management of lymphedema and is not indicated in patients with paraplegia. Weight shift techniques, skin care education, and customized wheel chairs are necessary in patients with paraplegia, which avoid the development of decubitus ulcers.

THOMAS H. FONG

DIRECTIONS   Each of the numbered items below is followed by lettered answers. Select the ONE lettered answer that is BEST in each case unless instructed otherwise.

QUESTIONS

Question 47.1.   Which of the following is NOT an element of valid informed consent?

    A. Competence or mental capacity
    B. Disclosure of information relevant to the decision
    C. Assurance of favorable outcome from treatment
    D. Voluntariness of choice, free from excessive pressure

Question 47.2.   Surrogates should decide which interventions to provide a patient who cannot give informed consent for himself/herself according to what standards?

    A. Substituted judgment (predicting patient's treatment preference, if competent)
    B. Best interest of the patient
    C. Best interest of the patient's family
    D. Both A and B

Question 47.3.   Institutional review boards review proposed clinical trials to ensure that research trials with human beings meet all of the following requirements, EXCEPT which one?

    A. Financial incentive for subject
    B. Scientific validity
    C. Favorable risk–benefit ratio
    D. Fair subject selection

Corresponding Chapters in *Cancer: Principles & Practice of Oncology,* Ninth Edition: 178 (Regulatory Issues), 179 (Health Disparities in Cancer), 180 (Cancer Information on the Internet), and 181 (Complementary, Alternative, and Integrative Therapies in Cancer Care).

Question 47.4.   Randomized controlled trials provide the highest level evidence for the efficacy and safety of a medical intervention. The ethical justification for these includes the concept of clinical equipoise, which is best defined in what manner?

A. Determination of physician to give best treatment irrespective of trial mandates
B. Uncertainty about the merit of a treatment versus the current standard of care
C. Valuation of societal benefit over individual patient outcome by the clinician
D. Ability of study subjects to withdraw from a clinical trial whenever desired

Question 47.5.   Conflict of interest is a potential risk when industry sponsors a clinical trial. Research shows that one of the most significant impacts of industry funding is which of the following?

A. Less rigorous methodology compared with nonindustry-sponsored research
B. Data interpretation that is favorable to the company instead of objective
C. Controlled reporting and dissemination of study results
D. Frequent ownership of stock by investigators of industry-funded trials

Question 47.6.   Which of the following statements regarding the Orphan Drug Act is NOT true?

A. Provides incentives for drugs intended to treat rare diseases.
B. Orphan drug designation can provide for 10 years of marketing exclusivity on drug approval.
C. Orphan drug designation could result in tax incentives and drug research grants to the manufacturer.
D. None of the above.

Question 47.7.   Which of the following is an example of nonvoluntary active euthanasia?

A. Provide a medicine that a patient can use to commit suicide.
B. Terminate life-sustaining treatments.
C. Administration of medications to cause death in a patient incapable of providing consent.
D. Intervention to cause death in a patient who is competent but did not sign the consent.

Question 47.8.   Which of the following types of euthanasia is considered universally unethical?

A. Passive euthanasia
B. Physician-assisted suicide
C. Voluntary active euthanasia
D. Involuntary active euthanasia

Question 47.9.   A 41-year-old woman is diagnosed with early-stage breast cancer. Genetic testing reveals that she is BRCA1 mutation positive. She has two younger sisters who are in their late 30s. What is the most appropriate action?

A. Call her sisters and request that they be tested for BRCA1 status.

B. Offer referral to a genetic counselor and provide informed consent for testing.

C. Order mammograms for her sisters.

D. Recommend prophylactic mastectomy for her sisters.

Question 47.10.   A study is undertaken to determine the timeliness of administration of intravenous antibiotics for patients with cancer with fever and neutropenia. This is an example of which type of quality measurement?

A. Process measure

B. Structural measure

C. Outcome measure

D. Technical measure

Question 47.11.   What sources of data may be used for quality assessment?

A. Medical records

B. Administrative databases

C. Cancer registries

D. All of the above

Question 47.12.   Strategies for implementing quality improvement include which of the following?

A. Use of evidence-based guideline recommendations in clinical practice

B. Improvement in documentation of cancer care

C. Implementation of health information technology

D. All of the above

Question 47.13.   Investigational New Drug (IND) applications are submitted to the Food and Drug Administration (FDA) for review at which phase of development?

A. Before phase I trials

B. Before phase II trials

C. Before phase III trials

D. After completion of a phase III trial demonstrating clear evidence of efficacy

Question 47.14.   Pharmaceutical companies submit a New Drug Application (NDA) to the FDA for approval of the sales and marketing of a new drug. These sponsors must provide evidence that the drug is safe and effective based on "adequate and well-controlled clinical investigations." Oncology drugs have been approved by the FDA on the basis of supporting clinical trials with which of the following primary end points?

A.   Overall survival or disease-free survival
B.   Tumor response rate
C.   Palliation
D.   All of the above

Question 47.15.   Expanded access protocols are designed with what goal in mind?

A.   Increasing the size of a clinical protocol for statistical robustness
B.   Enabling access to investigational drugs when no viable alternative is available
C.   Providing medications to patients unable to afford prescribed drugs
D.   Increasing market share of a newly approved medication

Question 47.16.   Which of the following statements regarding IND is NOT true?

A.   All studies for nonapproved drugs must be done under IND.
B.   Some studies on approved drugs may be exempted from IND requirement.
C.   The IND process spans the entire time of drug investigation.
D.   Sponsors may initiate the proposed study as soon as they receive the IND.

ANSWERS

Answer 47.1.   **The answer is C.**

Legal rulings have clarified that essential components of informed consent include competence (the mental capacity of a person to make health-care decisions), disclosure (information on the diagnosis, proposed intervention, potential risks and benefits, and alternative treatments), understanding (patient's grasp of information disclosed), and voluntariness (choice that is free from interference by others, such as coercion or excessive pressure).

Answer 47.2.   **The answer is D.**

There are two standard principles to guide surrogate decision makers for patients who cannot give informed consent: substituted judgment and best interests. Substituted judgment refers to the attempt to determine the incompetent person's preferences regarding a decision if that person were to be competent. The best interest standard refers to an objective evaluation of benefits and risks, and selection of the treatment in which benefit maximally outweighs the burdens of treatment of the individual patient.

Answer 47.3.   **The answer is A.**

Ethical requirements of clinical trials on human subjects are meant to minimize exploitation of research participants. These ethical principles, stated in guidelines issued by multiple agencies, include the principles of collaborative partnership, social value, scientific validity, fair subject selection, favorable risk–benefit ratio, independent review, informed consent, and respect for potential and enrolled subjects.

Answer 47.4.   **The answer is B.**

Clinical equipoise is present when there is a legitimate disagreement among clinicians about optimal treatment, particularly when there is lack of reliable data and genuine uncertainty about which treatment is best for a patient. When this principle is met, there is no violation of the physician–patient relationship, in which the physician is acting on behalf of the patient's best interest.

Answer 47.5.   **The answer is C.**

Studies sponsored by industry have been found to be at least as methodologically rigorous, if not more so, than nonindustry sponsored trials. Financial incentive for companies to avoid methodologic flaws that discredit study results has been suggested as the reason for this finding. There is little evidence to suggest that interpretation of data is frequently biased by financial considerations. Several studies point to the impact of industry funding on dissemination of trial results, including suppression of adverse findings, delayed or lack of publishing negative results, and multiple publications of results favorable to industry. Although personal stock ownership by clinical investigators is a common concern, this is rare in actual practice.

Answer 47.6.   **The answer is B.**

The Orphan Drug Act of 1983 provides financial incentives to promote the development of drugs for rare diseases including the potential for 7 years of marketing exclusivity on drug approval, tax incentives, and eligibility for orphan drug research grants.

Answer 47.7.   **The answer is C.**

Nonvoluntary active euthanasia is the intentional administration of medicine or other interventions in patients who are incompetent and unable to consent. Provision of a medicine that a patient can use to commit suicide, termination of life-sustaining treatments, and causing death in a competent patient who did not consent the procedure are examples of physician-assisted suicide, passive euthanasia, and involuntary active euthanasia, respectively.

Answer 47.8.   **The answer is D.**

Voluntary euthanasia and physician-assisted suicide are legal in Belgium and the Netherlands, with the latter also being legal in Switzerland and the US state of Oregon. Passive euthanasia is considered ethical but involuntary active euthanasia is considered unethical and is not known to be legal in any country.

Answer 47.9.   **The answer is B.**

Genetic testing may be advisable for people with increased susceptibility to cancer because of family history or other predisposing factors. Such information may help guide patients and their families to seek further interventions, such as early mammography or prophylactic mastectomy in patients with BRCA1 mutations. Testing may be associated with potential psychological, social, or economic harm, and a proper informed consent process should include discussion about the pros and cons. Genetic counselors may provide help in this process.

Answer 47.10.   **The answer is A.**

Quality measurement refers to the practice of evaluating care processes to bring about improvement and include structural, process, and outcome measures. Structural measures evaluate characteristics of providers or the care system, such as rates of board certification or volume of procedures. Process measures examine the actions taken by providers, such as delivery of a specific care component that has been demonstrated to be favorable for patient outcomes based on clinical trials or guideline recommendations. Outcome measures refer to patient results, including measures of quality of life, disease-free survival, and overall survival.

Answer 47.11.   **The answer is D.**

Quality data sources include medical records, patient surveys, administrative databases (e.g., Medicare claims), and registries. The National Cancer Data Base (NCDB) and the Surveillance Epidemiology and End Results (SEER) program of the National Cancer Institute (NCI) are examples of cancer registry programs in the United States. Each of these data sources may provide useful information for quality research.

Answer 47.12.   **The answer is D.**

All of the above measures are examples of strategies to improve quality of care delivered to patients with cancer. Guideline recommendations, such as the National Comprehensive Cancer Network (NCCN), may help to integrate evidence-based medicine into clinical practice. Improved documentation of cancer care can facilitate better care coordination, safety, and efficiency. Health information technologies, when implemented in the context of an overall process design, may improve efficiency and quality of care through measures such as point-of-service reminders or standardized order sets.

Answer 47.13.   **The answer is A.**

Investigational drugs must be administered under an IND application that is submitted to the FDA. The initial IND application typically consists of a proposed phase I clinical protocol and supporting data regarding safety. These data may include in vitro, animal, or human evidence describing drug toxicity and a predicted safe starting dose, as well as manufacturing data regarding the drug product. A panel of scientific reviewers from the FDA then determines if such data are sufficient to proceed with the proposed study without unreasonable risk of injury or harm.

Answer 47.14.   **The answer is D.**

From 1990 to 2006, 94 oncology drug marketing applications were approved by the FDA. End points supporting FDA approval included overall survival and disease-free survival, tumor response rates, response rate supported by additional data, and palliation or amelioration of symptoms (e.g., Neulasta, Leukine, and Ethyol approvals).

Answer 47.15.   **The answer is B.**

Expanded access protocols are designed to facilitate availability of investigational drugs when certain conditions are met: No satisfactory alternative treatment is available, the drug sponsor is pursuing marketing approval with due diligence, the drug is nearing the end of its development, and data support efficacy for use in the intended population. The NCI has provided expanded access to investigational drugs through an agreement with the FDA in these situations.

Answer 47.16.   The answer is D.

Unless in the case of an approved waiver, sponsors should wait 30 days after receiving the IND approval to initiate the study. All studies on non-approved drugs require IND, whereas studies on approved drugs may be exempted. The IND spans the entire process of drug investigation.

VAMSIDHAR VELCHETI • DANIEL MORGENSZTERN

DIRECTIONS   Each of the numbered items below is followed by lettered answers. Select the
ONE lettered answer that is BEST in each case unless instructed otherwise.

QUESTIONS

Question 48.1.   A 55-year-old African American woman was recently diagnosed with
metastatic carcinoma of the colon. She started first-line chemotherapy
with FOLFIRI (Irinotecan (CPT-11) and 5-fluorouracil and leucovorin).
She was advised by her aunt to take a herbal potion containing St. John's
Wort (*Hypericum perforatum*) for anxiety relief. Which one of these
responses is appropriate regarding the use of this herbal supplement during chemotherapy with irinotecan?

A. There is no scientific evidence supporting its anxiolytic effects.
B. St. John's Wort increases the side effects from treatment with irinotecan.
C. St. John's Wort results in more than 50% reduction in serum levels
of the active metabolite of irinotecan.
D. There is an increased risk of bleeding when used concomitantly with
irinotecan.

Question 48.2.   A 43-year-old premenopausal woman is on adjuvant tamoxifen therapy
for hormone-receptor positive breast cancer. She also uses herbal supplements including St. John's Wort for depression, and drinks three cups of
green tea daily. What would you recommend at this time?

A. Discontinue St. John's Wort
B. Discontinue green tea
C. Increase the dose of tamoxifen
D. Discontinue tamoxifen and start an aromatase inhibitor

Corresponding Chapter in *Cancer: Principles & Practice of Oncology*, Ninth Edition: 181 (Complementary, Alternative, and Integrative Therapies in Cancer Care).

Question 48.3.   A 58-year-old African American man was diagnosed with advanced unresectable squamous cell carcinoma of the head and neck (T4aN2Mo). He began concurrent chemoradiation with cisplatin and radiation ≥70 Gy planned over 7 weeks. He comes to your office for a prechemotherapy visit and enquires about the potential benefits from acupuncture therapy. Which of the following statements is true regarding acupuncture in the supportive care of patients with head and neck cancer?

A. Acupuncture reduces chemotherapy-induced nausea.
B. Acupuncture demonstrated significant reductions in pain, dysfunction, and xerostomia in patients with head and neck cancer undergoing radiation.
C. Both A and B.
D. There are no data from prospective trials suggesting clinical benefit.

Question 48.4.   A 39-year-old woman is on adjuvant tamoxifen therapy for breast cancer and is experiencing significant hot flashes. She is taking a herbal supplement which has been helping. Which of the following herbal medications may oppose the antitumor activity of tamoxifen, and should be avoided?

A. Tea tree oil
B. Fish oil (omega-3)
C. Soy supplements
D. Kava

Question 48.5.   A 70-year-old Caucasian man with refractory multiple myeloma was treated with lenalidomide plus dexamethasone. After two cycles the patient developed pulmonary embolism and deep vein thrombosis of the right leg. Chemotherapy was discontinued, and the patient was started on anticoagulation with home enoxaparin injections. He comes to your office for a scheduled visit and reports taking a herbal remedy containing Ginkgo extract to help his memory and cognitive function. Which of the following statement is TRUE regarding the effects of Ginkgo?

A. Increases the risk of serious bleeds
B. Will increase the metabolism of enoxaparin
C. Decreases the responsiveness of myeloma to further chemotherapy
D. May increase risk of infection from immunosuppression

Question 48.6.   A 60-year-old Hispanic man with early-stage squamous cell carcinoma of the lung has recently undergone surgical resection. He comes to your office for recommendations on adjuvant chemotherapy. He tells you that after his surgery he has been taking some herbal supplements "to fight his cancer," sent by his friend from Mexico. He has felt weak and anorectic for the past few weeks and experienced mild intermittent pain in the right upper quadrant of his abdomen. He takes no other medications, including over-the-counter medications. He does not use alcohol regularly and had no other known medical disorders. On examination of the patient, jaundice was noted, but no other significant findings were present. His initial laboratory test results revealed abnormal liver function tests, with total bilirubin 5.9 mg/dL, direct bilirubin 4.4 mg/dL, aspartate aminotransferase 52 U/L, alanine aminotransferase 272 U/L, total alkaline phosphatase 153 U/L, and γ-glutamyltransferase 226 U/L (0 to 45 U/L). The prothrombin time was normal. Which of the following herbal supplements has been associated with severe hepatotoxicity?

A. Mistletoe
B. Chaparral
C. Green Tea
D. Maitake

Question 48.7.   Which of the following herbal remedies has been widely used for treatment of prostate cancer?

A. Kava (*Piper methysticum*)
B. Ginger (*Zingiber officinale*)
C. PC-SPES
D. Alfalfa (*Medicago sativa*)

Question 48.8.   A 48-year-old Caucasian man with diffuse large B-cell lymphoma is receiving chemotherapy with R-CHOP. He bought a nutritional supplement containing Coenzyme Q10 from a health food store. He asks you if this would "improve tolerance for chemotherapy." Which of the following responses is most accurate regarding the use of Coenzyme Q10 supplements in patients undergoing chemotherapy?

A. Coenzyme Q10 reduces the cardiotoxicity from anthracyclines when administered for 3 weeks prior to start of therapy.
B. Coenzyme Q10 decreases chemotherapy-related fatigue.
C. There is slight increase in the hepatotoxicity when co-administered with anthracyclines.
D. There is no evidence from randomized controlled trials that Coenzyme Q10 has cardioprotective effects.

Question 48.9.   A 45-year-old African American man with locally advanced adenocarcinoma of the lung is currently undergoing concurrent chemotherapy with radiation. On one regular office visit, the patient reports taking Kava extracts (60 mg/d) to relieve his anxiety and insomnia. He tells you that it helped his symptoms very well and asks you if it is safe to continue taking this medicine. Which of the following responses is TRUE regarding Kava extracts?

A. There is no scientific evidence supporting the efficacy of Kava extracts in relieving anxiety and insomnia in patients with cancer.
B. Significantly reduces chemotherapy agents in the blood levels.
C. Increases the toxicity of chemotherapy
D. Kava extracts may cause severe hepatotoxicity.

Question 48.10.   A 50-year-old woman with metastatic breast cancer completed her fourth cycle of single-agent docetaxel 4 days ago. She now presents to the emergency department with severe nausea, vomiting, and diarrhea. Her laboratory test results reveal severe neutropenia with a total white blood cell (WBC) count of 400 cells/mm^3 and severe thrombocytopenia with a platelet count of 30,000 mm^3. She is admitted to the hospital, and with appropriate supportive care she recovers well from the episode and presents to your clinic for further chemotherapy. On careful history taking, she reveals that after her last cycle of chemotherapy she started taking grapefruit juice to relieve her heartburn symptoms from chemotherapy. Which of the following is the appropriate next step in her care?

A. Discontinue grapefruit juice and continue chemotherapy at scheduled dose
B. Discontinue grapefruit juice and delay the next dose of chemotherapy
C. Continue taking grapefruit juice and resume chemotherapy with a 25% dose reduction
D. Resume chemotherapy at the current dose as scheduled

Question 48.11.   A 59-year-old man is undergoing chemotherapy for pancreatic cancer and has constipation. He is interested in using a herbal treatment for constipation. Which of the following agents is a natural laxative?

A. Ispaghula
B. Flaxseed
C. Aloe vera
D. All of the above

Question 48.12.   Which of the following herbal supplements increases bleeding risk, and should be avoided in a patient with gastric cancer who is taking Coumadin for deep venous thrombosis?

A. Licorice
B. Red clover
C. Alfalfa
D. All of the above

Question 48.13.   A 69-year-old woman is on erlotinib therapy for metastatic lung cancer. She is using herbal supplements, including green tea, Kava, and saw palmetto. She has noticed yellow discoloration of her nails and skin. Which one of the following is the likely cause for the yellow discoloration?

A. Erlotinib
B. Green tea
C. Kava
D. Saw palmetto

Question 48.14.   A 55-year-old female with metastatic breast cancer is currently on hormonal therapy with anastrozole. She saw a commercial in a health magazine about shark cartilage supplements for patients with breast cancer. Which of the following responses is TRUE regarding use of shark cartilage supplements?

A. Shark cartilage supplements prolong survival in patients with metastatic breast cancer.
B. Shark cartilage supplements improve quality of life and may be useful adjuncts to chemotherapy.
C. There is no significant clinical benefit with shark cartilage supplements.
D. Shark cartilage supplements decrease risk for pathological fractures.

ANSWERS

Answer 48.1.   **The answer is C.**

St. John's Wort has been extensively studied in the treatment of mild-to-moderate depression and was found to be more effective than placebo and equally effective as tricyclic antidepressants (TCAs) in the treatment of mild-to-moderate major depression. However, because of multiple well-documented drug interactions, its use has been discouraged in patients. St John's Wort appears to inhibit the hepatic enzyme cytochrome P-4503A4. Irinotecan is metabolized via this pathway, and patients receiving irinotecan (CPT-11) have a greater than 50% reduction in serum levels of the active metabolite SN-38 after concomitant administration of St. John's Wort.

Answer 48.2.   **The answer is A.**

St. John's Wort may decrease levels of tamoxifen through its effects on hepatic metabolism. St. John's Wort should, therefore, be discontinued. Increasing the dose of tamoxifen, changing to an aromatase inhibitor, and discontinuing green tea are not appropriate in this setting.

Answer 48.3.   **The answer is C.**

Acupuncture is a safe and well-tolerated treatment. Several randomized controlled trials and meta-analysis support its efficacy for the treatment of acute and chronic pain. In addition, more recently acupuncture has also been studied in patients with cancer to reduce chemotherapy- and radiotherapy-induced nausea and vomiting, radiation-induced xerostomia, and for persistent chemotherapy-related fatigue. In a recently published randomized controlled trial, acupuncture produced improvement in xerostomia in patients treated with radiation for head and neck cancer (J Clin Oncol. 2010;28(15):2565).

Answer 48.4.   **The answer is C.**

Some women experience menopause-like symptoms with tamoxifen, including hot flashes and emotional changes. Phytoestrogens, such as genistein, are the major constituents of soy and exhibit selective estrogen-receptor modulator activity. Soy products are popular among women experiencing perimenopausal symptoms. However, in patients with breast cancer, genistein might antagonize the effects of tamoxifen, making it less effective and possibly helping proliferation of the breast cancer cells.

Answer 48.5.   **The answer is A.**

Herbs such as Ginkgo, feverfew, ginger, and garlic have anticoagulant effects and should be avoided by patients using warfarin, heparin, aspirin, and related agents.

Answer 48.6.   **The answer is B.**

Chaparral is a Native American herb that has purported anti-inflammatory and anticancer effects. There is no scientific evidence supporting the anticancer effects of chaparral. Numerous reports indicate hepatotoxicity after the use of chaparral and often severe fulminant hepatic failure requiring transplantation. Other common herbal supplements with significant hepatic toxicity include birch oil, blessed thistle, Kava, germander, dehydroepiandrosterone (DHEA), and turmeric.

Answer 48.7.   **The answer is C.**

PC-SPES is a herbal product that is a mixture of eight herbs: reishi mushroom, Baikal skullcap, Rabdosia, Dyer's woad, chrysanthemum, saw palmetto, Panax ginseng, and licorice. PC-SPES was a very popular herbal supplement to treat prostate cancer. Use of PC-SPES has demonstrated significant decreases in androgen and prostate-specific antigen (PSA) levels in humans. In vitro experiments revealed inhibition of growth and proliferation of human tumor cell lines, including androgen-sensitive and -insensitive prostate cancer.

Answer 48.8.   **The answer is D.**

Coenzyme Q10 (also known as Vitamin Q10, ubiquinone, or ubidecarenone) supplements are very popular among patients undergoing chemotherapy. There has been some suggestion that Coenzyme Q10 might reduce chemotherapy-induced fatigue and also has cardioprotective effect when used with anthracycline-based regimens. However, in double-blind, placebo-controlled trials in patients with breast cancer, use of Coenzyme Q did not show any clinically significant benefit from chemotherapy-related fatigue.

Although the use of Coenzyme Q for prevention of anthracycline-induced cardiotoxicity appears promising based on preclinical models, there is no strong evidence through randomized prospective trials. Two small prospective trials have suggested benefit; however, these had serious design flaws and no definitive conclusions could be drawn.

Answer 48.9.   **The answer is D.**

Kava extracts are commonly used by patients with cancer for anxiety and insomnia. Several randomized, controlled clinical trials have reported relief of anxiety and insomnia. However, numerous reports of severe hepatotoxicity have been reported. The use of Kava extracts has not been approved by the Food and Drug Administration for the above indication.

Answer 48.10.   **The answer is B.**

Grapefruit extracts inhibit cytochrome P450 isoenzymes and, therefore, affect serum concentrations of drugs metabolized by the cytochrome P450 3A4 system. Several chemotherapy agents, including docetaxel, paclitaxel, vincristine, vinblastine, vinorelbine, irinotecan, etoposide, and tamoxifen, are metabolized by the cytochrome P450 3A4 system, and concomitant use of grapefruit juice would decrease the clearance of these drugs and thus increase the toxicity from these drugs. Patients should discontinue grapefruit consumption for at least 96 hours before resuming chemotherapy.

Answer 48.11.   **The answer is D.**

Flaxseed and aloe vera are natural herbal laxatives. Ispaghula, another agent useful in the treatment of constipation, is also a bulk laxative.

Answer 48.12.   **The answer is D.**

Licorice inhibits platelet activity. Alfalfa and red clover are coumarin constituents. All of these agents can increase the risk of bleeding and should be avoided in a patient on anticoagulant therapy.

Answer 48.13.   **The answer is C.**

Use of Kava may be associated with abnormal liver function tests, including aspartate aminotransferase, alanine aminotransferase, alkaline phosphatase, and total and conjugated bilirubin. Patients taking Kava supplements should be monitored closely for signs of liver dysfunction.

Answer 48.14.   **The answer is C.**

Shark cartilage supplements are popular among patients with cancer. However, several clinical trials evaluating these supplements have not demonstrated any clinically significant benefit. In a randomized, placebo-controlled, double-blind, phase III clinical trial to determine whether a shark cartilage product improved overall survival or quality of life in patients with advanced breast and colon cancer, there was no evidence of benefit.

VISUAL QUICKSTART GUIDE

Macromedia Dreamweaver 8

FOR WINDOWS AND MACINTOSH

Tom Negrino
Dori Smith

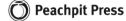 Peachpit Press

Visual QuickStart Guide
Macromedia Dreamweaver 8 for Windows and Macintosh
Tom Negrino and Dori Smith

Peachpit Press
1249 Eighth Street
Berkeley, CA 94710
510/524-2178
800/283-9444
510/524-2221 (fax)

Find us on the Web at www.peachpit.com
To report errors, please send a note to errata@peachpit.com
Published by Peachpit Press, in association with Macromedia Press
Peachpit Press is a division of Pearson Education

Copyright © 2006 by Tom Negrino and Dori Smith

Editor: Nancy Davis
Production editor: Lisa Brazieal
Proofreader: Liz Welch
Compositor: Kelli Kamel
Indexer: Julie Bess
Cover design: Peachpit Press

ISBN 0-321-35027-8

9 8 7 6 5 4 3 2 1

Printed and bound in the United States of America